CANADIAN NURSING

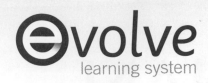

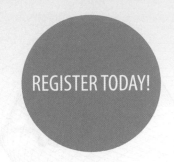

REGISTER TODAY!

To access your Student resources, visit:

http://evolve.elsevier.com/ Canada/Ross-Kerr/nursing/

Evolve® Student Learning Resources for Ross-Kerr & Wood, *Canadian Nursing: Issues & Perspectives,* 5th edition, offer the following features:

Student Resources

- Answer Key to Critical Thinking Questions from the textbook
- Appendices
- Examination Review Questions for practice and self-assessment, designed to reinforce content from each textbook chapter
- Key Points—available in printable format that you can use while on the go
- WebLinks let you link to numerous Web sites carefully chosen to supplement the contents of the textbook
- Content Updates include the latest information from the authors of the textbook to help you keep abreast of recent developments in select areas of study

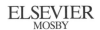

ELSEVIER
MOSBY

CANADIAN NURSING

ISSUES AND PERSPECTIVES

JANET C. ROSS-KERR, RN, BScN, MS, PhD
&
MARILYNN J. WOOD, BSN, MN, DrPH

FIFTH EDITION

ELSEVIER
MOSBY

ELSEVIER
MOSBY

Notice

Knowledge and best practice in this field are constantly changing. As new research and expertise broaden our knowledge, changes in practice, treatment, and drug therapy may become necessary or appropriate. Readers are advised to check the most current information provided (i) on procedures featured or (ii) by the manufacturer of each product to be administered, to verify the recommended dose or formula, the method and duration of administration, and contraindications. It is the responsibility of the practitioner, relying on their own experience and knowledge of the patient, to make diagnoses, to determine dosages and the best treatment for each individual patient, and to take all appropriate safety precautions. To the fullest extent of the law, neither the Publisher nor the Authors assumes any liability for any injury and/or damage to persons or property arising out of or related to any use of the material contained in this book.

The Publisher

Library and Archives Canada Cataloguing in Publication

Kerr, Janet C., 1940-
Canadian nursing: issues and perspectives / Janet Ross-Kerr & Marilynn J. Wood. — 5th ed.
  Includes index.
  ISBN 978-1-897422-10-6
1. Nursing—Canada—Textbooks. I. Wood, Marilynn J II. Title.
RT6.A1K47 2010   610.73'0971   C2010-900878-2

ISBN-13: 978-1-897-42210-6
ISBN-10: 1-897-42210-5

Vice President, Publishing: Ann Millar
Developmental Editor: May Look/Martina van de Velde
Managing Developmental Editor: Martina van de Velde
Managing Production Editor: Roberta Spinosa-Millman
Publishing Services Manager: Jeff Patterson
Copy Editor: Wendy Thomas
Cover, Interior Design: Kim Denando
Typesetting and Assembly: TnQ
Printing and Binding: Transcontinental

Elsevier Canada
905 King Street West, 4th Floor, Toronto,
ON, Canada M6K 3G9
Phone: 1-866-896-3331
Fax: 1-866-359-9534

Printed in Canada

1 2 3 4 5   15 14 13 12 11

▌▌▌CONTENTS

▌▌▌CONTRIBUTORS

Greta G. Cummings, RN, PhD
Professor, Faculty of Nursing, University of Alberta, Edmonton, Alberta
Principal Investigator, CLEAR Outcomes Program (Connecting Leadership Education & Research)
New Investigator, Canadian Institutes of Health Research
Population Health Investigator, Alberta Heritage Foundation for Medical Research

Susan E. French, BN, MS, PhD, RN
Professor Emeritus, School of Nursing, McMaster University, Hamilton, Ontario
Associate Dean and Director, School of Nursing, McGill University, Montreal, Quebec

Kathryn J. Hannah, RN, PhD
Health Informatics Advisor, Canadian Nurses Association

Margaret Ann Kennedy, RN, PhD
President, Kennedy Health Informatics Inc., Merigomish, Nova Scotia

Lori L. Kerr, BA, LLB, LLM
Barrister & Solicitor, The City of Calgary, Calgary, Alberta

June F. Kikuchi, RN (Ret.), MN, PhD
Professor Emeritus, Faculty of Nursing, University of Alberta, Edmonton, Alberta

Janice Lander, RN, PhD
Professor, Faculty of Nursing, University of Alberta, Edmonton, Alberta

Jane L. MacDonald, RN, BScN, MHSc
Vice President, Public Affairs and Community Engagement, VON Canada

Linda Ogilvie, RN, PhD
Professor, Faculty of Nursing
Co-Director, Prairie Metropolis Centre
University of Alberta, Edmonton, Alberta

Pauline Paul, RN, BSc inf, MSc(A), PhD
Associate Professor, Faculty of Nursing, University of Alberta, Edmonton, Alberta

Linda Reutter, RN, PhD
Professor Emeritus, Faculty of Nursing, University of Alberta, Edmonton, Alberta

Leslie J. Roberts, RN, BA, MHSc(A)
Retired from Health Sciences Centre, Winnipeg, Manitoba
Sessional Instructor, School of Nursing, McMaster University, Hamilton, Ontario

Eleanor Ross, RN, BScN, MScN
Nursing and Health Care Consultant, Toronto, Ontario
Adjunct Professor, Department of Nursing, Brock University, St. Catharines, Ontario

Janet C. Ross-Kerr, RN, BScN, MS, PhD
Professor Emeritus, Faculty of Nursing, University of Alberta, Edmonton, Alberta

Judith Shamian, RN, PhD, LLD (Hon.), DSc (Hon.), FAAN
President and CEO, VON Canada

Sally Thorne, RN, MSN, PhD
Professor and Director, School of Nursing, University of British Columbia, Vancouver, British Columbia
Fellow of the Canadian Academy of Health Sciences

Carol A. Wong, RN, PhD
Associate Professor, Arthur Labatt Family School of Nursing, Faculty of Health Sciences, University of Western Ontario, London, Ontario

Marilynn J. Wood, BSN, MN, DrPH
Professor Emeritus, Faculty of Nursing, University of Alberta, Edmonton, Alberta
Principal, Marilynn Wood Associates, Edmonton, Alberta

▋▋▋REVIEWERS

Catherine Aquino-Russell, RN, MN, PhD
Associate Professor, Faculty of Nursing, University of
New Brunswick, Moncton, New Brunswick

Dr. P.H. Bailey, RN, BN, MHSc, PhD
School of Nursing, Laurentian University, Sudbury,
Ontario

Dr. Wally J. Bartfay, RN, PhD
Associate Professor, Faculty of Health Sciences,
University of Ontario Institute of Technology
(UOIT), Oshawa, Ontario

Leslie Beagrie, RN, PhD
Director, School of Nursing, York University,
Toronto, Ontario

Doris Callaghan, RN, BSN, MCs
Associate Professor, School of Nursing, University of
British Columbia—Okanagan, Kelowna, British
Columbia

Kathy Crooks, RN, MN, PhD
Division of Health Studies, Medicine Hat College,
Medicine Hat, Alberta

Vicki Earle, RN, BN, MN
Centre for Nursing Studies, Canadian School of
Nursing, St. John's, Newfoundland and Labrador

Mary Elliott, RN, BScN, MEd
UNB–Humber Collaborative Bachelor of Nursing
Program, Toronto, Ontario

Josephine Etowa, PhD, MN, BScN, BN, RM, IBCLC
Assistant Professor, School of Nursing, Dalhousie
University, Halifax, Nova Scotia

**Linda Ferguson, RN, BSN, PGD (Cont. Ed.), MN,
PhD**
Professor, Director, Centre for the Advancement
of Study of Nursing Education and
Interprofessional Education, College of Nursing,
University of Saskatchewan, Saskatoon,
Saskatchewan

Sandra Filice, RN, BAAN, MEd
Program Coordinator, UNB–Humber Bachelor
of Nursing Program, Humber Institute of
Technology & Advanced Learning, Toronto,
Ontario

**Pasquale Fiore, RN, BScN, MSc Health Admin.,
Cert. Ed.**
Camosun College & School of Nursing, University of
Victoria, Victoria, British Columbia

Sandy Gessler, RN, BA, MPA
Program Coordinator & Instructor, Faculty of
Nursing, University of Manitoba, Winnipeg,
Manitoba

Sheila Heinrich, RN, BN, MHS
Program Leader & Instructor, Nursing Education
in Southwestern Alberta, Lethbridge Community
College, Lethbridge, Alberta

Vicki Holmes, RN, BScN, MScN
Assistant Professor, School of Nursing, Thompson
Rivers University, Kamloops, British Columbia

Lynette Leeseberg Stamler, RN, PhD
Associate Professor, College of Nursing, University of
Saskatchewan, Saskatoon, Saskatchewan

Jo-Ann MacDonald, RN, BScN, MN, PhD(cand.)
Assistant Professor, Faculty of Nursing, University
of Prince Edward Island, Charlottetown, Prince
Edward Island

Jane Moseley, RN, BScN, MAdEd
Assistant Professor, School of Nursing, St. Francis
Xavier University, Antigonish, Nova Scotia

Louise Racine, RN, BScN, MScN, PhD
Assistant Professor, College of Nursing, University of
Saskatchewan, Saskatoon, Saskatchewan

Lynn Rollison, RN, BSN, MA
School of Nursing, Malaspina University-College,
Nanaimo, British Columbia

Elaine Schow, RN, BScN, MN
Coordinator, Bridge to Canadian Nursing Program,
Mount Royal College, Calgary, Alberta

**Debbie Sheppard-LeMoine, MN, BN, RN,
PhD(cand.)**
Assistant Professor, School of Nursing, Dalhousie
University, Halifax, Nova Scotia

Nancy Walton, RN, PhD
Associate Professor, School of Nursing, Ryerson
University, Toronto, Ontario

▌▌▌PREFACE

At the time of the first edition of *Canadian Nursing: Issues & Perspectives,* there was no comprehensive written information that students could read to learn about a range of Canadian nursing issues. Since it is an impossible task for any instructor to present all the background on issues of concern to Canadian nurses by word of mouth, the idea for developing a text to serve as a resource on a whole range of issues emerged. Janet Ross-Kerr and Jannetta MacPhail, co-authors of the first three editions, and Janet Ross-Kerr and Marilynn Wood, co-editors of the fourth and fifth editions, have worked to identify and evaluate developments in the profession and to monitor the extent of progress over the 22 years since the first edition was published. Despite the fact that we would like things to move faster in some areas, it is evident that there has been steady and measurable progress over this relatively short period of time. Developments relative to the professional entry-to-practice goal have been impressive, and this process is virtually complete across the country. Also, the legal recognition of advanced practice nursing by skilled nursing practitioners has occurred in a number of provinces and territories, and the movement has gained considerable momentum. The emergence of 13 doctoral programs in nursing since January 1991 has also been a remarkable achievement. Nurses have been increasingly successful in using their political skills in the labour relations arena to serve the profession and its members. Our issues are being taken more seriously by politicians, employers, and institutions. In some cases, governments have been brought to their knees by the voices of nurses and forced to acknowledge important issues before them.

It is sometimes difficult to see where you are going and what you have accomplished "in the heat of battle"! Every nurse is a part of the action because each one of us contributes in a unique way to the development of the profession. There are matters of critical and fundamental importance to the provision of nursing and health system reform that require our careful attention. Although things may not always appear to be positive, and although progress often seems to be painfully slow and uneven, the pursuit of our goals is important to us, and in working for them individually and collectively, we can and do make a difference in the course of events over time. Nurses have been known both for their altruism and high standards of practice. The integrity of the individuals and the profession itself has been seen in the quality of the service provided and in the vigilance of the profession in ensuring that recognized standards are upheld.

Although disruptions to the nursing workforce have lessened as nursing unions have become stronger and more effective in lobbying for change, health system change has been necessitated by conditions of recession and financial insecurity nationally. Thus, recognition of the need for rationalizing and streamlining the health care system has underscored the mood for change nationally, and there have been a number of studies commissioned federally and provincially with a view to rationalizing services, maximizing care, and minimizing costs. It is apparent that the health care system of the future will look substantially different. Nurses are participating in a variety of ways as new and innovative models of health care emerge. It is clear to the authors of this book that, despite the complexity of the issues and the difficult problems presented by the changing nature of practice, the profession of nursing will survive and emerge stronger than ever. These and other developments have been explored in the fifth edition.

Features of the Fifth Edition

- Content in all chapters has been reworked and updated to reflect current developments in nursing and health care.
- New student-friendly pedagogy has been introduced, which includes the following:
  Chapter Objectives at the beginning of each chapter, to help students identify key content
  Canadian Research Focus boxes, highlighting current and relevant research in content areas specific to each chapter
  Reflective Thinking boxes for each chapter, to provide focused opportunities for reflection and discussion about chapter content
  Critical Thinking Questions at the end of each chapter, to help students apply learning to practice
  WebLinks at the end of most chapters, to provide information for relevant nursing and health care organizations
- **Chapter 7: Thinking Philosophically in Nursing** has been substantially revised to address the basing of nursing knowledge on conceptions of nursing, the downfall of conceptions of nursing, and new directions toward developing a sound philosophical nursing basis.
- **Chapter 8: Nursing Research in Canada** has been substantially revised and updated to include a section on funding nursing research, as well as a new discussion about advocacy for nursing research, landmark examples of cost effectiveness, and the emergence of advanced practice nursing.
- *New* **Chapter 9: Knowledge Translation and Evidence-Informed Practice** focuses on the significance of evidence-informed practice for nursing, discusses the process of innovation and barriers to the use of evidence, and explores factors that lead to clinical decision-making errors.
- *New* **Chapter 10: Health Informatics and Canadian Nursing Practice**, written by the foremost Canadian experts on this subject, provides an overview of the emergence of health informatics and how nursing data are represented in health care (e.g., Canada Health Infoway, Canada's e-nursing strategy, and the International Classification for Nursing Practice). This chapter also addresses privacy and confidentiality issues relating to health informatics. Since computerization and computer systems are increasingly an integral part of the nurse's world, this is a timely addition.
- **Chapter 11: Primary Health Care: Challenges and Opportunities for the Nursing Profession** has been completely revised to address health equity and the WHO's

Health for All initiative, discuss primary health care in the Canadian context, provide examples of primary health care initiatives in Canada, and present the challenges and complexities of reorienting the Canadian health care system to meet PHC goals.

- **Chapter 12: Quality of Care: From Quality Assurance and Improvement to Cultures of Patient Safety** has been updated with a new focus on patient safety and the patient safety movement, including a discussion about nursing-sensitive outcomes and best practice guidelines.
- **Chapter 13: The Practising Nurse and the Law** has been completely revised with a new discussion about the professional status of nurses, up-to-date coverage about negligence and documentation (including PIPEDA and electronic health records), and a focus on consent to nursing care.
- **Chapter 24: International Nursing: Looking Beyond Our Borders** has been completely revised to include detailed coverage of the main international health-related issues and events that have occurred since the year 2000.
- **Chapter 25: Internationalizing Nursing in Canada: Perspectives in Nursing Practice and Education** has been completely revised to include new discussions about the preparation of individual nurses, nursing recruitment, and international placements.
- The order of chapters has been modified. Most notably, the chapter on nursing theory now comes ahead of the chapter on thinking philosophically in nursing. Although you might think that this is placing "the cart before the horse," theoretical discussions actually preceded the philosophy movement in nursing, and we decided there was an advantage to presenting these chapters in an order that reflected the historical context.
- The chapter on the Canadian health care system has been reworked from the previous edition and now becomes the first chapter, providing an overall context for understanding developments in health care.
- Several chapters have been combined and shortened, most notably the chapters on nursing history. Originally comprising four chapters in the fourth edition, these have been streamlined into two chapters without losing sight of important developments in the evolution of nursing and nursing education. Two former chapters on nursing unions have also been combined and shortened into one chapter.
- Information about the role of the Canadian Nurses Association (CNA), previously confined to a single chapter, has now been integrated throughout the text where applicable.
- An accompanying **Evolve website** now offers additional student learning resources, including Answers to Critical Thinking Questions, Appendices, Examination Review Questions for each chapter, and printable Key Points for each chapter.

As always, we have attempted to place issues in historical context for enhanced understanding of the current situation. Nurses have been front row centre in the primary health care movement in Canada, and there have been positive steps forward in this area. It is also evident that nursing research has been enhanced by the quality of work done by an increasing number of nurses with research preparation. The success of the four previous editions confirmed that there was a tangible need for a resource book on issues and trends in contemporary Canadian nursing. The intent has been to provide a resource for nursing students as well as practising nurses, including those involved in direct care, education, research, and administering nursing systems. It is our hope that this book will inspire our colleagues to consider issues that will positively influence the health care of Canadians. The opportunity to step back, identify, and evaluate what has happened has given us satisfaction and pleasure. We hope that readers will be able to share with us a renewed appreciation of the accomplishments of nurses and the rewards of being involved in the evolution of our distinguished profession.

Winter, 2010

JANET C. ROSS- KERR, BScN, MS, PhD
Professor Emeritus, Faculty of Nursing, University of Alberta

MARILYNN J. WOOD, BSN, MN, DrPH
Professor Emeritus, Faculty of Nursing, University of Alberta
Principal, Marilynn Wood Associates, Edmonton, Alberta

CANADIAN NURSING

THE PROFESSION IN CANADA

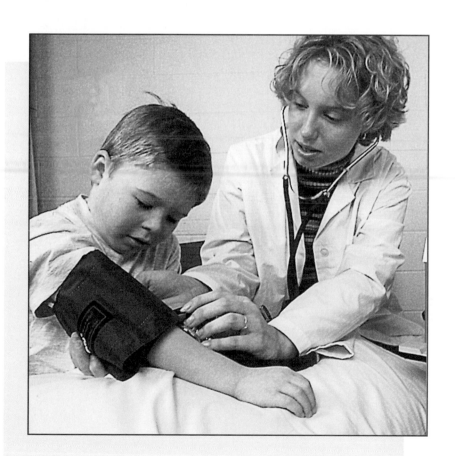

CHAPTER 1

The Canadian Health Care System

Janet C. Ross-Kerr

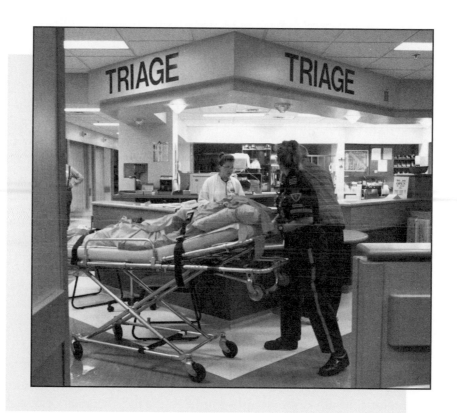

LEARNING OBJECTIVES

- To appreciate differences between the Canadian health care system and that of some other nations relative to the constitutional authority for health.
- To describe the historical development of a national system of Medicare in Canada.
- To understand the roots of Medicare in the early health insurance plans.
- To recognize how a universal system of national health insurance was developed in Canada.
- To identify the nature of federal legislation that found the basis of health care financing.
- To explain the provisions of the *Canada Health Act* of 1984.
- To identify the issues related to attempts to privatize health care in Canada.
- To interpret the philosophical basis of Canadian health care financing legislation.
- To describe the health care reform movement of the 1990s.
- To understand the issues in the retrenchment in health care financing in Canada exacerbated by the global economic recession.

THE HEALTH CARE SYSTEM: A COMPARATIVE VIEW

Since the *British North America Act* was passed at the time of Confederation, responsibility for health has rested with the provinces. The *Constitution Act* of 1982 confirmed the historical division of powers between the federal government and the provinces. Canada's arrangement is different from that of other nations with centralized health care systems, such as the United Kingdom, France, and Sweden, where authority for health care is vested in the federal government. Wallace (1980) observed that

> *the fathers of Confederation clearly thought they were assigning the provinces the less important and inexpensive functions of government, among which education, hospitals, charities and municipal institutions were then reasonably numbered. They could scarcely have foreseen the way in which time would reverse their expectations, so that the costliness of the responsibilities laid upon the provinces subsequently increased to the point where it was financially impossible to defray them. Within thirty years after Confederation social and economic conditions had so altered that public opinion was demanding government action on matters held in 1867 to be primarily personal and of no concern to the state. (p. 27)*

The constitutional division of authority and responsibility for health care also provides a partial explanation for the length of time it took to develop and implement a national health insurance program. Because jurisdictional responsibility for health lies with the provinces, achievement of uniform changes to benefit the entire country is a difficult task. Over the years, federal interest in this sector of provincial responsibility has been high because of the value placed on health and its importance in the life of society. The greater taxing power of the federal government in a publicly funded system has led the provinces to look to the federal government for help in financing health care.

The United States has not yet implemented a universal program of national health insurance, although national Medicare and Medicaid acts were passed during the tenure of President Lyndon Johnson. In his 1992 election campaign, former president Bill Clinton pledged to bring in health legislation so that the population would be covered by universal health care insurance. Although his legislative proposals were never passed, a debate in the United States about the merits of universal health insurance ensued and continues (American Public Health Association, 2001). Although the division of powers between federal and state or provincial governments in relation to health is similar in the United States and Canada, members of one party are not required to vote as a block in the US House of Representatives and the US Senate. This means that lobbying by interested individuals and groups must be directed toward individual members of these bodies as well as those who hold the reins of party power. The achievement of unanimity on a matter of national importance, such as a national plan of health insurance, is clearly more difficult because of the power held by individual elected members. These considerations, along with a value system centred on individual responsibility and free enterprise, explain why a form of Medicare in the United States has been achieved only for those over 65 years of age. In his 2008 presidential campaign, Barack Obama promised to bring universal national health insurance to the fore once again. Again, the difficulty of passing such legislation is evident as an emasculated version of his original proposals, which caused rancorous and partisan debate, was passed by a slim margin in the Senate and House of Representatives. Signed into law in March 2010, it ensured that over 30 million US residents who previously had no health insurance would be covered.

In contrast, the United Kingdom introduced its National Health Service in 1948, providing a model of health care financing for Commonwealth countries in particular. There were differences, however, in the national health plan adopted by the United Kingdom and that introduced in Canada. When legislation to establish Medicare in Canada was introduced, the approach was not to restructure the existing health care system. The Canadian legislation was simply an overlay on the existing system, providing a framework for financing it. A two-tiered system of health care financing has emerged more recently in the United Kingdom; the inefficiencies and shortcomings of the public system giving rise to a private one for those of means, complete with third-party insurance.

THE DEVELOPMENT OF A NATIONAL SYSTEM OF MEDICARE: A HISTORICAL PERSPECTIVE

Although universal health insurance was first suggested in 1919, it took a long time to implement the system. Taylor (1978) commented,

> Our heritage of the Elizabethan Poor Law had placed responsibility for the sick poor on local government, but many cities, towns and especially rural municipalities in Canada quickly reached the point of near or actual bankruptcy from the combination of declining revenues and expanding relief payments for food, clothing and shelter. Medical care, except in the direst emergency conditions, was a luxury that only few individuals or municipalities could afford. (p. 4)

The continuing financial problems facing hospitals during the early decades of the last century have been reported and analyzed. The struggle was greater in the voluntary hospital, but even among municipally owned institutions, the reluctance to provide adequate funds made financing a continuing nightmare for trustees and administrators (Agnew, 1974, p. 149). During the Depression years, a difficult situation deteriorated further until many hospitals had large deficits. In the 1930s, only 40 to 50% of the patient days in public hospitals had been paid in full by 55 to 60% of the patients. Eight percent of patients paid for part of their hospital stay, and one-third of those remaining were unable to pay their bill (Agnew, 1974, p. 151). In addition, "a fairly sharp division was usually drawn between paying and non-paying patients" (Agnew, 1974, p. 153), and extra payment for private accommodation was used to help offset deficits.

Physicians and professional nurses also experienced difficulties during this period. Since the proportion of patients unable to pay medical bills had escalated, many physicians had a difficult time financially. In Saskatchewan, "many in the medical profession . . . had suffered economic disaster along with the rest of the population during the 1930s, and many physicians received payments of $50 or $75 per month from the Saskatchewan Relief Commission" (*Report of the Saskatchewan Department of Public Health*, 1933, p. 7; as cited in Taylor, 1978, p. 83). Nurses also felt the pinch, and graduate nurses' positions in private-duty nursing evaporated with the stock market crash. In Calgary,

> General Hospital graduates, unable to get positions as special nurses, were glad to be taken on the hospital staff at a monthly salary of thirty dollars in addition to room and board. Many supervisory nurses, already on staff, had to take substantial salary reductions as the city slashed and re-slashed its hospital budget in a desperate attempt to make ends meet with the reduced taxes it was able to collect. (Agnew, 1974, p. 150)

Beginning in the 1920s, a number of small prepayment plans for hospital care were developed to provide for hospital services. Care was prepaid for all who were covered by the plan. There were many factors that encouraged thinking about using a system of insurance on a wider scale to create a health care system that would eliminate hardships for persons who became ill, allow hospitals to operate on other than a hand-to-mouth basis, and ensure that health care providers received remuneration for services provided. The Depression and, later, the World War II years were difficult for Canadians. In 1937, Canada ranked seventeenth in infant mortality among developed nations (Advisory Committee on Health Insurance, 1943; as cited in Taylor, 1978, p. 5). The views of politicians were also an important factor, particularly those of the party leader. Taylor (1978) has commented on this reference to the views of Prime Minister Mackenzie King:

> In the initiation of any government proposal, the personal objectives and commitment of the party leader who occupies the position of premier or prime minister at a particular juncture in history is frequently the most crucial factor in the decision to act or not to act. . . . But that his views were a powerful force in incorporating health insurance and other social security measures in the post-war reconstruction proposals is clear. (pp. 9–10)

EARLY HEALTH INSURANCE PLANS

Commercial insurance companies began developing plans in the 1930s, and publicly sponsored arrangements for prepaid care were initiated by municipalities, hospitals, and regional groups soon after. The first known voluntary plan for prepayment of hospital care in Canada was the Edmonton Group Hospitalization Plan, introduced by the four major general hospitals in that city in 1934. Initial efforts to establish a Blue Cross Plan in the province had met resistance from some institutions, so the four hospitals started their own small plan. This plan was extended to the rest of Alberta in 1948 as a Blue Cross Plan under the sponsorship of the provincial hospital association. Hospitalization benefits were provided when needed as prepaid fees for those who enrolled (Agnew, 1974).

The first province-wide Blue Cross Plan in Canada, initiated in 1937, was created by an act of the Manitoba legislature and administered by the Manitoba Hospital Service Association. Similar plans were implemented in other provinces: Ontario (1941), Quebec (1942), and Nova Scotia, New Brunswick, Prince Edward Island, and British Columbia (1943) (Agnew, 1974). Many of the provinces eventually added medical and surgical services to the plans they offered. Because different authorities were responsible for developing and maintaining plans offered in different provinces, there was considerable variation in benefits from plan to plan. The basis of most of the plans was payment of premiums by enrollees. A substantial segment of the Canadian population was not covered by any form of prepaid insurance owing to ineligibility for plans limited to specific groups of people or inability to pay the required premium.

THE ROAD TO NATIONAL HEALTH INSURANCE

Federal involvement in financing health care had been discussed since William Lyon Mackenzie King developed a proposal for universal health insurance in the platform of the Liberal Party in the election of 1919. In 1929, the Standing Committee on Industrial and International Relations of the House of Commons recommended that, "with regard to sickness insurance, the Department of Pensions and National Health be requested to initiate a comprehensive survey of the field of public health, with special reference to a national health programme" (Agnew, 1974, p. 165). The report was approved in 1933, and in 1935 the *Employment and Social Insurance Act* provided for collecting information and advising groups in provinces planning a health insurance program. Because the act was declared unconstitutional in the courts, it was not until 1942 that a federal committee on health insurance was established to study the issues. At that time the Canadian Medical Association (CMA) endorsed the principles of health insurance, and although it preferred fee for service as the method of payment for medical services, it indicated that a capitation, or salary, method of remunerating physicians might also be needed.

A federal–provincial conference, convened in 1945, "proposed universal health insurance with federal–provincial cost sharing" and "produced a model draft health care bill for the provinces" (Vayda, Evans, & Mindell, 1979, p. 218). Because of concern that such legislation would interfere with provincial autonomy and that Canada's health care facilities and personnel were inadequate to carry the load that health insurance would bring, the legislation failed. The province of Saskatchewan, under the leadership of Premier T.C. Douglas, instituted a hospital insurance plan financed entirely by the province in 1947. Payment of premiums was basic to this plan, and every Saskatchewan resident was required to register for it. The plan was subsidized from general revenues, and in 1948, the provincial sales tax was increased to help finance it. In 1949, a similar program was established in British Columbia.

FEDERAL LEGISLATION FOR HEALTH CARE FINANCING

The federal government's first foray into health care financing occurred in 1948 through the National Health Grants Program. Assistance was provided for hospital construction, public and mental health programs, and professional training to "gear up" for hospital insurance. At a federal–provincial conference held in 1955, agreement on the details of a national hospital insurance plan was translated into legislation in the form of the *Hospital Insurance and Diagnostic Services Act* of 1957. Provinces were given the option to join, with the federal government paying "an amount equal to 25% of its own per capita cost (less authorized charges) plus 25% of the national per capita cost multiplied by the number of insured persons" (Brown, 1980, p. 523). Programs were required to provide universal coverage, reasonable accessibility, portability of coverage from province to province, comprehensive coverage for all in-hospital care in general, and certain other designated care services; public, nonprofit administration of plans was mandatory (LeClair, 1975). The aforementioned principles are referred to as the five basic principles of health care. Administration of the plans was to be carried out by the individual provinces. All provinces had accepted the terms of the act by 1961 (Vayda, Evans, & Mindell, 1979).

The next struggle was to include medical care in the insurance plan. The Royal Commission on Health Services of 1964 emphasized the importance of including medical care in the national health insurance program. Again it took many years to reach agreement on the nature and form of the legislation, and the federal program was preceded by one developed by the province of Saskatchewan in 1962. Physicians opposed the Saskatchewan plan, and the 1962 Saskatchewan physicians' strike of 23 days will long be remembered. In 1968, the federal *Medical Care Act* was established to provide reimbursement to provincial health insurance plans for physicians' services. This was provided under the same cost-sharing conditions as assistance for hospital services. Again there was opposition from physicians, who feared interference in the physician–patient relationship and the possibility that the fee-for-service system of remuneration for physicians would be abandoned as the plan was implemented. New Brunswick was the last to join in 1971, and the provisions of the act were then applied in all provinces.

In the 1970s, the federal government became concerned about escalation in health care costs. With the unlimited 50–50 cost-sharing arrangement, there was no ceiling on the federal share of health care cost reimbursement. As the federal deficit increased, the government passed the *Fiscal Arrangements and Established Programs Financing Act* of 1977. The provisions of this act, which applied to hospital care, medical care, and post-secondary education, allowed for for block funding, reducing the federal contribution to health care to 25%, with additional federal contributions based on increases in the gross national product. Federal income taxes were decreased to allow the provinces to increase their taxes to offset the federal reductions. For the first time, funding was provided for extended and home care. In 1982, the federal government changed the method of calculating contributions through amendments to the health care financing legislation of 1977. This meant that provinces received considerably less federal assistance than before. The federal government responded to provincial objections to decreased funding by reiterating that decreases in federal income taxes had left room for increases in provincial income taxes.

The federal government was disturbed by the increasing incidence of extra billing and user fees in the provinces and by the premiums charged in some provinces. Brown (1980) has commented that, after the passage of the 1977 act, "user charges have increased both in prevalence and in amount. Extra billing by physicians over Medicare payments increased markedly during 1978 and 1979" (p. 522). Provinces had considerably more flexibility under the new rules for federal financing of health care: they could reduce their contributions to health care; to compensate, user charges for various health care services could be instituted. If provinces decreased funding of medical services relative to the fee schedule, the practice of extra billing was stimulated. According to Brown (1980),

> *Allowing doctors to extra-bill not only thwarts the social objective of free care, but also promotes a system under which total costs (public costs plus private costs) will be higher than they would be either under completely socialized medicine or under an unregulated market. Hospital user charges, on the other hand, suggest fewer problems because their development would not suggest a corresponding loss in government control over prices. (p. 531)*

THE *CANADA HEALTH ACT* OF 1984

Another confrontation between the federal government and the provinces occurred over the way health care dollars would be expended. The federal government took the position that extra billing and user fees were eroding Medicare and, further, that if those practices were allowed to continue and increase, a two-tiered system of health care would develop, one for the rich and another for the poor. There was a great deal of variation among the provinces in the extent to which user charges and extra billing were practised. Quebec had the most restrictive rules on extra billing: physicians who extra-billed were required to opt out of the plan and bill patients directly, and their patients could not seek reimbursement from the plan. A number of provinces—New Brunswick, Nova Scotia, Prince Edward Island, Saskatchewan, and Alberta—allowed physicians to extra-bill and remain in the plan. At the time the legislation was introduced, two provinces, British Columbia and Newfoundland, had user charges for daily stays in acute-care beds, and Alberta also had an admission charge. Chronic care patients were assessed a daily charge in some provinces: British Columbia, Alberta, Manitoba, Ontario, Quebec, and New Brunswick. Only British Columbia, Alberta, and Ontario charged premiums.

The Canadian Nurses Association (CNA) was strong in its representation to the federal government on its position that health care should be provided regardless of ability to pay; extra billing by physicians and user charges by health care agencies should be disallowed; health care providers should be remunerated on a salary-based system; and insured services should be extended to include community, home care, and long-term care services provided by qualified health care providers (CNA, 1983). The CNA also supported the idea of financial incentives for provinces that developed lower-cost health programs and services by using the skills of health care professionals more effectively.

> Basically, services are insured if they are delivered in one setting—hospitals, or provided by one kind of health professional—physicians. . . . A wide range and balanced system of services has not been fostered by the legislation; therefore, non-physician health professionals such as nurses have not been utilized to their potential and cost-effective alternatives to hospital care are underdeveloped. (CNA, 1983, p. 1)

The representation was vigorous and prolonged. Members of the CNA Board lobbied members of Parliament on several occasions in 1983 and 1984. Reports and analyses of individual meetings were published in bulletins and distributed to the membership. The CNA executive and staff held meetings with key members of the federal government and members of the civil service with responsibility for developing legislation. In a letter to members of the CNA Board, President Helen Glass (1983) urged:

> It's our responsibility to make nursing's voice heard—and soon. Even if you have already contacted your minister of health, we strongly urge you to keep up your lobbying efforts. Health department officials, leaders of opposition parties, opposition health critics and members of standing committees on health will be key targets. (p. 1)

The Honourable Monique Bégin, Minister of National Health and Welfare, faced the difficult task of drafting the legislation and shepherding it through committees of the cabinet and House of Commons before it could be introduced as a bill to be debated and acted on in the House of Commons. In her opening statement to the Conference of Federal and Provincial Ministers of Health in Ottawa in 1982, Bégin said:

> The health care system for which we are responsible is one of Canada's greatest social policy achievements. For Canadians it is the single most popular government program. To outside observers it is a source of great envy. . . . However, our commitment to health care insurance in Canada is no easy task. Our governments are faced with major problems of financing in tough economic times. . . . It is clear that Canadians today are particularly concerned about the future of their health care system. (pp. 1–4)

The pressure to implement more directly and carefully the five basic principles identified, but loosely applied, in initial health insurance legislation was intense, particularly with reference to user fees, access to health services, and opting out and extra billing by physicians (Bégin, 1982, p. 4).

The new legislation was passed in early April of 1984, amid intense publicity. Bégin became a high-profile figure, and the media focused on confrontations with health ministers in a number of provinces where elected officials considered the *Canada Health Act* an intrusion into the constitutional rights and powers of the provinces for health care. The CNA lobbied hard and was rewarded for its efforts with legislation that effectively ended the practices of extra billing and user fees and with the introduction of a statement that provided federal funding for services provided by "health practitioners." The door was thus open for the inclusion in provincial health plans of specialized nursing services that were eligible for reimbursement for the first time. The wording of the legislation could also apply to services provided by other health care providers. Clearly, this was the first step in achieving the stated CNA goals: better utilization of nurses and more cost-effective health care. The Canadian Medical Association lobbied equally hard against the legislation, but owing to the popularity of national health insurance, the unpopularity of extra billing and user fees, and strong political support for the legislation, it was unable to prevent the passage of the *Canada Health Act*.

PRIVATIZATION OF HEALTH CARE

Recession has led not only to a general shortage of resources and to retrenchment in the health care system but also to discussions of privatization of health care. The percentage of the gross domestic product (GDP) that Canadians spend on health care was substantially lower in 1998 at 9.2% than the 13% spent in the United States, but considerably higher than the 6.7% spent in the United Kingdom (World Bank, 2001). By 2007, Canadian health expenditures had risen to 10.1% of the GDP, while those in the UK constituted 8.4%, and US expenditures had risen to an astonishing 16% (OECD, 2009). According to the National Coalition on Health Care (2009), 47 million Americans under the age of 65 did not have health insurance coverage, an all-time high. The U.S. private sector is permitted to operate hospitals at a profit, even though their hospital costs are considerably higher than those of other developed countries (World Bank, 2001). A number of provinces have conducted experiments in privatization, contracting with private organizations to run hospitals. However, the results of these experiments have not been made public by the governments providing the financing. Many organizations, health analysts, and individuals were opposed to these ventures, as they appeared to violate, at least in spirit, one of the five basic principles on which health legislation in Canada was founded (i.e., public administration).

However, arguments in favour of allowing market forces to prevail in health care are not easily dismissed, as they are continually raised by supporters. Rachlis and Kushner (1994) have countered:

> *Explaining the basic economic principles affecting health care financing and delivery leads to conclusions that seem counter-intuitive: public health insurance is more efficient than private insurance; the knowledge gap between caregivers and patients almost eliminates price as an effective signal in the market. (p. 187)*

It is nevertheless likely that considerable opposition would surface if anything more than token experiments in privatization were undertaken. Despite its problems, most Canadians value their health care system, and most would not want the system of public financing to be significantly altered.

PHILOSOPHICAL BASIS OF HEALTH CARE FINANCING LEGISLATION

The combined effect of the provisions of the 1948 federal legislation supporting hospital construction and the 1957 hospital insurance legislation set in motion a system in which "hospital-based patterns of practice were solidified" (Vayda, Evans, & Mindell, 1979). The number of hospital beds increased at twice the rate of population increase between 1961 and 1971, and occupancy rates were around 80%. Since outpatient care was not eligible for federal cost sharing, there was an incentive for choosing more costly hospital care over outpatient or home care. Community health services were also excluded from federal financing, and provinces were required to finance the operation of such services without assistance.

Another point that pertains to nursing and the services offered by other health care providers is that medical-care insurance legislation provided federal cost sharing only for physicians' services. This constrained the development of the health care system by providing a financial incentive for the proliferation of physicians' services. Since these were the most costly services of all of the health professions, this decision had serious financial repercussions for the health care system.

> *One of the factors associated with the volume of health care services is the number of physicians. More surgeons are correlated with higher discretionary surgical rates and more physicians with an increased volume of medical services, just as more hospital beds are associated with greater bed use (Vayda, Evans, & Mindell, 1979, p. 220).*

Projections of the number of physicians needed to care for the Canadian population were grossly overestimated in the 1960s. The Royal Commission on Health Services Report of 1964 assumed there would be a shortage, based on its projections of 1961 patterns of health-services utilization, and failed to account for "changes in technology and productivity" (Vayda, Evans, & Mindell, 1979, p. 219). The ratio of physicians to population rose dramatically, from 1:850 in 1961 to 1:600 by 1973. This ratio continued to rise, and in 1998, it had reached 1:476 (World Bank, 2001), while in 2007 the ratio was 1:454 (OECD, 2009). The financial repercussions for a physician-driven system in which the skills of other health care providers are not effectively employed are obvious. As Vayda, Evans, and Mindell (1979) have pointed out, "There are dangers inherent in health care decisions that are predicated solely on financial considerations; yet now governments not only know what the total health care bill is, they also have to pay that bill and deal with the issues" (p. 230).

HEALTH CARE REFORM IN THE 1990s

There is ample evidence that, "although universal hospital insurance in Canada provided payment to hospitals, it did not mandate an organizational framework to deal with problems of efficiency or duplication of services" (Vayda, Evans, & Mindell, 1979, p. 219). When insurance for medical services was imposed on the existing structure of services, the environment for care was clearly the hospital. When new funding arrangements were implemented in 1977, the federal government attempted to stop open-ended health care financing by placing limits on total federal spending. Thus it sought to constrain its own financial commitment in a more predictable way, one that would encourage the provinces to manage their programs more efficiently (by removing any illusion that they were spending 50-cent dollars). The outcome was, predictably, a loss of federal control over health insurance programs. In retrospect it appears that the federal government was somewhat naïve in believing that the nature of Medicare and hospital insurance would make them immune to provincial government encroachment (Brown, 1980, p. 525).

It is not difficult to understand why restructuring and reorganizing the health care system were not included in federal legislative proposals for funding provincial health care services. The need for change had been recognized for some time. The Royal Commission on Health Services had recommended reorganization of health services in its 1964 report. Political considerations, the fierce determination of the provinces to retain their constitutional prerogatives for health care, and the opposition of powerful lobbyists were all factors that deterred needed change in the system. In the process of enacting new health care financing legislation, such as the *Canada Health Act* of 1984, the federal government encountered difficulty implementing even a few changes, as they were opposed by both physicians and provinces. The need for a new approach to health care remains and is more urgent than ever, but the agenda for legislative change is a political minefield. The federal government that next addresses the need for action in health care will require a firm commitment to change and the courage of its convictions in the presence of strong political opposition.

Canada cannot afford to continue to support a system in which the physician is the "gatekeeper" to virtually all health care services. Research indicates that using the services of nurses and other health care providers is a sensible and cost-effective approach to the provision of health care services. A study of nurses providing primary care in rural Newfoundland demonstrated that acute-care hospital services decreased by 5%, while in the control area there was a 39% increase in a physician-based, acute-care-centred system. The cost of providing services to the population in the experimental group was substantially lower (24%) than in the control group (Chambers, Bruce-Lockhart, Black, Sampson, & Burke, 1977, p. 971). An investigation in Manitoba demonstrated that physicians were less successful than nurse practitioners in helping comparable groups of patients control blood pressure and lose weight (Ramsay, McKenzie, & Fish, 1982). In a controlled trial, nurses were more successful in vaccinating elderly patients for influenza than were physicians — nurses immunizing 35% of patients compared with 2% by physicians (Hoey, McCallum, & LePage, 1982, p. 27). In Ontario, a study by the Institute of Clinical Evaluative Services provided evidence linking nursing knowledge to lower mortality rates in a group of 47,000 Ontario patients (Canadian Nurses Association, 2002). Nurse practitioners, or advance practice nurses, are being prepared in many provinces at both the master's and certificate level. Structural modifications in the organization of health services are gradually being made in most provinces and territories to accommodate them in the system. Until recently, Canada was one of few countries in the world where nurse midwives were not legally permitted to practise. Because midwives can offer basic services to maternity patients at substantially lower costs, the gradual development of provincial legislation to permit midwifery will facilitate effective and efficient use of professional personnel in the health care system.

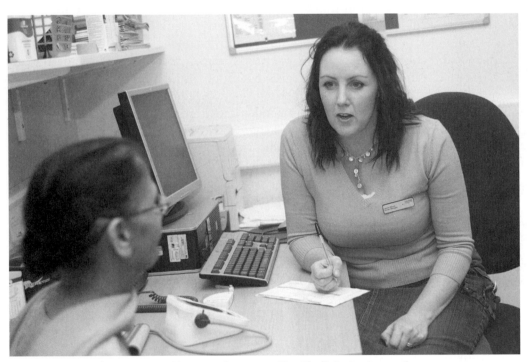

This nurse practitioner works at a rural health clinic that has no doctor.

By 2002, several studies of health care directed at remediating the system had been released. The first was the Mazankowski Report (Premier's Advisory Council on Health, 2002), an Alberta study that produced 44 recommendations, including limiting Medicare coverage by removing certain health services and blending private, public, and not-for-profit health providers, thus recommending a two-tiered system. The second study was conducted by the Senate of Canada under the direction of Senator Michael Kirby (2002). Its mandate was to review the state of the health system and the federal role. Its major recommendation was a tax that would raise $5 billion per annum to pour more money into the existing system. It also recommended changing the way in which hospitals and physicians are funded. The third study, the Commission on the Future of Health Care in Canada, was conducted by Roy Romanow (2002), a former provincial premier, and sought to put forward recommendations to preserve the long-term sustainability of Canada's health care system. Recommendations called for the federal government to increase its contribution to Medicare by $6.5 billion in 2005–2006 and follow that up with guaranteed minimum funding to the provinces in succeeding years, to ensure stable funding and allowing the provinces to plan. Romanow also recommended greater accountability by the federal government for Medicare funding, a limited system of pharmacare, better funding of home care, and limiting the role of the private sector. As a result of these recommendations, the federal government allocated considerably greater funding for Medicare than previously, specifically a 10-year, $41-billion transfer to the provinces in 2004.

REFLECTIVE THINKING

How would you describe the Canadian health system in terms of its mixture of public and private funding?

CANADIAN RESEARCH FOCUS

Laporte, A., Croxford, R., & Coyte, P.C. (2007). Can a publicly funded home care system successfully allocate service based on perceived need rather than socioeconomic status? A Canadian experience. *Health and Social Care in the Community, 15*(2), 108–119.

This Ontario study evaluated the extent to which socioeconomic status, rather than perceived need, was responsible for utilization of publicly funded home care. Using a large database of the Ontario Health Insurance Plan, utilization was measured by propensity to use services and actual use of services. Results demonstrated that the best predictors of receipt of service were age, sex, and co-morbidity. Propensity to use and actual use of services increased with lower socioeconomic status and decreased in regions with a larger proportion of new immigrants. Despite the fact that services were based on need without reference to ability to pay, there were barriers to utilization of services for those in areas where there was a high proportion of new immigrants.

THE HEALTH CARE SYSTEM IN THE FUTURE

Because physicians have in the past opposed efforts to include services provided by nurses among those eligible for direct reimbursement in provincial health care plans, it will not be easy to change existing provisions. Nevertheless, nurses provide a viable and cost effective alternative in delivering certain kinds of health care services, particularly those involving health promotion, health maintenance, and counselling activities in relation to health. In the mid-1990s, the health care environment was characterized by fiscal restraint that led to extensive layoffs of professional nurses and widespread salary reductions for health care providers and public-sector workers. This left the entire system in jeopardy, since the system lost legions of professionals and nonprofessionals alike. Seasoned health care providers warned of shortages looming in the future, and it was not long before there were desperate cries for personnel, particularly for nurses! At the moment, an all-out effort is being made to recruit new nurses from inactive ranks and from other countries and to increase the quotas of nursing students in basic educational programs in nursing.

The fact that downsizing of the system was carried out without making substantive changes in the way it was organized meant that the changes that might have occurred naturally in a free and open health care environment did not occur. To date, powerful physician-dominated lobby groups have successfully prevented major departures from the physician-centred health care system maintained through the force of health care financing legislation. Nurses are learning to develop effective lobby groups of their own to ensure that politicians understand the contribution nurses can make to the health care system. Governments will be forced to consider alternatives, despite the pressure to resist change, as the limits of the public purse and the demand for improved health services are recognized.

Despite the lack of planning for change at the system level, there have been some principles driving health care reform that have had some positive effects. These include the move toward more community-based services, attempting to provide care to people on either an outpatient or home-care basis, and placing more emphasis on health promotion at all levels. These kinds of changes have been needed for a long time in a system that was focused on acute care and on physician-centred and hospital-based care. When governments are able to summon up the political will to make structural changes to the system that will rationalize the delivery of health care provided by health care, the result will be both greater efficiency and effectiveness in health care provided to people.

CRITICAL THINKING QUESTIONS

1. Explain why Canada was able to develop a system of universal national health insurance in the twentieth century but, despite several attempts, the United States was not able to do so.
2. Discuss the five basic principles of health care that underlie federal health legislation in Canada, exploring the meaning of each.
3. Explore the relationship between the health care system and the economy with reference to nursing.

WEB SITES

Canada Health Act: http://www.hc-sc.gc.ca/hcs-sss/medi-assur/cha-lcs/overview-apercu-eng.php
Health Canada: http://www.hc-sc.gc.ca/index-eng.php

◤ REFERENCES

Agnew, G. H. (1974). *Canadian hospitals, 1920 to 1970: A dramatic half century.* Toronto: University of Toronto Press.

American Public Health Association. (2001). *Universal health care briefing—progressive caucus.* Report of a meeting held May 1, 2001, Washington, DC. Retrieved on March 26, 2002, from http://www.apha.org /legislative/universal_health_care_briefing.htm.

Bégin, M. (1982). *Opening statement to Conference of Federal and Provincial Ministers of Health.* Ottawa: Queen's Printer.

Brown, M. C. (1980). The implications of established program finance for national health insurance. *Canadian Public Policy, 3,* 521–532.

Canadian Nurses Association (CNA). (1983). *An information package on CNA's recommendations for the proposed Canada Health Act.* Ottawa: Author.

Canadian Nurses Association (CNA). (2002). *Press release: Canadian study provides evidence linking nursing knowledge to lower mortality rates.* Ottawa: Author.

Chambers, L. W., Bruce-Lockhart, P., Black, D. P., Sampson, E., & Burke, M. (1977). A controlled trial of the impact of the family practice nurse on volume, quality, and cost of rural health services. *Medical Care, 15*(12), 971–981.

Glass, H. P. (1983). Letter to Dr. Janet Kerr. *Provincial health insurance plans: Extra-billing/user charges by hospitals.* Ottawa: Health and Welfare Canada.

Hoey, J. R., McCallum, H. P., & LePage, E. M. (1982). Expanding the nurse's role to improve preventive service in an outpatient clinic. *Canadian Medical Association Journal, 127*(1), 27–28.

Kirby, M. J. L. (2002). *The health of Canadians—the federal role: Final report.* Ottawa: Government of Canada. Retrieved on October, 22, 2009, from http://www.parl.gc.ca/37/2/parlbus/commbus/senate/ com-e/SOCI-E/rep-e/repoct02vol6-e.htm.

LeClair, M. (1975). The Canadian health care system. In S. Andrepoulos (Ed.), *National health insurance: Can we learn from Canada?* (pp. 11–96). New York: John Wiley & Sons.

National Coalition on Health Care. (2009). *Health insurance coverage.* Retrieved on October 1, 2009, from http://www.nchc.org/facts/coverage.shtml.

Organization for Economic Development (OECD). (2009). *OECD health at a glance 2009: Key findings for Canada.* Retrieved on March 22, 2009, from http://www.oecd.org/document/51/0,3343, en_33873108_ 33873277_44220787_1_1_1,00.html.

Premier's Advisory Council on Health (Mazankowski Report). (2002). *A framework for reform.* Edmonton: Government of Alberta. Retrieved on October 22, 2009, from http://dsp-psd.pwgsc.gc.ca/Collection-R/ LoPBdP/BP/prb0133-e.htm.

Rachlis, M., & Kushner, C. (1994). *Strong medicine: How to save Canada's health care system.* Toronto: HarperCollins.

Ramsay, J. A., McKenzie, J. K., & Fish, D. G. (1982). Physicians and nurse practitioners: Do they provide equivalent health care? *American Journal of Public Health, 72*(1), 55–57.

Romanow, R. J. (2002). *Building on values: The future of health care in Canada.* Ottawa: Government of Canada. Retrieved on October 22, 2009, from http://www.collectionscanada.gc.ca/webarchives/ 20071122004429/http://www.hc-sc.gc.ca/english/pdf/romanow/pdfs/hcc_final_report.pdf.

Taylor, M. G. (1978). *Health insurance and Canadian public policy: The seven decisions that created the Canadian health insurance system and their outcomes.* Montreal: McGill-Queen's University Press.

Vayda, E., Evans, R., & Mindell, W. R. (1979). Universal health insurance in Canada: History, problems, trends. *Journal of Community Health, 4*(3), 217–231.

Wallace, E. (1980). The origin of the social welfare state in Canada, 1867–1900. In C. A. Meilicke, & J. L. Storch (Eds.), *Perspectives on Canadian health and social services policy: History and emerging trends* (pp. 25–37). Ann Arbor: Health Administration Press.

World Bank. (2001). *2001 world development indicators.* Retrieved on March 26, 2002, from http://devdata. worldbank.org/hnpstats/files/Tab2_15xls.

2

Nursing in Canada, 1600 to the Present:
A Brief Account

Pauline Paul and Janet C. Ross-Kerr

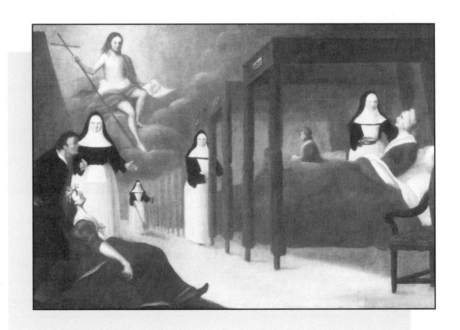

LEARNING OBJECTIVES

- To recognize the importance of considering historical factors when studying nursing trends and issues.
- To acquire fundamental knowledge about the history of nursing in Canada.
- To recognize the unique contribution of New France nurses to the development of nursing in Canada in the seventeenth century.
- To understand the role played by nurses in responding to health care needs of populations who migrated further west during the eighteenth and nineteenth centuries.
- To understand the link between modern nursing and the creation of national professional nursing organizations.
- To recognize the role played by Canadian nurses during the major armed conflicts of the twentieth century.
- To recognize that nurses have worked in the community and in hospital settings at various times in Canadian history.

Understanding the past, and particularly the history of nursing, reveals the contextual factors shaping contemporary nursing issues. Many important nursing issues today, even in a slightly different form, have been with the profession for decades, if not longer. As stated by the American Association for the History of Nursing (AAHN): "The social pressures that have shaped nursing in the past persist today in new forms. Today's challenges are not easily understood or addressed in the absence of such insight" (2001, p. 1). It is apparent that the attention paid to history in this text is useful to the understanding of nursing in the twenty-first century. This chapter provides a cursory review of the evolution of nursing in Canada, and a review of the development of nursing education is presented in Chapter 18. Additional historical insights in relation to the historical background of nursing and nursing education have been integrated into the more detailed analyses in other chapters of the major issues facing the profession in Canada.

NURSING IN NEW FRANCE: 1600 TO 1759

As a result of Jacques Cartier's numerous voyages across the Atlantic, including his 1535 landing on Newfoundland, France laid claim to the vast area along the St. Lawrence River that was to become Canada. Exploration and establishment of the first French settlement in the new land occurred over the next century. Samuel de Champlain established French settlements, including in 1608 one that became Quebec City; this sheltered and beautiful spot would serve as an ideal trading centre for the growing fur trade.

The story of the early colonization of New France parallels the development of nursing because the establishment of hospitals and a health care system preceded the general settlement of the colony. The development of health care in the new land was considered to be of prime importance in the civilization of the colony. At the outset, and for many years thereafter, human services, including health care, education, and social welfare, focused on the indigenous peoples —the numerous First Nations populating the region.

Spurred by religious fervour and zeal, nuns and priests made great efforts to befriend and subsequently convert Aboriginal peoples to Christianity. They and other early settlers endured considerable hardship and hazardous living conditions in the early years.

THE FIRST NURSES IN NEW FRANCE

The legacy of the first nurses in New France has received considerable attention as a result of their courage, sacrifice, altruism, and skill. It is noted that the several thousand Aboriginals living in the region before the Europeans had developed a system of health care characterized by numerous herbal remedies for particular ailments. The first nurses to tend the sick were male attendants at a "sick bay" established at the French garrison in Port Royal in Acadia in 1629 (Gibbon & Mathewson, 1947). Then the Jesuit priests who were missionary immigrants to New France found themselves caring for the sick in the course of their primary Christian mission. They "singly or in pairs travelled in the depth of winter from village to village, ministering to the sick and seeking to commend their religious teachings by their efforts to relieve bodily distress" (Parkman, 1897, p. 176).

MARIE ROLLET HÉBERT

The first laywoman who cared for the sick in homes in the community was Marie Rollet, married to the surgeon-apothecary, Louis Hébert. The Hébert family emigrated to Quebec in 1617 and Mme Marie Hébert thus became the first woman to emigrate from France (English, 2008, n.p.). In Quebec, Louis Hébert's "apothecary skill and his small store of grain were a godsend to the sick and starving winterers. In spite of the company's demands on his and his servant's time, he succeeded in clearing and planting some land" (English, 2008, n.p.).

"Marie Rollet aided her husband in caring for the sick" and shared his interest in the Aboriginal people (English, 2008, n.p). This was quite natural, as it was common for French wives of the early seventeenth century to collaborate with their husbands in their work. Of special attention was Mme Hébert's genuine concern for the indigenous people. The efforts of Mme Hébert and her husband to care for the Aboriginals and share health knowledge with them appear to have been welcomed (Thwaites, 1959). Although little is written, we know that settlers also learned from the Aboriginal peoples; for example, about the value of evergreen trees as a source of Vitamin C during the long winter months.

A CALL FOR NURSES

The people of France learned about the new colony through the *Jesuit Relations*, informative reports written regularly by the Jesuit missionary priests to spread word about colonial life and stimulate needed support. These were written over a 72-year period and provide a marvellous account of life in early Canada. "It was clear to the fathers that their ministrations were valued solely because their religion was supposed by many to be a 'medicine' or charm, efficacious against disease and death" (Parkman, 1897, p. 179). Thus they sent urgent requests for nurses to come to the colony to assist with their work. In 1634, Father LeJeune wrote in his *Relations*:

If we had a hospital here, all the sick people of the country, and all the old people, would be there. As to the men, we will take care of them according to our means; but, in regard to the women, it is not becoming for us to receive them into our houses. (Kenton, 1925, p. 49)

Questions of propriety, an important part of the culture of the times, made it a problem for the Jesuit priests to treat Aboriginal women who were ill on missionary premises. This presented another pressing reason for female members of a nursing order to come to Canada to assist with the work. It is somewhat curious to reflect on the fact that "Quebec, as we have seen, had a seminary, a hospital, and a convent, before it had a population" (Parkman, 1897, p. 259).

HOSPITALIÈRES DE LA MISÉRICORDE DE JÉSUS

The Duchesse d'Aiguillon, a niece of Cardinal Richelieu, read and was moved by the *Relations* and developed a plan to build the Hôtel-Dieu at Quebec. She used her influence to obtain a grant of land and arranged for the careful selection of three Augustinian nuns of the Hospitalières de la Miséricorde de Jésus, also known as Les Augustines, to go to Canada to establish the hospital. The three nuns, who all came from good families, were Marie Guenet de St. Ignace (later Mère de St. Ignace), Anne Lecointre de St. Bernard, and Marie Forestier de St. Bonaventure de Jésus. Aboard ship at Dieppe, the "hospital nuns" encountered three Ursuline nuns, whose mission was to teach the Aboriginal people, and Madame de la Peltrie, who intended to help establish a convent school for the Aboriginal children. The voyage was perilous, lasting from May to August 1639 (Juchereau & Duplessis, 1939), and upon their arrival the women began work immediately.

The Hospital Nuns arrived at Kebec on the first day of August of last year. Scarcely had they disembarked before they found themselves overwhelmed with patients. The hall of the hospital being too small, it was necessary to erect some cabins, fashioned like those of the [Aboriginal people], in their garden. Not having furniture for so many people, they had to cut in two or three pieces part of the blankets and sheets they had brought for these poor sick people. . . . The sick came from all directions in such numbers, their stench was so insupportable, the heat so great, the fresh food so scarce and so poor, in a country so new and strange. (Kenton, 1925, p. 157)

The smallpox epidemic, which was raging on the sisters' arrival and for a considerable length of time thereafter, also required the labours of the Ursuline nuns, whose school convent became a hospital, "and they found themselves nursing instead of teaching" (Millman, 1965, p. 424). Jamieson commented on the fact that the Ursulines used Aboriginal women for assistance in their hospitals and that "their teacher training was instrumental in providing the earliest instruction and supervision of nurses in America" (Jamieson, Sewall, & Gjertson, 1959, p. 196).

New recruits from Dieppe were sought, and the first two arrived the following summer. The nuns also moved their base of operations to Sillery, a settlement outside Quebec, in a more convenient location for the Aboriginal people. The structure in which the nuns had spent the first winter had proved inadequate to withstand the winter elements, and a new building was constructed in Sillery. Soon the hospital was inundated with Aboriginal patients, and many had to be cared for in adjacent cabins. With considerable regret, the nuns had to abandon their white habits for a more serviceable brown. The sisters also applied themselves to learning the language of the Hurons and Algonquins, for whom they cared (Gibbon & Mathewson, 1947).

In 1644, Governor de Montmagny implored the sisters to return to the safety of Quebec, because the Iroquois were reported to be threatening attack, and the sisters would be in danger by staying in Sillery. They returned and were lodged in temporary quarters while a new hospital was constructed. The latter was not completed until two years later, and during the smallpox epidemic of 1650, the number of patients received was so great that they could not all be accommodated in the hospital. The sisters also considered it their duty to assist new settling families in Quebec as much as they could. The archives of the Hôtel-Dieu de Québec contain a letter from Vincent de Paul written in April 1652. "I consider this enterprise as one of the greatest accomplished within fifteen hundred years" (Gibbon & Mathewson, 1947, p. 15). By 1671, the nuns were obtaining sufficient local recruits to the order and no longer depended on assistance from France.

In 1690, hostilities broke out once more between the British and the French, and the sisters of the Hôtel-Dieu de Québec found themselves in the middle of the conflict. It is reported that 26 cannonballs hit the hospital on one day of heavy fighting. The siege was over in four days, and the British withdrew. Epidemics followed from time to time, but the worst appears to have been a smallpox epidemic in 1703, when more than a quarter of the nuns died.

Our sisters fell ill in such numbers from the very first that there were not enough of those who were well to look after the infected cases in our rooms and wards. We accepted the offer of service from several good widows. (Gibbon & Mathewson, 1947, p. 35)

JEANNE MANCE

Born in 1606 to wealthy parents of 12 children in Langres, France, Jeanne Mance attended a girls' school and decided at an early age that she was going to devote her life to God. Following the death of her parents, she looked after her younger brothers and sisters. When an epidemic of plague came to Langres, Jeanne Mance assisted in caring for the sick along with other women in the community. She also gained experience nursing casualties of the Thirty Years' War. A cousin who was a Jesuit priest made plans to go to New France, and this interested Mance, who began to investigate how she could be of service in the New World.

La Société de Notre Dame de Jésus was composed of a group of philanthropists who wanted to establish a colony of a religious character to work with the Aboriginal people on the Island of Montreal. This was no easy matter because they had to secure the charter for the land and raise sufficient funds to send a carefully selected group of people to create the society they had in mind. They thought, however, the hospital might be begun at once. Mance had read the *Jesuit Relations* regularly and believed she had been called to serve in the New World. Through the wealth of Mme de Bullion, Mance was asked to take charge of building a hospital in the settlement that was to be established at Montreal. Thus she sailed from La Rochelle in 1641, along with three women and forty men, under the leadership of Paul de Chomédey, Sieur de Maisonneuve (Canadian Nurses Association [CNA], 1968). Their two ships arrived in Quebec, but their reception was not a welcoming one. They

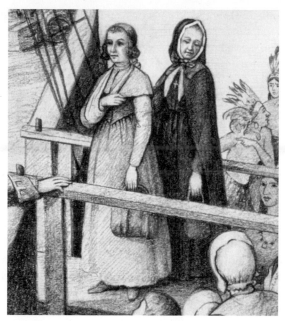

Marguerite Bourgeoys and Jeanne Mance, her broken arm in a sling, are depicted boarding a ship to France in 1657 to solicit funds for the struggling colony of Montreal.

arrived too late in the season to ascend to Montreal before winter. They encountered distrust, jealousy, and opposition. The agents of the company of the Hundred Associates looked on them askance; and the Governor of Quebec, Montmagny, saw a rival governor in Maisonneuve. Every means was used to persuade the adventurers to abandon their project, and settle at Quebec. (Parkman, 1897, p. 296)

Steadfast in his resolve to accomplish the mission to establish a settlement at Montreal, Maisonneuve "expressed his surprise that they should assume to direct his affairs. 'I have not come here,' he said, 'to deliberate, but to act. It is my duty and my honour to found a colony at Montreal; and I would go, if every tree were an Iroquois!'" (Parkman, 1897, pp. 296–297). The group had difficulty finding housing for the winter, but through the generosity of one colonist, they were housed at St. Michel. Jeanne Mance found that her neighbours were the hospital nuns who lived in their mission at Sillery, not far from Quebec. Here she spent a good deal of her time assisting in the work of the hospital, and this undoubtedly served her well as she ventured to Montreal as the only person with health care knowledge.

When on May 17, 1642, Maisonneuve and his followers landed at Montreal, the Associates of Montreal took possession of the land that "Champlain, thirty-one years before, had chosen as the fit site of a settlement" (Parkman, 1897, p. 302). They gave thanks and then proceeded to establish their settlement. The hospital was one of the first buildings constructed in the colony, although there were apparently some misgivings.

It is true that the hospital was not wanted as no one was sick at Ville Marie and one or two chambers would have sufficed for every prospective necessity; but it will be remembered that the colony had been established in order that a hospital might be built. . . . Instead then of tilling the land to supply their own pressing needs, all labourers of the settlement were set at this pious though superfluous task. (Parkman, 1897, p. 362)

The hospital was 46 m by 18.5 m and contained a kitchen, living quarters for Jeanne Mance and for the servants, and two large areas for the patients. "It was amply provided with furniture, linen, medicine and all necessaries and had two oxen, three cows and 20 sheep. A small oratory of stone was built adjoining it" (Parkman, 1897, pp. 362–363). A palisade was constructed around it because of the considerable danger of Iroquois attacks. "Here Mlle Mance took up her abode and waited the day when wounds or disease should bring patients to her empty wards" (Parkman, 1897, p. 363). All of the new settlers were committed to the objective of converting the Aboriginal people to Christianity and sought to gain their favour in whatever way they could. "If they could persuade them to be nursed, they were consigned to the tender care of Mlle Mance" (Parkman, 1897, p. 364). A year after its founding, Montreal became the target of the Iroquois, and Mance had

her hands full attending to men wounded by their arrows. She dressed wounds of all kinds. Chilblains and frostbite frequently required her attention. According to the Clerk of the Court, she had mortar, scales, a syringe with ivory tube, razors and lances. She had sufficient skill to compound her own medicines, and also had experience in blood letting. (Gibbon & Mathewson, 1947, pp. 25–26)

As she was soon in need of more help than the one young girl who had come with her, she enlisted the assistance of two others to cope with the patient load. Mance made three trips back to France, one four years after her arrival, one in 1657, and one in 1663. Her mission was to meet with members of the Associates of Notre Dame of Montreal and other benefactors to generate resources for her hospital. Worried about succession, she arranged for assistance from a nursing order in France in 1659, and three nuns of St. Joseph de la Flèche arrived thereafter to assist in nursing the sick in her hospital, of which she remained the administrator. By 1663, the Associates were bankrupt and could no longer continue their assistance to the colony and the hospital. They transferred their interests to the Gentlemen of Saint Sulpice, and Mance witnessed the transfer of ownership to this group. When she died in 1673, she was "universally respected and beloved by the Colony which she had helped to found" (Gibbon & Mathewson, 1947, p. 30).

Jeanne Mance is one of the most celebrated nurses in Canadian nursing history. Co-founder of the city of Montreal, she was held in high regard for the hospital she founded and the work she did ministering to Aboriginals and settlers alike. She was Maisonneuve's confidante, advisor, and accountant as well, and without her the colony would not have become as strong. Today, the highest award of the Canadian Nurses Association for contribution to the profession is named the Jeanne Mance Award.

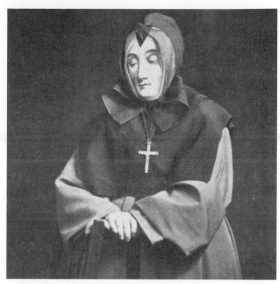

Canonized in 1990, Marguerite d'Youville, founder of the Grey Nuns, pioneered home visits and was renowned for her excellent care regardless of a patient's race, status, or religion.

THE GREY NUNS OF MONTREAL

Marie-Marguerite Dufrost de Lajemmerais was born in Varennes, Quebec. Niece of the famed explorer La Vérendrye, Marguerite d'Youville married a fur trader who was also notorious as a bootlegger and gambler and who died leaving his family in debt in less than a decade. After his death, Marguerite d'Youville drew on her religious faith and gathered a group of women of like mind to assist her. The Sisters of Charity of Montreal or les Soeurs Grises (the Grey Nuns), the nursing order of nuns she founded in 1736, are considered the first visiting nurses in Canada. The Grey Nuns order was the first noncloistered order to be established in Canada, patterned after the model initiated by St. Vincent de Paul. Madame d'Youville organized this group of women with charitable intentions, and they "agreed to combine their possessions in a house of refuge chiefly for the poor" (Gibbon & Mathewson, 1947, p. 45).

Life was by no means easy for them because they had to raise funds to subsist and carry on their work with the sick and the poor. For the purpose of raising money, wealthy paying guests were taken in, and the sisters did handiwork that they sold. Because the order was not cloistered, and because it took up the nursing of patients in their homes, something not previously done in Canada, there was originally some mistrust of its work and intentions. "Though they usually did their visiting in pairs for self-protection, the Grey Nuns were innovators and subject to misunderstanding" (Gibbon & Mathewson, 1947, p. 46). It is important to recognize that the other orders of nuns working in Canada, the Augustinians in Quebec and the St. Joseph's Hospitallers of Montreal, were cloistered and were not permitted to venture into the community except in an emergency by special permission of the bishop.

A fire in 1745 destroyed their house, and the Grey Nuns were forced to move from one place to another for the next two years to carry on their work. Then the Gentlemen of Saint Sulpice gave permission for d'Youville and the Grey Nuns to take over the General Hospital under a charter as the Soeurs de la Charité de l'Hôpital Général de Montréal. Their debts were so great that they had to resort to all sorts of new fundraising activities, including making military garments and tents, establishing a brewery and a tobacco plant, and operating a freight and cartage business. Patients who regained health as a result of the nuns' charitable efforts were put to work to aid in the fundraising effort (Gibbon & Mathewson, 1947, p. 47).

When war broke out between the British and the French in 1756, a section of the hospital called the Ward of the English was opened to care for the wounded English soldiers. The sisters were sufficiently generous of spirit to provide refuge to escaped English soldiers fleeing from the Aboriginals. "One of these English showed his gratitude, in 1760, by saving the hospital from the artillery fire of the army of invasion" (Gibbon & Mathewson, 1947, p. 48). In 1760, the transfer of authority over Montreal to the British brought with it statements testifying to the respect in which the sisters were held. General Amherst spoke

> of the goodwill I have to a Society so worthy of respect as that of the Monastery of St. Joseph de l'Hôtel-Dieu de Montréal, which can count so far as the British Nation is concerned on the same protection that it has enjoyed under French rule. (Gibbon & Mathewson, 1947, p. 48)

THE STATUS OF NURSING IN CANADA IN THE SEVENTEENTH AND EIGHTEENTH CENTURIES

There was a marked contrast between Canada and Britain in the status of nursing and the quality of care provided in the seventeenth and eighteenth centuries. Nursing in Britain had fallen into disrepute after Henry VIII's renunciation of the Catholic Church. The nursing orders of nuns, which had previously provided the nursing service in the large London hospitals, were expelled and replaced by those of the ilk of Charles Dickens's "Sairey Gamp." Gibbon and Mathewson (1947) recount a number of descriptions of such nurses in England, noting the negative effects on hospitals of incompetent staff more concerned about personal pleasure than the welfare of patients.

These conditions did not occur to any great extent in early Canada because of the historical fact that the first settlement at Quebec developed as a colony of France. In France, nursing did not undergo the regressive period that occurred in England. Young women of good character, who came from reputable families, were recruited to nursing in France—primarily under the auspices of the Catholic Church—throughout this period of time.

> If the settlements along the St. Lawrence River had been colonized in the seventeenth century by the English instead of by the French, the history of nursing in Canada might have been very different. Fate, however, decided in favour of the French, and that was fortunate both for the Huron and Algonquin Indians and for the white pioneers, since in the wake of the fur traders and coureurs de bois, came the Augustinian Hospitallers or Nursing Sisters of Dieppe to Quebec and the St. Joseph Hospitallers of La Flèche to Montreal on their missions of healing

and of mercy—missions which had no counterpart in the colonizing efforts of the Protestant
English in North America. (Gibbon & Mathewson, 1947, p. 1)

Health care in New France also developed with unique characteristics. From inception, the Hôtels-Dieu of New France were devoted to patient care and were more than
refuges for the poor. In contrast with the Hôtels-Dieu of France, they provided care to
patients of all social classes (Violette, 2005). The birth of the truly Canadian Grey Nuns
was also an important milestone since, as will be seen, they played a central role in the
development of health care in Western Canada.

The health care system that had developed in the colony was firmly established when the
English defeated the French in the battle of the Plains of Abraham in 1759. Undoubtedly,
factors such as the geographic separation from England and the political climate in North
America ensured the continuation of the French traditions of good nursing in Canada.

 ## SURVIVAL AND GRADUAL EXPANSION OF NURSING: 1763 TO 1874

After the war of 1756–1763, the transition to British rule was difficult for Quebec nursing
orders. The nuns received little or no financial support because their wealthy benefactors
had returned to France, and donations dwindled. Without a regular income, the nuns
were impoverished at the outset of the new regime. However, in correspondence with the
Duchesse d'Aiguillon, William Pitt, prime minister of Great Britain, stated that the com-
manding general of the British troops had "the satisfaction to be able to state that our
officers, who are very strong in their praises of the charitable care of our sick and wounded
by these nuns, have paid them every attention required by piety and misfortune" (Gibbon
& Mathewson, 1947, p. 52). In addition, there is a record of some financial assistance from
the British for the sisters. "By instruction of Pitt, General Murray relieved the Hôtel-Dieu
of a debt of taxes to the extent of 3389 livres, which had reverted to the British at the change
of the regime, and also paid £808 for rent of lodgings to the troops, and £3085 for the use of
furniture, laundry and utensils of the hospital" (Gibbon & Mathewson, 1947, pp. 52–53).
Nevertheless, all of the hospital systems remained in place at the transfer of power.

The next decades were tumultuous for the British colonies as Americans were seeking independence. From 1775 to 1776, during the American War of Independence, the
American attack on the Canadian border brought patients from each side of the battle
to the Hôtel-Dieu of Quebec, where all were cared for with warmth and humanity. An
American lieutenant recorded the following in his diary on March 10, 1776:

Was removed to the Hotel Dieu, sick of the scarlet fever, and placed under the care of the Mother
Abbess, where I had fresh provisions and good attendance. For several nights the nuns sat up
with me, four at a time, every two hours. Here I feigned myself sick after I had recovered, for
fear of being sent back to the Seminary to join my fellow-officers, and was not discharged until
I acknowledged that I was well. When I think of my captivity, I shall never forget the time spent
among the nuns who treated me with so much humanity. (Gibbon & Mathewson, 1947, p. 55)

Among other hospitals that also cared for the sick and wounded was the Hôtel-Dieu at Trois-Rivières, which had been established in 1697. The tradition of caring for all regardless of race, nationality, or creed was paramount, and preservation of human life and nourishment of the spirit through religious beliefs and practices remained central characteristics of their work.

EFFECTS OF IMMIGRATION ON NURSING

After the defeat of the French forces at the Plains of Abraham, the Treaty of Paris of 1763 established certain rules for the government of the colony of Quebec. Its thrust was anglicization to attract English-speaking settlers to help rebuild the shattered economy after the war. Although the British had imagined a flood of settlement would soon help anglicize Quebec, "in fact, few people came" (Morton, 1983, p. 23). Soon the people of Quebec were recognized as Canadians, and the *Quebec Act* of 1774 restored many of their former freedoms and rights. The act was also designed to win the support of these Canadians in the upcoming conflict with the Americans. With some difficulty, the British were able to hold Quebec in that conflict.

After the war, United Empire Loyalists, who wanted to remain loyal to Britain, immigrated to Canadian territory. Their numbers eventually totalled 50,000. These settlers were joined by large numbers of immigrants from Britain and Ireland. "Late Loyalists" followed during the early nineteenth century. There was also a sizeable increase in the French Canadian population, from 60,000 in 1760, to 110,000 by 1784, and 330,000 by 1860. The *Constitutional Act* of 1791 divided Quebec into Upper and Lower Canada, each with its own system of government, and confirmed the rights of French Canadians as laid down earlier in the *Quebec Act*.

The devastating effects of the Napoleonic Wars on trade in England led many from the British Isles to emigrate to overcome poverty. "Factory folk, miners, and farmers became equally distressed, and the British Government could do little more than divert the resulting emigration to countries where the British flag still flew" (Gibbon & Mathewson, 1947, p. 71). A majority of these immigrants were poorly nourished and travelled in "vessels which were overcrowded and unsanitary," so disease found easy prey among the new settlers.

The United Empire Loyalists did not have to travel in disease-infested vehicles or under unsanitary conditions and thus escaped the devastation that followed the voyages of the Europeans. Nevertheless, diseases brought by new arrivals spread rapidly among residents of the new colony. Dramatic increases in the population gave epidemic diseases more scope, and immigrants brought with them cholera, typhus, smallpox, and trachoma. In 1832, an epidemic of cholera wiped out one-seventh of the population of Montreal, or 4000 people (Gibbon & Mathewson, 1947). To protect the Canadian population, the British imposed health examinations for immigrants, and a quarantine station and hospital were established at Grosse-Île in the St. Lawrence River. This hospital was staffed by lay nurses, including Irish and French Canadian nurses and even a Norwegian nurse (Young & Rousseau, 2005).

The rapid increase in population in English-speaking Canada in the late eighteenth and early nineteenth centuries led to a shortage of health care facilities made necessary by persistent waves of epidemics. The dismal state of nursing in Britain was paralleled in new areas of the country opened up by the English and not served by the French nursing orders. It is noted that "nursing in English-speaking Canada remained primitive for many years" (CNA, 1968, p. 30). Laywomen attempted nursing in the hospitals that were established, but they were largely without the proper training and skill to do what was needed. The established French speaking sisterhoods expanded their work across the country and new English-speaking orders were formed.

Because so many of the arriving settlers were destitute and ill, they needed a great deal of assistance. The Female Benevolent Society was organized in Montreal in 1816 and was responsible for the establishment of what would be called the Montreal General Hospital. In Kingston, the Kingston Compassionate Society secured a grant of land from the government and constructed the first version of what would become the Kingston General Hospital. Likewise, in York, the Toronto General Hospital was founded by a philanthropic group with funds designated to buy medals for the War of 1812 (Gibbon & Mathewson, 1947). The introduction of lay nurses in areas previously served by nursing sisterhoods met with some opposition at first, but the needs of the sick and the poor had to be met. The influence of Florence Nightingale on the development of early nursing in Canada was important (see Box 2.1), and the principles she espoused were consistent with those of the French-Canadian nursing sisters.

BOX 2.1	The Influence of Florence Nightingale on Nursing in Canada

In 1854, Florence Nightingale set off with her small band of 38 carefully selected nurses to tend the British soldiers in the Crimea. Up to that time, British military hospitals had been staffed exclusively by male attendants. It had not been easy to secure permission to nurse the sick and wounded military personnel during the Crimean War. However, Nightingale came from a prominent and wealthy family and had connections with many powerful people. She had been well educated at home and had travelled widely before she set out to learn how to nurse the sick. She went first to Germany, where she stayed for some time at Pastor Fliedner's Lutheran hospital and later went to work with the nursing nuns at the Hôtel-Dieu in Paris. Upon her return to England, she obtained a position in charge of a private Harley Street hospital. When the Crimean War broke out, Nightingale managed not only to obtain permission to go to the Crimea but also to raise the British consciousness about the need for good nursing for the sick. "Her onslaught on the appalling lack of sanitation in the wards of the General and Barrack hospitals at Scutari contributed greatly to the reduction in the deaths of cases treated from 315 per thousand to 22 per thousand" (Gibbon & Mathewson, 1947, pp. 109–110). Recent scholarship (Gill & Gill, 2005) further confirms that Nightingale had a profound impact on the well-being of troops.

The outpouring of public support for Nightingale's cause was overwhelming, and a fund was established, even before she returned from the Crimea, to allow her to organize a training school for nurses (Nutting & Dock, 1937). At last nursing was to become a suitable occupation for women.

Mark what by breaking through customs and prejudices Miss Nightingale has effected for her sex. She has opened to them a new profession, a new sphere of usefulness . . . a claim for more extended freedom of action, based on proved public usefulness in the highest sense of the word (Gibbon & Mathewson, 1947, p. 110)

BOX 2.1	The Influence of Florence Nightingale on Nursing in Canada—cont'd

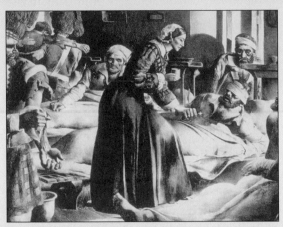

Florence Nightingale revolutionized nursing practice and training through her work with the British Army during the Crimean War, when many were "surviving the battles and being killed by the hospitals."

Florence Nightingale's influence was worldwide and reached Canada by way of both Britain and the United States when, during the American Civil War, there was an attempt to establish Nightingale's standard of nursing to minimize suffering. In 1873, training schools based on the Nightingale model were opened in three American hospitals: Bellevue in New York, Massachusetts General, and New Haven (Gibbon & Mathewson, 1947). Canadian hospitals, particularly the secular hospitals in English-speaking settlements, considered educating nurses to raise the standards of care, a direct result of Nightingale's influence. The establishment of schools of nursing is discussed in some detail in Chapter 18. However, it is important to recognize the profound influence that Florence Nightingale had on the initiation of an organized system of nursing education for lay nurses throughout the world.

In recent years, a number of scholars (for example, McDonald, 2001; Gill & Gill, 2005; McPherson, 2005; and Kudzma, 2006) have re-examined Nightingale's legacy, and as is the case for most historical figures of her stature, there are debates about the place she is given in history. It remains nonetheless that she is probably the most recognized name in nursing worldwide.

THE GREY NUNS AND THE OPENING UP OF THE WEST

On April 24, 1844, four Grey Nuns set out in long canoes bound for St. Boniface, Manitoba. The measure of courage required for the strenuous journey is difficult to appreciate in an age in which superhighways are commonplace. For example, on May 2, Sister Lagrave wrote:

> *What shall I tell you? I can hardly collect a few thoughts. I believe the high wind has scattered them over lake Huron, I sit on a rock: my head is spinning, my heart is fluttering. [. . .] I have not slept since our departure. [. . .] The bad weather is lasting and when the rain stops, contrary winds delay our progress. (Drouin, 1988, pp.170–171)*

They were greeted with a series of serious epidemics upon their arrival and found themselves stretched far beyond their capacity from the outset.

The onslaught of further epidemics in 1846 was a major challenge facing the nuns after their arrival. These epidemics were extremely serious, and the death toll was high. Sister Laurent has described how they coped with the patient load:

> *Each of us was appointed to do that which she was best fitted for. Some of us went into the houses where sick people were. They used to have measles and dysentery and inflammatory rheumatism, and smallpox sometimes. We had medicines from Montreal, but we also learned the uses of herbs that grew in this country, and how to help the sick people so as to ease their pain and aid them to get better. (Gibbon & Mathewson, 1947, p. 89)*

In Saskatchewan and Alberta, the Grey Nuns were again the pioneers who trekked west to establish health care facilities and systems for the populace. In 1859, after a long journey first from Montreal to St. Boniface, and then by ox cart to Lac Ste. Anne, in what is now Alberta, three Grey Nuns established their mission and began to minister to the Aboriginal peoples through nursing and teaching. Four years later, they moved to St. Albert. From the outset, they took the sick into their convent if they required constant care. In 1870, they built a hospital wing on their convent, and in 1881, they built a separate building. In 1860, three nuns of this order from St. Boniface arrived at Île à la Crosse, Saskatchewan, an Aboriginal settlement 200 miles north of Prince Albert. Arriving before most of the settlers, the sisters established systems of quality health care. The Grey Nuns performed a great deal of visiting nursing, regularly visiting the sick in their homes, working tirelessly as one epidemic after another devastated the local population. For example, in St. Albert, Alberta, Sister Emery wrote that during the last six months of 1870, the sisters had made 692 home visits, provided wound care to 22 patients, and had vaccinated 218 children and 133 adults against smallpox (Emery, 1871).

 REFLECTIVE THINKING

1. What was the effect on Canadian nursing of the fact that organized nursing in this country was established under a French regime?
2. Reflect on the contribution of Florence Nightingale to health care and nursing. Can you see examples of her influence in Canada?

THE ADVENT OF MODERN NURSING: 1874 TO 1914

The rise of the modern hospital, scientific developments, industrialization, and immigration were forces that changed the nature of nursing. With the advent of nursing schools, hospitals began to rely on nursing students for the provision of care (McPherson, 2005). During this period, English Canada embraced nursing, and nurses who were nuns were joined by lay nurses in shaping the future of the profession in Canada. Yet, nursing orders remained strong. The settling of Western Canada, particularly of Alberta and British Columbia, saw the arrival of other religious orders that would play significant roles in health services. Most of these were of French Canadian or British origin. A notable exception was the Sisters Servants of Mary Immaculate, who came from Ukraine in 1902 to provide nursing care to Ukrainian settlers of Alberta (Paul, 2005). As the network of hospitals gradually expanded, both religious and secular, nursing schools flourished and graduates began to seek recognition through organization.

ESTABLISHMENT OF NATIONAL PROFESSIONAL NURSING ORGANIZATIONS

A leading figure in British nursing was Ethel Bedford-Fenwick. Bedford-Fenwick was influential in the formation of the first nursing organizations and was editor of the forerunner of the *British Journal of Nursing*. Attending the 1893 Congress of Charities, Corrections, and Philanthropy in Chicago, Bedford-Fenwick met the leaders in American nursing: Isabel Hampton, Adelaide Nutting, and Lavinia Dock. Interestingly, of these three American leaders, two were Canadians living and working in the United States—Isabel Hampton and Adelaide Nutting. They discussed the need for a drive to secure legislation for the registration of nurses to raise the standard of professional nursing and to ensure those practising were qualified and able.

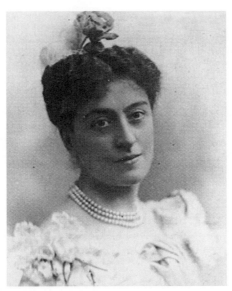

Ethel Bedford-Fenwick, 1857–1947, British nurse and lobbyist who conceived the idea of professional nursing organizations and helped form the International Council of Nurses.

Bedford-Fenwick had been struggling to achieve such legislation in Britain at the time and became convinced that, to succeed, nurses had to band together and form professional organizations. The three American leaders were so impressed with the case for establishing organizations that they immediately organized the American Society of Superintendents of Training Schools for Nurses of the United States and Canada, of which Isabel Hampton Robb became the first president. The major thrust of the organization never strayed from its original goal "to work for higher standards of nurse preparation." It was the forerunner of the National League for Nursing in 1912 (CNA, 1968, p. 35).

Soon after, alumnae associations were established at schools of nursing in the United States. In 1896, under the leadership of its first president, Isabel Hampton Robb, the Nurses' Associated Alumnae of the United States and Canada took root. Criteria for membership included graduation from a program at least two years in length and association with a 100 or more bed hospital. The organization, the forerunner of the American Nurses Association, first directed its efforts at improving the quality of educational programs, and then to pressing for legislation to ensure the registration of nurses. The *American Journal of Nursing* began to publish in 1900 and served as a way of communicating with nurses who could assist with the development of the organization (CNA, 1968).

One of Bedford-Fenwick's major goals was the formation of an international organization of nurses. She had initiated discussions about this with American nursing leaders in Chicago. The formation of national groups was the first priority. Although the North American organization had initially included both Canada and the United States, it was necessary to separate the organizations because of the concept of membership by country in an international organization. Since the responsibility for health care was vested at provincial and state levels, the campaign for registration of nurses was decentralized and separate national organizations were essential to pursue the goal of registering nurses. The International Council of Nurses (ICN) was formed in 1899 with Britain, the United States, and Germany as charter members. Canada was represented at this meeting by five nurses, and Mary Agnes Snively of Canada, superintendent of nurses at the Toronto General Hospital, became the first honorary treasurer of the fledgling organization.

In Canada, the Canadian Society of Superintendents of Training Schools for Nurses was the first completely Canadian national organization of nurses. It was formed in 1907 with Mary Agnes Snively as president. The next year the society invited representatives from all nursing organizations in Canada to meet and establish a national association of nurses. The result of the meeting was the inception of the Provisional Society of the Canadian National Association of Trained Nurses (CNATN), and Mary Agnes Snively was inducted as founding president. Initially, membership took place through member societies composed primarily of graduate nurse and alumnae associations. The first alumnae association in Canada had been founded in 1894 at the Toronto General Hospital (Gibbon & Mathewson, 1947). Nearly every school formed such an organization shortly thereafter, and many of these amalgamated with other groups regionally, and eventually provincially. The CNATN applied for membership in the ICN in 1908, and formal admission took place the next year at the international meeting in London. Because the CNATN had been organized somewhat hastily for the purpose of joining the ICN, a structure that would be suitable for the national organization and would recognize the historical division of powers between the provincial and federal governments had yet to be considered.

A full-time executive secretary, Jean Wilson, was appointed in 1923, and the first national office was opened in Winnipeg, moving later to Montreal and then to Ottawa. In the meantime, the *Canadian Nurse* had begun publication in 1905. Membership of affiliated organizations in the CNATN went from 28 in 1911 to 52 in 1924 when the association changed its name to the Canadian Nurses Association (CNA). In 1930, the organization became a federation of the provincial nurses associations that "made the provincial association the official representative of registered nurses in each province and automatically ensured that all members of the CNA were registered nurses" (CNA, 1968, p. 39).

Through its journal, the *Canadian Nurse*, CNA has a vehicle to reach nurses. In the early years, most articles were written by physicians, but it grew into a peer-reviewed journal, publishing research articles, general articles, columns, and professional information. The CNA also created the Canadian Nurse Portal in 2007—Nurse One, which provides access to search engines and other documents.

The Provisional Council of the Canadian Association of University Schools and Departments of Nursing held its first meeting in 1942 when representatives from eight university schools and departments of nursing met to respond to a proposed program of federal financial assistance for university schools of nursing. The organization was small for a considerable period of time after its founding, the work being carried out on a volunteer basis until 1970, when a part-time executive secretary was hired and the name changed to the Canadian Association of University Schools of Nursing (CAUSN). It was not until 1984 that the position of executive secretary became full-time. The name became the Canadian Association of Schools of Nursing (CASN) in 2002 to reflect the expansion of the membership to include schools in universities, university college partnerships, and colleges. Membership increased from 31 university schools in 1994 to 90 schools of all types in 2003. Responsibility for accreditation was incorporated into its mandate in 1973 and the first standards were published in 1987. In 2006 and 2007, a new accreditation program was initiated to reflect the various types of baccalaureate programs in nursing (CASN, 2009).

In 1962, the Canadian Nurses Foundation (CNF) was incorporated as an organization separate from the CNA to provide scholarships, bursaries, and fellowships for graduate study in nursing. Because the CNF was a charitable organization, donations could be accepted on a tax-exempt basis, thus facilitating the collection of funds for scholarships. A grant of $150,000 from the W.K. Kellogg Foundation in 1962 helped build the fund at its inception. Memberships, collected on a voluntary basis, provided the financial base. However, CNF has had continuing financial difficulty and later developed sophisticated corporate fundraising campaigns.

Initially, CNA and CNF operated autonomously, but developed closer links when it became clear that the financial structure of the CNF was not strong. The executive director of the CNA is the secretary-treasurer of the CNF, the CNF is housed in CNA House in Ottawa, and in the years of CNA biennial conventions, annual meetings of the CNF are held in association with the CNA meeting. Over time, CNF broadened its activities to work closely with the CNA on matters of importance to both organizations.

Although it is reported that provision was made in 1966 to include assistance for study at the baccalaureate level (CNA, 1968, p. 11), in practice, fellowships were awarded almost exclusively for master's and doctoral study. A resolution, passed at the 1982 annual meeting in St. John's, Newfoundland, provided a mandate to award one scholarship for baccalaureate study in each province or territory each year. Today, the CNF provides awards for study at the baccalaureate, master's, and doctoral levels. The number of awards varies from year to year, depending upon available funds. In the past, the CNF maintained a small research funding awards program. Now, through the Nursing Care Partnership Program the CNF provides one dollar for every two partner dollars of research funding (CNF, 2008).

NURSING IN TIMES OF CONFLICT: 1914 TO 1945

Nurses have played pivotal roles during military conflicts throughout Canadian history. The bipartisan role played by the nursing sisters of the Hôtel-Dieu hospitals in Quebec and Montreal during the hostilities between the French and English is legendary. During the Northwest Rebellion of 1885, a military request for nursing services shows the influence of Florence Nightingale and the experience gained during the American Civil War. "No volunteer nurses. If you can send an organized body under a trained head, they will be welcome" (CNA, 1968, p. 63). Two groups of nurses responded, one headed by Mother Hannah Grier from the Anglican order of St. John the Divine in Toronto, the other by Miss Miller, a head nurse at the Winnipeg General Hospital (CNA, 1968). In 1898, nurses with the Victorian Order of Nurses (VON) attached to the Yukon Military Force were praised for their efforts (Gibbon & Mathewson, 1947).

In 1899 an offer of a Canadian contingent of nurses for the Boer War was made by the Canadian government to Joseph Chamberlain, England's colonial secretary at the time. The first group of four nurses was sent to assist in South Africa under the leadership of Georgina Fane Pope, a Bellevue Hospital–educated nurse from Prince Edward Island. She described the conditions under which nursing took place:

> *We nursed in huts and found the work at times very heavy. . . . We received our first convoy of wounded a few days after the Battle of Maggersfontein and Modder River when the beds were filled with men of the Highland Brigade. . . . No. 3 General Hospital of 600 beds was pitched under canvas at Rondesbosch, a few miles away . . . having at times very active service; sometimes covered with sand during a "Cape South-Easter;" at others delayed with a fore-runner of the coming rainy season, and at all times in terror of scorpions and snakes as bedfellows. (Gibbon & Mathewson, 1947, pp. 290–291)*

The South African nursing experience was sufficient to persuade the Canadian Army Medical Corps that an army nursing service ought to be an integral part of the permanent corps. Georgina Pope and Margaret Macdonald were appointed to the staff on a permanent basis in 1906. When World War I broke out, the Army Nursing Corps consisted of five nurses. However, within three weeks of the declaration of war, thousands of nurses had volunteered for service overseas. Margaret Macdonald, who was appointed matron-in-chief of the Army Nursing Corps, described the first group of volunteers:

> *The selection, from coast to coast, of over one hundred nurses from thousands of applicants, the vast majority of whom were entirely unacquainted with Army Life and regulations, constituted somewhat of a problem. However, when all the formalities incident to the appointment of these Nursing Sisters were concluded, it was astonishing how quickly and naturally in becoming military minded they fell into place. Their example and esprit de corps became the pattern for the many hundreds that followed. (Gibbon & Mathewson, 1947, p. 296)*

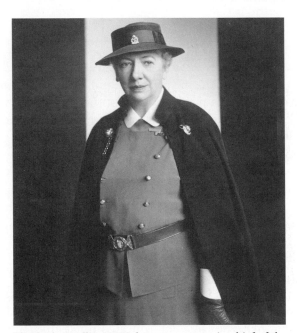

Elizabeth Smellie, VON, became matron-in-chief of the Army Medical Corps during World War II and was the first Canadian woman to reach the rank of colonel.

There are many accounts of the nature of service rendered by Canadian nurses during the war, all of which make note of the flexibility and devotion to duty that was required. Matron Macdonald described the introduction of the first group of nursing sisters to field nursing:

> *Their first introduction to Field Nursing began at Salisbury Plain in 1914; patients, many seriously ill, poured into huts that were ill-equipped to receive them. Cold, damp weather with continuous rain prevailed, adding much to the general discomfort. The sisters literally ploughed their way through mud and water from hut to hut; their living quarters left much to be desired. (Gibbon & Mathewson, 1947, p. 297)*

Major Margaret Macdonald was succeeded by Edith Rayside as matron-in-chief of the nursing service. In all, approximately 3100 nurses saw service during World War I, 47 losing their lives as a result of the conflict (Veterans Affairs Canada, 2002). Fourteen nurses perished in the sinking of the Canadian hospital ship *Llandovery Castle* (CNA, 1968). The significance of nurses' service during World War I led to the establishment of a permanent corps of nursing sisters by the Royal Canadian Army Medical Corps (RCAMC).

Matron-in-chief of the nursing service of the Army Medical Corps from 1940 to 1944 was Elizabeth Smellie. In civilian life, Smellie had been chief superintendent of the VON. She became the first Canadian woman to achieve the rank of colonel. The number of nurses who served during World War II was somewhat greater at 4473 than in World War I (Veterans Affairs Canada, 2002). However, the number of nurses who volunteered far exceeded the number of positions available (Toman, 2005). Twenty-four Canadian general hospitals were established to care for the wounded during World War II, compared with sixteen during World War I. In addition, there was a convalescent hospital in France, a neurologic and plastic surgery hospital in England, and casualty clearing stations, totalling 34 overseas hospitals. Sixty hospitals and two hospital ships were maintained in Canada, all staffed with nurses (Gibbon & Mathewson, 1947). In response to a request from South Africa, nurses under the leadership of Matron-in-Chief Gladys Sharpe were sent to care for wounded British soldiers.

For the major part of the war, Canadian nurses staffed the military hospitals in England and Canada and did not serve under battle conditions in Europe until 1943, when they were sent to assist after the invasion of Italy:

Canadian nurses were the first to reach Sicily after the invasion. . . . The unit was recruited largely from Winnipeg, and other Western cities, but the first girl ashore was Lieutenant Elizabeth Lawson of St. John, New Brunswick. . . . Lieutenant Trennie Hunter, of Winnipeg, was a close second. The Matron of this hospital is Miss Agnes J. MacLeod, of Edmonton. They were described as a "group of grimy, tin-hatted girls, perspiring in the terrific heat and burdened with cumbersome equipment." (Gibbon & Mathewson, 1947, p. 465)

Gladys Sharpe described conditions in South Africa and the response to their arrival:

Our beds filled rapidly, the first convoy via hospital train brought casualties from Burma, Madagascar, the Middle East and Singapore, at the rate of 257 admitted in just two hours— the highlight was the official opening ceremony at which Field Marshall Smuts took the opportunity of publicly thanking "Canada" for sending nurses. (Gibbon & Mathewson, 1947, p. 462)

Up to this point, nurses in military service held the relative rank of officers but did not actually have the official status or authority of officers. During the war, the Privy Council granted nurses commissions equivalent to those of other commissioned officers. In contrast, British and American nurses did not achieve this until the end of the war (CNA, 1968, p. 65).

THE EMERGENCE OF PUBLIC HEALTH NURSING

The development of public health nursing as both an area of specialization in nursing and an integral part of nursing in all settings is largely a process that occurred in the twentieth century. The idea of preventing illness and the spread of disease by educating people about beneficial health practices and lifestyle modifications was not recognized until the twentieth century. Further, it was realized that although good nutritional practices were important for all, these were essential to the health of young children and pregnant women. Some of the first public health nursing took place in the home, caring for patients with tuberculosis and teaching preventive measures.

The first school nurses were appointed in Hamilton, Ontario, in 1909, and Toronto in 1910. Lina Rogers, a graduate of the Hospital for Sick Children, had achieved international fame for her work correlating the absence of children from school with lack of medical care. Her appointment to the School Nursing Service of the Toronto Board of Education led to recruitment of a staff of nurses and dentists, with a mandate to teach children and their families hygienic practices to prevent disease. The Nursing Service was transferred to the health department several years later, providing a model for a system of public health nursing in each province (Gibbon & Mathewson, 1947).

The development of public health nursing has been a gradual process. The entrenchment of a hospital-based system of health care, encouraged by Canadian federal health legislation since 1948, undoubtedly retarded recognition of the need for preventive services, home-based services, and consumer involvement in health care. The Lalonde Report (1975) provided the first evidence of concern about disease prevention and health maintenance at the federal level. However, skyrocketing costs of care in hospitals focused attention on the need to care for people in different ways. Day surgery, ambulatory care, outpatient services, and home care are now being used extensively, with heavy reliance on nurses in each of these. Even though many of these services can be described as "illness care," the need to teach health practices for disease prevention and health maintenance is an important facet of nursing care. The continued emphasis of the Epp Report (1986) on prevention, poverty reduction, and enhancing people's ability to cope with their lives was further evidence of federal support for health promotion.

The Declaration of Alma-Ata adopted in 1978 at the International Conference on Primary Health Care jointly sponsored by the World Health Organization and UNICEF established a goal of health for all by the year 2000. This stimulated a strong thrust to promote health and prevent disease in Canada. Although past the initial target date of 2000, work continues on many of the initiatives. In 1994, the National Forum on Health was established under the direction of Prime Minister Jean Chrétien with a mandate "to consult with Canadians and advise government on innovative ways to improve the health of Canadians." The forum concluded its work in 1997, and a number of informative reports on its work are available on the Health Canada Web site. In view of the continuing debate about the future of Medicare and pressure by some provinces to move to privately funded health care, the Commission on the Future of Health Care in Canada chaired by Roy Romanow was appointed in 2001 by Prime Minister Chrétien. Its report recommended policies and measures to ensure the long-term sustainability of a universally accessible, publicly funded health care system (Romanow, 2002).

The initial impetus for the development of public health nursing took place at a time when there were no antibiotics and few immunizations to combat disease. Thus, good health practices to prevent the spread of infectious diseases were essential. As antibiotics and immunization against a number of diseases became available, the incidence and prevalence of communicable diseases subsided. This may have led to complacency on the part of governments and citizens. However, in the late twentieth and early twenty-first centuries, with the increasing incidence of AIDS, TB, and hepatitis C, and the emergence of SARS, it became clear that the battle against communicable diseases was far from over. Even if this was the case, and even if the official discourse has suggested that over the last 30 years health promotion would become more central, during the first decades of the twenty-first century, only 14.1% of registered nurses worked in the community (Canadian Institute for Health Information, 2008).

NURSING IN HOSPITALS

Prior to the 1950s, hospitals were primarily staffed by nursing students. Since the 1960s, hospitals have become the primary place of employment of registered nurses. In 2007, 63% of registered nurses in Canada worked in the hospital sector (Canadian Institute for Health Information, 2007). The last decades have been characterized by increased patient acuity and changes in technology. Hospitals are dependent on the availability of registered nurses and other nursing personnel. Currently, an acute shortage of nurses is fast becoming a national crisis. Major contributing factors include severe cuts to the health care system in the 1990s and the general aging of the nursing workforce. The challenge for the profession is to meet the shortage without compromising high standards of nursing and nursing education.

The history of nursing in Canada is long and distinguished. Nurses have been caring for people from the time of the earliest French settlements on the shores of the St. Lawrence. Likewise, nurses have been at the heart of new developments in high-technology acute care and have pressed for more emphasis on health promotion. Altruism has characterized nursing and nurses from the outset, and commitment to the public good has been a firmly entrenched principle guiding professional activities. Nurses will continue to meet the new and difficult challenges of the future successfully.

CRITICAL THINKING QUESTIONS

1. You may hear people say that nursing began with Florence Nightingale. Why do you think they say this? How would you explain to them that this is not the case? Give examples supporting your views.
2. Consider the nursing leaders described in this chapter. What characteristics were common to most, if not all of them? What lessons can today's nurses take from these characteristics?
3. Consider the historical aspects of the emergence of public health nursing and reflect on what you know about health care and priorities in the health care system of your province. Can you think of a few factors that explain why the proportion of nurses working in public health nursing continues to remain low?

WEB SITES

Canadian Association for the History of Nursing: http://www.cahn-achn.ca/
Library and Archives Canada: http://www.collectionscanada.gc.ca/

REFERENCES

American Association for the History of Nursing. (2001). *Position Paper—Nursing History in the Curriculum: Preparing Nurses for the 21st Century*. Retrieved on July 7, 2009, from http://www.aahn.org/position.html.

Canadian Association of Schools of Nursing (CASN). (2009). *Historic milestones*. Retrieved on July 7, 2009, from http://www.casn.ca/en/History_30.html.

Canadian Institute for Health Information (CIHI). (2008). *Regulated nurses: Trends, 2003 to 2007*. Retrieved on July 7, 2009, from http://secure.cihi.ca/cihiweb/dispPage.jsp?cw_page=PG_1710_E&cw_topic=1710&cw_rel=AR_2529_E.

Canadian Nurses Association (CNA). (1968). *The leaf and the lamp*. Ottawa: Author.

Canadian Nurses Foundation (CNF). (2008). *Nursing care partnership program*. Retrieved on January 31, 2008, from http://www.canadiannursesfoundation.com/apply.htm.

Drouin, C. (1988). *Love Spans the Centuries, Volume II: 1821–1853*. Montreal: Meridian Press.

Emery, Sister. (1871). Letter from Saint-Albert to Mother Slocombe at Montréal, 6 January 1871. In *Lettres de Saint-Albert, 1858–1877* (pp. 247–253). Montreal: Archives des Soeurs Grises de Montréal.

English, J. (Ed.). (2008). *Dictionary of Canadian biography online: 1000 to 1700* (Vol. 1). Retrieved on July 7, 2009, from http://www.biographi.ca/index-e.html.

Epp, J. (1986). *Achieving health for all: A framework for health promotion*. Ottawa: Health and Welfare Canada.

Gibbon, J. M., & Mathewson, M. S. (1947). *Three centuries of Canadian nursing*. Toronto: Macmillan.

Gill, C. J., & Gill, G. C. (2005). Nightingale in Scutari: Her legacy re-examined. *Clinical Infectious Diseases*, *40*, 1799–1805.

Jamieson, E., Sewall, M., & Gjertson, L. (1959). *Trends in nursing history*. Philadelphia: W.B. Saunders.

Juchereau, J.-F., & Duplessis, M.-A. (1939). *Les annales de l'Hôtel-Dieu de Québec: 1636–1716*. Quebec: l'Hôtel-Dieu de Québec.

Kenton, E. (1925). *The Jesuit Relations and allied documents*. New York: Vanguard Press.

Kudzma, E. C. (2006). Florence Nightingale and healthcare reform. *Nursing Science Quarterly*, *19*(1), 61–64.

Lalonde, M. (1975). *A new perspective on the health of Canadians*. Ottawa: Health and Welfare Canada.

McDonald, L. (Ed.). (2001). *Florence Nightingale: An introduction to her life and family*. Waterloo, ON: Wilfrid Laurier University Press.

McPherson, K. (2005). The Nightingale influence and the rise of the modern hospital. In C. Bates, D. Dodd, & N. Rousseau (Eds.), *On all frontiers: Four centuries of Canadian nursing* (pp. 73–88). Ottawa: University of Ottawa Press.

Millman, M. B. (1965). Nursing in Canada. In G. Griffin, & J. Griffin (Eds.), *Jensen's history and trends of professional nursing* (pp. 423–439). St. Louis, MO: C.V. Mosby.

Morton, D. (1983). *A short history of Canada*. Edmonton: Hurtig.

Nutting, M. A., & Dock, L. (1937). *A history of nursing*. (Vols. 1–4). New York: Putnam.

Parkman, F. (1897). *The Jesuits in North America in the seventeenth century*. Boston: Little, Brown.

Paul, P. (2005). Religious nursing orders of Canada: A presence on all western frontiers. In C. Bates, D. Dodd, & N. Rousseau (Eds.), *On all frontiers: Four centuries of Canadian nursing* (pp. 125–138). Ottawa: University of Ottawa Press.

Romanow, R. J. (2002). *Building on values. The future of health care in Canada*. Ottawa: Queen's Printer. Retrieved on January 31, 2008, from http://www.hc-sc.gc.ca.

Thwaites, R. G. (1959). *The Jesuit Relations and allied documents: Travels and explorations of the Jesuit missionaries in New France* (Vols. I–XII). New York: Pageant. Retrieved on July 7, 2009, from Library and Archives Canada http://epe.lac-bac.gc.ca/100/206/301/lac-bac/jesuit_relations-ef/jesuit-relations/h19-151-e.html.

Toman, C. (2005). "Ready, Aye Ready": Canadian military nurses as an expandable and expendable workforce (1920–2000). In C. Bates, D. Dodd, & N. Rousseau (Eds.), *On all frontiers: Four centuries of Canadian nursing* (pp. 169–181). Ottawa: University of Ottawa Press.

Veterans Affairs Canada. (2002). *Facts on Canada's nursing sisters*. Retrieved on December 19, 2007, from http://www.vac-acc.gc.ca/remembers/sub.cfm?source=history/other/Nursing/backgr.

Violette, B. (2005). Healing the body and saving the soul: Nursing sisters and the first Catholic hospitals in Quebec (1639–1880). In C. Bates, D. Dodd, & N. Rousseau (Eds.), *On all frontiers: Four centuries of Canadian nursing* (pp. 57–71). Ottawa: University of Ottawa Press.

Young, J., & Rousseau, N. (2005). Lay nursing from the New France era to the end of the nineteenth century (1600–1891). In C. Bates, D. Dodd, & N. Rousseau (Eds.), *On all frontiers: Four centuries of Canadian nursing* (pp. 11–25). Ottawa: University of Ottawa Press.

Janet C. Ross-Kerr

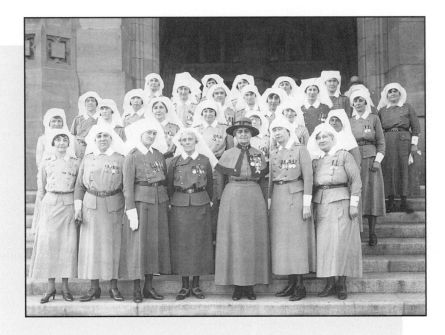

Nurses pose in front of the Parliament Buildings following the dedication of the Nurses Memorial in 1926.

LEARNING OBJECTIVES

- To recognize the characteristics of a profession.
- To identify changes in nursing education that have led to a more highly prepared workforce.
- To describe how the nursing profession has endeavoured to extend its knowledge base over the past century.
- To outline challenges the nursing profession has faced in its quest to raise its standards of education.
- To describe the nature of legislation governing nursing practice in each province and territory.
- To identify some contextual elements facilitating professional nursing practice today.

The evolution of nursing as a profession over almost four centuries in Canada is a story of courage, conviction, and altruism. In 1639, three Augustinian nuns arrived from France to provide nursing care to the small population at Quebec. From this humble beginning, nursing evolved as an essential service in the New World at a time when knowledge of disease was in a primitive state, technology was virtually nonexistent, and a few herbal remedies were the only drug therapies available. Over the centuries, the practice of nursing was refined and perceived as important to the health and well-being of the community. In the twentieth century, a concerted effort was made to develop educational standards and programs to prepare nurses for practice. Efforts were also made to gain control over the practice of nursing through registration of nurses and development of professional standards.

The process of professionalization, or the transition from an occupation to a profession, can be clearly seen and identified. However, there is considerable diversity of opinion about the characteristics of a profession and the extent to which particular occupational groups reflect or do not reflect these characteristics. The first two decades of the twentieth century signalled the beginning of the struggle to define the nature, scope, and object of nursing and the subsequent crusade for professional recognition and regulation. The latter movement has been worldwide, although its status varies widely from one country to another (Breda, 2009). Within Canada, there is relative uniformity, as nursing has been recognized as a self-governing profession established by mandatory registration in each province and territory.

DEVELOPMENT OF PROFESSIONS

Categorizing an occupation as a profession has traditionally been based on fairly standard criteria, developed by those with expertise in the study of professions. Although much time has been spent debating whether nursing is a profession or a semi-profession, it is important to recognize that the process of professionalization is a gradual one involving movement along a defined continuum, from an occupation at one end to a profession at the other. The measurement of progress along this continuum focuses on the extent to which an occupational group meets criteria deemed to characterize a profession. Despite

---

BOX 3.1   Flexner's Characteristics of a Profession

1. It is basically intellectual, carrying with it high responsibility.
2. It is learned in nature, because it is based on a body of knowledge.
3. It is practical rather than theoretical.
4. Its technique can be taught through educational discipline.
5. It is well organized internally.
6. It is motivated by altruism.

Source: Flexner, A. (1915). Is social work a profession? *Proceedings of the National Conference of Charities and Corrections* (pp. 578–581). Chicago: Heldermann.

---

the phenomenal changes in the nature and scope of nursing over the past two decades and progress along such a continuum, Schwirian (1998) concluded that nursing has not yet achieved full recognition as a profession.

The debate began shortly after the beginning of the twentieth century when Abraham Flexner (see Box 3.1) identified six characteristics of a profession based on his observations of the traditional professions of law, medicine, and theology.

These characteristics were presented to address the question of whether social work was a profession. Flexner (1915) observed that nursing did not appear to be a profession because "the responsibility of the trained nurse is neither original nor final" (p. 581). It should be noted that his assessment of how nursing met the stated criteria was made before the passage of laws regulating the practice of nursing in most provinces and before nursing education first appeared in a university prospectus in Canada. It also occurred at a time when women had yet to receive the vote and had not as yet been declared "persons."

An early analysis of the status of nursing as a profession was conducted by Bixler and Bixler (1945). In this classic study, they examined the extent to which nursing met the standard criteria for designation as a profession and reached the conclusion that although nursing was well into the process of professionalization, it had further to go before it could be described as a profession. Wilensky (1964) was the first to refer to the "natural history of professionalism" as a description of the milestones in the development of professions. Some of these milestones include the date the profession first became a full-time occupation, the date of the first educational program to prepare practitioners, and the date the first university school for the profession was established. Also included as significant events are the date the first national professional association was formed, the date of the enactment of the first provincial registration act, and the date of the development and adoption of a formal code of ethics. Although these events are static and finite, they allow for comparisons among professions and assessment of where a particular group stands in the process of professionalization.

Flexner (1915) saw the development of a formal base of knowledge, the first criterion, as the most central for professions. An articulated knowledge base is common to the vast majority of categorizations of professions. Since the knowledge needed to practise a profession is complex and cannot be mastered by the ordinary person, practitioners require a lengthy period of preparation and supervised practice before functioning competently on an independent basis. The educational process is considered important and complex enough that programs are offered within universities, and the first professional degree often follows a four-year university arts or science degree. The knowledge base of a profession is continually upgraded through research performed by members to expand and update knowledge for practice. Members also maintain control over educational standards for the admission of new practitioners into the profession and must use their knowledge to serve and benefit the public.

Because the professions are inherently important to the public, some form of licensing or registration of those qualified to practise is necessary. Control of this process, while vested in legislation, is normally left to the profession. Professions are organized for the purpose of regulating practice. Their associations seek to improve standards of practice and education, to register members and monitor professional conduct, and to judge the practice of professionals where disputes have arisen. Thus professions retain the authority to remove from practice those who are incompetent.

Professional commitment to the public is demonstrated by the development of a code of ethics, or statement of moral or ethical duty. A code of ethics is a code of behaviour for professionals, behaviour that is derived from principles that are set down as a code. Along with other professionals, nurses need to be accountable for their actions and those actions must be seen to be in the best interests of their patients. Because patients may be vulnerable due to the status of their health, nurses are ethically and morally bound to act in their best interests in all dimensions. Keogh (1997) refers to the need for professionals to take responsibility for their actions and be accountable to their patients. Patients should likewise be able to rest assured that nurses are worthy of their trust. Although codes of ethics are important for the health professions, there are limitations in that they are expressed as general principles and may not cover each and every issue that may arise in practice.

EVOLUTION OF NURSING AS A PROFESSION

In Canada, the nursing profession has been prominent in the life of society since the first nurses were encouraged to immigrate to the shores of New France. Later, in the nineteenth century, members of the Order of the Sisters of Charity of Montreal (the Grey Nuns) bravely set out, without benefit of reliable transportation, to provide needed health care to remote parts of the country where small settlements were opening.

Around the turn of the twentieth century, there was a movement to secure legislation to regulate nursing practice to differentiate qualified from unqualified practitioners. The first provincial statute governing the practice of nursing was passed in Nova Scotia in 1910. By 1922, with the passage of legislation in Ontario, there were statutes governing nursing in all provinces. The development of stronger legislation, which would differentiate the actual practice of nursing with the title of Registered Nurse (RN), occurred later, with the initial passage of legislation in Newfoundland in 1953. All provinces now have moved to mandatory forms of legislation governing nursing. Achieving exclusive right to practise, embodied in law, is an important step in professionalizing nursing. The profession in Canada has worked diligently to achieve acceptance of the need for such legislation.

Nursing education in Canada began in 1874 in St. Catharines, Ontario, after world-wide recognition of Florence Nightingale's efforts in nursing education. Nightingale believed that nurses needed to be educated to care for patients properly. She demonstrated her point by dramatically lowering mortality and morbidity rates of soldiers in the Crimea in 1856, when she and a small group of nurses provided care for wounded soldiers. Nursing education moved into the universities in 1918 when courses in public health nursing were given at the University of Alberta, and with the inception of the first degree program in nursing in Canada at the University of British Columbia under the direction of Ethel Johns. In 1959, master's degree education in nursing was initiated at the University of Western Ontario, and nursing research development began in earnest. Although initial preparation is now largely based in community colleges and universities across the country, the adoption and active promotion of the entry-to-practice position by the Canadian Nurses Association (CNA) and various professional associations served as a key force in promoting this change. The entry-to-practice position initially targeted the year 2000 as the date by which those entering the profession could qualify at the baccalaureate level. The process is complete in most areas of the country but continues in some provinces. Master's level preparation has been available since 1959 and has flourished, with many programs now accessible to students. The first doctoral program, at the University of Alberta, admitted students on January 1, 1991, and others followed so that doctoral preparation is available in all regions of the country.

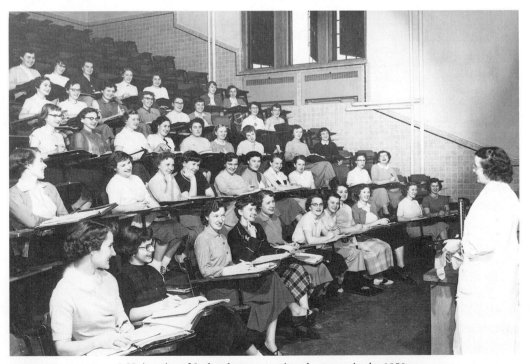

A University of Saskatchewan nursing classroom in the 1950s.

The development of a code of ethics normally occurs relatively late in the process of professionalization. "Toward the end, legal protection appears; at the end, a formal code of ethics is adopted" (Wilensky, 1964, pp. 143–144). A historical review indicates that this was the case for the nursing profession in Canada. The first North American code of ethics for nursing was published by the American Nurses Association in 1950; in 1953, the International Council of Nurses (ICN) approved a code of ethics. The latter was generally accepted and used by professional associations until 1980, when the first CNA code of ethics was developed. Disagreement about the wording of the initial code resulted in the development of a new code, adopted in 1985. The CNA reviews the code of ethics every five years, and the most recent code was approved in 2008 (CNA, 2008).

REFLECTIVE THINKING

How do you think nursing ranks currently among health care professions in respect of the extent to which it meets the criteria for professional status?

EMERGENCE OF A SCIENTIFIC KNOWLEDGE BASE FOR NURSING

Research to create and extend the knowledge base in nursing has been enhanced by the establishment of graduate programs in nursing at the master's and doctoral levels now distributed in all regions of the country. Many of these programs have a strong research thrust, and graduates of such programs are engaged in advancing the scientific basis of nursing.

The importance of studying nursing questions has been emphasized by leaders in the profession, who have stressed scientific testing of traditional nursing care practices. With the development and expansion of graduate programs, research in schools and faculties of nursing has increased exponentially. This has been accompanied by a movement to ensure evidence-informed practice, ensuring that nursing care is based upon the best possible evidence. Members of the public expect to receive high quality nursing care from practitioners based upon sound knowledge. Over the past several decades the movement to improve nursing care through the development of a knowledge base confirmed through research and other forms of evidence has gained prominence. A review of the chapters in Part II will help the reader gain an appreciation of the basis of professional nursing practice.

CANADIAN RESEARCH FOCUS

Estabrooks, C.A. (2004). Thoughts on evidence-based nursing and its science: A Canadian perspective. Worldviews on evidence-based nursing/Sigma Theta Tau International. *Honor Society of Nursing, 1*(2), 88–91.

The movement to develop the science of nursing through an evidence informed approach has been a critical step forward in the professionalization of nursing in the twenty-first century. Reference is made to the history of the evidence-based nursing movement in Canada and to international cooperation and networks that have developed in this field. The importance of this process in developing strong underpinnings for nursing practice through links with theory and research is underscored.

PROFESSIONAL EDUCATION FOR NURSING: ISSUES OF STATUS AND CONTROL

Nursing education has been the subject of considerable controversy. However, the entry-to-practice proposal has possibly engendered more heated debate than other issues in recent decades. Initially put forward in 1975 by a government-appointed committee in Alberta, the proposal stated that all nurses entering the profession should be qualified at the baccalaureate level by the turn of the century. The position was subsequently ratified by the CNA and provincial associations, and although the year 2000 has come and gone, all provinces are moving to implement the entry-to-practice position. However difficult it has been to implement the position, there has been tremendous progress as all provinces have made headway and some have been able to implement it completely.

A frequent argument against entry to practice by government officials and those who were opposed to it was that implementing entry to practice would result in higher costs. However, following cost-benefit analyses, the CNA suggested that it was unwise to assume the entry-to-practice proposal would result in higher costs.

The first development to facilitate implementation of the baccalaureate entry-to-practice standard occurred at the schools of nursing of the Vancouver General Hospital and the University of British Columbia when they initiated a collaborative degree program in 1989. This was followed by a program arranged collaboratively between the University of Alberta and Red Deer College in 1990. The program was extended to include the other four diploma schools of nursing in Edmonton in 1991. These developments were the first in a long series of arrangements in the provinces to implement the baccalaureate entry-to-practice standard (see Chapter 19 for a complete discussion of entry-to-practice developments).

The professional association monitors standards in initial programs of nursing education in all provinces except Ontario and Quebec (see discussion in Chapter 23). In the past, nursing has been different from most other professions with respect to this process, as most nurses graduated with diplomas rather than degrees. However, with the implementation of the baccalaureate entry-to-practice position, nursing is joining the ranks of established professions such as law, medicine, theology, pharmacy, engineering, and architecture, and all educational preparation is centred in the universities. When all practitioners enter the field of nursing as graduates from university programs in nursing, the monitoring function may no longer be necessary.

The nursing profession is bound to be preoccupied for some time with establishing educational programs within universities. This process is likely to extend over several decades because a major change in the educational requirements at the entry level takes time to implement completely. Since 1991, doctoral programs have prepared nurse researchers who have the expertise to undertake theory-building and theory-testing research. The placement of the professional program is likely to arise as an issue once initial programs of nursing education have been established and expanded within universities. It remains to be seen whether some university-level study in the liberal arts and sciences will be required before admission to the program.

CONTROL OF PROFESSIONAL NURSING PRACTICE

The first phase of the drive by nurses to gain control of professional nursing practice extended from the enactment of the first provincial legislation regulating nursing, in Nova Scotia in 1910, to the conclusion of the process, in Ontario in 1922. Prowse (1983) drew attention to the importance of "aspects of nursing legislation which (a) expedite effective utilization of nursing knowledge and expertise, (b) influence the supply of qualified competent nurses, and (c) ensure regulation and monitoring of both practice and practitioners" (p. 33).

The second phase of this process was the development of mandatory acts regulating nursing in each province. This ensured that the practice and practitioners would be more strictly regulated. Legislation incorporating mandatory registration requires a definition of nursing and a description of the scope of nursing practice. The first mandatory nursing legislation in Canada was enacted in 1953 in Newfoundland. Other provinces did not follow suit until Prince Edward Island passed such legislation in 1972, followed by Quebec in 1973 (with significant amendments in 1974). Legislation incorporating mandatory registration in Manitoba was enacted in 1999 and came into force in 2001. Alberta passed a mandatory Nursing Profession Act in 1983, and New Brunswick, Nova Scotia, and Saskatchewan and British Columbia followed suit in 1984, 1985, and 1988, respectively. Ontario passed the *Regulated Health Professions Act* in 1991 and incorporated a new approach, namely, regulating professional procedures. The legislation came into force in December 1993. These issues are discussed in more detail in Chapter 23.

The tremendous change in nursing roles over the past 25 years has altered the nature and scope of practice extensively. Specialization is almost a requirement because of changes in the knowledge required to practise in a specific area. Certification of practitioners in specialty areas is expanding to more and more areas. The trend toward increased specialization can be expected to strengthen as health care knowledge and technology continue to develop.

FACILITATING PROFESSIONALIZATION

It is likely that changes in the way in which nursing is practised will continue as society becomes more aware of the benefits of health promotion and the need to develop healthier lifestyles to prevent disease. Alternatives to hospitalization for tertiary and long-term care, in the form of home care and ambulatory care, appear attractive at both the personal and societal levels. Nurses have been preparing for their new roles in community and long-term care settings and have the knowledge and the communication and interactional skills to assist consumers in meeting health goals. They are thus well poised to serve society in a health system that is centred in the community and based on the primary health care model.

The initiation of doctoral education is an important milestone for the nursing profession because preparing nurses to contribute to the discovery of nursing knowledge through theory and research will lead to improved care. Increased availability of bacca-laureate programs in nursing, through collaborative arrangements between community colleges and universities as well as entirely through universities, will provide a stronger basis for the practice of nursing. Dynamic leadership is required to provide direction to new generations of skilled practitioners and to ensure that their talents are used to the fullest extent for the benefit of the public.

 REFLECTIVE THINKING

Reflect on the progress of nursing in the last century in improving its standards of education and practice.

CRITICAL THINKING QUESTIONS

1. How would you distinguish a profession from an occupation?
2. Why is a code of ethics important for a profession such as nursing?
3. Explain why nursing has faced so many challenges in implementing university-level education for members of the profession.

WEB SITES

Canadian Nurses Association. (2008). Code of Ethics for Registered Nurses: http://www.cna-aiic.ca/CNA/practice/ethics/code/default_e.aspx

REFERENCES

Bixler, G. K., & Bixler, R. W. (1945). The professional status of nursing. *American Journal of Nursing, 45*(9), 730–735.

Breda, K. L (2009). *Nursing and globalization in the Americas: A critical perspective.* Amityville, NY: Baywood.

Canadian Nurses Association. (2008). *Code of ethics for registered nurses.* Ottawa: Author.

Flexner, A. (1915). Is social work a profession? In *Proceedings of the National Conference of Charities and Corrections* (pp. 578–581). Chicago: Heldermann.

Keogh, J. (1997). Professionalization of nursing: Development, difficulties and solutions. *Journal of Advanced Nursing, 25,* 302–308.

Prowse, A. J. (1983). *Nursing legislation in Canada: An overview for health services administrators.* Edmonton: Department of Health Services Administration and Community Medicine, University of Alberta.

Schwirian, P. M. (1998). *Professionalization of nursing: Current issues and trends.* Philadelphia: J.B. Lippincott.

Wilensky, H. L. (1964). The professionalization of everyone? *American Journal of Sociology, 70*(2), 137–187.

4

The Professional Image: Impact and Strategies for Change

Marilynn J. Wood

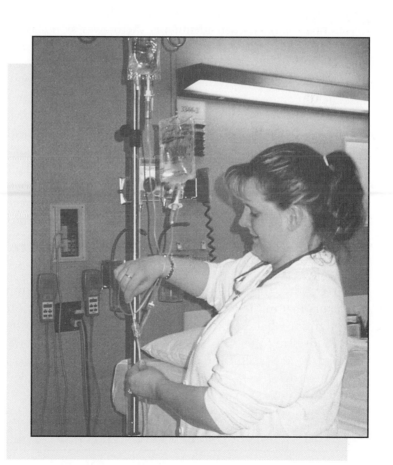

LEARNING OBJECTIVES

- To understand why the image of nursing is important to the profession.
- To appreciate the role played by the mass media in shaping the public image of nursing.
- To recognize the impact of a negative image on recruitment.
- To understand how the self-image of nursing affects the profession.
- To identify strategies for changing the image of nursing.

The image of nursing has been the centre of much attention in nursing literature and within professional associations because of its impact on recruitment. It is of concern to nurse educators seeking to attract the best students into nursing, to nurse administrators trying to staff health care agencies, to nurse researchers who encounter difficulty in explaining nursing research to others, and to all nurses who encounter negative or indifferent responses when identifying themselves as nurses in social situations. Currently, Canada faces a worsening shortage of nurses that creates many problems for nurses, including staffing shortages that make it difficult to meet the needs of patients and lead to dissatisfaction with nursing (Miller & Cummings, 2009). In addition, the health care system is changing to one in which innovation and creativity are required of all workers, technology is ever increasing, and roles of health care providers are shifting for economic reasons (Miller & Cummings, 2009). Now, more than ever before, the nursing profession needs bright, articulate leaders who can pave the way to success in resolving these issues.

In a systematic review of research on the career influences and aspirations of gifted high school students, these students were found to choose careers that fit their personal self-concept and their ideas of what was needed to succeed in a profession. They were most likely to choose careers with high prestige, education, and pay. Nursing was not seen as a career choice by these gifted students, the very ones that the nursing profession would like to recruit (Miller & Cummings, 2009). Surely now is the time to address changing the image of nursing.

In addressing the issue of the image of nursing, it is important to reflect on historical factors that influence the image of nurses and nursing. Such a perspective is needed to determine what can be done to enhance the image and who might or should be involved in addressing this important issue. In recent years, however, the topic of the nursing shortage has taken over as the top priority for nursing organizations. It may be shortsighted to overlook the image of nursing in the present world and to assess its impact on building a workforce of high quality, competent nurses.

EXTERNAL AND INTERNAL IMAGES

One often hears or reads about the image of nursing as if there were only one image. Nursing actually has many images, because nurses relate to a variety of audiences. For example, the image presented to attract students or to recruit nurses in health care agencies is different from the image presented to legislators, whose main concern is cost-effectiveness. These are external images; internal images are the views that nurses have of themselves as individuals and of the profession. There was much interest in studying nursing images in the 1960s. In examining studies of nursing images conducted through 1964, Simmons and Henderson (1964) found two popular and competing images of the nurse.

> At one pole is the image of the humanitarian and altruistic person, more or less competent and endowed with sympathy, compassion, and exceptional capacities for establishing rapport—one who gives of herself. At the other pole is the image of the professional, well-trained, technically efficient and cool-headed individual who can be relied upon for able performance within her specialty, and relatively independent of feeling components—one who may seem to keep herself out of her work. (p. 222)

Probably few nurses can be classified at the two extremes; most fit at various points between the two poles.

In the time of the Romans, those identified with the nurse role were wealthy Roman matrons who gave nurturance, self-sacrifice, and mothering. Nursing continues to be sex stereotyped, even though those who cared for the injured during the Crusades were men. Today, some men are entering nursing. The proportion of male nurses in Canada and the United States continues to be very limited, at 5.8% (CNA, 2007) and 5.8% (HRSA, 2007), respectively. In Canada, this is a slight increase from the 4.8% reported for 2000 (CNA, 2007).

Images of any profession or work group are influenced by the values and orientations learned from family and friends, and by individuals' experiences with particular members of a profession. Images are also influenced by the mass media, particularly with today's media. Two studies of the public's perception of nurses and nursing found that respondents' views were strongly influenced by personal contact with nurses or the experiences of others (Lippman & Ponton, 1989; Giovannetti, 1990; Payne, Cook and Associates, 1990). Hence, observational learning is an important means of developing images of various professions, including nursing. Such learning promotes a concept of a particular profession and has great impact on how a profession is regarded by members of society and how attractive the profession is to individuals.

THE MASS MEDIA AND THE IMAGE OF NURSES AND NURSING

Kalisch and Kalisch (1982) surveyed mass media products pertaining to nursing from the past century and a half. These included "the print media (200 novels, 143 magazine short stories, poems and articles and 20,000 newspaper clippings), as well as the newer non-print media (204 motion pictures, 122 radio programs, and 320 television episodes)" (p. 5). From these products they classified the image into five dominant types characterizing five successive time periods.

The "Angel of Mercy" image of the nurse was portrayed "as noble, moral, religious, virginal, ritualistic and self-sacrificing" (Kalisch & Kalisch, 1982, p. 7). Although it has been said that Florence Nightingale epitomized this image, she was also a scholar and has been termed the first nurse researcher. Nightingale's achievements were astounding. She saved the lives of many wounded soldiers during the Crimean War; she restored order from chaos by assuming responsibility for the soldiers' environment as well as nursing care, despite strong resistance from the physicians in charge; and she brought innovation and advancement to the fields of nursing, health, and hospital planning. Nightingale was of high social class and well educated. If her model for nursing had been followed, the nursing profession would be in a much more advantageous position today. The "Angel of Mercy" image, as identified by Kalisch and Kalisch, existed from 1854 to 1919. It continued when nurses were presented by the media as noble and heroic. A typical film from that period portrayed the nurse enlisting in the service to be near her sweetheart, finding him wounded, and restoring him to health (Kalisch & Kalisch, 1982).

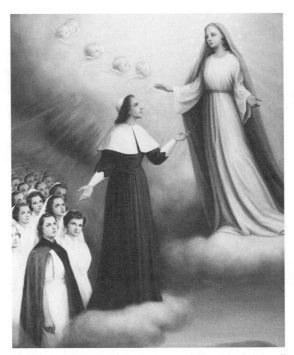

The virginal image of the nurse as an "angel of mercy," as exemplified by this painting of Jeanne Mance, persisted from the time of Florence Nightingale to the end of World War I.

The next image, "Girl Friday," existed from 1920 to 1929; it was very different and reflected considerable deterioration. The nurse was portrayed as "subservient, cooperative, methodical, dedicated, modest, and loyal" (Kalisch & Kalisch, 1982, p. 11). In essence, she served as a handmaiden, an image that grew out of the deprofessionalization of nursing that occurred in the 1920s with declining standards of nursing education. The decline was the result of a proliferation of hospitals accompanied by schools of nursing to staff them, as well as poor working conditions and the ruthless exploitation of students. Some of these conditions continued into the 1940s, although the image of the nurse as portrayed by the media changed.

The third image, "The Heroine," existed from 1930 to 1945, when the media portrayed the nurse as "brave, rational, dedicated, decisive, humanistic, and autonomous" (Kalisch & Kalisch, 1982, p. 11). Motion pictures in the 1930s and 1940s depicted this image. Biographies were written about heroines such as Florence Nightingale; Edith Cavell, who was shot by a German firing squad during World War I for helping wounded soldiers escape; and Sister Kenney, whose treatment of poliomyelitis victims enabled many to recover muscular function at a time when the victims were being kept immobilized by the medical profession. Adventure dramas about air or sea travel involved nurse heroines. Airlines required flight attendants to be graduate nurses. Delivering babies, assisting in emergency surgery, and even landing the plane safely when pilots were disabled were among the heroic acts of flight attendants portrayed in movies and other media (Kalisch & Kalisch, 1982). World War II intensified the "Heroine" image; nurses were portrayed very positively on recruitment posters. Many volunteered for military service and were highly regarded by society. When television became available in the mid-1950s, the "Heroine" image was portrayed to a larger audience.

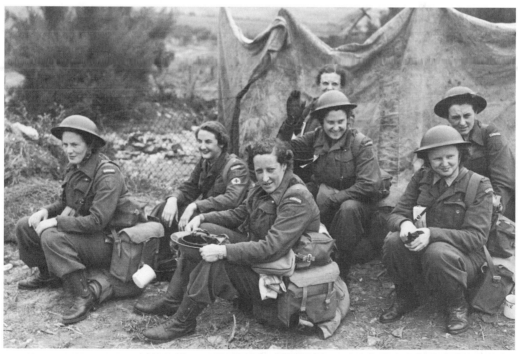

Nursing Sisters of No. 10 Canadian General Hospital, R.C.A.M.C., France, July 23, 1944. (L R): Lieuts: Jean Scrimageour, Susan Edwards, Neta Moore, Leona Whitmore, Margaret Stewart, Jean Lawson, and Irene Stephenson.

The fourth image, "The Mother," existed from 1945 to 1965. It seems almost incredible that women went home to function as wives and mothers after enduring the hardships of war, but they did. At that time the place for married women was perceived to be in the home, and society frowned on working mothers. Although nursing remained a high-status occupation for women, nurse characters were portrayed by the media as "maternal, nurturing, sympathetic, passive, expressive, and domestic" (Kalisch & Kalisch, 1982, p. 15).

As this image faded in the mid-1960s, the most negative media image of the nurse since Dickens's imbibing Sairey Gamp developed—the nurse as "Sex Object." This negative image, which portrayed the nurse as "a sensual, romantic, hedonistic, frivolous, irresponsible, promiscuous individual" (Kalisch & Kalisch, 1982, p. 17), continues today on television and particularly in movies. This image is readily identified in older television programs such as *M*A*S*H*. The nurse was depicted as a sex object with no evidence of intellectuality or professionalism. She is also often depicted as a sex object on greeting cards and in advertisements. More recent programs, such as *ER, Grey's Anatomy*, and numerous reality TV shows, sometimes depict nurses in a more positive and realistic light, for the most part, as these storylines focus attention on medicine rather than on nursing.

The ideal image, proposed by Kalisch and Kalisch (1982), is "The Careerist," "an intelligent, logical, progressive, sophisticated, empathic, and assertive woman or man who is committed to attaining higher and higher standards of health care" (p. 21). This image is timeless and is as relevant today as it was when Kalisch and Kalisch proposed it in 1982. Most of the recent research supports the work of Kalisch and Kalisch, thus encouraging us to conclude that not much has changed over time. Several recent analyses have been carried out on motion pictures (Bayer, 2007; Gordon & Johnson, 2004; Rasmussen, 2001). These authors concluded that nurses are generally depicted as "heroic angels" or something much more negative, giving a warped view of the image of nurses. Gordon and Johnson (2004) noted that nurses could be described as "the good, the bad and the crazy" (p. 16). However, a comprehensive study by Stanley (2008) concludes that filmmakers are starting to see nurses as "intelligent, strong and passionate characters and are increasingly turning to nursing characters who offer a broader, deeper and authentic representation of modern nurses and nursing" (p. 94). This is encouraging indeed, as it has been demonstrated repeatedly that media image has a strong impact on how nurses see themselves (Ward, Styles, & Bosco, 2003; Meadus & Twomey, 2007; Hereford, 2005).

One bright light in current literature is the inclusion of Madam Pomfrey in the series of books about Harry Potter (Freda, 2006). Madam Pomfrey is the nurse at Hogwarts School for Wizards, and she is depicted as an intelligent, powerful, and independent professional—a good role model for children. Otherwise, the prevalent image projected by the media as reflected in the literature, in motion pictures, and on television over the past 30 years has been primarily negative. This image is bound to have negative implications for the profession of nursing in the recruitment and retention of nurses. The recent trend toward a more reality-based image is very encouraging in light of warped views from the past.

CANADIAN RESEARCH FOCUS

Stanley, D.J. (2008). Celluloid angels: A research study of nurses in feature films 1900–2007. *Journal of Advanced Nursing, 64*(1), 84–95.

The purpose of this study was to assess how nursing and nurses are portrayed in feature films from 1900 to 2007, in cases where a nurse was a principal character and the storyline related directly to nursing.

The researchers used quantitative analysis to identify the number of films with nurses as main characters. Over 36,000 film synopses were reviewed, as well as an Internet search of many databases in order to identify an initial 827 films, from which 280 were found to support the research aims. These were assessed for country, genre, storyline, and other details. They were then analyzed and coded to identify concepts such as doctor–nurse relationship or zombie nurse films. The majority of films were produced in either the United States or the United Kingdom, and they covered a wide range of story types. Themes that emerged were self-sacrifice/care, the Heroine, sex object, romantic/feminine, intelligence, strong woman, the "Dark nurse," and victim. These themes varied over time, with early- and middle-decade films focusing on self-sacrifice, and other themes appearing occasionally throughout. Films from the 1970s tended to depict nurses as sex objects. Themes relating to intelligence, strong woman, dark nurse, and victim were found predominantly in recent decades.

The authors concluded that more recent films represent nurses as "more than angels and devils, doormats and divas" and that nurses are increasingly seen as "intelligent, strong and passionate characters who offer a broader, deeper and authentic representation of modern nurses and nursing."

PUBLIC PERCEPTION OF NURSES AND NURSING

Nurses have become increasingly concerned about their image and its effect on recruitment into nursing programs and the retention of nurses in the workforce. Studies have supported the idea that a negative image is a barrier to recruitment of talented individuals into the profession (Brewer, Zayas, Kahn, & Siendiewicz, 2006; Brodie, Andrews, Andrews, Thomas, Wong, & Rixon, 2004; Miller & Cummings, 2009).

At a time when the shortage is expected to have a longer duration than we have experienced in the past, nursing's image in the public eye becomes crucial. Ward, Styles, & Bosco (2003) found that the image of nurses continues to be influenced by the media, and that nurses' self-image is more negative than that of other health care providers.

A positive image is also seen as a form of power that brings respect and enables nurses to create changes to improve conditions for their patients (Roberts & Vasquez, 2004). How to create and support a positive image of nursing is a challenge we all face if we are to succeed as a profession.

Lippman and Ponton (1989) conducted a survey of faculty in all disciplines in 19 northeastern US universities with accredited baccalaureate degree programs in nursing. They obtained perceptions of nurses and nursing from a random sample of 535 faculty members, 11% of whom were nursing faculty. The findings reflected a different and more positive view of nursing than that presented by the media. Nurses were perceived as "educated, autonomous and compassionate individuals whose role is vital to health care" (Lippman & Ponton, 1989, p. 27). They were viewed as knowledgeable about good health and as good sources of information about health and its promotion. The majority did not perceive nurses as handmaidens to physicians and believed nurses should be treated as equals to physicians. Most were not averse to their daughters entering nursing, although 18% stated that "bright young women should study medicine rather than nursing." The investigators indicated that the responses may have been influenced by the personal contact the respondents had had with nurses. It is also possible that nursing faculty had communicated effectively about nursing and nursing education within the 19 universities from which the sample was drawn. This type of study has not been repeated, but it would be interesting to see if these same findings would occur today among faculty members in other disciplines.

Over time, concerns about the nursing shortages and how to attract more people to nursing have stimulated research into the public's attitudes, values, and beliefs about nursing as a career. A study of college freshmen (27.1%), students in Grades 6 through 12 (29.6%), and "enablers" (those who had potential to influence career selection) is one such survey. The findings indicated that, for these respondents, nursing and the ideal career were similar in "opportunities for employment, use of intellectual abilities, caring for people as a career attribute, need for academic achievement, and scholastic achievement as a prerequisite for career development" (May, Austin, & Champion, 1988, p. 7). However, an ideal career was viewed as "more financially rewarding, more respected, more appreciated, and more powerful," providing "more opportunities for leadership, more safety in the workplace, more opportunities for making decisions, and more opportunities for obtaining and applying knowledge," and involving "less emphasis on manual skills, less utilization of high technology, lighter workload, and easier work" (May, Austin, & Champion 1988, p. 7). Based on the findings, a number of recommendations were made to enhance the positive attitudes and improve the negative perceptions, including ways to increase respect and appreciation for nurses, reduce workloads, promote more autonomy in practice and more safety in the workplace, achieve more competitive salaries, increase leadership opportunities and empowerment of nurses, and place less emphasis on manual skills and high technology in publicity materials. Many of the recommendations reiterate strategies that nurses have advocated for years, both as individuals and as members of study commissions established to address the problems of recruitment and retention in nursing.

A more recent study of the public image of nursing indicates that not much has changed since the 1980s, when most of the previous studies were published. A sample of 3000 college students in science and math courses were asked for their perceptions of nursing as a career. Their perceptions were quite favourable, and more than two-thirds saw nursing as interesting, with good job security and income. However, they perceived nurses to have less independence in the workplace than other occupations, and nursing was more likely to be viewed as a women's occupation (Seago, Spetz, Alvarado, Keane, & Grumbach, 2006).

In the late 1980s, the AARN (Alberta Association of Registered Nurses), now renamed the College and Association of Registered Nurses of Alberta (CARNA), commissioned a large-scale study to assess public attitudes about nursing in Alberta. This is the largest survey of its kind ever carried out in Canada. The study sample included 1087 adults, randomly selected from all regions of Alberta. Respondents were asked to describe in their own words their perception of the nursing profession. More than 87% of the responses were positive, using descriptors such as caring, compassionate, knowledgeable, intelligent, helpful, devoted, dedicated, professional, responsible, and hard-working. The few negative images pertained to nursing being a hard, tough, and demanding job, and nurses being overworked and underpaid. Although the media influenced about 60% of the respondents' images of nursing, more than 80% formed their opinions through personal contact with nurses or experiences of others with nurses. Response to items rated on a five-point Likert scale indicated that respondents viewed nursing as mentally and physically demanding and as requiring special people. Most also viewed it as challenging and interesting, and for the most part, nursing was highly respected. "Despite the fact that 91% of the respondents believed nursing is a highly respected profession, only 76% would recommend nursing as a career" (Giovannetti, 1990, p. 7). Support for nursing as a career was found to be lowest among persons under age 25 and persons with some postsecondary education, two groups from which potential nursing students could be recruited and who are likely to have strong peer influence. As the level of income of respondents increased, positive views of nursing as challenging and interesting decreased, and strong support for nursing as a career decreased. Also disconcerting was that 79% of the respondents believed nurses should always consult a physician before administering client care, and 72% perceived physicians as having total authority over patient care. These attitudes were less prevalent among the younger persons, the more highly educated, and those with higher incomes.

On a more positive note, most respondents perceived nurses as accountable for their own practice and conduct and as having a role in client education. Moreover, the majority supported nurses' involvement in research to improve practice and believed that nurses should be required to upgrade their education continually. On the controversial issue of nurses being allowed to strike, 47% were firmly opposed, although almost 70% conceded that strike action might be necessary to keep nurses' salaries on a par with those of other professions (Payne, Cook and Associates, 1990). This is interesting because the province of Alberta has experienced four nurses' strikes since 1977. Because of these study findings, the AARN undertook a province-wide public education campaign to enhance the image of nurses and nursing, but the success of this campaign has not been determined.

Others have examined the relationship between the image that nurses perceive the public to have, and nurses' own self-image. Takase, Maude, and Manias (2006) examined this relationship and then looked at it in relation to job performance and turnover. Their subjects rated their aptitude for leadership as higher than they perceived the public viewed them. However, they rated their caring image less negatively than their perceived public image. Job performance was predicted by self-image relating to leadership aptitude. On the other hand, the relationship between self-image and perception of the public image as being caring predicted job performance. Intention to quit the job was related to a negative image in both these areas.

The Internet has transformed our very way of life in a very short time. We have become a society of "Googlers" who think nothing of looking up anything we want to know on the Web. A newer study by Kalisch, Begeny, and Neumann (2007) looks at the nurses' image on the Internet. Content analysis was done of 144 Web sites in 2001 and 152 in 2004. A content analysis tool was developed and tested to measure the image of nursing on Internet Web sites. Sample selection utilized search engine technology to select sites with high exposure to the public. In 2001, 144 sites were chosen.

By 2004, major changes had taken place in the technology of searching, confounded by the disappearance of some search engines and the appearance of new ones. The process was altered to account for these changes. In 2004, there were 122 sites selected from Google, 41 from Look Smart, 17 from Ovature, 25 from TEOMA, and 7 from Infospace. When duplicates were eliminated, the sample size was 152.

The findings from this study showed a positive image of nursing on the Internet. Around 70% of the sites depicted nurses as intelligent and educated, and 60% as respected, accountable, committed, competent, and trustworthy. In addition, the specialized knowledge and skills of nurses were depicted in the majority of Web sites. Doctorally prepared nurses were evident in 19% of the Web sites in 2001 and in twice that many in 2004. It is clear that the Internet could be an excellent vehicle through which to effect change in the public's image of nursing.

SELF-IMAGE OF NURSING

Nurses' view of themselves may be referred to as self-image or internal image. Self-image is vitally important because people's perception of nurses and nursing is influenced by their interactions and experiences with nurses. The studies cited indicated that these interactions were considerably more influential in shaping images of nursing than were the media.

Nurses have been criticized in the literature for having low self-esteem. This may be reflected in appearance, approach to patients, relationships with other health care providers, and behaviour in the community. Many factors contribute to the development of self-image, including the values and attitudes one brings to a profession. These values and attitudes are influenced by life experiences before entering the educational system to prepare for the profession. The educational system then influences the learner's concept of nursing practice, the role of the nurse, relationships with other health care providers, and professional responsibilities as a member of the profession and the community.

Nurse educators can help change the self-image of nursing through their teaching and role-modelling. They may also contribute unknowingly to some negative aspects of image development. The importance that they attach to the individual nurse and to the work of nursing can have a major effect on how the students view themselves for many years. Students are also strongly influenced by the nurses—practitioners, administrators, researchers—with whom they interact in clinical practice settings, and by the relationships they observe between nurses and other health care providers.

Nurses have the opportunity to effect changes now and assume responsibility for the future of nursing. Individuals can affect the image of nursing through their daily performance in nursing practice and their reactions to various publics—patients, family members, friends, students, potential recruits, other professionals, legislators, policymakers, or colleagues. As indicated by the studies cited, these interactions contribute to other people's views of nursing. Moreover, one's personal experiences as a nurse and one's own perception of nursing have a great impact on daily encounters with the public. Styles (1982) points out that we must view nursing with a sense of collegiality and collectivity, thus sharing responsibility and authority for nursing and working together to preserve the wholeness of the profession. Achieving unified action is difficult, however, because of the disparity in nursing over issues such as educational preparation for nursing; preparation for specialty practice; unionism; research to improve practice; and allocation of funds among practice, education, and research. It is well known that others can use such disparities to deter or defeat efforts to make constructive and desirable changes that will help achieve unity.

Nursing is more complex than most people think. Developing the knowledge, skills, attitudes, and values needed to practise nursing is a very complicated undertaking. The list of the knowledge and skills needed is endless. Differentiating nursing from medicine, nurses often cite the focus of nursing as "care," whereas "cure" is viewed as the focus and end goal of medicine. Perhaps the essence of nursing practice is caring, and caring is not easy. Diers (1984) pointed out that it is not easy to care for people—any people—anytime, anywhere. It is especially difficult when there are no ties of blood or common interest that bind the nurse and the patient. In nursing, caring requires authentic altruism that must be titrated precisely so as not to overwhelm on the one hand, nor be lost on the other. Caring takes enormous energy, even when genuine liking is present, for it is impossible to care equally for and about everyone. Yet that is precisely the role nurses have assumed.

The self-image of nursing affects how nurses think students should be educated; whether they encourage others to enter nursing, particularly daughters or sons; the importance they attach to nursing research; how they think nursing services should be organized; how they view nurses' strikes; the importance they attach to helping people take responsibility for their own health; and how much influence they think people should have in decisions about their own care. Although nurses do not have to agree on everything, they should agree on basic goals and have sound rationales to support their positions. Too much internal disparity weakens the profession and undermines the power of nurses, which is potentially great because the number of persons in the nursing profession far exceeds that of any other health care profession.

REFLECTIVE THINKING

How do you see the quality of leadership in nursing affecting nurses' self-image? Could this concept be at the basis of nursing's problems with image?

STRATEGIES FOR CHANGING THE IMAGE

Because of the negative image of nurses and nursing that continues to exist, it is important to identify strategies that may be undertaken by individuals and the profession, through professional associations, to help enhance the image. A basic requirement is to change the self-image held by a nurse if it is a deterrent to developing the positive image nurses wish to portray. A change in the self-image would logically begin with nursing education promoting the "careerist" image projected by Kalisch and Kalisch (1982). Although this is presumably the objective of all nursing programs, nurse educators need to examine their teaching strategies to ensure that they indeed do promote the "careerist" image of nursing.

The nursing educational system is generally held responsible for promoting nursing's self-image in a positive way. However, the nursing practice setting where students gain experience in caring for patients is equally responsible for providing a positive practice environment and for providing students with constructive feedback.

Buresh and Gordon (2000) have highlighted specific strategies that nurses and groups of nurses can use to help improve public images of nursing. Other methods of changing the image of nursing during the process of education pertain to the attributes or characteristics of a profession that students learn during their basic education. Students are not always taught that the profession has its own body of knowledge, defined through research. Research is not emphasized in diploma programs because it is not a component of the programs, but it is important that students know about research development and recognize its importance in advancing nursing knowledge and improving nursing practice. Educators can help students develop research awareness and understand the importance of applying valid and reliable research findings in practice.

Recently, the Canadian Nurses Association (2009) published *The Next Decade,* which describes future roles of nurses and recommends a strong focus on the development of leadership by nurses within the health system. Since good leadership is strongly related to a positive self-image (Miller and Cummings, 2009), it makes sense that this should be the focus of any strategies to improve nursing's image.

Since mass media influence the public's image of nursing, it is important that nurses be alert and educated to assess the media for the type of images portrayed. Kalisch and Kalisch (1987) advocate a deliberate process of intervention that "involves four key steps: (1) getting organized; (2) monitoring the media; (3) reacting to the media; and (4) fostering an improved image" (p. 187). The "media watch" has been promoted and implemented by professional nursing associations in Canada and the United States. Nurses are encouraged to assess the media for the portrayal of undesirable images and take action by identifying the inadequacies to the producers (Evans, Fitzpatrick, & Howard-Ruben, 1983; Kalisch & Kalisch, 1983; Kalisch & Kalisch, 1987). An example of a positive result from media watch is the organized protest by many nurses and the professional organizations in 1989 to the National Broadcasting Corporation's television series *Nightingales.* The series portrayed an extremely demeaning and grossly outdated image of nurses and nursing students. The result of a mass letter-writing campaign, organized by professional nursing associations, and meetings with the producers was a victory for nursing: the series was cancelled and the producers and the public became keenly aware of the reasons for nurses' protest. They also became aware of the image that nursing wishes to convey and its importance in attracting and retaining nurses to provide quality health care.

Current television programs such as *ER* and *Grey's Anatomy* have presented both positive and negative images of nurses at times, although for the most part nursing is not featured by these programs. The main characters are physicians. Other television series, such as *House*, rarely mention nurses, and when they do, nurses are depicted as handmaidens.

For the past few years, the Centre for Nursing Advocacy, based in Maryland, has served to monitor the media and to spearhead protest efforts when nursing is depicted incorrectly or in a negative way. It has made a valuable contribution in documenting all media genres in their portrayal of nursing. However, the Web site currently states that the board of directors of the centre has recommended its closure.

One approach that has been used with considerable success by professional organizations is presenting awards for media presentations that portray the most positive images of nursing. This strategy was implemented by the CNA in 1988, when three awards and five certificates of merit, in the areas of television, radio, and journalism, were presented by the Minister of Health and Welfare at a dinner organized by the CNA (CNA Connection, 1988). In 1989, five award recipients and five certificate-of-merit recipients were selected from 29 entries, including national newspapers and magazines, private and public radio and television, and individual publications (CNA Connection, 1989). The CNA's media awards have become an annual event, initially during Nurses' Week in May but changed to March, and then February to help increase visibility and impact when parliament is likely to be in session. The importance of the awards to the media is reflected in an increase in entries from 29 in 1989 to 69 in 1992, when six awards of excellence and six certificates of merit were awarded. That year, CNA president Alice Baumgart "noted that many entries looked at the support system consumers have developed to help them face the difficulties of disease and handicaps. A number also dealt with the funding crisis in the health care system" (CNA Connection, 1992, p. 14). These awards have continued to the present time and are a significant part of the public image strategy of the CNA. In 2002, sixteen awards were given; ten were awards of excellence, and six were awards of merit (CNA, 2002). In 2006, "8 awards were presented for news and in-depth categories in print, radio and television, along with online and international health reporting, in addition to the Newsmaker of the Year" (CNA, 2006). These awards are now presented jointly with the Canadian Medical Association to honour outstanding journalism that enhances understanding of health, the health system, and the role of health care providers. In 2009, eight awards were presented to a variety of media. In addition to helping to foster greater public understanding of health care issues, the media awards have a positive effect on the image of nurses and nursing.

Public opinion surveys are important to enhancing the image of nursing. The samples used must be random and of sufficient size to allow generalization, and instruments must be tested for validity and reliability. The results of such surveys should be used in marketing the nursing profession to the public as the CARNA has done. The younger age groups should be targeted, not only to increase recruitment into nursing, but also to ensure favourable public opinion in the future. Reichelt (1988) emphasizes the importance of regular assessment of public opinion of nursing, both to formulate marketing strategies and to assess the results of the strategies that are implemented. Since there is no real up-to-date information available in Canada today, it is clear that this should be a priority for the profession.

Recruitment materials, both to attract persons into nursing and to attract nurses into positions in health care agencies, must be scrutinized carefully for the image presented. They should apply to both men and women. To attract staff in times of scarce resources, health care agencies often use gimmicks that promote a negative and sexually oriented image by emphasizing nonprofessional aspects of the place of employment. An example is advertisements emphasizing the advantages of social life in a particular setting rather than the challenges of professional practice. Another means of promoting the positive and careerist image of nursing has been to eliminate some of the traditions and rituals of graduation ceremonies. The graduation ceremony for nursing students in university and college programs should be the same as for other students, not set apart for long-standing rituals. Similarly, the language used in educational programs and among nurses themselves must be changed to eliminate sexist and paternalistic phrases, such as "the girls." Most institutions now use their Web sites for student recruitment. These can be very effective in presenting a positive image to prospective students. Nursing institutions must ensure that their Web sites are picked up by the major search engines in order to hit as broad a public group as possible. A search using Google.ca on the term "nursing, Canada" brings up thousands of Web sites. Many of these are prospective employers, and they include most of the Canadian nursing schools. It also brings up Wikipedia (the free encyclopedia), which provides a description of nursing as a profession. These sites on the Internet are an excellent opportunity to present nursing to the public.

In all public presentations, the practice of nursing should be envisioned and interpreted as primarily independent and interdependent, with some dependent aspects pertaining to the prescription of therapies. The focus of practice should be on the promotion and maintenance of health, not only illness care, with the goal of helping people attain, maintain, and regain their optimal levels of health and function. Nurses should be portrayed as being in interdependent practice, where they have an important role in collaborative decision making and in making independent decisions related to nursing care. They should also be depicted as playing an active role in making policies that pertain to health care and financing of health care, not merely serving in a reactive manner. In an effort to portray the desired image of nurses as intelligent, capable, and equal partners in health care delivery, a number of universities, as well as organizations such as the Registered Nurses' Association of Ontario (RNAO) and the Canadian Nursing Students Association, have produced videos to assist with the recruitment of students into the profession. The videos depict nurses as caring and articulate professionals working as key members of the health care team.

Nurses can play a key role in explaining the image of nurses and nursing to society in general and to the other health care providers with whom they work on a daily basis. The image of nursing held by practitioners themselves is of vital importance, as is their skill at communicating that image to others. Unless nurses have a concept of the professional "careerist" image, as originally proposed by Kalisch and Kalisch (1982), nursing will not succeed in changing the image and developing a cadre of intelligent, sophisticated, assertive, competent, empathic, and supportive nurses whose major goal is to assist individuals in assuming increased responsibility for their own health.

CONCLUSION

In spite of the huge advances in technology and health care that have taken place over the past 30 years, not much has changed in the way nurses are perceived, both within and outside the profession. Although the image of nurses and nursing may be changing to overcome the sex-object image that still exists in mass media, the challenge for nurses is to change both the internal and external images of nursing to promote a professional image. Only nurses can change the image, and change will be effected only by commitment on the part of individuals and the profession as a whole. The priority given to enhancing the image of nurses and nursing by professional associations needs to be continued. In addition, individual nurses need to accept the challenge of promoting the ideal professional image of nurses, which will help attract the kind of person needed to develop the potential of nurses to advance knowledge and improve practice, and to be known as persons committed to knowing and especially to doing. By taking every opportunity to promote professional nursing as well as the diversity of opportunities available to nurses, we can ensure that the potential impact of the Internet is maximized. Meanwhile, we must keep up efforts to monitor the other media through programs such as the Media Awards of the Canadian Nurses Association, and most of all, we must ensure that nursing students are socialized into a professional role, within nursing and in interdisciplinary practice. Knowing the importance of our image to addressing issues such as the nursing shortage will keep us on track.

CRITICAL THINKING QUESTIONS

1. Why should nurses be concerned about the image of nursing portrayed by television?
2. What impact can the actions of individual nurses have on the public image of nursing?

REFERENCES

Bayer, B. E. (2007). *From angels to devil: Images of nurses on film*. Retrieved on April 23, 2008, from http: www.nursevillage.com/nv/content/personalside/entertainment/nursesinfilm.jsp.

Brewer, C. S., Zayas, L. E., Kahn, L. S., & Siendiewicz, M. J. (2006). Nursing recruitment and retention in New York State: A qualitative workforce needs assessment. *Policy, Politics & Nursing Practice, 7*(1), 54–63.

Brodie, D. A., Andrews, G. J., Andrews, J. P., Thomas, G. B., Wong, J., & Rixon, L. (2004). Perceptions of nursing: Confirmation, change and the student experience. *International Journal of Nursing Studies, 41*(7), 721–733.

Buresh, B., & Gordon, S. (2000). *From silence to voice: What nurses know and must communicate to the public.* Toronto: HarperCollins.

Canadian Nurses Association. (2002). *2002 Media Awards for excellence in health care reporting.* Retrieved on February 7, 2008, from http://www.cna-nurses.ca/CNA/news/releases/public_release_e.aspx?id=42.

Canadian Nurses Association. (2006). *2006 Media Awards.* Retrieved on February 7, 2008, from http://www.cna-nurses.ca/CNA/news/releases/public_release_e.aspx?id=197.

Canadian Nurses Association. (2007). *2007 Workforce Profile of Registered Nurses in Canada.* Retrieved on October 18, 2009, from http://www.cna-aiic.ca/CNA/resources/bytype/statistics/default_e.aspx.

Canadian Nurses Association. (2009). *The next decade: CNA's vision for nursing and health.* Retrieved on October 30, 2009, from www.CNA-aiic.ca/CNA/resources;next-decade/.

Connection CNA. (1988). CNA media awards a hit. *The Canadian Nurse, 84*(7), 6.

Connection CNA. (1989). Media excellence. *The Canadian Nurse, 85*(7), 9.

Connection CNA. (1992). Media awards. *The Canadian Nurse, 88*(7), 14.

Diers, D. (1984). To profess—to be a professional. *Journal of the New York State Nurses' Association, 15*(4), 22–29.

Evans, D., Fitzpatrick, T., & Howard-Ruben, J. (1983). A district takes action. *American Journal of Nursing, 83*(1), 52–59.

Freda, M. C. (2006). Nurses in the strangest places. *MCN: The American Journal of Maternal-Child Nursing, 31*(4), 214.

Giovannetti, P. (1990). News release. *AARN Newsletter, 46*(1), 7.

Gordon, S., & Johnson, R. (2004). How Hollywood portrays nurses: Report from the front row. *Revolution,* March/April, 15–21.

Hereford, M. (2005). *Exploring the real image of nursing: How movies, television and stereotypes portray the nursing profession.* PhD Thesis pp. 232. University of Idaho.

HRSA. (2007). *The registered nurse population: Findings from the 2004 national sample survey of registered nurses.* US Department of Health and Human Services. Retrieved on January 29, 2008, from http://bhpr.hrsa.gov/healthworkforce/rnsurvey04/appendixa.htm.

Kalisch, B., Begeny, S., & Neumann, S. (2007). The image of the nurse on the Internet. *Nursing Outlook, 55*(4), 182–188.

Kalisch, B., & Kalisch, P. (1982). Anatomy of the image of the nurse: Dissonant and ideal models. In C. Williams (Ed.), *Image-making in nursing* (pp. 3–23). Kansas City, MO: American Academy of Nursing.

Kalisch, B., & Kalisch, P. (1983). Improving the image of nursing. *American Journal of Nursing, 83*(1), 48–52.

Kalisch, P., & Kalisch, B. (1987). *The changing image of the nurse.* Toronto: Addison-Wesley.

Lippman, D. T., & Ponton, K. S. (1989). Nursing's image on the university campus. *Nursing Outlook, 37*(1), 24–27.

May, F., Austin, J. K., & Champion, V. (1988). *Attitudes, values and beliefs of the public in Indiana toward nursing as a career: A study to enhance recruitment into nursing.* Indianapolis, IN: Sigma Theta Tau International Honor Society of Nursing.

Meadus, R. J., & Twomey, J. C. (2007). Men in nursing: Making the right choice. *Canadian Nurse, 103*(2), 13–26.

Miller, K., & Cummings, G. (2009). Gifted and talented students' career aspirations and influences: A systematic review of the literature. *The International Journal of Nursing Education Scholarship, 6*(1), Article 8.

Payne, Cook and Associates Inc. (1990). *Insight: The 1989 provincial public opinion study of nursing in Alberta.* Available from CARNA, 11620 168 St., Edmonton, AB T5M 4A6.

Rasmussen, E. (2001). Picture imperfect: From Nurse Ratched to Hot Lips Houlihan, film/TV portrayals of nurses often transmit a warped image of real-life RNs. *Nurse Week,* May 7. Retrieved on April 23, 2009, from http:www.nurseweek.com/news/features/01.05/picture.html.

Reichelt, P. A. (1988). Public perceptions of nursing and strategy formulation. *Western Journal of Nursing Research, 10*(4), 472–476.

Roberts, D., & Vasquez, E. (2004). Power: An application to the nursing image and advanced practice. *AACN Clinical Issues, 15*(2), 196–204.

Seago, J. A., Spetz, J., Alvarado, A., Keane, D., & Grumbach, K. (2006). The nursing shortage: Is it really about image? *Journal of Healthcare Management, 51*(2), 96–108.

Simmons, L. W., & Henderson, V. (1964). *Nursing research: A survey and assessment.* New York: Appleton-Century-Crofts.

Stanley, D. J. (2008). Celluloid angels: A research study of nurses in feature films 1900–2007. *Journal of Advanced Nursing, 64*(1), 84–95.

Styles, M. M. (1982). *On nursing: Toward a new endowment.* Toronto: C.V. Mosby.

Takase, M., Maude, P., & Manias, E. (2006). Impact of the perceived public image of nursing on nurses' work behavior. *Journal of Advanced Nursing, 53*(3), 333–343.

Ward, C., Styles, I., & Bosco, A. M. (2003). Perceived status of nurses compared to other health care professionals. *Contemporary Nurse, 15*(1–2), 20–28.

5 Issues of Gender and Diversity in Nursing

Janet C. Ross-Kerr

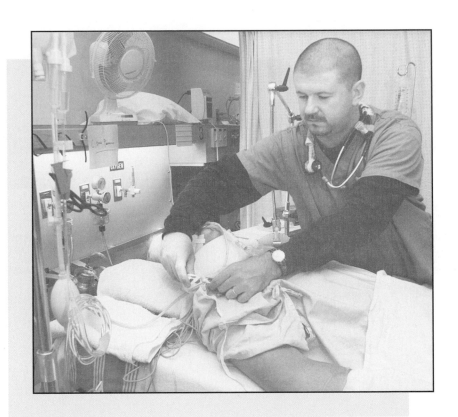

⬛ LEARNING OBJECTIVES

- To recognize the contribution of feminism and feminist thinking to women's health.
- To describe the various philosophical views of feminism.
- To comprehend the nature of the relationship between feminism and nursing.
- To understand the impact of feminism in nursing on women's health.
- To recognize research findings from studies on feminism in nursing.
- To describe workforce statistics relative to the representation of men and women in nursing.
- To understand the nature of the barriers to men entering the nursing profession and ways of overcoming these.
- To recognize research findings from studies of men in nursing.
- To comprehend the issues for students from diverse populations in entering the nursing profession as well as strategies to reduce existing barriers to taking up a career in nursing.

Understanding issues of gender and diversity is fundamental to appreciating the nature and origins of the nursing profession, as well as its evolution over time. Gender issues have been prominent since the first formal arrangements to care for the sick. Historically, nursing had its roots in the work of Roman matrons who provided care and nurturance for the sick poor in their own homes. Fabiola and others were well known for their work, possible because of their wealth and altruism. Care of the sick continued to be carried out by women with the advent of the religious orders of nuns.

During the Crusades in the eleventh century, men tended the sick and injured. This pattern was repeated when Canada was first explored and settled as New France. As mentioned in Chapter 2, the first nurses who came from Europe to serve as nurses were male attendants at Port Royal and later Jesuit priests at Quebec. The impropriety of male priests' caring for sick women led in 1639 to the emigration from France of three nuns, who were nurses, to establish the first hospital at Quebec. A pattern thus developed that continued for four centuries, whereby female religious orders built and operated hospitals to care for the sick, prevent illness, and promote health. Later, they took on the added responsibility of training nurses to staff the hospitals. After the middle of the twentieth century, religious orders began to withdraw from nursing education and management of hospitals, and secular health agencies prevailed as hospital operations became more expensive and moved into the public sector.

Wars influenced who attended the sick and injured and who was recruited into nursing. Societal attitudes were at the basis of military policy permitting only men to go to war, based on the view that it was considered appropriate for men both to kill others and to die in defence of their country. This was apparent in the seventeenth-century battles with Aboriginal peoples and in wars and conflicts until recent years. During World War I, only men in the Medical Corps were permitted to serve on the front lines of battle, while female nurses, also members of the Medical Corps, staffed Canadian base hospitals caring for the wounded, but were not permitted on the front lines. In both World Wars, women were recruited in great numbers to staff civilian hospitals because many nurses left to enter the Nurse Corps of the three armed services divisions, and many men volunteered for, or were conscripted into, the services. This increased the number of women entering nursing and decreased the number of men entering nursing, as they were needed for battle.

The practice of having only male attendants care for the sick and injured prevailed until Florence Nightingale, with her small band of nurses, went to the Crimea, where she worked to improve the care of wounded soldiers. Although Nightingale was only grudgingly accepted by the heads of the army, she saved many lives and improved the environmental conditions during recovery through her strong determination, expert knowledge, and nursing skill. She overcame barriers to women's involvement in nursing the sick and wounded during war and later challenged and finally overcame Victorian barriers to women working outside the home. Later, when the first nursing school was established at St. Thomas's Hospital in London in 1860, only women were accepted as applicants. The school was organized separately from the hospital, thus creating an opportunity for women to work outside the home and promoting a separate environment for women to work. In the process of overcoming societal pressures for women to conform to Victorian beliefs and customs, Nightingale also excluded men from nursing.

Currently, nursing is a profession in transition from one that has historically been predominantly female in character to one that is gender balanced. Societal values about the capabilities of men to assume a nurturing role both in the family and outside the home have been changing over the past several decades, and it has become more and more acceptable for men to enter nursing. In order to develop an understanding of the whole gamut of gender-based issues facing the nursing profession, it is necessary to have some knowledge both of feminism and of issues related to men. Consequently, a review of feminism and feminist issues in relation to health will be followed by a review of those issues relating to men and men in nursing and of those pertaining to diversity in nursing.

INTRODUCTION TO FEMINISM

Feminism is an outgrowth of reactions against forms of social organization in which women are not valued as highly as men. The norms of such a system condone systematic bias toward women. Although feminism is commonly thought of as a movement that grew out of the 1960s, feminist ideas are reflected in writing by women in the seventeenth century. In more recent history, the suffragette movement of the late nineteenth and early twentieth centuries had a powerful impact on society and resulted in important changes in the treatment of women. Nightingale's work in this era is "recognized by feminist scholars as reflecting remarkable feminist insight" (Chinn & Wheeler, 1985, p. 74).

Nurses were profoundly influenced by the thinking of the women suffragists and were in an important position to demonstrate women's capabilities. Nursing had recently gained respect as a profession and was one of few careers open to women. Politically active nursing leaders were able to accomplish critical professional goals that would allow their profession remarkable development throughout the twentieth century. The entrenchment of nursing registration in legislation in Canada and other countries during this period was a victory and an important step forward for the status of women.

Feminist methods were suggested as a framework for research by MacPherson (1983). Then, four philosophical views of feminism were put forward by Chinn and Wheeler (1985), including the liberal feminist stance, in which women are seen as an oppressed group who will be aided by equalizing opportunities for women. According to Marxist feminist thinking, capitalism and the acquisition of property has created a class system that favours men, and resolution of the inequality is seen as an important consequence in a society in which materialism and capitalism are rejected for a system of collective organization and ownership. Socialist feminist ideas derive from analyses of socio-cultural phenomena and institutions where "the oppression of women and socio-economic class oppression are equally fundamental and mutually reinforcing" (p. 75). In contrast, radical feminist theory emphasizes the importance of defining issues from a female approach to the world. In this stance, attention is not focused on the relation of women to men, as in some other perspectives, but on viewing and valuing women separately from the male world.

The eco-feminist framework is seen as liberating nursing from the narrow environment of the individual and family to the environmentally conscious setting of the larger world where women are liberated from patriarchal oppression and can relate differently to patients and others (Kleffel, 1991, p. 16). Pohl and Boyd (1993) explored liberal feminist claims that progress can be made while acknowledging no influence on the power structure. Kushner and Morrow (2006) extended thinking about the generation of knowledge using feminist methods and proposed a "critical feminist grounded theory methodology" (p. 30).

The ideology of feminism is threatening to some, undoubtedly because its framework represents a radical departure from traditional thinking. Although feminism may be seen as a movement that opposes both men and traditional institutions such as the family, its fundamental ideas espouse valuing both women and men. Systems and institutions favouring one sex over the other are targets of feminist criticism. Feminists also model behaviour that may not be thought of as feminine, undoubtedly unsettling to some. In this respect, modern feminists share some characterizations of the early suffragists in the way their ideas are presented. Independent thought and action, straightforward and hard-hitting commentary on issues of concern, and generally assertive behaviour characterize the feminist *modus operandi*.

THE RELATIONSHIP BETWEEN FEMINISM AND NURSING

The relationship between feminism and nursing has been somewhat tenuous or uneasy in the modern era, but this was not always the case. Although nursing was at the forefront of the women's movement early in the twentieth century, predominantly male professions have been the focus of recent feminist concern. This has largely been a successful thrust because women are now entering nontraditional professions in greater proportions than ever. Sex-stereotyped views of nursing emphasize subservience, lack of assertiveness, and domination of nurses, who are primarily female, by physicians, who are primarily male. The real status of modern nursing may be difficult to appreciate from a view outside the profession. Technological advances and increases in health care knowledge heightened performance expectations and had a phenomenal impact on nursing in general, leading to new and independent roles in many areas. However, as a predominantly female profession in the modern era, nursing has been undervalued when measured by the contributions made by its members to society and has sometimes been invisible in the social and professional policy making arena. Further, feminists have tended to fall prey to sexist stereotypes and have discounted nursing as a legitimate professional domain for highly educated women (Mason, Leavitt, & Chaffee, 2002).

Persuasive arguments suggesting that nurses can be categorized as an oppressed group are provided in a classic article by Roberts (1983). The discussion is an illuminating one and provides some intriguing explanations for characteristic behaviour observed in nurses. For example, of some interest is the low value some nurses place on participation in professional organizations. Emanating from a low degree of esteem for the profession, such behaviour is thought to be based on fear that associating with others who are oppressed may not be in one's best interest.

The implications of a feminist view of practice, education, and research in nursing are important and require a shift in thinking and new approaches to care. The challenge to traditional patriarchal family structures represents an inherent challenge to nursing theories and conceptual frameworks as well, because many of these have "underlying patriarchal assumptions about human experience" (Chinn & Wheeler, 1985). By advocating the same treatment for men and women in society, feminists have been tremendously successful in challenging traditional roles of men and women. In health care, as in other areas, new approaches to care and treatment and to education in the health professions are resulting in a total restructuring because of the influence of new ideas from the women's movement. For example, women's health is designated as a service department in many health care agencies, and the federal government has funded several research "centres of excellence for women's health" across the country.

The changes that are occurring are nothing short of revolutionary, and the system that results will look very different from the one that existed before feminist ideas were widely known and appreciated. Baer (1991) has sounded a note of caution, however, about the directions of feminism: "Feminism will have succeeded not only when females have equal access to all fields but also when traditionally female professions, such as nursing, gain the high value and solid respect they deserve" (p. 121).

A FEMINIST APPROACH TO WOMEN'S HEALTH

The women's movement has had considerable impact on the ways that nurses have conceptualized health:

> *Nursing's contributions . . . over the past 30 years have redefined women's health; proposed new frameworks for understanding [it]; provided review of the women's health literature across disciplines; developed communities of nurse scholars and researchers focused on new areas of women's health research; generated and expanded the knowledge base for women's health practice and education; promoted a global view of women's health; and proposed new models for women's health care delivery. (Taylor & Woods, 2001)*

Baumgart (1999) underscored the essence of the struggle for recognition of the nursing profession and its unique contribution to health in a historical context:

> *Not since the struggle for registration at the turn of the century has political action assumed so high a priority on the agenda of organized nursing groups. Fuelled by social and political forces such as the women's movement and the shift from entrepreneurial to political power in Canadian health services, organized nursing associations in Canada have begun to define themselves as political pressure or interest groups having a direct, continuous, and active role in influencing health policy. (p. 131)*

Historically, the health problems emphasized in most nursing curricula have been male-biased; for example, cardiac disease, which was previously thought to be primarily a male medical problem, received far more attention than depression, which was thought to affect primarily women. Challenges have arisen to the traditional areas of focus in health largely because of the women's movement. There is new attention to women's overall health problems (as opposed to reproductive health only), such as osteoporosis, depression, rape, premenstrual syndrome, and menopausal difficulties. The women's and consumers' movements have jointly influenced the role of the health care client and have legitimized an active role.

Delineation of patients' rights in health care (see Chapter 14) has led to the consensus that a patient has a right to information and should participate in decision making about care because there are often options for treatment. Consumers, including women, are asking for clear statements of these options so that they can be informed participants in the decision-making process. For many years, nursing curricula have emphasized the importance of communication, interpersonal skills, and health assessment skills, as well as community assessment and development. Nurses thus have a strong foundation for interacting with consumers about their health and for working with them to improve conditions for health, both individually and at the community level. An icon of the nursing profession, the late Virginia Henderson, is noted for her early emphasis upon the importance of assisting people to regain abilities and resume usual activities when she wrote that nurses should seek to assist patients "to gain independence as rapidly as possible" (Henderson, 1961, p. 42). Since many of the directions the women's movement has taken coincide with those being taken by the nursing profession, women's health stands to benefit.

Analysis of the impact of feminists and feminism yields some interesting perspectives. As the strident years of the early feminism of the 1960s gave way to the more reflective feminism of the 1980s, Malka posits her thesis that it was the "second wave" or later style of feminism that had a profound impact on the nursing profession. New value was placed on nursing and, as a result, nurses were empowered to seek higher education to become specialized professionals, they began to collaborate with other health disciplines on a more collegial level, and nurses achieved greater independence in all aspects of their work in practice, education, and research (Malka, 2007).

RESEARCH AND FEMINISM

Nursing research that focuses on women's issues may or may not take a feminist stance. A paradigm shift is necessary because previous theories and conceptual frameworks used in research did not view women's health from a female perspective and were therefore incomplete.

> These [new] theories have a dual function: they offer descriptions of women's oppression and prescriptions for eliminating it. They are empirical insofar as they examine women's experience in the world, but they are political insofar as they characterize certain features of that experience as oppressive and offer new visions of justice and freedom for women. (MacPherson, 1983, p. 19)

Feminist research is characterized more frequently as qualitative rather than quantitative. The emphasis on describing the meaning of women's health experiences leads frequently to the use of qualitative approaches. Such research tends to be exploratory and may encompass field studies and participatory action research. Quantitative approaches need to be used to gather basic data that have been unavailable in areas that have received little attention. "Because we have undervalued women's and nursing's 'ways of knowing,' we have unwittingly abrogated a powerful influence for change and in so doing deprived society of our strength" (Sohier, 1992, pp. 64–65).

While it is clear that both qualitative and quantitative approaches are likely to be useful in the long run, the problem for women's health is that there has been little exploratory work in some areas. Nursing researchers have become increasingly conversant with qualitative methods, and many studies reported in journals use qualitative methods. Health problems of concern to women are receiving considerable attention from nursing researchers, as evidenced by publications in the nursing research journals (Wuest, 2006; Norris & King, 2009).

The interpretation of results in research investigations has been the focus of attention by feminists. There is a concern that feminist values may bias the interpretation just as male values have historically biased the interpretation of previous research. "There needs to be an ongoing struggle to conduct research without allowing feminist values to become prisms that distort or bend the truth, or blinders that hide the truth entirely" (MacPherson, 1983, p. 24). Thus open and truly objective approaches are desirable for scholarly work. Undoubtedly, when the framework through which the data are viewed is broader and encompasses human values, the possibility that new interpretations will be derived is enhanced.

Public concern about studies that have used only men as research subjects with the result that the conclusions are generalizable only to men has led to a perception of the need to broaden the subject base for investigations in general and to use women as well as men in a number of areas. There is also a need to communicate results of studies to consumers so that all women can benefit.

Nursing research has much to offer in the area of women's health, and a feminist perspective can be very useful to nursing researchers who wish to go beyond the traditional biomedical model, which is "reductionistic and contradictory to nursing's holistic mission" (Morse, 2000). One means of encouraging such research would be to employ feminist ideals and pedagogy throughout the nursing curriculum, rather than classifying women's health as a separate entity. "This approach would provide a mechanism to explore women's health issues that were previously minimally addressed at best, or not addressed at all" (Morse, 2000). Nurses have just begun to recognize the challenges and to make a commitment to carry out meaningful work in these areas.

 REFLECTIVE THINKING

What questions might a nurse ask about women's health outcomes using a feminist perspective?

MEN IN NURSING

Despite an increase in the number of men in nursing during the past two decades, men still constitute an insignificant proportion of the registered nurse population in Canada. This is remarkable at a time when the proportion of women in traditionally male-dominated professions has increased at a phenomenal rate. Areas now opened to women include business, dentistry, law, medicine, and pharmacy because of pressure from women's groups, whose allegations of sexism have led to changes in recruitment policies and affirmative action. Thus, as many as half of the admission placements in these disciplines are available to women. At the same time, there have been notable increases in the number of men entering other traditionally female-dominated professions, such as teaching and librarianship.

Why has the proportion of men in nursing increased so slowly? What factors have influenced the entry of men into nursing? Will these factors continue to exert the same influence? What are the advantages of having more men in nursing? What has the nursing profession done or not done to change the proportion of men entering its ranks? What implications does the Charter of Rights have for the continuation of a predominance of women or men in any profession?

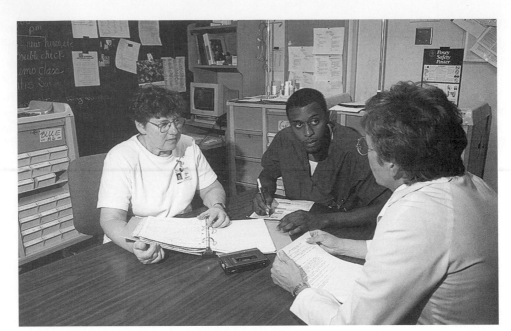

Nurse giving a change-of-shift report.

PROPORTION OF MEN AND WOMEN IN NURSING

The proportion of men in nursing in Canada has increased slowly since the 1960s, as shown in Table 5.1. Even though the number of men employed in nursing in Canada has increased exponentially since 1966, the current proportion of male nurses still represents only 5.8% of the total nurse population, a slight increase over the 4.7% it made up in 2000. If segregated by sex and compared with other health care groups, the male registered nurse population is one of the smallest professional groups in the health care system (Canadian Nurses Association, 2009). To consider gender differences in nursing, one must examine factors that influence the entry of men into a traditionally female-dominated profession.

BARRIERS TO MEN ENTERING NURSING

One of the major barriers to men's entering the nursing profession is societal attitudes about work that is appropriate for men or women. In general, nursing has not been considered an appropriate career choice for men because of its characteristics of nurturance, gentleness, and caring. Men are supposed to be strong and powerful and not show emotions. Negative and discouraging reactions from others, including family members, have been reported by male nurses. Undoubtedly, these young men had to be very determined and committed to persist in their efforts to pursue a career in nursing. Male nurses encountered similar reactions from other health care providers

| TABLE 5.1 | Comparison of Female and Male Nurses Employed in Canada, 1966–2007 | | | | |

YEAR	TOTAL NO. RNs EMPLOYED IN NURSING	FEMALE		MALE	
		NUMBER	%	NUMBER	%
1966	82 917	82 545	99.55	372	0.45
1975	144 193*	142 095	98.55	2 098	1.45
1986	204 571*	199 085	97.32	5 486	2.68
1992	234 128*	225 910	96.49	8 218	3.51
2000	254 628	242 497	95.24	12 131	4.72
2005	251 675	237 668	94.4	14 007	5.6
2007	257 961	242 959	94.2	15 002	5.8

*Remainder employed in other than nursing or not employed or not stated.
Sources: Canadian Institute for Health Information (CIHI), 2000; CIHI, 2005; CIHI, 2007; Statistics Canada, 1994.

when medicine was predominantly male. Indeed, such reactions were not uncommon within the profession of nursing itself; some female nurses tended to regard men who selected nursing as not "real men." Dyck, Oliffe, Ogubbet, & Garrett (2009) have underscored the continuing challenges faced by men entering a profession that is viewed as feminine by both men and women and where roles and identity tend to support that view (Meadus and Tworney, 2007). There are other difficulties for men "within this milieu including perceptions that male nurses are gay or are failed physicians who in undertaking nursing automatically fall short of masculine ideals" (Dyck et al., 2009, p. 650).

Men were not accepted readily in nursing schools for many years. Initially, most of those accepted entered schools of nursing connected with mental hospitals, because of the belief that men were physically better able to deal with violence. Strength was considered so important in psychiatric nursing that this specialty did not become a required part of basic nursing education in Canada until the 1950s and even the 1960s in some schools. Until the 1960s and 1970s, male nursing students were not permitted to study theory and practice in obstetric and gynecological nursing; they devoted that time to urologic nursing, caring for male patients only. Evans (2004) reported that differential barriers to residential accommodation, separate and weaker educational programs for male nursing students, and difficulty securing positions following graduation were historical deterrents for men entering the profession.

For many years, another barrier to the admission of men to nursing programs was an economic one, as nurses were paid poorly in comparison to those in many other occupations. As a result, men who may have been interested in nursing chose not to enter because of the societal expectation that they should be the "breadwinners." Male nurses have sometimes been criticized for aspiring to high positions as administrators in order to earn enough to support a family.

CANADIAN RESEARCH FOCUS

Dyck, J.M., Oliffe, J., Phinney, A., & Garrett, B. (2009). Nursing instructors' and male nursing students' perceptions of undergraduate, classroom nursing education. *Nurse Education Today, 29*, 649–653.
  This study was conducted in two large Canadian baccalaureate nursing schools and was motivated by the need to understand the male experience in nursing in order to encourage male students to enter the profession. Using a qualitative, ethnographic, interpretive methodology, interviews were conducted with male nursing students and their female instructors. Findings uncovered continuing dominant feminization of nursing that made it difficult for male students in the educational setting. Also difficult for the students were public attitudes that typically stereotyped men in nursing as feminine and gay. Even though the male students were part of the nursing unit where they gave care as students, they felt they were dealt with ineffectively and did not feel totally integrated into its culture.

RESEARCH ON MEN IN NURSING

In his seminal review of research on men in nursing, Christman (1988) found a dearth of studies and identified many inadequacies in the methods of investigation used and interpretation of results. The research he reviewed included six survey studies, two studies using focused interviews, and five studies using standardized test batteries to assess personality, intelligence, and attitudes. The questionnaires used in the survey research had not been tested adequately for validity and reliability. In general, study samples were small and not representative of the population being studied, which can "result in sampling bias and incomplete knowledge of the phenomenon under study" (Christman, 1988, p. 198). Christman concluded: "If clarification of the male role in the nursing profession was a goal of the research done so far, then there are major shortcomings in both the research and the outcomes of research" (1988, p. 202). He questioned the utility of studies that elicited opinion and argued against doing more of them. Instead, he suggested building on the beginnings of two studies by Brown and Stones (1972) and Holtzclaw (1981), both of which used standardized test batteries. He also emphasized obtaining larger multi-site and more representative samples. In a more recent review of men in nursing, O'Lynn and Tranbarger (2006) have discussed communication problems, reverse discriminatory practices, and gender-based barriers for male students in nursing. The historical struggle by male nurses to achieve equality with their female counterparts in the Canadian military is documented in a fascinating study by Care, Gregory, English, and Ventakesh (1996). The study by Dyck et al. (2009) sought to shed some light on the experiences of male students in nursing programs using an interpretive ethnographic approach. Interviews with male students and their female instructors revealed that "men saw themselves as accommodated but not integrated" into the nursing education environment. This study provides some understanding of the difficulties faced by men in nursing and their higher attrition rates.

  Finally, there is no doubt that many factors have deterred men from entering and remaining in nursing and that some of the negative influences in society are slowly beginning to change. Factors such as cultural influences may serve to attract or discourage young people, particularly men, from choosing nursing as a career. The increasing number of Canadian immigrants coming from Asian and Latin-American countries, where men have not been a part of nursing, is one such factor. Another factor to be considered is that many fields, such as medicine, dentistry, business, law, and pharmacy, are now available to women. As more women are attracted to these fields, there may well be a reverse effect of attracting more men to nursing, particularly since there has been some, albeit gradual, increase of men in the profession over time (see Table 5.1), indicating greater acceptance of men in the profession.

To attract more men to nursing, educators and administrators must work together to correct the myths and overcome barriers that deter them. Hospitals and other health care agencies and nursing schools need to portray men in the role of nurse in their publicity materials to help change the public's perception of nursing. Evans (2004) cites examples of recruitment efforts that used posters downplaying feminine images of nursing and putting forward more masculine male images that focus on their abilities to do nursing. As a result of their study conducted in two large Canadian schools of nursing offering baccalaureate preparation, Dyck et al. (2009, p. 653) recommended supporting nursing instructors to develop "teaching strategies and approaches to better engage and avoid pressuring, privileging or alienating male students." The Registered Nurses Association of Ontario offers a special-interest group on men in nursing. The advantages of increasing the proportion of men in nursing are considerable and this is clearly being recognized by the nursing profession.

REFLECTIVE THINKING

Do you think that the profession has been successful in trying to overcome traditional stereotypes about men in nursing that have served as barriers to their entry? Explain the reasons you took the stance you did.

DIVERSITY IN NURSING

Canada has become a highly multicultural society. Immigration from countries other than those of the British Isles has increased exponentially in the last quarter of the twentieth century and into the twenty-first as Canada began to realize that its immigration policies had been highly biased in favour of immigrants from predominantly Anglo-Saxon countries. The increase in racial, ethnic, and cultural diversity among citizens of Canada meant that these new citizens would permeate the ranks of every major population and occupational group. The benefit to Canada of the new racial, ethnic, and cultural diversity is inestimable and provides a far richer background for local, national, and international relationships.

Some groups have been under-represented in the professions, including nursing, as compared with their representation in the population. Recognition of the contributions of other groups to the cultural mosaic in Canadian society has been slow in coming, for

Aboriginal societies preceded the European settlement that began in the seventeenth century. Villeneuve decried the fact that the majority of nurses in Canada remain white and female, a situation that is common in the health professions (2002–3). A study by Gibbs and Waugaman (2004) found cultural and racial differences in professional socialization and career commitment in an advanced practice role; they suggested that this issue needs to be considered carefully by those in education and practice in order to enhance and improve programs to encourage nurses with minority cultural and racial backgrounds to enter such programs and remain committed to their choices. These findings would appear to be corroborated by research by Gates (2007), which found that the greater the perceived increased difference between a staff nurse and others in the setting, the weaker was the intent to remain on the job. The development of shared value systems was seen as critical to retain staff, along with defined strategies to enhance recruitment, retention, and management. Gilchrist and Rector (2007) studied strategies to recruit and retain nursing students from diverse populations and concluded that it is important to begin early in elementary and high schools to plant seeds encouraging these potential students to consider nursing. Tours and clear information about entry requirement and benefits offered by a nursing career were seen as important strategies; further, once students are in school, support groups and peer mentors as well as curriculum support were found to be essential to retaining these students. Culturally sensitive practice is an issue that faces the nursing profession. Some have argued that the problem in educating nurses to engage in culturally sensitive practice rests with the fact that such education has not been based to a sufficient extent in a sociopolitical context (Clark & Robinson, 1999). This has meant that health outcomes from traditionally under-represented groups have not been sufficiently positive pointing to the need for improvements in nursing education and staff-in-service training programs. Aboriginal groups in Canada have been traditionally under-represented in all the health professions. Martin (2006) studied Aboriginal nursing students' experiences in two Canadian schools of nursing and found that tension between students and faculty centred on lack of understanding of their needs and of content that would promote Aboriginal health. These students also experienced considerable difficulty because of inadequate band and Canada Student Loans funding and lack of social support because of geographic distance from their families and friends. The need for change is apparent in order to ensure that recruitment and retention of Aboriginal nurses is enhanced and that this group is empowered to assist in improving the health of Aboriginal peoples in Canada.

CONCLUSION

Gender has exerted a powerful influence in the nursing profession over time. The foregoing discussion confirms that the issues pertain both to women and to men. Even though the profession has been largely female in character, this is changing gradually with a shift in public attitudes concerning the roles of men and women in society as well as concerning the nature of nursing and the kind of individuals required to provide high-quality nursing care (Anonson, Karkanis, & McDonnell, 2000). More recently, the need to move to a workforce more diverse in race, ethnic origin, and culture has been recognized. The diversity of the population that is increasingly reflected in the nursing workforce is also an important factor relative to offering culturally sensitive care to patients. The change that has occurred to date is remarkable and there can be no doubt that this will continue. The nursing profession stands to gain much as it moves in the direction of a culturally diverse and gender-balanced workforce. However, the pace of change is likely to continue to be slow and steady.

CRITICAL THINKING QUESTIONS

1. Describe the impact of feminism on nursing and women's health over the past half century.
2. Why has nursing in modern times been practised primarily by women?
3. Are men able to pursue satisfying careers in nursing today?
4. What kinds of strategies are needed to attract those from diverse ethnic backgrounds into nursing?

WEB SITES

Aboriginal Nurses Association of Canada: http://www.anac.on.ca/
Canadian Men in Nursing Group of the Canadian Nurses Association:
  http://www.nursesentry.com/men-in-nursing.html
Men in Nursing Interest Group of the Registered Nurses Association of Ontario: http://www.rnao.org/Page.asp?P
  ageID=924&ContentID=1725

REFERENCES

Anonson, J., Karkanis, A., & McDonnell, P. (2000). Recruiting nurses for the new millennium. *Canadian Nurse, 96*(5), 31–34.

Baer, E. D. (1991). Even her feminist friends see her as "only" a nurse. *International Nursing Review, 38*(4), 121.

Baumgart, A. J. (1999). Nurses and political action: The legacy of sexism. *Canadian Journal of Nursing Research, 30*(4), 131–141.

Brown, R. G. S., & Stones, R. H. W. (1972). Personality and intelligence characteristics of male nurses. *International Journal of Nursing Studies, 9*(8), 167–177.

Canadian Institute for Health Information (CIHI). (2000). *Supply and distribution of registered nurses in Canada, 2000.* Retrieved on September 27, 2009, from http://secure.cihi.ca/cihiweb/dispPage.jsp?cw_page=AR_20_E.

Canadian Institute for Health Information (CIHI). (2005). *Workforce profile of registered nurses in Canada, 2005.* Retrieved on September 27, 2009, from http://secure.cihi.ca/cihiweb/dispPage.jsp?cw_page=statistics_results_topic_nurses_e&cw_topic=Health%20Human%20Resources&cw_subtopic=Nurses.

Canadian Institute for Health Information (CIHI). (2007). *Workforce profile of registered nurses in Canada. 2007.* Retrieved on September 27, 2009, from http://secure.cihi.ca/cihiweb/dispPage.jsp?cw_page=statistics_results_topic_nurses_e&cw_topic=Health%20Human%20Resources&cw_subtopic=Nurses.

Canadian Nurses Association. (2009). *Workforce profile of registered nurses in Canada.* Retrieved on March 25, 2010, from http://www.cna-aiic.ca/CNA/documents/pdf/publications/2007_RN_Snapshot_e.pdf.

Care, D., Gregory, D., English, J., & Venkatesh, P. (1996). A struggle for equality: Resistance to commissioning of male nurses in the Canadian military, 1952–1967. *Canadian Journal of Nursing Research, 28*(1), 103.

Chinn, P., & Wheeler, C. E. (1985). Feminism and nursing: Can nursing afford to remain aloof from the women's movement? *Nursing Outlook, 33*(2), 74–77.

Christman, L. P. (1988). Men in nursing. In J. J. Fitzpatrick, R. L. Taunton, & J. Q. Benoliel (Eds.), *Annual review of nursing research* (Vol. 6) (pp. 193–205). New York: Springer.

Clark, C., & Robinson, T. M. (1999). Cultural diversity and transcultural nursing as they impact health care. *Journal of National Black Nurses' Association, 10*(2), 46–53.

Dyck, J. M., Oliffe, J., Phinney, A., & Garrett, B. (2009). Nursing instructors' and male nursing students' perceptions of undergraduate, classroom nursing education. *Nurse Education Today, 29*, 649–653.

Evans, J. (2004). Men nurses: A historical and feminist perspective. *Journal of Advanced Nursing, 47*(3), 321–328.

Gates, M. G. (2007). *Demographic diversity, value congruence, and workplace outcomes in acute care.* Unpublished Ph.D. dissertation. Chapel Hill, NC: University of North Carolina.

Gibbs, D. M., & Waugaman, W. (2004). Diversity behind the mask: Ethnicity, gender and past career experience in a nurse anesthesiology program. *Journal of Multicultural Nursing and Health, 10*(1), 77–80.

Gilchrist, K. L., & Rector, C. (2007). Can you keep them? Strategies to attract and retain nursing students from diverse populations: Best practices in nursing education. *Journal of Transcultural Nursing, 18*(3), 277–285.

Henderson, V. (1961). *Basic principles of nursing care.* London: International Council of Nurses.

Holtzclaw, B. J. (1981). *The man in nursing: Relations between sex-type perceptions and locus of control.* Dissertation Abstracts International, 4202A. (University Microfilms No. 81-16, 752).

Kleffel, D. (1991). An ecofeminist analysis of nursing knowledge. *Nursing Forum, 26*(4), 5–18.

Kushner, K. E., & Morrow, R. (2006). Grounded theory, feminist theory, critical theory: Toward theoretical triangulation. *Advances in Nursing Science, 26*(1), 30–43.

MacPherson, K. I. (1983). Feminist methods: A new paradigm for nursing research. *Advances in Nursing Science, 5*(2), 17–25.

Malka, S. G. (2007). *Daring to care: American nursing and second wave feminism.* Urbana and Chicago: University of Illinois Press.

Martin, D. E. (2006). *Aboriginal nursing students' experiences in two Canadian schools of nursing: A critical ethnography.* Unpublished Ph.D. dissertation. Vancouver: University of British Columbia.

Mason, D. J., Leavitt, J. K., & Chaffee, M. W. (2002). *Policy and politics in nursing and health care.* St. Louis, MO: Elsevier.

Meadus, R. J., & Tworney, C. (2007). Men in nursing: Making the right choice. *Canadian Nurse, 103*(2), 13–16.

Morse, G. G. (2000). Reframing women's health in nursing education: A feminist approach. *Nursing Outlook, 42*, 273–277.

Norris, C. M., & King, K. (2009). A qualitative examination of the factors that influence women's quality of life as they live with coronary artery disease. *Western Journal of Nursing Research, 4*, 513–524.

O'Lynn, C., & Tranbarger, R. (2006). *Men in nursing: History, challenges and opportunities.* New York: Springer.

Pohl, J. M., & Boyd, C. J. (1993). Ageism and feminism. *Image: Journal of Nursing Scholarship, 25*(3), 199–203.

Roberts, S. J. (1983). Oppressed group behaviour: Implications for nursing. *Advances in Nursing Science, 5*(4), 21–30.

Sohier, R. (1992). Feminism and nursing knowledge: The power of the weak. *Nursing Outlook, 40*(2), 62–66, 93.

Statistics Canada. (1994). *Registered nurses management data.* Ottawa: Author, Health Statistics Division.

Taylor, D., & Woods, N. (2001). What we know and how we know it: Contributions from nursing to women's health research and scholarship. *Annual Review of Nursing Research, 19*, 3–28.

Villeneuve, M. J. (2002–3). Healthcare, race and diversity: Time to act. *Hospital Quarterly, 6*(2), 67–73.

Wuest, J. (2006). Towards understanding women's health through a social determinants lens. *Canadian Journal of Nursing Research, 38*(1), 3–5.

NURSING KNOWLEDGE

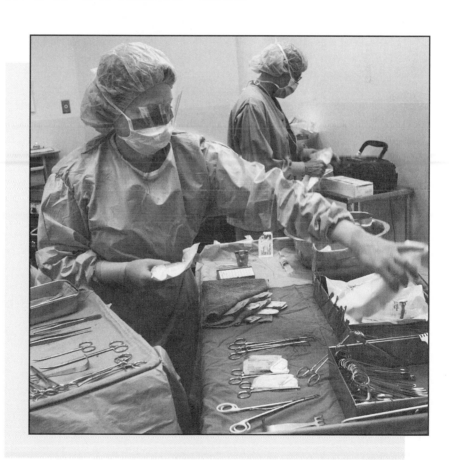

6

Theoretical Issues in Nursing

Sally Thorne

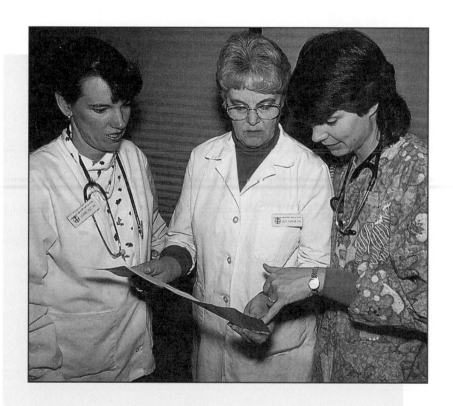

LEARNING OBJECTIVES

- To recognize social and historical conditions that contributed to the nursing profession as we now know it.
- To appreciate the characteristics of nursing that make it so difficult to define.
- To understand the role of conceptual models within the historical context of nursing knowledge development.
- To recognize the scientific context within which theorizing was understood to serve the interests of the advancing nursing profession.
- To understand the historical tradition of systematic thinking in nursing.
- To appreciate the contribution that theorizing made to an understanding of the complexity inherent in excellent clinical reasoning within nursing.
- To interpret the role of early theorizing on the expanded roles and conceptualizations into which it evolved.
- To recognize basic commonalities and variations among and between theoretical models for nursing.
- To understand the resistance of practising nurses to widespread implementation of formal theoretical models.
- To identify recent health care trends that are influencing the emergence of new forms of theoretical activity to serve the needs of the discipline.
- To interpret the implications of current theoretical debates within nursing.
- To appreciate the role of nursing theorizing in setting the stage for modern approaches to philosophical and scientific thinking in nursing.

The central paradox of nursing is that it is a professional-practice discipline at once so mundane that some of its technical aspects can be performed by almost anyone yet so cognitively sophisticated and mysterious that its excellent application requires advanced education, extensive reflective clinical practice, and an ongoing commitment to inquiry. In this context, nursing theory can be understood as a conceptual mechanism by which nursing scholars attempted to define the essence of the discipline, to place its practices within an intellectual context, and to explain what it is that we mean by our standards of excellence.

THE CONTEXT OF EARLY NURSING THEORIZING

Although the idea that nursing might represent a particular form of practice excellence has been documented throughout recorded history (Yura & Walsh, 1983), Florence Nightingale (1946/1859) is often cited as the person who formalized the knowledge and practice of nursing into a professional context, popularizing nursing for the modern era. As one of the discipline's early theorists, she rejected the traditional social role available to aristocratic women in Victorian times by mobilizing nurses to care for British soldiers injured in the Crimean War and, subsequently, by creating systems for the education of nurses and the delivery of nursing care. This was a time of considerable change within both society and science, bringing improved sanitation systems and systematic recording of clinical and public health data (de Graaf, Mossman, & Slebodnick, 1986). Recognizing that the epidemiological patterns of sickness and disease pointed to the need for public as well as individual health principles, Nightingale was an active participant in a massive reform of the health care delivery system, shifting the primary location of nursing from the private home to the hospital setting (Casteldine, 2007).

Over the following century, professional nursing evolved, its fortunes shifting with the sands of social change. During periods between the various feminist movements, for example, nursing work was rendered invisible (as was all of women's work), and nurses' formal authority within health care decision making was eroded. In contrast, during wartime, the social status of nurses tended to be elevated and their contributions to key processes and decisions highly regarded. In the Nightingale tradition, many nurse leaders resisted and challenged the systems in which they operated, while others worked more quietly, using any available means, to develop and expand nursing knowledge and practice for the benefit of patients and society (Libster, 2008). This quiet commitment to professional service by the larger community of nurses, catalyzed from time to time by public challenges of the occasional assertive and proactive leader, characterized the discipline until the conclusion of World War II.

When major advances in science and technology developed for wartime purposes were redirected within society at large, health care and nursing were among the primary beneficiaries. The explosion of knowledge within all the health sciences during the 1950s and 1960s created a climate in which nursing leaders were motivated to theorize and conceptualize the scientific basis of their practice and to distinguish the structure of nursing's knowledge from that of the more traditionally dominant health disciplines. In this context, it became increasingly important to conceptualize nursing and nursing science as having a character and nature all their own and not simply as applications of the knowledge generated by other disciplines. Nursing theory became the mechanism by which the discipline attempted to organize and understand the infinitely complex and dynamic body of knowledge, both borrowed and unique to nursing, that would be required for accountable, defensible, and excellent clinical practice (Beckstrand, 1978).

DEFINITIONS OF NURSING

As illness care became more complex and diverse, nursing roles more technologically and organizationally sophisticated, and physicians more politically powerful in shaping the organization and structure of health-service delivery, nurse leaders became increasingly aware of the need for common conceptual definitions to articulate the nature of their discipline (Chinn & Kramer, 1999; Newman, 1972). Among those most active in this theoretical explosion were nurse educators, who reasoned that the traditional apprenticeship model, augmented by occasional lectures by physicians, was insufficient and inappropriate to prepare a new generation of professional nurses capable of holding their own in the changing times. To justify the major curriculum changes they envisioned, they engaged in inspired theorizing about the distinct nature of nursing knowledge so as to articulate the unique aspects of nursing practice and the knowledge required to enact them (Orem & Parker, 1964; Torres, 1974).

These early definitional theories took the form of "theoretical frameworks" to organize the concepts that were central to nursing practice and around which nursing school curricula might be built. The conceptual frameworks organized the informational and decisional processes that would not only identify the core categories of nursing knowledge but also structure its application into the context of individual practice (Ellis, 1968; Johnson, 1974a; McKay, 1969; Wald & Leonard, 1964). The usual term by which these frameworks were known was "nursing theory," which made sense at the time because more sophisticated ways of conceptualizing knowledge and its workings were not yet available, especially within the scientific community. By calling their conceptual frameworks "nursing theories," early scholars simultaneously created a context in which nursing knowledge could be advanced and a language that legitimized nursing within the scientific community (Cull-Wilby & Peppin, 1987; Jones, 1997). However, because these nursing theories were not amenable to traditional proofs and did not articulate causal relationships in the manner of more traditional scientific theories, they also inadvertently created an uncomfortable situation within mainstream nursing practice in which the relevance of nursing theories was never well understood or accepted (Levine, 1995).

EARLY THEORETICAL CHALLENGES

For many nurses, the fundamental clinical decision-making structure upon which all nursing theory was built was the "nursing process" first articulated by Orlando in 1961 (Yura & Walsh, 1983). This systematic process of assessing, planning, intervening, and evaluating the impact of that intervention created a theoretical structure within which the knowledge available to nurses could be applied in an infinite variety of individual contexts (Field, 1987). Intended as a dynamic and iterative process, but amenable to systematic thinking and sufficient rigour for testing, the nursing process became the essential problem-solving approach by which nurses applied general knowledge into specific clinical situations (Carnevali & Thomas, 1993; Henderson, 1966; Torres, 1986).

In the late 1960s and into the 1970s, the conceptual framework builders, now referred to as "the nursing theorists," began to publish their models for how various forms of knowledge (both "borrowed" and unique) could be applied to practice using the nursing process. Nursing leaders were often impressed with the way in which expert nurses could systematically attend to and organize complex bodies of knowledge so as to appreciate the unique nature of an individual patient's situation and determine appropriate strategies by which the nurse might effectively and appropriately act to restore health and ameliorate or prevent disease (Orem & Parker, 1964; Barnum, 1994; Meleis, 2007). In developing conceptual models, they were attempting to capture the complexity of excellent nursing reasoning by shifting away from the more simplistic linear, logical, cause-and-effect reasoning processes that were easier to explain, and toward intellectual processes that were much more difficult to articulate (Benner, Tanner, & Chesla, 1996). Their idea was that, if neophyte nurses could have educational and practical experiences in which these expert analytic processes were systematically encouraged, they might be able to develop the capacity for such reasoning much more efficiently and rapidly than their predecessors, who were forced to learn it through reflection, trial, and error (Raudonis & Acton, 1997).

Each of these early conceptual frameworks attempted to depict the theoretical structures by which a nurse could fully grasp all the things that might happen in any clinical situation and to appreciate the larger implications of the available nursing care decisions. Thus, a major focus of their theorizing was to create a conceptual model of the person that would allow nurses to ask appropriate questions in order to develop the most comprehensive understanding possible about each patient encountered. According to the way in which it conceptualized the person for the purpose of nursing, each model called for nurses to assess each unique case to make sense of the patient's biological, social, and psychological situation in relation to any particular health or illness experience, to sort and organize that data, and to interpret the major issues of concern at that point (Barnum, 1994). On the basis of analyzing and interpreting this information, nurses arrived at a conclusion or "nursing diagnosis" as to the appropriate focus of attention in that particular clinical situation (Durand & Prince, 1966). They would then use the individualized data obtained about that particular patient to plan care, attending to interrelationships among and between the various forms of data that had been gathered. When that plan was enacted, the framework provided a similarly systematic structure within which to evaluate the impact of each intervention, including not only its intended effect but also any unintended or coincident effect upon the whole person. Thus, the conceptual frameworks created an analytic structure to enact the systematic reasoning of the nursing process.

Because it was a logical and useful way to describe basic problem solving and to guide nursing decisions about any particular patient's situation (Henderson, 1982), the nursing process initially received wide acceptance among nurse educators and practitioners. Although some interpreted it as a strictly linear process (Varcoe, 1996), most practising nurses quickly adapted the nursing process to denote a continuous cycling of relevant clinical information through the phases of the process according to the variations of the context (Meleis, 2007). Although rigid adherence to "the nursing process" or to specific conceptual models is no longer popular in the current era, the basic idea of a systematic problem-solving approach to gathering and using knowledge and accounting for an infinite range of variations within a generally recognized scope of practice is as relevant now as it was in Orlando's day. More recently, nursing theoretical literature tends to rely on terms like "clinical judgement," "critical thinking," and multiple "ways of knowing" to reflect the complex intellectual and conceptual processes that excellent clinical decision making in nursing entails (Alfaro-LeFevre, 1995). However, the theoretical origins of each of these ways of understanding nursing reasoning owe a tremendous debt to those early theorists.

THE METAPARADIGM CONCEPTS IN NURSING THEORY

As has been noted, each of the model builders of the nursing theory era attempted to create a conceptual structure for the person that represented the primary focus of nursing's attention. In addition, each attended to three further definitional aspects of the unique role of the nurse by attempting to depict the additional concepts of nursing, health, and environment. In time, these four concepts came to be recognized as essential building blocks for any theoretical representation of nursing and became known as nursing's "metaparadigm concepts" (Fawcett, 1984) (See Table 6.1).

Because it was clearly recognized that nursing's expanding role extended beyond those who were hospitalized, many of the early conceptual frameworks began to refer to the person who was the focus of nursing care as nursing's "client," rather than the traditional "patient." This term was intended to signify a range of health states, including both sick and well, and a less patriarchal relationship between the care and the individual toward whom it was directed. Concurrently, nursing was increasingly aware of its potential to deliver care beyond the individual level—to families, groups, and even communities. Although this expanded client focus led to significant theoretical developments in the role of nursing families and communities, most of the early conceptual models continued to focus attention on the individual person as the primary client of nursing.

To help nurses systematically gather, organize, and interpret the vast body of information that might be relevant to any individual client, the early models explicitly included conceptual definitions of that person. Some understood the person as a system comprising interacting parts (Auger, 1976; McKay, 1969; Putt, 1978). Some saw the person as an entity composed of competing basic human needs or drives (Henderson, 1966). And others more generally recognized that human experience had biological, psychological, social, and spiritual dimensions (Fuller, 1978). Despite these apparent differences, each framework focused nursing's attention toward interactions among multiple aspects of the human person so that each health and illness experience could be understood for its uniqueness. In their different ways, each of these models attempted to provide the nurse with a holistic appreciation of the individual so that the implications of any possible supportive action or intervention could be understood as completely as possible and care decisions individually tailored (Hawley, Young, & Pasco, 2000).

TABLE 6.1	Nursing's Metaparadigm Concepts	
	CONCEPT	DEFINITION
1.	Person	The individual, family, group, or community that is the recipient of nursing care.
2.	Environment	The social environment (client's family, friends, significant others) and the physical environment (surroundings).
3.	Health	The client's state of wellness/illness.
4.	Nursing	The actions taken by the nurse on behalf of (or in conjunction with) the client.

Source: Fawcett, J. (1984) The metaparadigm of nursing: Present status and future refinements. *Image, 16*(3), 84–87.

The conceptual frameworks also reflected an understanding that each person is intricately embedded within a complex familial, social, geographical, and political environmental system. Although many of the early theorists encountered difficulty articulating this conceptual aspect of the nursing role, each attempted to orient the nurse to an appreciation of the larger world within which every health and illness experience takes place. Thus, these early conceptual frameworks included an envisioned future in which nursing was enacted at the level of social and health policy, in population health promotion, and in community development (Thorne, Canam, Dahinten, Hall, Henderson, & Kirkham, 1998). Although many of these ideas seem embryonic as they are depicted in these early models, the inclusion of environment as a fundamental metaparadigm concept for nursing created the platform upon which to build the socially relevant thought characteristic of modern nursing scholarship.

Because nursing always recognized a moral and ethical component to its social mandate, the model builders all struggled to conceptualize that which nursing was directed toward. They all recognized that an appropriate conceptualization of health had to extend beyond a mere absence of disease so that it could inspire nurses to work toward some kind of ideal state both for individuals and for the societies in which they lived (Ballou, 2000). These ideal states were distinguished from more concrete notions of bodily health through such terms as "optimal health," "high-level wellness," or "total well-being," and included social, emotional, and even spiritual dimensions of the quality of life. These creative ways of conceptualizing health allowed the model builders to define nursing in such a manner that it had application for all clients, sick or well, and created a visionary objective to guide the evolving roles and functions that nursing took on during this era.

Reflecting these subtle distinctions in conceptualizing the person, the environment, and health, each model articulated a unique definition of nursing as a professional ideal within a social context. Because each conceptual framework drew from distinct bodies of borrowed knowledge, used language differently, and articulated relationships between these metaparadigm concepts in a unique manner, each of the models came to be understood as a distinct coherent belief system about nursing and its practice. (See Table 6.2.)

AN ERA OF MODEL BUILDING

During the era of model proliferation, several different species of models began to emerge, signalling the efforts of various nursing theorists to locate the problems of nursing within a larger context (see Table 6.3). Several of the earliest models had tried to conceptualize nursing as an interaction between a patient and a nurse, each engaged with the other in a complex human relationship in pursuit of a valued objective (e.g., Orlando, 1961; Peplau, 1952; Travelbee, 1966). Others depicted the client of nursing as an entity driven by efforts to satisfy basic human needs, and positioned nursing care as a particular response to those needs (e.g., Henderson, 1966; Orem, 1985). Following on the early leadership of Dorothy Johnson (1974b), other model builders explicitly worked with General Systems Theory (von Bertalanffy, 1968) to create models in which

TABLE 6.2	The Nursing Metaparadigm in Selected Conceptual Models			
MODEL	PERSON	ENVIRONMENT	HEALTH	NURSING
Nightingale, 1859	An individual with self-recuperative powers	External conditions (e.g., air, warmth, light, odours, diet) that affect life	Absence of disease; ability to realize one's potential, including healing	A profession distinct from medicine that uses nature's laws to optimize conditions for healthy living
Henderson, 1966	A unique individual with 14 basic needs	Not specified	Achievement of the person's desired level of independence	A helping profession working with or on behalf of the person to assist health, recovery, or a peaceful death
Parse, 1981	An individual or family in constant interchange with the environment, having free choice within health situations	A constantly changing universe with which the person coexists and which is an integral part of being	A unique, continuously changing process of becoming	An art/science focusing on the person's living unity and achievement of wellness through system stability
Neuman, 1982	A dynamic "open system" with 5 interacting variables: physiological, psychological, socio-cultural, developmental, and spiritual	Includes internal and external components (e.g., economic/educational status, family, lifestyle, coping patterns)	System stability	A unique profession working on the total person or system to promote system stability
Campbell, 1987	An individual using a range of coping behaviours to satisfy 9 basic needs	Anything lying outside the system's boundaries	Highest perceived level of system stability achievable	A nurturing profession that supports the person during critical periods in the life cycle so that coping behaviours may be developed and needs may be met

all aspects of the human person were understood to be in constant interaction, both with each other and with the environment around them (e.g., Neuman, 1982; Roy, 1976). In these instances, the role of the nurse was to be conscious of the implications of any action or interaction upon all other aspects of the human system. Finally, a fourth major type of model emerged, which distinguished itself from the other types in attempting to depict an irreducible abstract conceptualization of "unitary human beings" inherently holographically connected with a universal environment (e.g., Parse, 1981; Rogers, 1970; Watson, 1979). Proponents of this later group of theories referred to them as

TABLE 6.3	Theoretical Underpinnings of Major Conceptual Models
THEORETICAL ORIENTATION	**NURSING MODEL**
Practice-Based	Nightingale's Notes on Nursing
	McGill Nursing Model
	Hall's Core, Care and Cure Model
Basic Human Needs	Henderson's Principles & Practice of Nursing
	Orem's Self Care Deficit Theory
	Abdellah's Patient-Centred Care
Interaction	Peplau's Interpersonal Relations Model
	Orlando's Dynamic Nurse–Patient Relationship
	Travelbee's Human-to-Human Relationship Model
	Adam's *To Be a Nurse*
General Systems Theory	Johnson's Behavioural Systems Model
	UBC Model for Nursing
	Neuman's Systems Model
	Roy's Adaptation Model
	King's Open Systems Model
	Levine's Conservation Model
Simultaneity	Rogers's Science of Unitary Human Beings
	Parse's Human Becoming School of Thought
	Paterson & Dzerad's Humanistic Nursing Theory
	Watson's Caring Theory
	Newman's Health as Expanding Consciousness

"simultaneity theories" and began to refer to all other theories as representing a "totality" paradigm (Newman, 1992; Parse, 1987). The presence or absence of fundamental distinctions between these simultaneity/totality paradigm groupings continues to be one of the most contentious and fascinating debates in nursing theory.

Although much of the scholarly activity that has come to be known as "nursing theory" represented the work of individual theorists from the United States, Canadian nurse scholars of the time were also actively involved in theory building. Working from lecture notes from the early classes of Dorothy Johnson, a team at the University of British Columbia led by Margaret Campbell developed a systems model known as the UBC Model for Nursing (Campbell, 1987; Campbell, Cruise, & Murakami, 1976). (See Box 6.1.) This model was developed and widely applied, particularly within Western Canada, for a period lasting two decades (Thorne, Jillings, Ellis, & Perry, 1993). Margaret Campbell was also a member of a group of six Canadian nursing leaders who were actively involved in the development of another distinct nursing model that was commissioned by the Canadian Nurses Association (CNA) to guide the conceptualization of its testing service. The CNATS Model, as it came to be known, organized substantive knowledge for national licensure exams and therefore became a popular theoretical structure for nursing curricula across the country (Canadian Nurses Association Testing Service, 1981).

Basing her conceptualizations on the pioneering work of Virginia Henderson, Evelyn Adam of the Université de Montréal (1979, 1980) considered nursing as a helping

BOX 6.1 Margaret Campbell and the UBC Model Committee

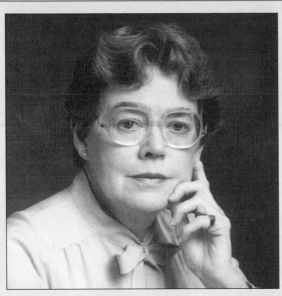

Margaret Campbell.

Dr. Margaret Campbell (1923–1992) was a major figure in Canadian nursing theorizing. Among the earliest group of Canadian nurses to obtain a doctoral degree at Teachers College, Columbia University (1970), she returned to the faculty at the University of British Columbia during a time of great enthusiasm for theoretical developments in the discipline. Chairing a faculty committee that included an exceptional group of academic nurse leaders (Janet Gormick, Helen Shore, Rose Murakami, and Mary Cruise), Campbell developed Canada's first nursing model, based on ideas about basic human needs gleaned from Virginia Henderson's writings, as well as lecture notes on behavioural systems that had been taken by Cruise and Gormick during their time in Dorothy Johnson's theory class at UCLA. The committee further developed the first nursing curriculum based entirely on a theoretical framework for nursing. In their 1994 history of the school, Zilm and Warbinek note that an entire 1976 issue of Nursing Papers (forerunner of the *Canadian Journal of Nursing Research*) was devoted to articles about the UBC Model and its implementation. In addition to explaining its influence on nursing curriculum, these articles included descriptions of a companion framework on loss, study modules, tools for clinical evaluation, and research into student satisfaction with the new program—all innovations considerably in advance of their time.

process, in which the nurse complemented a patient's strength, knowledge, and will. Her model, published in both French and English, achieved wide recognition (Creekmur, DeFelice, Hodel, & Petty, 1986). Finally, another university faculty group, this time from McGill University, worked collaboratively to develop a model for nursing that derived not from borrowed theories but from an in-depth analysis of nursing practice knowledge (Gottleib & Rowat, 1987). The McGill Model (see Box 6.2) conceptualized nursing as health promotion, primarily at the family level. Although the Canadian models were used across Canada, they tended not to be widely popularized beyond Canada's borders. To some extent, this may be a product of their generally being collaborative achievements, rather than the property of an individual theorist, by whose

BOX 6.2   Moyra Allen and the McGill Model

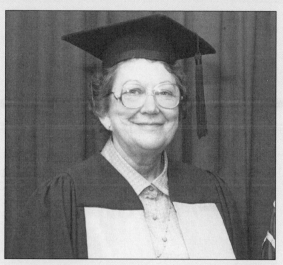

Moyra Allen's groundbreaking McGill Model inspired The Health Workshop, a community health facility managed by nurses and committed to long-term family health.

Dr. Moyra Allen (1921–1998) is widely considered to be one of the architects of modern Canadian nursing. An eminent scholar, she was among the first group of nurses in the country to earn a doctoral degree. She became a prominent nursing researcher and was one of only two nurse recipients of the prestigious scientist award of the National Health Research and Development Program over a 35-year period. Dr. Allen was respected as a creative and independent thinker who embraced challenge in the cause of furthering the nursing profession. For example, she lobbied hard early in her career for collective bargaining rights for nurses and had the distinction of being elected the founding president of the United Nurses of Montreal.

A graduate of the Montreal General Hospital School of Nursing, Dr. Allen earned a bachelor of nursing degree from McGill University, a Master of Arts degree from the University of Chicago, and a doctor of philosophy degree from Stanford University. She was a founding member of the Accreditation Committee of the Canadian Association of University Schools of Nursing, which developed the criteria for accreditation of schools of nursing. Allen served the World Health Organization, designing a model for evaluation of schools of nursing and carrying out evaluations in South America, India, and Ghana. She was appointed to the faculty of the School of Nursing at McGill in 1954 and was named professor emeritus in 1985 upon her retirement from the university.

In demonstrating her model of nursing, now known as the McGill Model, Dr. Allen established The Health Workshop, a community health facility where she put into practice a developmental concept of health and nursing as a prototype of primary health care. Supported by the McGill University School of Nursing and the National Health Research and Development Program, The Health Workshop opened in 1977. The facility, viewed as complementary to existing services, was staffed by nurses, a community development officer, and a health librarian. It was located in a modestly affluent suburban community where physicians and other health care providers were in abundant supply. The purpose of the project was to demonstrate the validity of a local health resource managed by nurses that was directed toward long-term family health. As such, it was an innovative strategy to provide the resources that families require to gain competence in coping with the situations of daily living, including illness and disease, and thereby improve their health status.

As the founder of *Nursing Papers*, renamed the *Canadian Journal of Nursing Research*, Dr. Allen enhanced and facilitated the quality of nursing research in Canada. In view of her important contributions

BOX 6.2	Moyra Allen and the McGill Model—cont'd

to nursing research and scholarship in Canada, the CNA honoured her with its highest award, the Jeanne Mance Medal. The Order of Nurses of the Province of Quebec conferred upon her the Order of Merit, and the Canadian Association of University Schools of Nursing awarded her the Ethel Johns Award. In 1987, the Governor General of Canada invested her as a member of the Order of Canada, the highest honour the country can bestow upon its citizens who have made outstanding contributions in their lives.

name the theory was generally known, and who typically took responsibility for leading the promotional efforts. Thus, Canadian models emerged for similar purposes to those in the United States, but tended to follow a different trajectory in their evolution as practice resources. Interestingly, beyond the borders of Canada and the United States, there is very little evidence of formal models or model building ever taking hold within nursing scholarship.

THE MODEL DEBATES

From the late 1960s through the mid-1980s, at least 20 distinct theoretical models for nursing were published. Some of the earliest were articulated in the form of general systems of belief about nursing, but a particular structure and style, developed by Dorothy Johnson (1974a) at the University of California, San Francisco, came to represent nursing's standards for what a conceptual model ought to look like. Because it was assumed that each model represented a distinct and coherent orientation to nursing, and that the profession would be disadvantaged by undue theoretical division, many leaders of the model-building era assumed that one model would eventually surpass its competitors and become the dominant (if not the exclusive) conceptual framework for nursing (Choi, 1986). To gain prominence over others, proponents of the different models developed clinical practice resources, curricular applications, and research programs intended to test the application of each of these models in both nursing practice and educational contexts. Communities of theorists and scholars aligned themselves with one nursing theory or another, and the theoretical development climate took on an atmosphere of rather intense competition and marketing.

While some nurse scholars were invested in advocating for the increasingly widespread application of certain conceptual models, others began to notice the rather rigid and codified thinking that some application strategies entailed. Within many of the application initiatives, the efforts drifted off course from inspiring systematic thinking within nursing practice toward such concrete manifestations as using language in prescribed ways or filling out assessment forms according to fixed categorizations. Predictably, many of the nurses caught up in this implementation frenzy found that such rigid application of frameworks inhibited rather than supported their systematic and critical thinking, and considerable debate appeared within the nursing literature as to the relevance of the model-building enterprise and the usefulness of conceptual frameworks as the theoretical foundation for nursing (Holden, 1990; Engebretson, 1997). Thus, in this contentious and often heated context, many nurses developed an understandable distaste for what they understood "nursing theory" to represent.

REFLECTIVE THINKING

1. What might motivate a nursing theorist to advance a particular framework as inherently preferable to all others?
2. What theoretical problems within nursing may be resolved in the foreseeable future, and which ones are likely to remain permanently in a state of uncertainty?

THE CHANGING THEORETICAL CLIMATE

During the period in which the various models were being developed and published, other significant trends influenced the discipline's understanding of its theoretical foundations. Although the model movement represented an attempt to conceptualize, theorize, and philosophize about the nature of nursing, it was not always apparent to nurses what relevance such theorizing might have for the practical business of planning, intervening, and evaluating nursing care. In a process distinct from model building, and in response to the terminological variations and theoretical disputes that the world of nursing theory seemed to epitomize, another group of nursing leaders in the early 1970s began to recognize the importance of a precise language to categorize and taxonomize nursing diagnoses (Warren & Hoskins, 1990). Following a series of consensus conferences, the North American Nursing Diagnoses Association (NANDA) was formed, and the process of generating a fixed list of potential diagnoses for which nursing care might be indicated was launched. As several authors have noted (Fitzpatrick, 1990; Roy, 1982), the motive underlying this initiative was to standardize nursing care across settings and contexts, which represented a diametrically opposite conceptualization from the infinite individualization that the model builders were striving to support. With the advent of computerized databases within health care systems, the expediency of fixed categories of clinical decisions became apparent, and many organizations looked to the NANDA taxonomy of nursing diagnoses as a way of standardizing nursing service allocations (Warren & Hoskins, 1990). Thus, the information-technology revolution began to privilege ways of thinking about nursing that were amenable to coding and computation.

Another feature of the changing intellectual climate over the last two decades of the twentieth century was the general trend within society and the sciences away from logical positivism as a strategy for advancing epistemological claims and toward postmodernist thinking, in which multiple forms of knowledge may be equally credible. When the modern era of nursing theorizing began several decades ago, there was a general consensus among scholars that theories ought to take the form of logical propositions that could be rigorously tested and proven to answer or not answer the questions of a discipline. T.S. Kuhn's work, originally published in 1962 but achieving increasing levels of popular appeal through the 1980s, created a language for conceptualizing scientific knowledge that illuminated many more options than those to which the early nursing theorists had access (Kuhn, 1962). Kuhn's reframing of scientific advancement discounted the traditional idea that science operated according to an evolutionary series of discoveries that emerged in an orderly progression, one upon the next. Instead, using examples from the history of science in many fields, he argued that major developments in science were characterized by ways of thinking about problems that were so radically different from the traditional taken-for-granted knowledge that they constituted an entirely distinct world view, or paradigm. From this perspective, scientists within a discipline could be characterized as either "old paradigm," whose efforts perpetuated the models that were entrenched within the discipline's history, or "revolutionary," having escaped the trap of traditional thinking to approach the discipline's problems using an entirely distinct paradigmatic world view. As this model of thinking about science filtered into nursing scholarship, it convinced some nurses that the nursing models and theoretical frameworks were not simply alternative conceptualizations of nursing's metaparadigm concepts, but in fact represented entirely distinct paradigms for approaching the complexities inherent in a science of nursing (Fry, 1995). Further, the fundamental understanding of what nursing knowledge might entail shifted dramatically from a shared belief that there were common truths that nurses ought to know toward recognition of multiple coexisting and competing realities within which no singular form of knowledge ought to claim authority.

These trends in thinking have more recently bumped up against a new trend in health care toward evidence-informed practice, privileging that which can be measured against that which is known by other means. The tension between a conventional definition of "evidence" and the essential structure of excellent nursing reasoning has become a more recent hot debate within the discipline (French, 2002; Romyn et al., 2003; Rycroft-Malone et al., 2004).

🔍 CANADIAN RESEARCH FOCUS

Romyn, D.M., Allen, M.N., Boschma, G., Duncan, S.M., Edgecombe, N., Jensen, L.A., Ross-Kerr, J.C., Marck, P., Salsali, M., Tourangeau, A.E., & Warnock, F. (2003). The notion of evidence in evidence-based practice by the nursing philosophy working group. *Journal of Professional Nursing, 19*(4), 184–188.

Canadian nurses have often taken an important lead in asking penetrating questions about the nature of nursing knowledge and the manner in which the profession can advance its public-service objectives through philosophical interpretation of current trends. In this 2003 example, a group of seasoned and early-career-stage Canadian scholars gathered to think through issues associated with the nature and proper ends of nursing within the current evidence-informed health care context. A distinctive feature of Canadian nursing theorizing and philosophizing has been its capacity to attend to a diversity of world views as fundamental to an understanding of what nursing ought to strive toward, rather than advancing the position that any one view ought to prevail. It is interesting to think about whether there may be something in the underlying structure of Canadian society that explains why Canadian nurses have been at the forefront of shaping the philosophical thinking of the discipline internationally.

NURSING'S ONGOING PARADIGM DISPUTES

As scientists across disciplines struggled with the implications of these new ways of philosophizing about science, nurses began to engage in new forms of scholarship that were more explicitly philosophical than conventionally theoretical. They began to conceptualize nursing not only as a science, but also as an art and a practice (Sarter, 1990; Johnson, 1991; Rodgers, 1991). Among many nurse scholars, the conceptual models came to represent an embarrassing aspect of nursing's history, representing little relevance for the fundamental problems facing the discipline (Engebretson, 1997). However, as many nursing leaders clearly recognized, the original challenges had not been resolved. Nurses still needed to learn how to organize and make sense of all the possible bodies of knowledge that might help them respond intelligently to the unique context of any individual clinical encounter and to develop systematic mechanisms for interpreting the concepts of concern to the discipline (Thorne, 2005).

In this context, a general agreement emerged that the traditional expectation that nurses ought to adopt a single nursing model had become indefensible, and nurses instead began to focus their attention on articulating debates between groups of models. By categorizing the nursing models originally derived from theories of basic human needs, human development, and general system theory as reductionistic and anti-holistic, one group of theorists began to advocate acceptance of what they conceptualized as the alternative paradigmatic position—simultaneity theory. Advocates of the simultaneity paradigm positioned their theories as philosophically sophisticated and modern alternatives to the traditional forms of thought characteristic of models they depict as deriving from a totality paradigm (Nagle & Mitchell, 1991; Newman, 1992; Cody, 1995; Parse, 1987).

By framing these debates as a basic philosophical difference between simultaneity and totality, reductionistic thinking and holism, modernism and postmodernism, some theorists constructed a climate that discounted all but adherents of simultaneity models as legitimate contributors to the science of nursing (Nagle & Mitchell, 1991; Cody, 1996). Identifiable through such linguistic cues to their theoretical allegiance as "unitary-transformative" (as compared to "particulate-deterministic") (Newman, Sime, & Corcoran-Perry, 1991), "human science" (Mitchell & Cody, 1992), and "human becoming" (Cody, 1995; Parse, 1992), some of these authors attributed a range of negative characteristics to what they referred to as totality theories, including a desire to control variables, to reduce holistic contexts into fragmented pieces of information, and to impose objectively derived expert solutions on subjectively experienced human problems (Edwards, 2000). Drawing on Kuhn's notion that traditional world views of a science can create a theoretical blindness among adherents until such time as they make the dramatic shift to a new paradigm, they set up a logic whereby theoretical challenges could be dismissed on principle without serious consideration (Cody, 2000; Parse, 1998). As a result of this division within thinking, exacerbated by popular ideas about how science evolves, discourse across the paradigm divide deteriorated to such a degree that it became extremely difficult to conduct a thoughtful theoretical debate within the discipline (Thorne, Henderson, McPherson, & Pesut, 2004; Thorne, Reimer Kirkham, & Henderson, 1999).

FORGING NEW THEORETICAL DIRECTIONS

The theoretical work that has characterized recent decades in nursing is the conceptual foundation for the scientific and philosophical work that challenges the discipline today. Although some nurse scholars have tried to discredit the model-building era of nursing theory as an irrelevant intellectual exercise, others who revisit the same fundamental questions that those early nurse theorists first sought to answer actually find a great deal of theoretical sophistication in those early attempts. In an era prior to such ideas as "complexity science" and postmodern thinking, the early theorists were trying to capture and guide the intricate reasoning processes with which general substantive knowledge about such things as disease, bodies, culture, and societies could be transformed into a comprehensive, individualized plan for each client in need of nursing care. Excellent clinical reasoning remains our common goal, and the problem of understanding how nurses can be guided toward such complex intellectual processes is far from resolved, especially in the context of an increasing emphasis on interdisciplinarity in both education and practice (Sullivan-Marx, 2006). We still have much to gain from reflecting on the basic values and guiding principles that shape our conception of nursing (Meleis, 2007).

Although much of the nursing theorizing that has occurred over the past several decades has confused rather than clarified our thinking (Kikuchi, 1999), nursing scholars are increasingly embracing philosophical inquiry in addition to scientific methods as strategies with which to strive toward disciplinary conceptual clarity (Silva, Sorrell, & Sorrell, 1995). For example, Liaschenko (1997) has oriented our theorizing toward three levels of abstraction—knowing the case, the client, and the person in any given clinical encounter. Watson (1990) has challenged us to consider nursing as a moral enterprise, and Yeo (1989) has examined nursing theory as an ethical reasoning process. Campbell and Bunting (1991) have encouraged theorists to apply critical social and feminist theories toward an emancipatory theory for nursing. In the following chapter, June Kikuchi, one of the foremost leaders in Canadian philosophical theorizing, will provide further examples of the range and scope of this intriguing work.

These newer species of philosophical theorizing all capitalize on the dialectic between knowledge and practice that has been termed "nursing praxis" (Reed, 1995; Clarke, James, & Kelly, 1996; Starzomski & Rodney, 1997). By focusing our philosophical lens on the practice of nursing at its best, and continuing to theorize about how it got to be that way, the new generation of nurse scholars will create philosophical structures within which we can integrate an infinite range of new knowledge and new ideas (Flaming, 2004).

Nursing philosophical theorizing will continue to explore the blend between bold new thinking and the everyday practices of excellent nurses. The complexities of nursing in all its infinite variations will continue to fascinate us, and the mysterious processes by which nurses organize, sort, and use knowledge will remain a focus of our thinking for a long time to come. Those of us who claim to know nursing intimately will always recognize it as a mysterious and complex intellectual, spiritual, and embodied phenomenon and certainly one most worthy of a few more generations of thoughtful contemplation.

CRITICAL THINKING QUESTIONS

1. How did nursing evolve from a relatively unappreciated activity within society toward attaining professional status?
2. What is the importance of defining nursing?
3. What attributes of nursing make a theoretical description of it so challenging?
4. What purpose does each of the four metaparadigm concepts play in shaping an understanding of nursing?
5. How have evolving notions of science shaped theoretical debates within nursing?

WEB SITES

Nursing Theory Page (University of San Diego): http://www.sandiego.edu/academics/nursing/theory/
The Collected Works of Florence Nightingale: http://www.sociology.uoguelph.ca/fnightingale/

REFERENCES

Adam, E. (1979). *Être infirmière.* Montreal: Editions HRW.

Adam, E. (1980). *To be a nurse.* Philadelphia: W.B. Saunders.

Alfaro-LeFevre, R. (1995). *Critical thinking in nursing: A practical approach.* Philadelphia: W.B. Saunders.

Auger, J. R. (1976). *Behavioral systems and nursing.* Englewood Cliffs, NJ: Prentice-Hall.

Ballou, K. A. (2000). A historical-philosophical analysis of the professional nurse obligation to participate in sociopolitical activities. *Policy, Politics & Nursing Practice, 1*(3), 172–184.

Barnum, B. J. S. (1994). *Nursing theory: Analysis, application, evaluation* (4th ed.). Philadelphia: J.B. Lippincott.

Beckstrand, J. (1978). The notion of a practice theory and the relationship of scientific and ethical knowledge to practice. *Research in Nursing & Health, 1,* 131–136.

Benner, P., Tanner, C. A., & Chesla, C. A. (1996). *Expertise in nursing practice: Caring, clinical judgment, and ethics.* New York: Springer.

Campbell, J. C., & Bunting, S. (1991). Voices and paradigms: Perspectives on critical and feminist theory in nursing. *Advances in Nursing Science, 13*(3), 1–15.

Campbell, M. A. (1987). *The UBC model for nursing: Directions for practice.* Vancouver: The University of British Columbia School of Nursing.

Campbell, M. A., Cruise, M. J., & Murakami, T. R. (1976). A model for nursing: University of British Columbia School of Nursing. *Nursing Papers, 8*(2), 5–9.

Canadian Nurses Association Testing Service. (1981). *A model for nursing.* Ottawa: Canadian Nurses Association.

Carnevali, D. L., & Thomas, M. D. (1993). *Diagnostic reasoning and treatment decision making in nursing.* Philadelphia: Lippincott.

Casteldine, G. (2007). Florence Nightingale, a force to be reckoned with: The BJN over 100 years ago. *British Journal of Nursing, 16*(9), 525.

Chinn, P. L., & Kramer, M. K. (1999). *Theory and nursing: Integrated knowledge development* (5th ed.). St. Louis, MO: Mosby.

Choi, E. C. (1986). Evolution of nursing theory development. In A. Marriner (Ed.), *Nursing theorists and their work* (pp. 51–61). St. Louis: Mosby.

Clarke, B., James, C., & Kelly, J. (1996). Reflective practice: Reviewing the issues and refocussing the debate. *International Journal of Nursing Studies, 33,* 171–180.

Cody, W. K. (1995). About all those paradigms: Many in the universe, two in nursing. *Nursing Science Quarterly, 8*(2), 144–147.

Cody, W. K. (1996). Occult reductionism in the discourse of nursing theory. *Nursing Science Quarterly, 9,* 140–142.

Cody, W. K. (2000). Paradigm shift or paradigm drift? A meditation on commitment and transcendence. *Nursing Science Quarterly, 13*(2), 93–102.

Creekmur, T., DeFelice, J., Hodel, A., & Petty, C. Y. (1986). Evelyn Adam: Conceptual model for nursing. In A. Marriner (Ed.), *Nursing theorists and their work* (pp. 131–143). St. Louis, MO: Mosby.

Cull-Wilby, B. L., & Peppin, J. C. (1987). Toward a coexistence of paradigms in nursing knowledge development. *Journal of Advanced Nursing, 12,* 515–521.

de Graaf, K. R., Mossman, C. L., & Slebodnick, M. (1986). Florence Nightingale: Modern nursing. In A. Marriner (Ed.), *Nursing theorists and their work* (pp. 65–79). St. Louis, MO: Mosby.

Durand, M., & Prince, R. (1966). Nursing diagnosis: Process and decision. *Nursing Forum, 4,* 50–64.

Edwards, S. D. (2000). Critical review of R.R. Parse's *The Human Becoming School of Thought*: A perspective for nurses and other health professionals. *Journal of Advanced Nursing, 31,* 190–196.

Ellis, R. (1968). Characteristics of significant theories. *Nursing Research, 17*(3), 217–222.

Engebretson, J. (1997). A multiparadigm approach to nursing. *Advances in Nursing Science, 20*(1), 21–33.

Fawcett, J. (1984). The metaparadigm of nursing: Present status and future refinements. *Image, 16*(3), 84–87.

Field, P. A. (1987). The impact of nursing theory on the clinical decision making process. *Journal of Advanced Nursing, 12,* 563–571.

Fitzpatrick, J. J. (1990). Conceptual basis for the organization and advancement of nursing knowledge: Nursing diagnosis/taxonomy. *Nursing Diagnosis, 1*(3), 102–106.

Flaming, D. (2004). Nursing theories as nursing ontologies. *Nursing Philosophy, 5*(3), 224–229.

French, P. (2002). What is the evidence on evidence-based nursing? An epistemological concern. *Journal of Advanced Nursing, 37*(3), 250–257.

Fry, S. T. (1995). Science as problem solving. In A. Omery, C. E. Kasper, & G. G. Page (Eds.), *In search of nursing science* (pp. 72–80). Thousand Oaks, CA: Sage.

Fuller, S. S. (1978). Holistic man and the science and practice of nursing. *American Journal of Nursing, 26,* 700–704.

Gottlieb, L. N., & Rowat, K. (1987). The McGill model of nursing: A practice based model. *Advances in Nursing Science, 9,* 51–61.

Hawley, P., Young, S., & Pasco, A. C. (2000). Reductionism in the pursuit of nursing science: (In)congruent with nursing's core values? *Canadian Journal of Nursing Research, 23*(2), 75–88.

Henderson, V. (1966). *The nature of nursing.* New York: Macmillan.

Henderson, V. (1982). The nursing process: Is the title right? *Journal of Advanced Nursing, 7,* 103–109.

Holden, R. J. (1990). Models, muddles and medicine. *International Journal of Nursing Studies, 27,* 223–234.

Johnson, D. E. (1974a). Development of theory: A requisite for nursing as a primary health profession. *Nursing Research, 23*(5), 372–377.

Johnson, D. E. (1974b). The behavioral system model for nursing. In J. P. Riehl, & C. Roy (Eds.), *Conceptual models for nursing practice.* New York: Appleton-Century-Crofts.

Johnson, J. L. (1991). Nursing science: Basic, applied, or practical? Implications for the art of nursing. *Advances in Nursing Science, 14*(1), 7–16.

Jones, M. (1997). Thinking nursing. In S. E. Thorne, & V. E. Hayes (Eds.), *Nursing praxis: Knowledge and action* (pp. 125–139). Thousand Oaks, CA: Sage.

Kikuchi, J. F. (1999). Clarifying the nature of conceptualizations about nursing. *Canadian Journal of Nursing Research, 30*(4), 115–128.

Kuhn, T. S. (1962). *The structure of scientific revolutions.* Chicago: University of Chicago Press.

Levine, M. E. (1995). The rhetoric of nursing theory. *Image: Journal of Nursing Scholarship, 27*(1), 11–14.

Liaschenko, J. (1997). Knowing the patient? In S. E. Thorne, & V. E. Hayes (Eds.), *Nursing praxis: Knowledge and action* (pp. 23–38). Thousand Oaks, CA: Sage.

Libster, M. M. (2008). Elements of care: Nursing environmental theory in historical context. *Holistic Nursing Practice, 22*(3), 160–170.

McKay, R. (1969). Theories, models, and systems for nursing. *Nursing Research, 18*(5), 393–399.

Meleis, A. I. (2007). *Theoretical nursing: Development and progress* (4th ed.). Philadelphia: Lippincott, Williams & Wilkins.

Mitchell, G. J., & Cody, W. K. (1992). Nursing knowledge and human science: Ontological and epistemological considerations. *Nursing Science Quarterly, 5,* 54–61.

Nagle, L. M., & Mitchell, G. J. (1991). Theoretic diversity: Evolving paradigmatic issues in research and practice. *Advances in Nursing Science, 14,* 17–25.

Neuman, B. M. (1982). *The Neuman systems model: Application to nursing education and practice.* Norwalk, CN: Appleton-Century-Crofts.

Newman, M. A. (1972). Nursing's theoretical evolution. *Nursing Outlook, 20*(7), 449–453.

Newman, M. A. (1992). Prevailing paradigms in nursing. *Nursing Outlook, 40*(1), 10–13, 32.

Newman, M., Sime, A., & Corcoran-Perry, S. (1991). The focus of the discipline of nursing. *Advances in Nursing Science, 12*(1), 1–6.

Nightingale, F. (1946/1859). *Notes on nursing: What it is and what it is not.* Philadelphia: Lippincott.

Orem, D. E. (1985). *Nursing: Concepts of practice* (3rd ed.). New York: McGraw Hill.

Orem, D. E., & Parker, K. S. (1964). *Nursing content in preservice nursing curriculums.* Washington, DC: Catholic University of America Press.

Orlando, I. J. (1961). *The dynamic nurse–patient relationship: Function, process, and principles.* New York: G.P. Putnam's Sons.

Parse, R. R. (1981). *Man-living-health: A theory of nursing.* New York: Wiley.

Parse, R. R. (1987). *Nursing science: Major paradigms, theories, and critiques.* Philadelphia: W.B. Saunders.

Parse, R. R. (1992). Human becoming: Parse's theory of nursing. *Nursing Science Quarterly, 5,* 35–42.

Parse, R. R. (1998). The art of criticism. *Nursing Science Quarterly, 11*(2), 43.

Peplau, H. E. (1952). *Interpersonal relations in nursing.* New York: G.P. Putnam's Sons.

Putt, A. M. (1978). *General systems theory applied to nursing.* Boston: Little, Brown.

Raudonis, B. M., & Acton, G. J. (1997). Theory-based nursing practice. *Journal of Advanced Nursing, 26*(2/1), 138–145.

Reed, P. G. (1995). A treatise on nursing knowledge development for the 21st century: Beyond postmodernism. *Advances in Nursing Science, 17*(3), 70–84.

Rodgers, B. L. (1991). Deconstructing the dogma in nursing knowledge and practice. *Image: Journal of Nursing Scholarship, 23*(3), 177–181.

Rogers, M. E. (1970). *An introduction to the theoretical basis of nursing.* Philadelphia: F.A. Davis.

Romyn, D. M., Allen, M. N., Boschma, G., Duncan, S. M., Edgecombe, N., Jensen, L. A., Ross-Kerr, J. C., Marck, P., Salsali, M., Tourangeau, A. E., & Warnock, F. (2003). The notion of evidence in evidence-based practice by the nursing philosophy working group. *Journal of Professional Nursing, 19*(4), 184–188.

Roy, C. (1976). *Introduction to nursing: An adaptation model.* Englewood Cliffs, NJ: Prentice-Hall.

Roy, C. (1982). Historical perspective of the theoretical framework for the classification of nursing diagnosis. In M. J. Kim, & D. A. Moritz (Eds.), *Classification of nursing diagnoses: Proceedings of the third and fourth national conferences held in St. Louis, MO, in 1978 and 1980* (pp. 235–246). St. Louis, MO: McGraw-Hill.

Rycroft-Malone, J., Seers, K., Titchen, A., Harvey, G., Kitson, A., & McCormack, B. (2004). What counts as evidence in evidence-based practice? *Journal of Advanced Nursing, 47*(1), 81–90.

Sarter, B. J. (1990). Philosophical foundations of nursing theory: A discipline emerges. In N. L. Chaska (Ed.), *The nursing profession: Turning points* (pp. 223–229). St. Louis: Mosby.

Silva, M. C., Sorrell, J. M., & Sorrell, S. C. (1995). From Carper's patterns of knowing to ways of being: An ontological philosophical shift in nursing. *Advances in Nursing Science, 18*(1), 1–13.

Starzomski, R., & Rodney, P. (1997). Nursing inquiry for the common good. In S. E. Thorne, & V. E. Hayes (Eds.), *Nursing praxis: Knowledge and action* (pp. 219–236). Thousand Oaks, CA: Sage.

Sullivan-Marx, E. M. (2006). Directions for the development of nursing knowledge. *Policy, Politics & Nursing Practice, 3*(3), 164–168.

Thorne, S. (2005). Conceptualizing in nursing: What's the point? (guest editorial). *Journal of Advanced Nursing, 51*(2), 107.

Thorne, S., Canam, C., Dahinten, S., Hall, W., Henderson, A., & Kirkham, S. (1998). Nursing's metaparadigm concepts: Disempacting the debates. *Journal of Advanced Nursing, 27,* 1257–1268.

Thorne, S., Jillings, C., Ellis, D., & Perry, J.-A. (1993). A nursing model in action: The University of British Columbia experience. *Journal of Advanced Nursing, 18,* 1259–1266.

Thorne, S. E., Henderson, A. D., McPherson, G. I., & Pesut, B. K. (2004). The problematic allure of the binary in nursing theoretical discourse. *Nursing Philosophy, 5,* 208–215.

Thorne, S. E., Reimer Kirkham, S., & Henderson, A. (1999). Ideological implications of paradigm discourse. *Nursing Inquiry, 6,* 123–131.

Torres, G. (1974). Curriculum process and the integrated curriculum. In National League for Nursing (Ed.), *Unifying the curriculum: The integrated approach.* New York: National League for Nursing.

Torres, G. (1986). *Theoretical foundations of nursing.* Norwalk, CN: Appleton-Century-Crofts.

Travelbee, J. (1966). *Interpersonal aspects of nursing.* Philadelphia: F.A. Davis.

Varcoe, C. (1996). Disparagement of the nursing process: The new dogma? *Journal of Advanced Nursing, 23*(1), 120–125.

von Bertalanffy, L. (1968). *General systems theory: Foundations, development, application.* New York: George Braziller.

Wald, F. S., & Leonard, R. C. (1964). Toward development of nursing practice theory. *American Journal of Nursing, 13*(4), 309–313.

Warren, J. J., & Hoskins, L. M. (1990). The development of NANDA's nursing diagnosis taxonomy. *Nursing Diagnosis, 1*(4), 162–168.

Watson, J. (1979). *Nursing: The philosophy and science of caring.* Boston: Little, Brown.

Watson, J. (1990). Caring knowledge and informed moral passion. *Advances in Nursing Science, 13*(1), 15–24.

Yeo, M. (1989). Integration of nursing theory and nursing ethics. *Advances in Nursing Science, 11*(3), 33–42.

Yura, H., & Walsh, M. B. (1983). *The nursing process: Assessing, planning, implementing, evaluating.* Norwalk, CN: Appleton-Century-Crofts.

Zilm, G., & Warbinek, E. (1994). *Legacy: History of nursing education at the University of British Columbia 1919–1994.* Vancouver: UBC Press.

Thinking Philosophically in Nursing

June F. Kikuchi

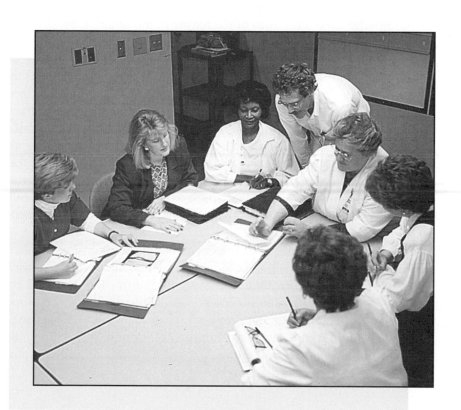

LEARNING OBJECTIVES

- To appreciate the development of conceptions of nursing from a historical perspective.
- To distinguish between a scientific and a philosophical conception of nursing.
- To understand the philosophical basis and implications for nursing thought and action of a sound conception of nursing and of nursing knowledge.
- To understand what philosophical thinking in nursing demands of the inquirer.
- To identify pivotal assumptions and values that promote or impede philosophical thinking in nursing.
- To think creatively of ways and means to advance philosophical thinking in nursing.

During the last quarter of the twentieth century, many in the nursing profession were involved in an ambitious enterprise: to base the development of a body of nursing knowledge on conceptions of the nature of nursing. Today, the buzzwords (e.g., "conceptual models of nursing" and "grand nursing theories") reflective of that enterprise are rarely heard. They have been replaced by buzz words (e.g., "evidenced-informed practice" and "knowledge transfer") reflective of a new enterprise: to base nursing practice on scientific evidence. As this new enterprise has come to the foreground, the earlier one has receded into the background. Concomitantly, nurses have become less concerned about specifying the nature of nursing and of nursing knowledge and developing a body of nursing knowledge. If their concern continues to dissipate, the nursing profession may lose itself before it finds itself. Does this mean that the profession should revive its earlier enterprise? The purpose of this chapter is to suggest another option: to develop a sound conceptual nursing basis by thinking philosophically (i.e., to develop a clear, coherent, and comprehensive philosophical conception of nursing and of nursing knowledge).

The chapter begins with a brief overview of the enterprise to base nursing knowledge on conceptions of the nature of nursing. Then, the downward spiral of that enterprise and of nurses' concern about specifying the nature of nursing and of nursing knowledge and developing a body of nursing knowledge are depicted. The proposal is then put forward that nurses think philosophically to develop a sound philosophical nursing basis. A conception of the nature of philosophical thinking and some major impediments to such thinking in nursing are enunciated. Finally, the recent growth of philosophical thinking in nursing is described.

BASING NURSING KNOWLEDGE ON CONCEPTIONS OF NURSING

The enterprise to base the development of a body of nursing knowledge on conceptions of the nature of nursing was initiated in the late 1960s in response to a problem identified by nurse educators. In the absence of knowledge of the nature of nursing, nurse educators were finding that they could not determine what to include within a nursing curriculum as nursing knowledge. Thinking that the problem could be solved by developing conceptions of the nature of nursing, nurse scholars set about developing them (Kikuchi, 1997).

When the enterprise was initiated, science reigned supreme and nurses' preparation in research was primarily scientific in nature. Consequently, conceptions of the nature of nursing were erroneously assumed to be scientific rather than philosophical in nature and there was a tendency to derive them from one or another scientific theory of such basic disciplines as psychology, physiology, and sociology, to characterize them by the levels and ranges attributed to sociological theories; and to assign purposes to them as per basic scientific theories (i.e., to describe, explain, and predict). Initially, the enterprise went well. For the most part, nurses eagerly adopted the various conceptions that were put forward. Soon, however, as the conceptions began to be labelled variously as conceptual models of nursing, conceptual nursing frameworks, and nursing theories, confusion set in about the nature of the conceptions. Were they models, frameworks, or theories (Kikuchi, 1997)?

Over time, with some conceptions being based on scientific theories and/or philosophical theories but considered to be nursing science, confusion increased. It did not help that the methods used to develop the conceptions were not always explicitly stated. Scepticism about their worth grew, fuelled by nurses' complaints that they were difficult to understand, too abstract, and far removed from the particulars of everyday practice. By the 1990s, the conceptions were being characterized as useless, impractical, and unnecessary (Thorne, 2003).

 REFLECTIVE THINKING

Why do you think that nurses are so willing to proceed without a clear, coherent, and comprehensive conception of nursing to guide them?

DOWNFALL OF CONCEPTIONS OF NURSING: ITS AFTERMATH AND IMPLICATIONS

In their heyday, the extant conceptions of nursing were taught in nearly every undergraduate and graduate nursing program in Canada and the United States. That is no longer the case. Many schools of nursing have dropped them from their curricula. Chinn (2001) has called for their reinstatement, warning that, if nurses do not learn to apply them and continue to take on doctoring activities, nursing will find itself once again serving as a handmaiden to doctoring, but her call has yet to be taken up. Further, as nurses' confidence in the power and necessity of conceptions of nursing has spiralled downward, so too has their concern about specifying the nature of nursing and of nursing knowledge and developing a body of nursing knowledge. For example, nurses are tending not to base their research on any conception of nursing (Kikuchi, 2003b; Spear, 2007). In the nursing theoretical literature on evidenced-informed practice, little or no mention is made of basing nursing practice on a conception of nursing or of developing a body of *nursing* knowledge. Similar manifestations are apparent in recent Canadian nursing association publications.

In the document *Toward 2020: Visions for Nursing*, prepared for the Canadian Nurses Association by Villeneuve and MacDonald (2006), it is said that, by the year 2020, registered nurses should be doing much of what general practitioners currently do. Further, they should be acting as coordinators, educators, consultants, and advocates in the health care system, leaving the provision of direct nursing care mainly to others. Also, asserting the necessity of fluid professional boundaries and of not focusing on profession-specific activities such as the development of nursing research, Villeneuve and MacDonald forecast that, by 2020, generic terms will have replaced profession-specific terms such as "nursing diagnosis" and "nursing care plans." Conceptions of nursing and of nursing knowledge are not mentioned in the document and none is identified as underpinning it. Rather, the efficient use of human health care resources drives the forecasted scenarios.

Along similar lines, the College and Association of Registered Nurses of Alberta has proposed that the activities of ordering and applying X-rays and of prescribing specified medications be included within the legislated scope of restricted activities of registered nurses and that nurse practitioners be allowed to order radiation therapy. It is maintained that, with nurses taking on some of the activities currently done by doctors, the efficiency of the health care system will improve and nurses will be able to enact the full scope of nursing practice (Phillipchuk, 2006, 2007). The proposal is related to a conception of nursing, but it is so all-encompassing that it could apply to almost all health care professions, rendering it essentially a conception of nursing in name only.

If nurses continue not to be concerned about specifying the nature of nursing and of nursing knowledge and developing a body of nursing knowledge, nursing stands in great danger of losing itself and, in the process, not meeting its potential but rather that of other professions, particularly that of doctoring. As Gottlieb and Gottlieb (2007) state, if nursing is to become a profession in its own right and to provide the kind of care that the public deserves, it must differentiate itself and develop its own body of knowledge. Further, it must differentiate itself as a profession that complements rather than competes with other professions. The need for the nursing profession to attend to these matters is brought home by White et al.'s (2008) research study of Western Canadian nurses' perceptions of their scopes of practice.

In their study, White et al. (2008) found that the practice and morale of all groups of nurses (registered nurses, licensed practical nurses, and registered psychiatric nurses) were being negatively affected by unclear intraprofessional and interprofessional scopes of practice. Based on their findings, they state,

> *Clearly defining and articulating the role of nurses, and clarifying what is unique to nursing practice and what is shared with other healthcare professionals, pose significant challenges to the profession at this time. We must be able to describe nursing practice in terms of the knowledge and principles that underpin nurses' roles. If nurses are unable to explain the theoretical*

basis for their practice, they may find themselves unable to articulate what motivates their actions. It is difficult indeed to document accountability for one's practice without an explanatory framework within which to evaluate practice. (p. 54)

So, then, ought the profession to revive the enterprise of developing a body of nursing knowledge using extant conceptions of nursing?

ANOTHER WAY FORWARD

Aside from the earlier mentioned problems, the aforementioned enterprise per se has serious foundational problems of an epistemological nature that make it an untenable option. One such problem is its assumption that conceptions of the nature of nursing are to be developed using scientific means. Another is its adherence to the idealist thought that reality conforms to the mind—the world and all that exists in it are a reflection of the mind. Consequently, conceptions of the world and all that exists in it are characterized as ideologies. As such, they lie in the realm of taste and are beyond the realm of reason, argumentation, and questioning. They are chosen on the basis of preference and become dominant by might rather than by reason (Adler, 1990; Kikuchi, 2003a).

If revival of the enterprise is not a real option and if the current trend not to specify the nature of nursing and of nursing knowledge is also not an option, are there any other options? A sound one would be for the nursing profession to get its bearings by reaffirming the truth of the following philosophical proposition, upon which the enterprise of the 1960s was based: a conception of the nature of nursing is necessary to define a body of knowledge as a body of nursing knowledge. However, to avoid the aforementioned foundational problems of that enterprise, it would then proceed on a different footing: on the moderate realist tenets that the mind conforms to reality, philosophical thought focuses on that which is immaterial (i.e., the nonphenomenal and therefore nonobservable), and philosophical knowledge is attainable in the form of probable truth or truth beyond a reasonable doubt (Adler, 1965; Maritain, 1959). On that footing, a conception of nursing would be developed by thinking philosophically about aspects of nursing that are nonphenomenal or nonobservable (e.g., the end goal of nursing practice). In contrast, a conception of nursing developed using scientific means is a conception of the phenomenal or observable aspects of nursing as they existed at the time of observation (Kikuchi, 1997).

THINKING PHILOSOPHICALLY IN NURSING

Basically, thinking philosophically, or philosophizing, entails asking questions about the nature of that which exists and happens in the world and about what humans ought to seek and do. In the pursuit of truth, as answers are proposed, ever more penetrating questions are asked and answered in a contingent, logical, and rational manner (Adler, 1965; Phenix, 1964). For example, suppose we were asked, "What is good nursing care?" In attempting to answer it, we would likely soon find ourselves having to answer more basic and penetrating questions such as "What is the nature of that which is good?" As the dialogue proceeds, we will likely find that "good" has been defined in a moral sense (as that which is morally sound) and in an artistic sense (as that which is artistically sound). We will then have to consider if by "good nursing care" we are referring to nursing care that is good in the moral sense, in the artistic sense, or in both senses. Sooner or later, we are apt to come face to face with such questions as these:

- What is the nature of nursing?
- What is the nature of care or caring?
- What is the nature of the nurse–patient relationship?
- What is the nature of human beings?

All the aforementioned questions are philosophical questions. As such, they can be answered only by philosophizing. However, as Pieper (1952) reminds us, philosophizing entails more than just asking and answering philosophical questions. He cautions that, if we ask and answer questions in the absence of wonder, we are not truly or genuinely philosophizing. In this case we are operating as technicians, treating philosophizing as a skill that can be acquired in the way that we can acquire any skill. Philosophizing is a matter of skill, but only in a skeletal sense. Principles and rules for asking and answering questions that have the capacity to deepen our understanding of the world (e.g., asking questions that call for other than a "yes" or "no" answer) can be learned or taught, but to think philosophically, we must acquire such skills within the context of wonder. It is wonder that will give our question asking and answering its philosophical character of "searching for the truth" (p. 103).

Pieper describes the philosophical act, or philosophizing, as "a full, personal attitude which is by no manner of means at the sole disposal of the ratio" (p. 18). In other words, reason alone cannot dictate the philosophical act, since a particular attitude toward the world is necessary—one of standing in wonder before the world as it exists and longing to understand it. This approach to the world is the exact opposite of one more familiar to us: relating to things only from the perspective of our pragmatic interests so that we ask questions only for the purpose of determining how to use them to our advantage or to solve a problem. According to Pieper,

> *To philosophize is to act in such a way that one steps out of the workaday world… the world of work, the utilitarian world, the world of the useful, subject to ends,… a world in which there is no room for philosophy or philosophizing. (pp. 70-71)*

Pieper (1952) emphasizes that, in stepping out of or transcending the workaday world, we do not leave it behind us nor consider it as nonessential. Rather, the opposite is the case. We back away from the usual way we look at the things of our everyday lives—of our workaday world—to see them for what they really and ultimately are. We cannot, however, just tell ourselves to step out of the workaday world. It is not that simple. Pieper says that a shock—one that stuns and shakes us—is necessary to "pierce the dome that encloses the… workaday world" (pp. 72–73). It is comparable to the spiritual awakening that one experiences on coming face to face with that which is awesome, such as the birth of a baby. It can happen when we encounter questions of the sort that Socrates posed—questions with the capacity "to strip things of their everyday character" (p. 98) so that we realize we do not know of what we speak and are no longer as complacent as we were. Because his questions had this effect, Socrates "compared himself… to an electric fish that gives a paralyzing shock to anyone who touches it" (p. 98). In the nursing world, the question mentioned earlier—"What is good nursing care?"—holds the potential to have this kind of effect on nurses who think they know the answer, only to find that the opposite is the case.

The shock that stirs us from our complacency is described by Pieper (1952) in relation to wonder, since wonder moves and shakes us to the point where "the ground quakes beneath [our] feet,… [our] whole spiritual nature, [our] capacity to know,… is threatened" (p. 101). He attributes this effect to the fact that "wonder signifies that the world is profounder, more all-embracing and mysterious than the logic of everyday reason had taught us to believe" (p. 102). Although wonder is often said to be the beginning of philosophy, Pieper asserts:

> Wonder is not just the starting point of philosophy… [but also its] lasting source…. The inner form of philosophizing is virtually identical with the inner form of wonder…. To wonder is not merely not to know; it means to be inwardly aware and sure that one does not know, and that one understands oneself in not knowing. And yet it is not the ignorance of resignation. On the contrary, to wonder is to be on the way, in via; it certainly means to be struck dumb, momentarily, but equally it means that one is searching for the truth. (p. 103)

Given its essential role in philosophizing, it is clear that, if nurses are to philosophize, they must develop their sense of wonder. But that is easier said than done. Wonder is an innate human capacity that, like any of our other innate capacities, can be developed to the degree to which we possess it, under beneficial circumstances (Adler, 1978; Pieper, 1952). The circumstances, however, under which nurses are educated and practise are still such that they impede rather than facilitate not only the development of wonder but also the kind of questioning that it engenders.

REFLECTIVE THINKING

What do you think it will take for nurses to realize the need to think philosophically in nursing?

IMPEDIMENTS TO WONDERING AND PHILOSOPHIZING IN NURSING

Most of the impediments to the development of nurses' capacities to wonder and philosophize have been, and continue to be, built into the nursing curricula. Hockey (1990), a British nurse, asserts that basic nursing programs, including the baccalaureate, "are too tightly packed with essential information and the crucially important measures to ensure safe practice, to allow critical enquiry into everyday phenomena, which must be the essence of philosophy" (p. 49). Similarly, Levine (1995), an American nurse, eloquently states:

> *Nursing is a humanitarian enterprise. The emphasis placed on scientific and technical knowledge is indispensable to the development of the craft—but it is imperfectly achieved without the intellectual skills that are the special province of the humanities…. Racing through curricula which seek to be all-inclusive, there is seldom time for courses in philosophy or literature, or history or music…. [Consequently,] nurses… do not have the language and reading and thinking skills that are the basis of a liberal education. This failure… ultimately limits the depth and meaning of the profession itself. (p. 19)*

Dellasega, Milone-Nuzzo, Curci, Ballard, and Kirch (2007) agree. Given the unprecedented rate at which scientific and technological knowledge is now becoming available and being included in nursing curricula, they assert that it is more urgent than ever for nursing students to be exposed to the humanities.

Stinson (1990), a Canadian nurse, relates the almost exclusive emphasis of nursing curricula on scientific knowledge and inquiry to another concern: the lack, in Canada and elsewhere, of nursing faculty who are adequately prepared in philosophy and history. Although the number of faculty with such preparation is increasing, it continues to be insufficient and, as Stinson says, "there is often a lack of due recognition and support given to the few who are adequately prepared in such areas" (p. 3). The seriousness of these problems is reflected in Levine's (1995) description of American nursing faculty who have never studied philosophy and think of it merely "as the preamble to the curriculum required for accreditation by the National League for Nursing" (p. 21). Levine maintains that, in outnumbering faculty schooled in philosophy, they are able to perpetuate the notion that philosophy is what they have produced: "a mundane listing of 'We believe…'" (p. 21).

Another continuing impediment to the development of nurses' capacities to wonder and philosophize is apparent in Hockey's (1990) declaration that "by and large, philosophy tends to be a fringe subject in nursing courses… and so-called philosophical pronouncements are often little more than disguised policy statements, dictated by exigencies and need rather than developmental thought" (p. 49). Here, Hockey is bringing our attention not only to the fringe status of philosophy in nursing programs, but also to an ever-increasing problem: mere pragmatic concerns of special-interest groups, including those of political bodies, dictating what the preparation of nurses, and what adequate nursing care, shall entail.

By responding as they have to the demands of political and economic factions, universities are fast becoming part of the workaday world. Half a century ago, Pieper (1952) expressed concern that the workaday world "is becoming our entire world and threatens to engulf us completely… [to the point where] philosophy—inevitably—becomes more and more distant, strange and remote; [and] even assumes the appearance of an intellectual luxury" (p. 71). It would appear that Pieper had every reason to be concerned.

Increasingly, university students are choosing their courses and careers almost purely for pragmatic reasons. Wonder and inquisitiveness are taking a back seat. Similarly, faculty members' choices of research projects and careers are being driven more by what the universities reward (e.g., large grants from prestigious funding sources and publications in renowned journals) than by intellectual matters. Unfortunately, graduate students are being socialized by their faculty mentors to do likewise (Meleis, 2001). Within such a climate, philosophical endeavours that are driven by a sense of wonder, take considerable time to complete, and can be undertaken without large grants fare poorly.

As Maben, Latter, and Macleod Clark's (2007) study has revealed, the practice-setting climate is not any better. Historically, nurses have been taught to follow the directions of "authorities" (e.g., other health care providers, particularly physicians) and not to ask questions. Recognizing the ominous potential consequences of nurses continuing to behave in that manner, the nursing profession is encouraging nurses to become independent thinkers. However, with other professionals still tending to view them mainly as receivers and implementers of their orders and with the current lack of clarity about the nature of nursing practice, nurses find it tough to question the directions of "authorities." They discover that doing so usually results in negative consequences (e.g., they are reprimanded). Consequently, they are apt to do so only if serious harm is likely to follow from their not doing so. Otherwise, they tend to be acquiescent and to carry out the orders of other health care providers even if, in so doing, nursing care is compromised. For example, to get patients to a particular place at a particular time as ordered, nurses still tend to hurry them through their meals or baths, or skip these entirely. The ongoing financial cutbacks to health care and shortage of health care providers are making it harder than ever for nurses to do otherwise or to stand back and reflect on what is happening (Rankin & Campbell, 2006).

Clearly, the circumstances under which nurses are learning and practising are not conducive to wondering and philosophizing. Changing them, however, will not be a simple matter mainly because of the special-interest groups that have a vested interest in maintaining the status quo. For example, by preserving society's current conception of nursing work as work requiring little more than some practical skills and a willingness to follow directions, governments can keep nursing education and health care costs down and other health care providers can continue to have passive nursing staff do their bidding. So, given the current circumstances, how is the nursing profession to develop a sound philosophical conception of nursing and of nursing knowledge? The answer lies in wisely using a scarce but growing nursing resource: nurses who are developing their capacities to think philosophically despite the existing impediments to wondering and philosophizing in nursing.

TOWARD A SOUND PHILOSOPHICAL NURSING BASIS

Against all odds, philosophical thought is starting to flourish in nursing, thanks largely to nurse educators' fairly recent recognition that not only knowledge of research methods but an understanding of their philosophical underpinnings is required to develop nursing science. Subsequently, with philosophy of nursing science courses being included in most if not all doctoral nursing programs, a growing (albeit still small) number of nurses are managing to develop their philosophical capacities and helping to increase awareness of the need for nurses to wonder and philosophize about various aspects of their profession and discipline. They are participating in philosophical discussions at conferences and online and contributing substantively to the nursing literature.

In the 1980s, few papers of a philosophical nature appeared in nursing journals. Today, such papers appear regularly in such prestigious nursing journals as the *Journal of Advanced Nursing and Nursing Inquiry*. Also, with the growing interest in nursing philosophy, the *Canadian Journal of Nursing Research* devoted an issue, in 1995 and 2000, to the topic "Philosophy/Theory." As well, in 1999, the journal *Scholarly Inquiry for Nursing Practice* published a special issue entitled "Philosophy of Nursing: Emerging Views." Then, in 2000, the journal *Nursing Philosophy* was established. Also, books pertaining specifically to nursing philosophy are becoming available—for example, *Philosophic Inquiry in Nursing* (Kikuchi & Simmons, 1992), *Philosophy for Nursing* (Reed & Ground, 1997), *Philosophy of Nursing* (Brencick & Webster, 2000), and *Philosophy of Nursing* (Edwards, 2001).

The growing philosophical nursing knowledge literature has been helpful in creating an atmosphere conducive to wondering and philosophizing in nursing, as have infrastructures such as the Institute for Philosophical Nursing Research (IPNR), established in 1988 at the University of Alberta, and the International Philosophy of Nursing Society (IPONS), established in the United Kingdom in 2003. The nursing philosophy conferences organized by the IPNR, the IPONS, and other institutions, such as Laval University, are helping to meet nurses' need to come together and philosophize.

🔍 CANADIAN RESEARCH FOCUS

Kikuchi, J.F. (2003). Nursing knowledge and the problem of worldviews. *Research and Theory for Nursing Practice, 17*, 7–17.

Kikuchi's philosophical examination of conceptions of nursing based on the idea of worldviews identifies their ontological and epistemological underpinnings and implications for nursing knowledge development and practice.

Rankin, J.M., & Campbell, M.L. (2006*). Managing to nurse: Inside Canada's health care reform.* Toronto: University of Toronto Press.

Rankin and Campbell's book, based on a sociological study of the reforming of health care in Canada in the 1990s, sheds light on how that reformation has affected nurses' control over nursing practice, including that of nursing thought.

Reimer-Kirkham, S., Varcoe, C., Browne, A.J., Lynam, M.J., Basu Khan, K., & McDonald, H. (2009). Critical inquiry and knowledge translation: Exploring compatibles and tensions. *Nursing Philosophy, 10,* 152–166.

Reimer-Kirkham et al.'s philosophical examination of their attempts (as Canadian nurse researchers) to translate their work in critical inquiry raises questions about whether and how disparate philosophical stances can be accommodated.

White, D., Oelke, N.D., Besner, J., Doran, D., McGillis Hall, L., & Giovannetti, P. (2008). Nursing scope of practice: Descriptions and challenges. *Canadian Journal of Nursing Leadership, 21*(1), 44–57.

White et al.'s scientific study of Western Canadian nurses' perceptions of their scopes of practice brings home the need for a clear, coherent, and comprehensive conception of nursing to guide the development of nursing practice.

Although the number of nurses who are now thinking philosophically is still small, it is getting to the point where removal of the impediments to wondering and philosophizing and development of a sound philosophical conception of nursing and of nursing knowledge are no longer fantastical goals. Consequently, at this time, we would do well to begin thinking about what we could be doing to work toward them. We need to think about how to develop more nurses who can truly do what Smadu (2007), past president of the Canadian Nurses Association, asks: "As nurses we need to lead the discussions about what nursing is, in language that is clear, forthright and complete—neither minimizing nursing work, nor taking for granted that others know what we are and do" (p. 3). Here, we would do well to bear in mind that this endeavour is not a simple one to execute, given the growth of diverse philosophical stances among nurses. While generative, it has also made for challenging dialogue (Reimer-Kirkham et al., 2009).

Finally, it would certainly be unrealistic to expect that *all* nurses would do *all* the work necessary to develop a sound philosophical nursing basis. A more realistic expectation is that nurses would contribute to that development in whatever ways they can. For example, those with the necessary philosophical preparation could take responsibility for the project and do the in-depth philosophical analysis, while those without such preparation could contribute in their own ways (e.g., by sharing their thoughts regarding those aspects of the scope of nursing practice that need to be clarified). Dialoguing together, each group could benefit from the expertise of the other not only with regard to gained insights but also with regard to development of their capacities to wonder and philosophize.

REFLECTIVE THINKING

1. At what stage of their education ought nurses be introduced to philosophical inquiry?
2. What case, if any, can be made for *not* introducing nurses to philosophical inquiry?

CONCLUSION

With the need for a sound philosophical conception of nursing and of nursing knowledge, the path that has been cleared thus far to advance philosophical thought in nursing is very encouraging. Indeed, it is remarkable, given the impediments to wondering and philosophizing that continue to exist both within and outside of nursing educational and practice settings. Much more work lies ahead and needs to be done, if the profession is not to lose itself before it finds itself, because, already there are signs that the nursing profession may be on the way to becoming an amorphous entity.

CRITICAL THINKING QUESTIONS

1. What is an essential difference between a conception of nursing developed using scientific means and one developed using philosophical means based in moderate realism?

2. What are some fundamental implications of grounding nursing practice in a conception of nursing based on idealism? Based in moderate realism?

3. What differentiates thinking philosophically from critical thinking?

4. What pivotal assumptions and values underlie the impediments to wondering and philosophizing in nursing? Underlie genuine wondering and philosophizing in nursing?

WEB SITES

International Philosophy of Nursing Society: http://www.ipons.dundee.ac.uk/
The International Centre for Nursing Ethics (ICNE): http://www.nursing-ethics.org/
A Philosophy of Nursing Forum: http://caring-matters.blogspot.com/

REFERENCES

Adler, M. J. (1965). *The conditions of philosophy*. New York: Dell.

Adler, M. J. (1978). *Aristotle for everybody*. New York: Macmillan.

Adler, M. J. (1990). *Intellect: Mind over matter*. New York: Macmillan.

Brencick, J. M., & Webster, G. A. (2000). *Philosophy of nursing*. New York: State University of New York Press.

Chinn, P. L. (2001). Where is the nursing in nursing education? [Editorial]. *Advances in Nursing Science, 23*, v–vi.

Dellasega, C., Milone-Nuzzo, P., Curci, K. M., Ballard, J. O., & Kirch, D. G. (2007). The humanities interface of nursing and medicine. *Journal of Professional Nursing, 23*, 174–179.

Edwards, S. D. (2001). *Philosophy of nursing*. Hampshire, UK: Palgrave Macmillan.

Gottlieb, L. N., & Gottlieb, B. (2007). The developmental/health framework within the McGill Model of Nursing: "Laws of nature" guiding whole person care. *Advances in Nursing Science, 30*, E43–E57.

Hockey, L. (1990). The philosophical underpinnings of doctoral education. In P. A. Field (Ed.), *Advancing doctoral preparation for nurses: Charting a course for the future* (pp. 45–53). Edmonton: Faculty of Nursing, University of Alberta.

Kikuchi, J. F. (1997). Clarifying the nature of conceptualizations about nursing. *Canadian Journal of Nursing Research, 29*(1), 97–119.

Kikuchi, J. F. (2003a). Nursing knowledge and the problem of worldviews. *Research and Theory for Nursing Practice, 17*, 7–17.

Kikuchi, J. F. (2003b). Nursing theories: Relic or stepping stone? *Canadian Journal of Nursing Research, 35*(2), 3–7.

Kikuchi, J. F., & Simmons, H. (Eds.). (1992). *Philosophic inquiry in nursing*. Newbury Park, CA: Sage.

Levine, M. E. (1995). Discourse: On the humanities in nursing. *Canadian Journal of Nursing Research, 27*(2), 19–23.

Maben, J., Latter, S., & Macleod Clark, J. (2007). The sustainability of ideals, values, and the nursing mandate: Evidence from a longitudinal qualitative study. *Nursing Inquiry, 14*(2), 99–113.

Maritain, J. (1959). *The degrees of knowledge* (G.B. Phelan, Trans.). New York: Charles Scribner's Sons.

Meleis, A. I. (2001). Scholarship and the R01 [Editorial]. *Journal of Nursing Scholarship, 33*, 104–105.

Phenix, P. H. (1964). *Realms of meaning*. New York: McGraw-Hill.

Phillipchuk, D. (2006). The time has come: Describing and shaping RN Practice. *Alberta RN, 62*(7), 6–8.

Phillipchuk, D. (2007). CARNA supports revisions to restricted activities for RNs. *Alberta RN, 63*(9), 12–13.

Pieper, J. (1952). *Leisure: The basis of culture* (A. Dru, Trans.). New York: Pantheon Books.

Rankin, J. M., & Campbell, M. L. (2006). *Managing to nurse: Inside Canada's health care reform*. Toronto: University of Toronto Press.

Reed, J., & Ground, I. (1997). *Philosophy for nursing*. London: Edward Arnold.

Reimer-Kirkham, S., Varcoe, C., Browne, A. J., Lynam, M. J., Basu Khan, K., & McDonald, H. (2009). Critical inquiry and knowledge translation: Exploring compatibilities and tensions. *Nursing Philosophy*, *10*, 152–166.

Smadu, M. (2007). We must use our voices and speak up about nursing. *The Canadian Nurse, 103*(2), 3.

Spear, H. J. (2007). Nursing theory and knowledge development: A descriptive review of doctoral dissertations, 2000–2004. *Advances in Nursing Science, 30*, E1–E14.

Stinson, S. M. (1990). Prologue. In P. A. Field (Ed.), *Advancing doctoral preparation for nurses: Charting a course for the future* (pp. 1–5). Edmonton: Faculty of Nursing, University of Alberta.

Thorne, S. (2003). Theoretical issues in nursing. In J. C. Ross-Kerr, & M. J. Wood (Eds.), *Canadian nursing: Issues and perspectives* (4th ed.) (pp. 116–134). Toronto: Mosby.

Villeneuve, M., & MacDonald, J. (2006). *Toward 2020: Visions for nursing*. Ottawa: Canadian Nurses Association.

White, D., Oelke, N. D., Besner, J., Doran, D., McGillis Hall, L., & Giovannetti, P. (2008). Nursing scope of practice: Descriptions and challenges. *Canadian Journal of Nursing Leadership, 21*(1), 44–57.

8 Nursing Research in Canada

Janice Lander

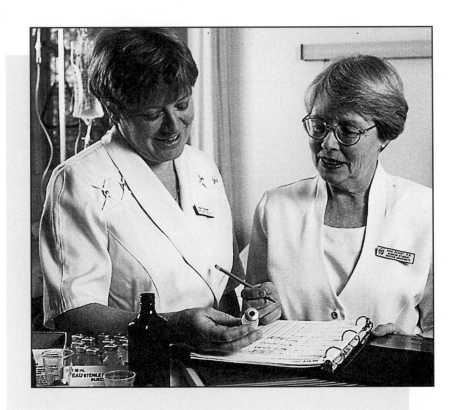

LEARNING OBJECTIVES

- To understand the development of Canadian nursing research.
- To be aware of the obstacles faced by nursing researchers to acquire research funds.
- To be able to describe the connection between research and practice and the barriers.
- To understand issues related to nursing outcomes.
- To recognize the value of the collaborative partnership involved in research-based practice.
- To be aware of what is required to implement research into nursing practice.

EVOLUTION OF CANADIAN NURSING RESEARCH

Research in nursing has developed gradually as a result of a slowly enlarging pool of nurses with research expertise. This development parallels the evolution of graduate education in nursing because this is where research skills are learned. Graduate students are taught research methods, and they conduct research investigations to fulfill thesis requirements as part of their education. Since graduate education in nursing was established, nursing research activities have increased in scope and number. Although master's programs provide the background in research needed for doctoral work, few Canadian universities offered master's degrees before the early 1980s. University administrations in some Canadian institutions were reluctant to approve and fund the programs. Symons (1975) commented: "The slowness in developing graduate schools of nursing in Canada has, in turn, adversely affected the amount of research undertaken in this field. Little support has been available for publication, or for investigating problems in nursing and health care of particular interest to Canadians" (p. 212).

When master of nursing programs became widely available in Canada, the next challenge was to establish doctoral nursing education in Canada. The first funded doctoral program began at the Faculty of Nursing, University of Alberta, in January 1991, when the first students were admitted to the program. Doctoral programs in nursing began in earnest thereafter. From 1991 to 2007, another 14 doctoral programs were established in Canadian universities. Opportunities for graduate education are now available across the country, and although admission is competitive, accessibility presents less of a problem than it once did. However slow the basic development of research and graduate study in nursing was, there is little doubt that the process will continue.

The lack of a Canadian doctoral program in nursing until 1991 forced nurses to be resourceful and to find alternatives that enabled them to develop research skills. These alternatives included entering doctoral programs in nursing in other countries, most notably the United States, and seeking admission to doctoral programs in other disciplines. The development of Canadian doctoral programs in nursing has increased access to doctoral programs for nurses. It has also resulted in the development of postdoctoral research fellowships for Ph.D. graduates, something that was virtually unknown in Canadian nursing before 1991.

RESEARCH SUPPORTED BY UNIVERSITY SCHOOLS OF NURSING

From a very small endeavour in just a few schools, nursing research has become a more broadly based and better financed undertaking. From the rather bleak levels of research funding reported for the 1965–66 fiscal year (Griffin, 1971; Imai, 1971; Poole, 1971) to the vastly increased amounts reported in later years, it is evident that funding for nursing research in university schools of nursing has entered a new era. Undoubtedly, this change has been predicated on new expectations for faculty performance in research; without the development of research expertise among faculty, it would not have been possible. Essential to the transition was the appointment of members of faculty qualified at the doctoral level who were prepared to undertake research.

NURSING RESEARCH IN HEALTH CARE AGENCIES

In the 1980s, nursing research became a growth activity in health care agencies because of increasing recognition of the importance of nursing research to health care and increasing the availability of research support. Many large teaching hospitals appointed nursing researchers to formulate and conduct research initially within the nursing department. These individuals often toiled alone. By the end of the decade, research activities were having a significant impact on nursing practice, and the research programs and spirit of inquiry that had evolved were the envy of many, including other disciplines. Collaboration between nursing researchers in health care agencies and those in university schools of nursing was mutually beneficial. Joint appointments of researchers to these organizations facilitated the investigation of nursing research problems. This collaborative work undoubtedly resulted in important outcomes in the nature of research questions asked and the quality of the research effort.

By the early 1990s, many of the hospital-based nursing research positions were being phased out or significantly changed in response to a perceived need for fiscal restraint. Remaining positions were reconfigured to emphasize responsibilities for measurement and evaluation on a hospital-wide basis. This drastically decreased research involvement by hospital nurses for several years. When funding of hospital-based nursing research resumed in the late 1990s, research had shifted from a discipline-based endeavour to a multidisciplinary one. Academic health centres established multidisciplinary research divisions for research administration and support. It seems unlikely that hospital-based nursing research departments will make a comeback.

BREADTH OF NURSING RESEARCH

In the absence of Canadian master's and doctoral nursing programs, many nurses received their graduate education from the social sciences. Others embarked on graduate study in a faculty of education or in epidemiology in a faculty of medicine. Rarely, some nurses undertook graduate studies in the biological sciences. Wherever nurses studied, their early research training socialized them to the ways and topics of interest of other disciplines, including the research methods common to those fields. It is that exposure to a breadth of research methods that accounts for such diversity in research methods used by Canadian nursing researchers. No other discipline is as varied in the methods used in research nor as respectful of the value of all research methods in advancing knowledge.

FUNDING NURSING RESEARCH

The first national conference on nursing research in Canada was held in Ottawa in 1971 under the auspices of the University of British Columbia, with federal assistance from the National Health Research and Development Program (NHRDP). As this was a "first" for the nursing profession in Canada, historical overviews were presented on the kinds of nursing research projects conducted over the years by governments, service agencies, professional associations, and universities (Griffin, 1971; Imai, 1971; Poole, 1971). These overviews documented that most studies in nursing had been undertaken since 1965, and some were funded by a variety of sponsoring agencies.

The first centre for nursing research in Canada was established at McGill University in 1971 with federal support from Health and Welfare Canada. Until funding for nursing research became readily available as an integral part of the terms of reference of the NHRDP of Health Canada, there were few sources of funds other than the limited resources of the Canadian Nurses Foundation (CNF) and those of private foundations and voluntary organizations. The 1971 documentation provided by Griffin reveals that research funding was not secured for many projects:

> It must be underlined that, to date, a substantial portion of Canadian nursing research has been done by graduate students at their own expense, and by nursing faculty and health agency members, often on their own time, and on a non-funded basis. As such, direct cost figures give us only a hint of the time, equipment, supplies, and publication costs of all the nursing research being done. (p. 22)

Slowly, almost imperceptibly, new sources of funding for nursing research have been opening up for nurses since the 1970s. Some of these sources are provincial organizations, whereas others are federal ones. The four primary areas for which external research support is sought are research projects, research training, infrastructure (space and equipment) for conducting research, and salary support for the researcher (career research awards).

Canadian nurses have struggled to obtain an equitable share of external research support. The process used by research funding agencies to distribute grant funds is complex. Researchers who need financial support to complete a research project must apply to an appropriate agency and the topic must fit funding priorities of the agency. The researcher prepares a detailed application outlining the research and describes qualifications and experience. Most decisions at agencies that fund research are arrived at with input from scientists. Funding agencies strike review committees of researchers from various disciplines that have been funded by the agency. This creates a Catch-22 situation for nursing. To be represented on review committees, nurses must submit applications to the agency and be funded. However, without nurses on the committee, no one is able to speak to the applications submitted by nurses. Merit scores given by reviewers, therefore, may not be high enough for the application to be funded. Another issue was that some of the review committees were familiar with only a narrow type of research method (in particular, not qualitative methods). Many applications submitted by nurses using alternative methods were not funded.

🔍 CANADIAN RESEARCH FOCUS

Dr. Janice Morse arrived in Canada in 1982 from New Zealand via the United States to begin her career as a nursing researcher at the University of Alberta. She held graduate degrees in both anthropology and nursing. Her training in anthropology helped shape the research questions she posed and the research methods used to address those questions. She primarily used qualitative research methods to study *comfort*—a topic of central concern to nursing. Her plan was to study comfort from various perspectives, including those of nurses, patients, and families, ultimately to develop a theory that would guide research and nursing practice.

When she sought funding for her research, her methods were heavily criticized by biomedical reviewers who were unfamiliar with this research approach. She faced the same criticisms locally and nationally and was unable to secure major funding that would provide financial support for her research and students. When the Medical Research Council (MRC) and NHRDP development grants were established to encourage nursing research in Canada, Morse was one of the recipients of the award. This award increased her eligibility for other major Canadian research funding. With the broadening of the mandate of MRC/CIHR in the late 1990s and the infusion of public funds into research, Morse applied for and received further grants.

Morse has made significant contributions to the development of qualitative research. Her research ingenuity led to improved scientific methods and analyses. Students around the world have used her research methods books (Morse & Field, 1995; Richards & Morse, 2006) to learn about qualitative research. Numerous Canadian nursing researchers received training in Morse's lab, which they put to use to address questions of interest to nursing.

Janice Morse is one of many of the early generation of Canadian nursing researchers who have helped shape research in general or in particular fields. The pathway for many of these individuals was similar to that taken by Morse. The current and next generation of Canadian nursing researchers will have improved access to research funds so that they can advance nursing knowledge.

The process of obtaining research support was disheartening. Many nursing researchers stopped seeking funds. Others supported their research by cobbling together small grants from a variety of small funding agencies. From the granting agencies' perspectives, Canadian nurses were complaining about not being funded but were not submitting many applications, and those submitted were flawed. Many applicants were, in fact, in early stages of their careers and lacking good role models to help them become competitive in seeking grant funds.

In response to the efforts of the Canadian Nurses Association (CNA) to communicate nurses' concerns about the low level of federal funding for nursing research, the Medical Research Council (MRC) established the Working Group on Nursing Research in 1982. Final recommendations in the report of the Working Group in 1985 referred to the need to designate funds for nursing research within MRC's structure and the need to assist in creating opportunities for the establishment of doctoral nursing programs across the country. No federal action was taken on the recommendations until early 1988, when MRC announced its decision to collaborate with NHRDP to make separate funding available for nursing research development on a competitive basis. University nursing programs were invited to submit proposals, to be considered in the same manner as were development grants and program grants of MRC, for funding over five years. Almost all university schools of nursing submitted letters of intent to the first round of this competition. Less than half were invited to submit full proposals, and only five institutions across the country received funding, a result that did not please the nursing community. A second round of the competition resulted in the funding of another handful of nurse researchers, after which the program was suspended pending evaluation.

The nursing community accelerated its lobbying efforts, and in 1994 the government announced that the mandate of MRC would be broadened to include health research. It was also to be transformed into the Canadian Institutes for Health Research in 2000. The resulting new programs of MRC (CIHR) did serve to increase the funding of nursing research projects and to integrate nursing research into the mainstream of health research in Canada. For the first time, the full range of research methods suitable for health research questions was proposed and funded. CIHR funding of nursing research rose from $2.3 million in 2000 to $11.6 million in 2005 (Gottlieb, 2007).

The federal government also established the $25-million 10-year Nursing Research Fund (NRF) in 1999. The impetus for this decision came from the Canadian Nurses Association, which had lobbied extensively for a dedicated source of funding for the development of nursing research. The association envisioned that the MRC program would be the model for the NRF program, by funding salaries of researchers and supporting their research project costs. When the government gave the Canadian Health Services Research Foundation (CHSRF) responsibility for administering the NRF funds, a model of funding emerged that ultimately displeased many in the nursing community. The mandate of the CHSRF, which is health services research, did not represent the broad research interests of nurses, particularly those engaged in clinical research. Where NRF had at first appeared to be a windfall for nursing research, it now seemed to be inaccessible to many nursing researchers who worked in fields outside the CHSRF mandate. The other issue was that CHSRF required the applicant to obtain partnership funding in the amount of 60% of the request. The requirement of partnership funding creates hurdles for researchers and lengthens the time spent seeking funds for research. Many researchers, even those who fit the health services mandate of CHSRF, were discouraged from applying because of the partnership funding requirement.

After several years of lobbying, CHSRF transferred some funds to the Canadian Nurses Foundation in 2003 for support of clinical nursing research. The Nursing Care Partnership Program (NCP), as it came to be known, received a $2.5-million five-year award from the CHSRF. One limitation of this award was that funds given by NCP were to be augmented by another agency, as NCP contributes only one dollar for every two partner dollars. The initial funding for NCP was for 2003 to 2007. In 2008, CHSRF provided just over $1 million in funding for 2008–2009. It was unclear in early 2010 whether the program would continue beyond 2010.

The 1990s produced a funding boom in Canada. This development occurred for two reasons: lobbying by researchers across disciplines, and the economic and political climate of the time. Several new research foundations or agencies were created in addition to NRF and CHSRF. The Canadian Foundation for Innovation was established in 1997 in order to fund research infrastructure so that research capacity could be built in universities, research hospitals, and research institutes. The fund supports equipment, buildings, laboratories, and databases required to conduct research. The millennium Canada Research Chairs program was established in 2000 to recruit and retain researchers to help universities and research hospitals to become world-class centres of research and research training. A total of 2000 Chairs were to be awarded from 2000 to 2008. Chairs enable researchers to dedicate their time to research and graduate student training. Although nurses were slow to take advantage of this program, nursing researchers from across the county now hold Canada Research Chairs, which were awarded for 7- or 10-year periods. The effect of the development of new funding sources was to increase funding of nursing research. The amount of funding held by nurses tripled from 1998 to 2001 (Pringle, 2006).

Many of the new research programs and foundations were established for specific intervals of time and funded by the federal government. Many are nearing the end of their initial funding period. Whether they will continue to receive funds from the government will depend on the political and economic climate existing at the time of renewal and on their initial successes.

ADVOCACY FOR NURSING RESEARCH

The events of the 1990s drew attention to the benefits of a united voice when advocating for nursing research. The Office of Nursing Policy at Health Canada took the initiative to bring together policymakers and researchers in 2002 to consider the future of nursing research in Canada. Out of this initiative came the recommendation to create the Canadian Consortium for Nursing Research and Initiative (CCNRI), which is a collaboration of key nursing organizations. Among its priorities is advocating for research funding (Health Canada, 2006). The Canadian Association for Schools of Nursing (CASN) is a member of CCNRI. It commissioned a report on the status of nursing research in Canada, carried out by Jeans (2008) for the purpose of determining nursing research capacity and productivity. This information is useful for advocating for funding of nursing research.

WHO SETS THE AGENDA?

As with many of the health professions, nursing found that the research agenda was not always set by the discipline (Jeans, 2005). This trend began in the 1970s when NHRDP introduced strategic funding priorities. After investing millions of dollars in health research, NHRDP had been unable to find evidence that research had improved the health of Canadians or met the needs of the federal and provincial health departments. Until this time, research had been exclusively investigator-driven, meaning that researchers decided what research questions needed to be asked based on their knowledge of the field. Along with funding investigator-driven research, NHRDP began dedicating a significant portion of its funding budget to strategic priorities that were important to federal and provincial health departments. The earliest strategic health research priorities were in the areas of aging and AIDS. By the late 1990s, even the very traditional Canadian funding agencies, including the MRC, had made the transition to strategic funding priorities. This recent change in funding was stimulated by the federal government who, before approving more health research funding, asked for accountability for the funds that had previously been approved for research—what was the impact of their investment on the health of Canadians?

The setting of strategic priorities by funding agencies was a first step in a new direction in research policy. Some of the directions set by funding agencies and other organizations had an enormous and beneficial impact on health research. One example is the focus on interdisciplinary work. Granting agencies now favour interdisciplinary approaches to research. They have used proposal review criteria and funding incentives to increase the amount of interdisciplinary research and change the focus from discipline-based to patient-based research. Nursing research was perhaps not quite ready for the increased emphasis on multidisciplinary teams, but such great strides have been made in this area that nurses now play an important partnership role in most multidisciplinary health research. Another example is the focus on knowledge transfer, also called research utilization. Granting agencies concluded that one reason research was not having an impact on the health of Canadians was that researchers were not effectively disseminating their findings to policymakers, the public, and practitioners. Most researchers believed their target audience was other researchers. NHRDP, which was the first granting agency to ask researchers to describe their plans for knowledge transfer, was interested in knowledge being transferred to policymakers first, followed by practitioners and the public. CIHR and CHSRF followed NHRDP's suit by requiring that researchers outline knowledge transfer plans. CIHR also established specific funding envelopes for knowledge transfer research whereas CHSRF focused on knowledge transfer training. Overall, these changes in research policy were particularly significant for practice-based disciplines such as nursing.

The environment for nursing research in Canada has never been more promising than it was in the first decade of the new millennium. For the first time in history, there is adequate funding available, and nursing is in the mainstream and not excluded from eligibility. Nurses in increasing numbers are being trained in Canadian universities to conduct high-quality research into issues of interest to the profession and of benefit to the public. These nurses are equipped to be leaders in interdisciplinary health research.

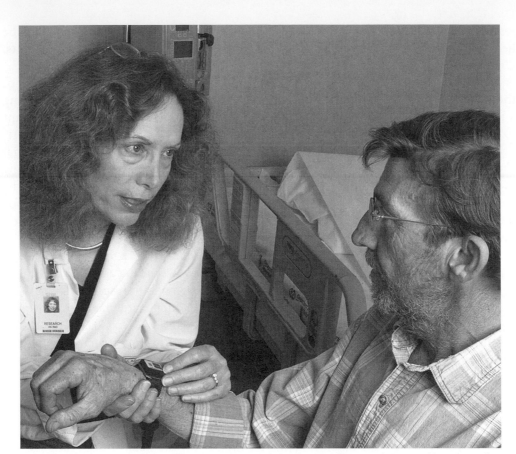

Research participants are selected based on factors such as age, gender, condition, and location. They must then be informed about certain aspects of the proposed research in order to make a decision about participating. That decision, which is written and signed, is known as "informed consent."

RESEARCH AND PRACTICE: BRIDGING THE GAP

The everyday decisions that nurses make are complex and require accurate, reliable information upon which to predict patient, family, and health-system outcomes of specific nursing interventions. Research is the means by which this vital nursing knowledge is generated and validated, but the research process cannot stop with the conduct of research. It also includes dissemination of findings and their use and evaluation. Research utilization is the "use of research as a means of verifying or as a basis for changing nursing practice . . . [and] the purpose of such . . . is to substantiate or improve the quality of nursing practice" (Horsley, 1985, p. 135). Research-based nursing includes both research utilization and the conduct of research to investigate nursing problems.

The suggestion that nursing practice should be research based is not a new one. Florence Nightingale viewed research as an integral part of nursing and believed that nursing practice should be generated from confirmed facts and epidemiological data (Nutting & Dock, 1907). More than 100 years later, the issue of research-based practice is receiving attention from the nursing profession, with more nurses questioning whether their practices are based on science, or whether they are based on ritual, tradition, intuition, or outdated teachings.

Good clinical judgements can be made only when nurses possess the necessary facts. Professional nursing requires that we discard unsubstantiated tradition and allow research evidence to challenge practice. To meet current and future health care needs, nursing practice must not be based purely on beliefs, traditions, and rituals but rather on knowledge that is susceptible to change as a result of new information and new ideas. One source of such new information is research.

Promoting and implementing research-based nursing practice is not a simple task, nor does it rely only on nurses in the clinical area. At the health care system level there are both macro- and micro-level hindrances—costs to the system and agency, and the need for supportive infrastructures—particularly within health care agencies. Within the profession of nursing, there are perceived, if not real, barriers to the development of collaborative partnerships within and across agencies and to the acceptance and integration of innovations in clinical practice.

COSTS OF RESEARCH-BASED NURSING PRACTICE

There are both hidden and visible costs associated with research-based nursing practice. Visible costs include salary for nurse researchers and research staff, computers or other equipment costs, computer time, and consultation fees. Hidden costs are associated with time of researchers, staff, and secretaries applied to reviewing the literature; development of a research proposal or nursing protocol; analysis of the data or evaluation of patient outcomes; written reports; and dissemination of results. As well, there are hidden costs of professional development and change implementation.

RESEARCH-BASED NURSING PRACTICE: AN INVESTMENT

In her review of the economic value of conducting and applying nursing research, Fagin (1982) found that the return on investment from nursing research far exceeded what she cited as acceptable to the investment community. The review demonstrated the cost-effectiveness of primary nursing, innovative staffing plans, research-based patient teaching plans, and nurse-delivered primary care to both home care patients and public school patient populations.

Overall, the benefits of implementing research-based nursing practice can be shown to far outweigh the visible and invisible costs. In a research-friendly environment, staff will begin to question their practice and systematically document the problems of greatest concern. This fosters a sense of accountability and professionalism, which itself leads to increased job satisfaction and lower staff turnover (Hinshaw, 2006). For nurse managers and administrators, research-based nursing practice provides reliable data to describe the effectiveness and significance of nursing interventions or programs, to allocate or reallocate their resources, and to participate in health policy formulation. Research-based nursing practice ensures that the quality and cost-effectiveness of nursing care will be the best possible.

 REFLECTIVE THINKING

Has the face of Canadian nursing research changed over the past 30 years?

COSTS AND BENEFITS

One of the reasons it has been difficult to sway decision makers—especially those in health care agencies—about investing in nurses and the research process is the overriding notion that "worth" or "payoff" is determined by cost-benefit analysis rather than cost-effectiveness analysis. The cost-benefit approach focuses solely on monetary aspects and neglects the essential human and social costs and benefits; it weighs the inherent worth of a program in costs and benefits that are expressed in numerical terms, usually dollars (Fordyce, Mooney, & Russell, 1982). This is the "whether" of decision making: whether the costs are justified by the benefits. Cost-effectiveness analysis is the "how" of decision making; it weighs the relative merit of one program against another, given an already established objective. Outcomes or consequences are not always measured in monetary terms and can include considerations such as preventing death, reducing disability, and improving patient activity levels (Fordyce, Mooney, & Russell, 1982).

In promoting research-based nursing practice, it is imperative that the cost-effectiveness of the process be considered, rather than merely its cost-benefit ratio. Recent attention to outcomes research, both in nursing and health care in general, supports a cost-effectiveness perspective that includes measures of effectiveness (the degree to which an action can accomplish a purpose or help bring about an expected outcome) and efficiency (the ability to accomplish a task within a minimum expenditure of time and effort).

LANDMARK EXAMPLES OF COST-EFFECTIVENESS

A frequently cited meta-analysis that compared patient outcomes resulting from research-based nursing care with those resulting from routine, procedural nursing care validated the effectiveness of research-based care. The analysis showed that not only did more patients in the research-based intervention group have better outcomes than those who received routine nursing care, but also the magnitude of improvement was greater. The results were both statistically and clinically significant (Heater, Becker, & Olson, 1988). The patient-related outcomes that were measured included changes in observed behaviour; changes in cognitive level of understanding; changes in health or normal functioning, such as heart or respiratory rate as compared with a baseline measure; and changes in the manner of relating to self and to others.

A second meta-analysis undertaken by Olson, Heater, and Becker (1990) evaluated the effectiveness of research-based nursing interventions used with children and their parents. Once more it was found that subjects receiving specified research-based nursing interventions benefited more often and to a greater extent than did those receiving standard or routine nursing care. Better patient outcomes in this study included improvement in self-care practices, reduction in anxiety for children and their parents, and increased clinical improvement for premature infants.

Although neither of the meta-analyses included monetary outcomes, it can be argued that these positive patient outcomes resulted in monetary gains. For example, improved clinical outcomes for premature infants would lead to reduced acuity of illness and lower levels of required staffing; increased self-reliance in health behaviours of patients would eventually lead to reduced reliance on costly episodic or emergent care; psychosocial gains could be shown to lead to reduced need for mental illness interventions as well as reduction in social problems, such as family violence and substance abuse. These short- and long-term outcomes could be translated into cost savings for the health care system and patients.

A landmark study by Brooten and her colleagues (1986) demonstrated that, with the care provided by a nurse specialist, low-birth-weight infants could be safely discharged home an average of 11 days earlier, at a cost savings to the health care system of $10,560 (in 1986 US dollars) for each infant. Another study, a clinical trial involving patients with peripheral vascular disease, showed that the group that received "traditional" nursing care had more inpatient days at a higher cost per day than did the experimental group that was on a research-based exercise plan (Ventura et al., 1984). At the end of the 26-week data-collection period, the combined cost of the experimental intervention plus the research project was found to be significantly lower than the cost of traditional care.

Agencies that support research-based nursing practice improve nurses' work satisfaction (Kenneth & Stiesmeyer, 1991). Hinshaw (2006) believes that creation of a research environment serves as a major retention strategy in the clinical setting because it involves nurses. According to Gortner (1986), research-based practitioners learn "the joy of discovery" in their everyday practice (p. 554). When asked which elements were most significant to quality work life, nurses indicated that intellectually challenging work, creative problem solving, and an opportunity to grow and be in touch with new ideas were essential (Attridge & Callahan, 1987). Additionally, Attridge and Callahan found that nurses tend to equate power with their ability to apply knowledge. Research becomes powerful when the knowledge generated is utilized. Enhanced power increases nurses' credibility, supports their autonomy, and ideally encourages a more balanced relationship between nurses and physicians. If research-based nursing practice improves satisfaction, and thereby reduces turnover, it reduces costs for the institution and improves the efficiency of the health care system.

NURSING: THE INVISIBLE PROFESSION

The term "minimum data set" (MDS) refers to standardized data that are extracted from all hospital patient records. Included here are things like admitting diagnosis, surgeries performed, complications, discharge diagnosis, cause of death, and so on. If these sound very medical in nature, the reader has hit on the problem. None of the variables in the MDS are nursing variables. None of the nursing problems, nursing interventions, or nursing contributions to patient care is included in the MDS. In spite of efforts over the past two decades to rectify this situation, no real change has occurred. This creates a significant problem when trying to document the impact of nursing on patient outcomes and makes discussions with policymakers about nursing research difficult (Werley, Devine, Zorn, Ryan, & Westra, 1991; Huston, 1999). Whereas mortality rates are easily compiled for any patient grouping, they are hard to relate to particular nursing care variables. When decision makers ask, "What difference does nursing make to the outcome?" the answer is difficult to produce.

In the past, nurses have avoided using MDS outcome measures such as mortality and morbidity in relation to nursing care, feeling that these variables are mainly affected by medical care rather than nursing. Recently, however, some nurse researchers have looked at the effect of nurse staffing patterns, intensity of nursing, and professional levels of nurses on outcome measures such as mortality rates and have found startling results. Mortality is indeed affected by nursing care. Tourangeau et al. (2007) found that lower patient mortality rates in Ontario hospitals were linked to increased levels of nursing preparation (staffing with more registered nurses and baccalaureate-prepared nurses) and also linked to greater use of care maps or patient care protocols. These results support the value of nursing care. Having results about the outcomes of nursing care will enhance communication with policymakers and health care administrators.

MEASURING OUTCOMES

In the past, nursing has experienced limitations in clearly defining and measuring outcomes, monetary or otherwise. A glance through the nursing research literature reveals that research on nursing interventions rarely addresses the efficacy of a given intervention—that is, its capacity to produce specific effects. Also, the term "nursing outcome" as it has been used is not particularly useful and should be replaced with "patient outcome" (Shamian, 1992). Debate about this and the development of nursing-sensitive outcome measures has centred on the issue of the impact of other disciplines' interventions on nursing interventions and patient and system outcomes. Any single discipline's approach is too narrow and limited to address the wide variety of structures and interventions that influence outcomes (Shamian, 1992). It is contradictory for nurses to advocate a holistic perspective while practising from an exclusionist point of view. Undoubtedly, the public interest is best served in multidisciplinary, holistic approaches, where the impact of multiple interventions and providers can be studied. Nursing must be a central part of that movement. For this to happen, however, nurses must agree on the major outcomes relevant to nursing.

The International Council of Nurses (ICN) defines nursing-sensitive outcomes as "changes in health status upon which nursing care has had a direct influence." The type of patient outcomes that are nursing-sensitive indicators include patient complications (such as urinary tract infection, nosocomial infection, pressure ulcer, deep vein thrombosis) and morbidity; surgical complications (such as wound infection and metabolic imbalances); and health system indicators (such as length of stay) (ICN, 2008).

Despite its limitations, nursing research has demonstrated the effectiveness of nursing care in relation to patient satisfaction. It has also demonstrated that high-quality research-based care can be delivered at reduced cost to an agency even though an explicit cost-benefit analysis is not done. The following three major categories of effectiveness outcome indicators have been used in nursing research (Marek & Lang, 1992; Shamian, 1992):

1. *Patient-related indicators*—physiological, psychosocial, and functional measures (behaviour, knowledge, symptom control, and resolution of nursing diagnoses or nursing problems)
2. *Consumer- and environment-related indicators*—quality of life, home functioning, family and caregiver strain, goal attainment, and patient satisfaction
3. *Organization-related indicators*—service utilization and safety

WORK ENVIRONMENT

A supportive work environment is necessary for research utilization to occur in an organization (Kenrick & Luker, 1996; Gifford, Davies, Edwards, Griffin, & Lybanon, 2007). This includes the necessary infrastructure to promote easy access to research results. Infrastructure can be defined as those structures, policies, and facilities in a health care agency that support specific activities, such as research and utilization of findings in practice. Basic organizational elements supportive of research activities include key administrative positions that include responsibility for research leadership within the agency and provide liaison with academic nurse researchers who may be employed by universities. Other essential elements include services (space, secretarial assistance, computers), time (release time), communication (channels and a climate to facilitate two-way dialogue between researchers and consumers), and consultation (methods, design, and grantsmanship). Research promotion activities may include presenting research findings, publishing a research newsletter, consulting on research proposal writing, promoting or providing research education, and liaising between the staff and the research program (Gething & Leelarthaepin, 2000).

Consultation within an agency relies on all other elements being in place. For successful implementation of research-based practice, the services of consultants may be required in the areas of content, statistics, research design, and grantsmanship. These consultants may be shared among the many disciplines involved in patient care within the agency.

Clinical nurse scientists, if present in a health care agency, can create an organizational environment that supports the conducting and use of nursing research. According to Knafl, Bevis, and Kirchoff (1987), a clinical nurse scientist is a doctorally prepared nurse employed by a health care agency to foster and coordinate nursing research using research and grantsmanship skills, an astute understanding of nursing practice, and leadership abilities. The role has been created to bring nursing research and practice into closer alignment. Positions for clinical nurse scientists can vary greatly from one agency to another. Some are hired by the agency for particular positions. In other cases, the scientist may be a faculty member who is jointly appointed to the clinical agency for the purpose of conducting research in the agency. The University of Toronto has been the recipient of several endowed chairs in nursing research, including the first in Canada that allowed a senior nurse researcher to set up a research program in maternal–child nursing within one of the major academic health centres in Toronto. These positions are proving to be highly successful partnerships between academic nursing research and the clinical setting.

Eagle, Fortnum, Price, and Scruton (1990) describe the clinical nurse scientists' responsibilities as the following:

1. Education of general staff, educators, and management nurses in the areas of research design, methodology, data analysis, critical appraisal of research studies, and the value of translating valid research findings into new clinical practice
2. Leadership of the nursing research committee and implementation of its terms of reference
3. Consultation on all phases of the development of educational research, clinical research, administrative research, internal projects, grant proposals for external funding, and on the development of nurses' skills in the areas of design, measurement, data analysis, and research finding reports (written or oral)
4. Liaison with appropriate groups (senior nursing administrators, nursing unit managers, and clinicians) to discuss current nursing issues and develop potential research questions

For over 20 years, researchers and administrators have been describing a type of work environment in which nurses thrive, referred to as the magnet hospital, one that attracts nurses to work in it (Scott, Sochalski, & Aiken, 1999; Hinshaw, 2006). Excellent nurses can be recruited and retained. The quality of care in magnet hospitals is excellent and the work environment satisfying and harmonious. One of the reasons for quality care is that staff nurses are engaged in shaping research-based practice. Hospitals with magnet hospital characteristics are located in urban Canadian regions and in northern and rural regions (Smith, Tallman, & Kelly, 2006).

PROFESSIONAL ROLES IN THE PRACTICE OF NURSING

PARTNERSHIPS

The research process does not end with completion of the study or dissemination of results. It also involves assessment of findings for clinical application, utilization of findings to improve nursing care, and evaluation of the clinical outcomes of research-based practice. Who is responsible for this complex set of activities? In addition to researchers, there is the need for nurses in administration, education, and clinical practice roles to have specific and critical responsibilities that may be best actualized in collaborative partnerships. Although interdisciplinary collaboration is often desirable, harmonious partnerships within nursing are the crucial first steps.

ADMINISTRATORS

At the senior management level, nursing administrators are responsible for ensuring that the corporate philosophy is integrated into daily operations. They actualize a philosophy that places value on research-based nursing practice by setting nursing policies and procedures that are based on nursing research findings, developing job descriptions for staff that include research responsibilities, and making infrastructure support available within and beyond the agency.

At the operational level, nursing unit managers anchor the organizational efforts for research utilization. They are responsible for establishing a climate that encourages inquiry and change. Such a climate is established by identifying clinical problems, organizing release time for staff nurses to read and critique research, assisting with the selection and critique of studies, and encouraging application and evaluation of valid and reliable findings. Other supportive nurse manager activities include managing resources, appraising staff performance, networking, and collaborating.

Administrators and unit managers must work together to create a research environment. Their collaborative efforts can ensure that

- nurses feel free to question practice;
- consultation is available to support their efforts;
- time is provided for research activities and professional development;
- agency resources are allocated to research-based nursing practice;
- opportunities are provided to incorporate research findings into practice and evaluate clinical outcomes;
- staff members who undertake nursing research receive due recognition for their endeavours.

Many staff nurses do not perceive that they have a supportive research climate in their agencies, but identify such support and commitment as critical to facilitating nursing research. In a multiple-case study of eight clinical units of a tertiary care setting, Pepler et al. (2005) examined research utilization (RU) on the units, using a variety of sources and perspectives. They found unit culture to be the principal factor, with themes within the cultures linking to RU. "Unit culture was defined as the beliefs, values, and practice norms on a given unit" (Pepler et al., 2005, p. 73). It was made up of several interdependent factors, including the level of understanding of research and RU, work and communication patterns, the decision-making pattern, and the process of facilitation on the unit, as well as characteristics of the nurses. Elements of the unit culture that were linked to high RU were the belief that nursing practice can be built on research, the learning environment, level of questioning, and critical inquiry; mutual respect and interdisciplinarity; a sense of unit identity; pride in expertise and a desire to share it; and an orientation toward goals and future achievements. In addition, leadership was linked to RU, including the valuing of and support for the use of research.

EDUCATORS

Other partners in research-based nursing practice are nursing educators, those who teach in schools of nursing, and those who instruct in the clinical area. University faculties are the primary source of nurse researchers, yet these academics have not always collaborated with practitioners in planning and carrying out their work. It makes sense that effective partnerships between these two groups will surely produce the best, most relevant results. Team-building for research must be a priority both within nursing and among disciplines. Within nursing, joint appointments can be an effective way of promoting collaboration, as they give each group the opportunity to become familiar with each other's potential contribution to research and patient care.

Unit-based clinical instructors, whose responsibility is continuing education and in-service education for nursing staff, may not share the same sense of alienation that faculty educators experience. However, they do face the challenge of encouraging staff nurses to incorporate nursing research into their practice. How can this be accomplished? It has been noted that the major reason nurses do not apply research findings in clinical practice is that the unit culture does not support them to do so (Pepler et al., 2005). Clinical educators can have a significant role in offering programs designed to enhance or impart the framework and skills required to utilize nursing research and support the nursing department's philosophy and objectives.

ADVANCED PRACTICE NURSES

Advanced practice nursing (APN) is a term used to describe an advanced level of nursing practice that extends the scope of practice. Clinical nurse specialists, clinical nurse educators, and nurse practitioners are all APNs. According to the CNA (2002), the characteristics of advanced nursing practice include the following:

- *is expert and specialized practice grounded in knowledge that comes from nursing theory and other theoretical foundations, experience and research;*

- *involves the deliberate, purposeful and integrated use of in-depth nursing knowledge, research and clinical expertise. It also involves integration of knowledge from other disciplines into the practice of nursing;*
- *requires a depth and breadth of knowledge that enables the nurse to provide an ever-increasing range of strategies to meet the complex needs of clients;*
- *includes the ability to explain the theoretical, empirical, ethical and experiential foundations of nursing practice;*
- *contributes to the understanding and development of evidence-informed nursing knowledge through involvement in research and the evaluation and utilization of relevant research findings; influences the practice of nurses by facilitating the integration of research-based knowledge into practice;*
- *involves planning, coordinating, implementing and evaluating programs to meet client needs through partnerships and intersectoral collaboration;*
- *involves the ability to critically analyze and influence health policy;*
- *reflects substantial autonomy and independence, with a high level of accountability.*

The difficulties that APNs experience in meeting the research expectations of their roles are well documented. Their greatest constraint is time. Gortner (1986) identifies the need for a high degree of organizational support for research and fulfillment of the nursing research responsibilities of the CNS role, as well as developing partnerships with staff nurses and managers.

A vitally important player in the research partnership is the staff nurse. Staff nurses may raise questions from practice that provide impetus for research studies (Kirchoff, 1991). They are in an excellent position to collaborate with researchers in nursing and other disciplines and implement changes in practice that will have a positive impact on the quality, efficacy, and cost of health care (Alcock, Carroll, & Goodman, 1990). Successful collaboration between nursing researchers and staff nurses requires that they meet on common ground to establish research priorities leading to meaningful and applicable outcomes. The way to begin to develop this type of collaboration is to create opportunities for staff nurses to be contributors to ongoing nursing research endeavours. Involving staff nurses in research activities has been found to increase their attitude toward research, which in turn, increases their research utilization (Tramner, Lochhaus-Gertach, & Lam, 2002).

RESEARCH-MINDEDNESS: IMPLEMENTING RESEARCH IN NURSING PRACTICE

We are in an era in which research is visible to us every day. In Canada, the federal government provides an unprecedented level of financial support for research, and universities demand high research productivity from academic staff. In health care, government ministries promote research, health care agencies support research departments, nursing faculties have made great strides in the development of nursing research, and students are exposed to research throughout their educational process. Why, then, are the results of research still seldom reflected in nursing practice?

Part of the problem may be that most nurses are unsure about the applicability of published research findings in their practice. They do not know when research findings are ready to be used in their particular setting. Nurses are perfectionists, with a tendency to look for absolute proof of the facts before considering research findings useable (Wood, 1992). Applying research findings in nursing practice usually requires adopting an innovation such as a new idea, a different way of thinking about an issue, and a change in behaviour.

Some activities that might facilitate the research process include the following:

- Funding key research positions
- Creating institutional infrastructures, including resources needed to access summarized evidence
- Encouraging and assisting nurses to attend practice-based research workshops and conferences
- Providing continuing education courses to assist nurses in critiquing research
- Creating a reward system within the agency for research utilization in practice
- Promoting collaborative efforts between agency personnel and other health care agencies or educational institutions
- Establishing a means for nurses to access research reports relevant to their practice
- Promoting demonstration projects that illustrate the cost-effectiveness of changing from a traditional, intuitively based practice to one that is research-based
- Ensuring that research utilization is a role expectation for all nursing positions (management, educational, and clinical) and that it is reinforced in job descriptions, agency policy, and the institution's philosophy of nursing

Diagnosing barriers and planning and implementing strategies to overcome them are challenges. The first challenge is to demonstrate the cost-effectiveness of nursing research and to justify the allocation of resources and personnel to create the necessary infrastructures. The second challenge is to reduce the time gap between when knowledge is developed and when it is used. The third challenge is to create agency infrastructures that will support the transformation of nursing practice from a ritual base to a research base. Efforts to address these challenges require partnerships among practitioners, researchers, administrators, and disciplines.

CRITICAL THINKING QUESTIONS

1. What is a magnet hospital?
2. What is a minimum data set (MDS)?
3. Is the MDS useful for nursing?
4. What was the significance of the 1971 national nursing research conference in Canada?
5. What is the benefit of research-based nursing practice?

WEB SITES

Canadian Journal of Nursing Research: http://cjnr.mcgill.ca/

REFERENCES

Alcock, D., Carroll, G., & Goodman, M. (1990). Staff nurses' perceptions of factors influencing their role in research. *Canadian Journal of Nursing Research, 22*(4), 7–18.

Attridge, C., & Callahan, M. (1987). *Women in women's work: An exploratory study of nurses' perspective of quality work environments.* Victoria, BC: University of Victoria, Faculty of Human and Social Development.

Brooten, D., Kumar, S., Brown, L., Butts, P., Finkler, S., Bakewell-Sachs, S., Gibbons, A., & Delivoria-Papadopoulos, M. (1986). A randomized clinical trial and home follow-up of very-low-birth-weight infants. *New England Journal of Medicine, 315*(15), 934–939.

Canadian Nurses Association (CNA). (2002). Position statement on Advanced Nursing Practice. Retrieved on February 4, 2008, from http://www.cna-nurses.ca/CNA/documents/pdf/publications/PS60_Advanced_Nursing_Practice_June_2002_e.pdf.

Eagle, J., Fortnum, D., Price, P., & Scruton, J. (1990). Developing a rationale and recruitment plan for a nurse researcher. *Canadian Journal of Nursing Administration, 3*(2), 5–10.

Fagin, C. (1982). The economic value of nursing research. *American Journal of Nursing, 12*(12), 1844–1849.

Fordyce, J. D., Mooney, G. H., & Russell, E. M. (1982). Economic analysis in health care. *Health Bulletin, 39*(10), 21–38.

Gething, L., & Leelarthaepin, B. (2000). Strategies for promoting research participation among nurses employed as academics in the university sector. *Nurse Education Today, 20*(2), 147–154.

Gifford, W., Davies, B., Edwards, N., Griffin, P., & Lybanon, V. (2007). Managerial leadership for nurses' use of research evidence: An integrative review of the literature. *Worldviews on Evidence-Based Nursing, 4*(3), 126–145.

Gortner, S. (1986). Research for a practice profession. In L. Nichols (Ed.), *Perspectives on nursing theory* (pp. 549–555). Toronto: Little, Brown.

Gottlieb, L. (2007). Canadian nursing scholarship: A time to celebrate, a time to stand guard. *CJNR Editorial, 39*(1).

Griffin, A. (1971). Nursing research in Canadian universities. *National conference on research in nursing practice.* Ottawa: School of Nursing, University of Ottawa.

Health Canada. (2006). *Nursing issues: Research.* Retrieved on February 1, 2008, from http://www.hc-sc.gc.ca/hcs-sss/pubs/nurs-infirm/onp-bpsi-fs-if/2006-res_e.html#fn_3.

Heater, B., Becker, A., & Olson, R. (1988). Nursing interventions and client outcomes: A meta-analysis of studies. *Nursing Research, 37*(5), 303–307.

Hinshaw, A. S. (2006). Keeping patients safe: A collaboration among nurse administrators and researchers. *Nursing Administration Quarterly, 30*(4), 309–320.

Horsley, J. (1985). Using research in practice: The current context. *Western Journal of Nursing Research, 7*(1), 135–139.

Huston, C. J. (1999). Outcomes measurement in healthcare: New implications for professional nursing practice. *Nursing Case Management, 4*(4), 188–194.

ICN. (2008). *Nursing matters.* Retrieved on February 17, 2008, from http://www.icn.ch/matters_indicators.htm.

Imai, H. R. (1971). Association and research activities. In *National conference on research in nursing practice.* Ottawa: School of Nursing, University of Ottawa.

Jeans, M. E. (2005). Shared leadership for nursing research. *Nursing Leadership, 18*(1), 20–23.

Jeans, M. E. (2008). *Nursing research in Canada: A status report*. Retrieved on October 19, 2009, from http://www.chsrf.ca.

Kenneth, H., & Stiesmeyer, J. (1991). Strategies for involving staff in nursing research. *Applied Nursing Research, 10*(2), 103–107.

Kenrick, M., & Luker, K. A. (1996). An exploration of the influence of managerial factors on research utilization in district nursing practice. *Journal of Advanced Nursing, 23*, 697–704.

Kirchoff, K. (1991). Who is responsible for research utilization? *Heart and Lung, 20*(3), 308–309.

Knafl, K., Bevis, M., & Kirchoff, K. (1987). Research activities of clinical nurse researchers. *Nursing Research, 36*(4), 249–252.

Marek, K. D., & Lang, N. M. (1992). Nursing-sensitive outcomes. In *Papers from the Nursing Minimum Data Set Conference* (pp. 100–120). Ottawa: Canadian Nurses Association.

Morse, J. M., & Field, P. A. (1995). *Qualitative research methods for health professionals.*. Thousand Oaks, CA: Sage.

Nutting, M. A., & Dock, L. L. (1907). *A history of nursing*. New York: Putnam & Sons.

Olson, R., Heater, B., & Becker, A. (1990). A meta-analysis of the effects of nursing interventions on children and parents. *Maternal Child Nursing, 15*(2), 104–108.

Pepler, C., Edgar, L., Frisch, S., Rennick, J., Swidzinski, M., White, C., Brown, T., & Gross, J. (2005). Unit culture and research-based nursing practice in acute care. *Canadian Journal of Nursing Research, 37*(3), 66–85.

Poole, P. E. (1971). Research activities conducted or sponsored by government or service agencies. In *National conference on research in nursing practice*. Ottawa: School of Nursing, University of Ottawa.

Pringle, D. (2006). Realities of Canadian nursing research. In M. McIntyre, E. Thomlinson, & C. McDonald (Eds.), *Realities in Canadian nursing* (2nd ed.), (pp. 262–281). Philadelphia: Lippincott, Williams & Wilkins.

Richards, L., & Morse, J. M. (2006). *README FIRST for a user's guide to qualitative methods*. Thousand Oaks, CA: Sage.

Scott, J., Sochalski, J., & Aiken, L. (1999). Review of magnet hospital research: Findings and implications for professional nursing practice. *Journal of Nursing Administration, 29*(1), 9–19.

Shamian, J. (1992). Response to K.D. Marek's and N.M. Lang's paper on nursing sensitive outcomes. In *Papers from the Nursing Minimum Data Set Conference* (pp. 121–126). Ottawa: Canadian Nurses Association.

Smith, H., Tallman, R., & Kelly, K. (2006). Magnet hospital characteristics and northern Canadian nurses' job satisfaction. *Canadian Journal of Nursing Leadership, 19*(3), 73–86.

Symons, T. H. B. (1975). *To know ourselves: The report of the Commission on Canadian Studies*. (Vols. I–II). Ottawa: Association of Universities and Colleges of Canada.

Tourangeau, A., Doran, D., McGillis-Hall, L., O'Brien Pallas, L., Pringle, D., Tu, J., & Cranley, L. (2007). Impact of hospital nursing care on 30-day mortality for acute medical patients. *Journal of Advanced Nursing, 57*(1), 32–44.

Tramner, J. E., Lochhaus-Gertach, J., & Lam, M. (2002). The effect of staff nurse participation in a clinical nursing research project on attitude towards, access to, support of and use of research in the acute care setting. *Canadian Journal of Nursing Leadership, 15*(1), 18–26.

Ventura, M., Young, D., Feldman, M., Pastore, P., Pikula, S., & Yates, M. (1984). Cost savings as an indicator of successful nursing intervention. *Nursing Research, 34*(1), 50–53.

Wood, M. (1992). Shaping practice through research. *Clinical Nursing Research, 1*(2), 123–126.

Werley, H. H., Devine, E. C., Zorn, C. R., Ryan, P., & Westra, B. L. (1991). The nursing minimum data set: Abstraction tool for standardized, comparable, essential data. *American Journal of Public Health, 81*(4), 421–426.

Knowledge Translation and Evidence-Informed Practice

Janice Lander and Marilynn J. Wood

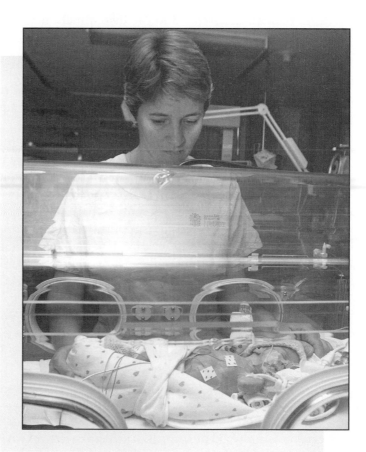

Moncton Hospital neonatal clinical resource nurse Delcia LeBreton and others in the department provide care for at-risk infants using the latest incubators and other equipment.

LEARNING OBJECTIVES

- Describe evidence-informed practice and understand its significance for nursing.
- Understand the process of innovation and diffusion and barriers to use of evidence.
- Describe stakeholders in evidence-informed practice and their roles.
- Understand the factors that lead to clinical decision-making errors.
- Distinguish filtered from unfiltered evidence and know how to locate filtered evidence.

In recent years, much has been written about the importance of increasing the use of research in nursing practice because research is needed to advance knowledge and improve patient care. Considerable attention also has been given to problems and inadequacies related to the dissemination and application of research findings in practice. Attempts to advance "evidence-informed" practice have increased in recent years in all health professions. Many factors contribute to this state of affairs (see Chapter 8), but the central issue is the necessity to create the research-minded-ness among nurses that would make utilization of research findings a natural part of practice. This is a complex issue that must be addressed at all levels of nursing practice.

In the past, for research to be incorporated into the everyday practice of nurses, it had to be part of their knowledge base. Nurses were expected to know almost every-thing they needed to know to give good care. A "good nurse" was one who always knew what to do in any situation. Nurses were expected to learn everything they needed to know during their basic programs. What they learned in the classroom was put into practice through service they supplied to their training institutions. With this combi-nation of instruction and practice, most senior nursing students were expected to take charge of a hospital unit and function almost as well as veteran nurses. However, an explosion of knowledge occurring in the past 30 years has made us aware of the hope-lessness of trying to acquire all knowledge to provide care. Research and technological development make yesterday's knowledge obsolete. Nowadays, nurses strive to develop skills for lifelong learning, including skills needed to find new knowledge and evaluate its quality.

WHAT IS EVIDENCE-INFORMED PRACTICE?

Using the best evidence to plan and provide care for individuals is what we mean by evidence-informed practice. Best evidence refers to what we know about the efficacy and safety of particular therapies or management strategies. Best evidence supports the use of one therapy or strategy over others. Evidence-informed practice utilizes not only evi-dence from research but also evidence stemming from clinical practice and from patient preferences (Blizz-Holtz, 2007).

EVIDENCE-INFORMED PRACTICE: A GOAL FOR NURSING

Striving to achieve evidence-informed practice is a major goal for nursing, one that is expressed in provincial and territorial standards of nursing practice as well as the Canadian Nurses Association *Code of Ethics.* All Canadian nursing professional associations list it somewhere on their Web sites as a priority, yet there is some lack of clarity in our understanding of what it is. We have trouble agreeing on the right terms for the processes associated with evidence-informed practice. The terms "knowledge transfer," "knowledge translation," and "research utilization" are sometimes used synonymously with evidence-informed practice. Research utilization seems to be too narrow, as some knowledge that could be used in practice is not research-based. Knowledge transfer and translation give the impression of processes involving passive or compliant and uninformed audiences. Evidence-informed practice is more complex than one might think, since practice involves clinical decision making, which is prone to bias.

THE EVIDENCE-INFORMED PRACTICE MOVEMENT

Although the term "evidence-informed practice" is recent, the issue has been around since the eighteenth century (Goodman, 2003). Florence Nightingale was the first nurse to advocate for a type of practice that today would be referred to as evidence-informed (LoBiondo-Wood & Haber, 2006, p. 11). Nevertheless, the 1970s are regarded as the beginning of the modern evidence-informed practice movement. This was the time when a large nursing research utilization project was carried out in the United States (Conduct and Utilization of Research in Nursing [CURN]) (Horsely, Crane, & Bingle, 1978). However, it was a Scottish physician by the name of Archie Cochrane who is regarded as a pioneer of the modern evidence-informed practice movement. He observed that health care providers were not able to gain access to evidence needed to provide good care. Cochrane was subsequently funded by the National Health Service in the United Kingdom to make evidence accessible. He believed that preparing reviews and summaries of research in all areas of health care and making them readily available would put evidence within reach of practitioners. This led to the formation of the Cochrane Collaboration, an affiliation of skilled clinician-researchers who generate reviews of research in various areas of health care and maintain them in databases that are made available to practitioners and the public. Nursing in Canada has been influenced by the Cochrane Collaboration and has been urged to become an evidence-informed profession (Estabrooks, 1998).

The evidence-informed practice movement has been embraced by many practice disciplines, including nursing, and by government agencies. The Canadian government has made a significant investment in evidence-informed practice by creating new funding agencies that have an emphasis on translating or transferring knowledge from the researcher to the policymaker (see Chapter 8 for details). The government has also invested in technology to support evidence-informed practice. These inducements have been effective in persuading the Canadian health care system and health care professions, including nursing, to adopt evidence-informed practice.

SPREAD OF NEW KNOWLEDGE: INNOVATION AND DIFFUSION

Rogers (2003) provides a useful framework for viewing the process of research utilization. He refers to the new knowledge generated from research as the "innovation" and the process of implementing the innovation as "diffusion." Diffusion of an innovation (new knowledge) occurs in five stages: awareness (or knowledge), persuasion, decision, implementation, and adoption (Rogers, 2003). According to Rogers, diffusion is a process of moving an innovation from an idea to a reality in practice. The process starts with the discovery of the innovation, and then looks at the communication channel or means by which the innovation is shared. Another element is the time it takes for an individual to move from the point of discovery to the adoption or rejection of the innovation. Another factor is the social system involving the particular set of interrelated units that jointly engage in problem solving to accomplish a common goal: implementing the innovation. This complex process occurs every time a potential adopter considers a new idea, and it includes forming an attitude, whether positive or negative, about the idea; experimenting with the idea; and finally, choosing to adopt or reject it. It is estimated that it takes 8 to 15 years from creation of new knowledge until it is used in practice (Dobbins, Ciliska, Estabrooks, & Hayward, 2005). The development of one innovation (penicillin) and its diffusion illustrate this complex process (Box 9.1).

BARRIERS TO UTILIZATION OF EVIDENCE

Not having access to evidence is a significant barrier for evidence-informed nursing practice. Most rural nurses reported having no access to evidence (O'Lynn et al., 2009) or lacked skills for finding evidence (Winters et al., 2007). Clinical nurses have difficulty finding relevant studies (Pank, Rostron, & Stenhouse, 1984; Haughey, 1988; Funk, Champagne, Wiese, & Tornquist, 1991) if they look for them at all (Pravikoff, Tanner, & Pierce, 2005). They find that much of the literature includes findings with little relevance to the clinical situation, or if relevant, studies are presented in an unusable form. On the other hand, advance practice nurses do use the research literature for decision making (Profetto-McGrath, Smith, Hugo, Taylor, & El Hajj, 2007). One of the problems with the primary research literature is that researchers often present findings in tentative terms and discuss results as they relate to theory and the need for further inquiry. They may use standard research jargon and emphasize methodological or statistical issues instead of implications for practice. Although sometimes appropriate among researchers, this style of communication provides little on which practitioners can base their care. To overcome this barrier, it is suggested that researchers make the practice setting the focus of their scientific inquiry and disseminate their findings to practitioners in a comprehensible and

BOX 9.1	The Spread of an Innovation

The story of Sir Alexander Fleming's 1928 discovery of the first antibiotic agent, penicillin, is fairly well known. However, the story of how penicillin came to be used is not.

During World War I, Fleming noticed that many soldiers died from relatively minor wounds that became infected. He began to search for a means of preventing such deaths—an antibacterial. Fleming, bemoaning the extra work he'd had to do since his lab assistant's departure, considered a stack of Petri dishes that had yet to be cleaned. There was something strange about one dish, however. A mould had grown on the dish and had killed the *Staphylococcus aureus* that had been growing there before.

Fleming isolated the "mould juice," naming it "penicillin," and proceeded to publish papers and give lectures about its virtues. No one seemed to care. Fleming received no fame and fortune for his discovery. People could understand cleaning and sterilizing a wound, but injecting people with mould to cure infection did not make sense. Fortunately, one man listened.

A former student of Fleming's, Cecil Paine, was intrigued by Fleming's paper and began to experiment with penicillin. Although the experiments worked—he successfully treated two cases of eye infection—Paine did not disseminate his results. He did, however, discuss his work with Professor Howard Florey.

In 1938, Florey was conducting bacteriology research when Fleming's work was again brought to his attention. Florey was rather indifferent, but his colleague Ernst Chain was fascinated by penicillin. The two, in their experiments, established both that penicillin could combat infections and that it was safe to use on humans. The scientific community began to take notice. Then World War II broke out; once again, wounded soldiers would die of infections. In 1941, Florey and an assistant moved to the United States from Europe in order to continue the research and development of penicillin.

There, they developed a method by which penicillin could be produced in far greater quantities. By the end of the war, enough penicillin was produced per year to treat seven million patients. Deaths due to infection dropped dramatically among soldiers, while hospital patients were quickly and effectively cured of ailments like strep throat, scarlet fever, and various venereal diseases.

Fleming was finally acknowledged when in 1943, along with Howard Florey, he was knighted and later, in 1945, when he received the Nobel Prize alongside Florey and Chain. Though he is widely credited with penicillin's discovery, it took Florey and Chain to turn his discovery into a safe, usable medicine.

The chain of discovery, dissemination, uptake of knowledge, and development of production methods took nearly 30 years.

relevant manner. A number of professional organizations have taken the initiative to produce summarized evidence for practitioners. They provide clear statements of research findings that are relevant to clinical practice, often referred to as *the clinical bottom line*.

The persuasion phase of a new innovation or knowledge can be influenced by many factors (Dobbins et al., 2005). They can be grouped into four categories related to the innovation, the organization, the environment, and the individual. Any of these factors or combinations of them can determine if the innovation is adopted or not. Communication has been cited as a major barrier (King, Barnard, & Hoehn, 1981; Chambers, 1989; Bock, 1990; Repko, 1990). Other barriers to research utilization include cost and time constraints, negative attitudes toward research, the quality and relevance of the research, lack of time to read and implement research, and a variety of organizational and workplace limitations (Kajermo, Nordstrom, Krusebrant, Bjorvell, & Nilsson-Kajermo, 1998; Carroll et al., 1997; Karkos & Peters, 2006). Hospital policy, policy and procedure manuals, and the opinions of other professionals also affect research use. Brett (1987) found that it was perceived rather than actual hospital policy about research-based nursing

TABLE 9.1	What Influences the Adoption of New Knowledge?

CATEGORY	CHARACTERISTIC
Innovation or Knowledge	• The innovation is an improvement • It is acceptable to nurses • It is easy to understand • It can be tried on a small scale first • It can be evaluated
Organization	• Structure of the organization (size, number of departments, number of managers, number of services) • The value the organization places on research • Success of communication • Support of research by leadership and resources
Environment	• Location—urban or rural • Financial resources of the region • Peer pressure to adopt the knowledge • Degree of competition for resources • The reputation of the organization compared to others in the region
Individual (the nurse)	• Attitudes to research • Ability to make changes to practice

Source: Dobbins, M., Ciliska, D., Estabrooks, C., & Hayward, S. (2005). Changing nursing practice in an organization. In A. DiCenso, G. Guyatt, & D. Ciliska (Eds.), *Evidence-based nursing: A guide to clinical practice.* St. Louis, MO: Mosby.

practice that influenced the adoption of innovations among her sample of nurses. Policy and procedure manuals that support the use of research findings are reviewed and revised frequently and substantiated with research references.

Negative opinions or perceptions from other health care colleagues deter nurses' passing through the persuasion stage (Alcock, Carroll, & Goodman, 1990; RNABC, 1993). Nurses may perceive that they lack authority and do not have the administrative support to change nursing practice. Whether or not this is the case, it is the perception that inhibits adoption of innovations. The factors influencing adoption of knowledge are summarized in Table 9.1.

Using knowledge generated from research is generally not a natural element of everyday nursing practice. Although nurses agree that they need information to make good decisions about patient care, the most often used source of information is not evidence from research, but rather consultation with colleagues (Pravikoff et al., 2005) or experience (Estabrooks, 1998). Nurses with responsibility for promoting research-based nursing practice may find it helpful to address issues concerning the availability of research-based knowledge to practising nurses, the ability of nurses to read and interpret research findings, the credibility of the research, the relevance of the findings to practice, and the support for applying them in practice. The principles of research utilization can be found in Box 9.2.

BOX 9.2   Principles of Research Utilization

1. Research utilization depends on the interest, commitment, and expertise of nurses in all areas and cannot be achieved by any one individual working in isolation.
2. Success of research utilization requires that it be proactive, deliberate, and systematic, addressing the process of adopting innovation.
3. Research-utilization frameworks provide guides for nursing practice, research, and educational and administrative systems.
4. Relevant research-utilization frameworks include phases aimed at identifying the problem, critically reviewing the literature, translating findings to practice, implementing the new practice, and evaluating the outcome.

CANADIAN RESEARCH FOCUS

Estabrooks, C. (1999). The conceptual structure of research utilization. *Research in Nursing & Health, 22*(3), 203–216.

Estabrooks, C., Thompson, D., Lovely, J., & Hofmeyer, A. (2006). A guide to knowledge translation theory. *The Journal of Continuing Education in the Health Professions, 26*, 25–36.

Estabrooks (1999) surveyed Alberta nurses to determine how much they used research and what influenced the extent of their research use. The model tested by Estabrooks established three kinds of research use: (1) direct or instrumental, (2) indirect or conceptual, and (3) persuasive or symbolic. Instrumental use involves the direct application of the research in a form such as a protocol or care map. Conceptual use refers to a situation in which research changes people's thinking, even though it may not affect their practice, whereas persuasive use is political in nature and tries to influence policy or practice. Estabrooks identified the following characteristics of the practitioner that significantly influenced overall research utilization: a positive attitude toward research, the number of in-services attended, and a willingness to change strongly held beliefs. She also found that nurses used experiential knowledge to a far greater extent than they used research in their practice. Estabrooks has also analyzed the history of knowledge translation and the theories that have been developed to explain it (Estabrooks et al., 2006).

STAKEHOLDERS IN BEST PRACTICE

Nurses and other health care providers are not the only stakeholders in evidence-informed practice. Manufacturers, policymakers, media, and the public are also stakeholders.

BUSINESS AND MANUFACTURING

In health care, new knowledge often means that new products and drugs will become available for the treatment or improvement of health. One of the earliest stages of achieving best practice, then, is transferring knowledge from the research laboratory to the manufacturer so that products can be developed, marketed, and distributed. However, simply having products available does not guarantee use. It takes the combined efforts of many stakeholders.

In recent years, the pharmaceutical industry has taken an active role in knowledge transfer. Once a product has been developed, the pharmaceutical industry invests heavily in advertising so that the product will be used (and profits made). The target audience is typically physicians, pharmacists, and hospitals. Increasingly, pharmaceutical companies have been advertising directly to the public as a strategy for indirectly influencing physicians to prescribe their products.

EVIDENCE-INFORMED POLICYMAKING

One outcome of the evidence-informed practice movement is the evidence-informed policy movement. A goal of the health care system is making sure that practice is the best that can be achieved with safe, effective, and cost-efficient interventions. One of the best ways to achieve this is to make sure that health care policy decisions are based on best evidence. In spite of this, few policy decisions seem to be based on evidence. This ought not to be a surprise as policymaking is a complex matter in which evidence is only one of the factors to be considered. An example of breast cancer screening illustrates some of that complexity (Gray, 1998). The US National Institutes of Health (NIH) convened a consensus conference to look at the evidence for or against routine mammography screening of women aged 40 to 49. Based on the evidence, the panel recommended that screening of women before 50 years of age was not necessary, a recommendation that is consistent with those made in Canada and Great Britain. Led by the *New York Times*, the press launched a vicious attack on the NIH experts, whom they accused of killing American women. This hyperbole attracted the attention of Congress, which applied pressure to the National Cancer Institute (NCI). Members of the NCI Advisory Board subsequently overruled the Consensus Panel decision, recommending routine mammographic screening for women in the United States beginning at age 40. They opted for values over evidence.

Smoking offers another example in which evidence has been available for some time about its hazards and those of exposure to second-hand smoke. However, many of the Canadian bylaws that restrict smoking in public places have only recently been enacted. Best evidence was ignored by government and nongovernment organizations for a long time while they grappled with making decisions that could infringe on the rights of smokers and potentially anger their constituents or clients.

ROLE OF THE PUBLIC

The public includes the community (also patients and their families) and the media. These groups, which have a powerful influence on the use or non-use of health care therapies and practices, are often the groups that are most disadvantaged when it comes to dealing with science and evidence. They lack technical knowledge about research and the health disciplines. They trust researchers and health care professionals to supply them with the facts (and not with biased or inaccurate information).

As the above example about mammography demonstrates, the public and media have important roles in decisions about what interventions will be available or used. They can push an innovation into the marketplace or pull it back into obscurity. In 2002, the media reported early results from one study about adverse events associated with combined progesterone-estrogen hormone replacement therapy (Health Canada, 2004).

Women taking any kind of hormone replacement therapy abandoned their drugs virtually overnight, without medical supervision. In another historic case, the public successfully pushed to have an innovation made available that practitioners were not convinced was safe or efficacious (Box 9.3).

AN EXAMPLE OF ADOPTION OF POOR EVIDENCE

In the late 1990s, rumours had been circulating about a possible link between the vaccine for measles, mumps, and rubella (MMR) and the development of autism in children. Then a fatally flawed British study was published in *The Lancet* in 1998 (Wakefield et al., 1998). A group of 12 children had been selected to participate in a study because they had two

---

BOX 9.3	The Public Push

At the beginning of the 1800s, Joseph Priestly tested the effects of various gases on animals and humans, measuring their therapeutic effects. At the same time, an American chemist named Humphrey Davey conducted many experiments to determine the effects of inhaling various gases in different quantities, including oxygen, hydrogen, nitrous oxide, and carbon dioxide. He noted the power of nitrous oxide to calm the pain of a bad toothache and headache. At the time, nitrous oxide was primarily used as an attraction at travelling shows; patrons could choose to inhale the gas and experience its effects—euphoria and laughter. On one occasion, a group of patrons, who accidentally inhaled too much of the gas, went into a deep sleep.

Following one such exhibition, a dentist named Horace Wells supposed that nitrous oxide could be used to suppress pain during tooth extraction. He believed this so strongly, in fact, that in 1844, he extracted one of his own teeth while under the influence of nitrous oxide. He was subsequently embarrassed when, at a public demonstration, his "anaesthetized" patient cried out in pain—perhaps he had not used a high enough dose.

At around the same time, the American surgeon William Crawford Long was experimenting with the use of ether as an anaesthetic. His experiments, performed largely on himself and his assistants, culminated in the first use of anaesthesia for surgery. In March 1842, he removed a tumour from the neck of a patient. The patient had been anaesthetized with ether and felt no pain whatsoever. Long did not make this information public. However, in 1846, eminent surgeon John Warren held a public demonstration, much as Wells had. His presentation went far better, though, as the patient anaesthetized with ether felt no pain when a tumour was surgically removed from his cheek. People began to take note of anaesthetics.

At the time, ether was held in far higher esteem than nitrous oxide. Nitrous oxide was, after all, essentially a sideshow attraction at travelling circuses, known more for its ability to induce laughter than its effectiveness at reducing pain. Ether, on the other hand, was already in common use as a medical agent—though not yet as an anaesthetic.

In 1847, Wells travelled to the Académie de médecine in Paris to propose the use of nitrous oxide and ether as anaesthetics. This, combined with news of the surgery performed by Dr. Warren, brought a debate into being in the Académie de médecine and academies of sciences. While some doctors were quick to praise the virtues of anaesthesia, others, most notably Dr. François Magendie, fought against it. How were surgeons to work without the cries of the patient to guide them? How would an unconscious patient know when the surgeon was making mistakes or being too heavy-handed?

Despite these objections, news of anaesthesia soon found its way into the press. The public avidly supported the idea of painless surgery, and the press, of course, catalyzed their hopes. The public's impatience, bolstered by continuing accounts of the wonders of anaesthesia, led to enormous pressure on the scientific community. Thus, both ether and a new substance, chloroform, were quickly incorporated into standard surgical practice.

syndromes: bowel symptoms and autistic-like behaviour (there was no control group). The children ranged in age from 3 to 10 years. Parents were asked to recall if the onset of behavioural symptoms occurred after vaccination. The potential for recall errors and biased responses was high. Some parents had to think back a long way, and all parents knew they were participating in a study about the link between autism and MMR vaccination.

The tone of the *Lancet* article suggested a relationship between these syndromes and MMR vaccination even though the authors said, "We did not prove an association between measles, mumps and rubella vaccine and the syndrome described." In the last paragraph of the article, the researchers said, "Onset of symptoms was after measles, mumps, and rubella immunisation." When the article was released, the media picked it up as a potentially hot story given recent rumours and parents' natural fears about their children. At a press conference, the lead researcher stepped outside the limits of the research and announced that MMR should not be given to children.

The story received worldwide attention and created confusion and paranoia. Shocking details about the research emerged for many years afterward. Wakefield, the lead investigator, was accused of taking money to find a link between MMR and autism—the money was alleged to have come from a legal group that wanted to sue the drug manufacturer. He was also accused of wanting to discredit the MMR vaccine so that he could develop his own vaccine. The research did not receive peer review to see if it adhered to ethical guidelines, a step that may have uncovered the financial relationship and other conflicts of interest. Whether these conflicts of interest influenced data analysis or not is unclear; however, the data were incorrectly interpreted to suggest a link between MMR and autism. As the controversy grew, Wakefield's co-investigators and *The Lancet* distanced themselves from the research. Eventually, Wakefield faced a disciplinary hearing by the medical association. *The Lancet* published its regrets and other medical journals published position statements in an attempt to offset the negative effects of the news stories.

Public paranoia was fuelled inadvertently by Prime Minister Tony Blair and his office. When the media asked Blair if his young son had received the MMR vaccine, he would not answer (citing privacy issues). This made parents even more suspicious about the vaccine.

The result of the media attention was a significant drop in MMR vaccinations as well as an outbreak of measles and measles-related deaths. This is a good example of poor research that should not have been published and should never have influenced practice or behaviour. It is also a good example of the power of the media.

Annual seasonal influenza immunization sparks similar confusion as well as claims of a conspiracy between drug companies and government. Despite being members of a high-risk group, many nurses avoid immunization for seasonal influenza. For example, only 42% of all health care workers in acute-care settings in Toronto had seasonal influenza immunization in the 2008–2009 season (Toronto Public Health, 2009). The objections of health care workers, including nurses, to requirements that they be vaccinated against the H1N1 influenza virus were widely reported by the media in 2009.

Many nurses are unable to determine best practice because they do not know how to find good quality evidence or know how to evaluate it. Without an understanding of the science, the roles of various stakeholders in best practice, and clinical judgement errors, nurses may not make informed decisions about their own health or may not properly advise the public. Stories in the media and a lack of high-quality information from health care providers and government health agencies led to public fear about H1N1 followed by confusion, then a drop in anticipated rates of vaccination, and ultimately changes to seasonal influenza vaccination policy for 2009.

REFLECTIVE THINKING

The example of adoption of poor evidence (MMR and autism) and the discussion about influenza immunization raise questions about what nurses can and should do when these situations arise. What are the responsibilities of the individual nurse and of our nursing associations when adoption of poor evidence threatens public health?

CLINICAL DECISION MAKING

Having access to best evidence is no guarantee that it will be used. In the end, the practitioner must make a clinical judgement, one that can be contrary to the evidence. Many clinical decisions are complicated and must be made under difficult conditions, in noisy environments, by fatigued or distracted practitioners. The complexities of the decisions plus the conditions under which they are made lead to errors in judgement. We are all susceptible to certain biases that cause errors (Tversky & Kahneman, 1974). These errors can interfere with our ability to achieve evidence-informed practice or policy.

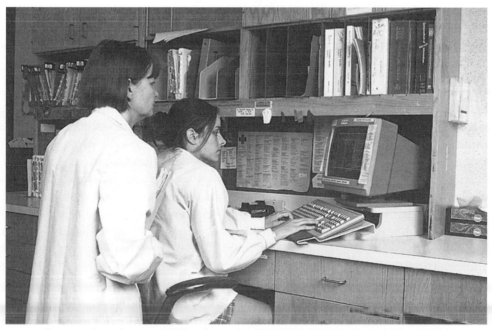

All nurses share the responsibility for implementing the findings of nursing research.

"MAN-WHO" METHOD

We have a tough time relating to research findings as typically presented by researchers. A publication of research begins with a review of the past literature and statement of the problem. The methods of the study are described in meticulous detail followed by statistical reports of the results. The discussion is often protracted and inevitably a main conclusion of the researcher is the need for more research.

Scientific evidence is bland and too often forgettable. Alternatively, information acquired through the "man-who" method is vivid and memorable. This approach for sharing information typically begins with "I know a man who…" (e.g., "I know a man who smoked his whole life and lived to be 98"). These stories offer vivid details and easy-to-recall information that can take on the status of bona fide evidence. Even in the face of best evidence, we may place our faith in this type of vivid information although the case may well represent an outlier (an extreme case that is atypical).

UNDERSTANDING PROBABILITY

The prevalence of health-related events has been established for many treatments or illnesses. Prevalence is the frequency of occurrence of an event for a set number of cases. When it is known, prevalence can be used to estimate the probability of an event, illness, or outcome. For example, if we know that the rate of serious adverse events associated with a particular surgery is 1 per 10,000 people, then we can estimate the likelihood that a patient will run into problems. Statements about probability are used to fully inform patients who are making treatment choices.

The trouble is that many of us are not very good at understanding probability and odds. Some built-in imperfections in our cognitive reasoning processes contribute to errors in the use of probabilities. Strangely enough, probability estimates can be biased by the ease with which we can bring occurrences to mind (Tversky & Kahneman, 1982). Rare events that receive a great deal of attention can make us believe that the probability that an event will occur is greater than it really is simply because we can recall the information easily. For example, we heard a great deal about death occurring during the 2003 SARS outbreak in Toronto. Many came to assume that death was nearly certain once SARS was contracted because the media focused on these cases. This misperception affected nurses' decisions to go to work during the crisis and decisions people made about travel to the Toronto area.

Probability estimates can also be affected by recent events, which can be recalled more easily than distant events. If a patient we cared for recently suffered a 1 in 10,000 adverse surgical event, we will believe that the probability of the same event is much higher for a subsequent patient. If we have seen a particular outcome recently, we likely will overestimate the probability of it occurring.

The prevalence of various decision biases in health care is unknown (Chapman & Elstein, 2000). Little has been done to find strategies for correcting clinical decision biases.

PROBLEMS INTERPRETING RESEARCH

It has been estimated that less than 25% of medical decisions are based on evidence (Haines & Donald, 1998). This means that most medical practitioners have inadequate justification for their interventions. It does not, however, follow that their interventions are faulty. Conversely, using evidence does not make the decisions correct. For example, a single study (or several studies conducted in a similar manner) may have produced erroneous findings. The findings of one study might apply narrowly in a nearly identical situation, but it is generally accepted practice to expect to see the compilation of results from a number of studies leading to similar conclusions about a particular intervention before it could be considered something to lead to a change in practice.

When researchers speak about one intervention being significantly different from another, they do not mean that all patients who received one intervention had clinical outcomes that exceeded those who did not get the intervention, as the public may be inclined to interpret a significant difference. In the real world, some people who received the better intervention will have worse outcomes than those who received no intervention or the less desirable intervention. It is useful to have researchers express their findings in ways that throw light on the situation. One of these is *number needed to treat* (NNT). This is a statistic that describes the magnitude or impact of an intervention in terms of the number of people who have to be treated to prevent one additional event. For example, a new vaccine has been developed for prevention of herpes zoster (also known as shingles). This troubling disorder can occur in adults who have a reactivated varicella zoster virus that had been lying dormant in nerve fibres following childhood chicken pox. This is a potentially painful disorder that can become chronic and unremitting. The cost of immunizing all adults would be high. How effective is the vaccine in terms of NNT? In order to prevent one case of shingles, 64 people have to be vaccinated. We need to take into account the fact that only a percentage of the study participants would have come down with shingles without the vaccine. Therefore, this NNT of 64 tells us that the vaccine is effective. Generally, the smaller the NNT, the greater will be the impact of the intervention.

STRATEGIES TO ENHANCE ACCESS TO EVIDENCE

With two million health care publications distributed annually (Haines & Donald, 1998), clinicians are unable to read everything published that relates to their practice area, no matter how small the field. As mentioned, Archie Cochrane argued that it is not the volume of available research, but the practitioners' access to it that is the problem. For that reason, many of the strategies that have been developed to enhance evidence-informed practice improve practitioners' access to evidence.

Most health disciplines have taught emerging practitioners to approach learning about new knowledge the same way they have taught researchers. This process involves a lengthy search of *unfiltered* research evidence, reading many articles, integrating the findings into a coherent piece, and then forming conclusions that can be applied. The evidence is referred to as unfiltered because the practitioner reads all of the literature. Although this may have worked in a time when knowledge was produced slowly, it has not worked with the knowledge explosion. It is impossible for a practitioner to read everything as it is published in a field or to catch up on what has been published already.

While educators have been emphasizing the importance of evidence-informed practice, they have not yet adjusted their educational approaches. Instead of teaching practitioners the same methods as one would teach researchers, they need to teach them how to find *filtered* evidence. The evidence is referred to as filtered because primary publications have been reviewed and summarized in a form that can be used by practitioners. Filtered evidence lessens practitioners' workloads. Several sources of filtered evidence are available, including systematic reviews, synopses, and clinical practice guidelines (DiCenso, Ciliska, Dobbins, & Guyatt, 2005).

It is important to choose reliable sources to be sure to find best evidence. There are also some strategies for assessing the quality of the filtered evidence (DiCenso et al., 2005).

SYSTEMATIC REVIEWS

One approach for making evidence available to practitioners is the systematic review. This approach consists of a rigorous method for reviewing primary research on a specific topic. Strategies are used to surmount biases that can arise during the various stages of a systematic review. Although these methods were originally developed for randomized controlled trials, they are being used for nonrandomized quantitative research (Ciliska, DiCenso, & Guyatt, 2005) and for qualitative research (often referred to as meta-synthesis) (Paterson, Thorne, & Canam, 2001).

The stages of a systematic review include posing the question, finding the research, applying inclusion and exclusion criteria, abstracting the data, assessing it, and having it approved by peers (Ciliska et al., 2005). In some systematic reviews, the data from a number of studies may be combined and reanalyzed through a process referred to as meta-analysis. The advantage of meta-analysis is that data from small-sample studies can be combined to give a better estimate of the effect of a treatment than that which could be obtained from individual studies. What is also produced is a concise, reader-friendly statement of conclusions about particular interventions that can be applied to practice, saving the practitioner much work.

One example of a systematic review deals with topical anaesthetics for relieving needle puncture pain in children. Two of these drugs that nurses can apply using a standard order are EMLA and Ametop. If a practitioner searched the literature to find out which of these two drugs is more efficacious, the literature would not give a clear answer since some studies say that EMLA is better while others say that Ametop is better and still others say there is no difference. However, a systematic review and meta-analysis determined that Ametop is the better drug (Lander, Weltman, & So, 2006). This review can be found in the Cochrane Collaboration database (http://www.cochrane.org).

The Cochrane Collaboration contains systematic reviews on many topics. They also include a record of reviews conducted and published outside of the collaboration. Quality systematic reviews that have been peer reviewed can also be located in health care journals. In recent years, many systematic reviews have been completed on topics of interest to nurses and by nurses. The systematic review is a method that has found its way into thesis and dissertation research conducted by nurses.

SYNOPSES OF INDIVIDUAL STUDIES AND SYSTEMATIC REVIEWS

Another approach for helping practitioners gain access to research is to have experienced researchers evaluate published articles or systematic reviews and prepare a summary for practitioners. This is an approach used by the journal *Evidence-Based Nursing* and by a number of online databases such as *Clinical Evidence* (http://www.clinicalevidence.com), *ACP Journal Club, DARE* (Database of Abstracts of Reviews of Effectiveness), and *Evidence-Based Medicine*. These are synopses of individual articles or individual systematic reviews that can ease the practitioner's load. One can subscribe to many of these online and receive information in one's own field.

CLINICAL GUIDELINES

The clinical practice guideline is another document that is useful for practitioners. Guidelines consist of reviews of evidence that culminate with clinical recommendations. Because the clinical recommendations are only as good as the guideline, it is important to evaluate it. Who participated in the development of the guideline (experts, clinicians, consumers)? Who is sponsoring the guideline (industry, a special-interest group, government or nongovernment agency)? Is the description of the method comprehensive (including the search for evidence)? Has the guideline been peer reviewed?

There are several online sources for clinical guidelines. The National Guideline Clearinghouse is a reliable site that can be accessed free of charge. It contains many relevant clinical guidelines. The Registered Nurses' Association of Ontario (RNAO) Web site includes nursing best-practice guidelines (http://www.RNAO.org).

REMOVING SOME BARRIERS TO EVIDENCE

Because of the importance of evidence-informed practice to nursing, some investment has been made in developing new approaches to help nurses. These include providing access to resources and providing educational programs.

SEARCH CANADA

SEARCH Canada was a program that was developed in 1996 to enhance health care research and its utilization in Alberta. It became available nationwide and operated until late 2009. The programs were offered in partnership with health authorities.

Approximately half of the participants were nurses. Its aims were to increase the use of evidence, develop collaborative networks, disseminate research, promote research that influences policy, and contribute to new health research. Participants attended formal classes, took part in a supportive network, and used Internet-based resources to learn about evidence-informed practice. Although this program has come to an end, it initiated a tradition of evidence-informed nursing practice.

CENTRE FOR HEALTH EVIDENCE

The Centre for Health Evidence is a nonprofit organization based at the University of Alberta that is committed to helping organizations and professional associations improve best practice. The centre creates decision-support tools and helps professionals find and apply best evidence.

RNAO BEST NURSING PRACTICE GUIDELINES

The RNAO Web site (http://www.RNAO.org/bestpractices/) was developed in 1999 with funding from the Ontario government. It identifies and offers clinical guidelines that are of interest to Canadian nurses. Some of the guidelines can be accessed from a personal digital assistant (PDA), which makes them available at or near the bedside.

NURSEONE: THE CANADIAN NURSES ASSOCIATION PORTAL

The Canadian Nurses Association has developed an Internet site that can be used by all active members of the CNA and by nursing students. This is a portal to many free resources that are useful for evidence-informed practice. These include the National Guidelines Clearinghouse, the RNAO Best Practice Guidelines, and useful e-journals and e-books. The CNA has also subscribed to other resources, making them available to nurses at no personal cost. These include EMSCO, Medline, CINHAL, DARE, Cochrane database, and STATREF (which gives access to the ACP Journal Club and other useful resources). The portal also provides links to some useful Web sites such as the Canadian Health Network, the Canadian Institute for Health Information, Centre for Health Evidence, and some university libraries. Some tools are provided, including teaching materials from the Centre for Health Evidence.

MULTIDISCIPLINARY EVIDENCE REPOSITORIES

Many new sources for filtered evidence are being developed each year. They are not all equally reliable or useful. Some sites offer filtered evidence that is valuable for nurses. Bandolier, ACP Journal Club, Bugs 'n Drugs, *UpToDate*, *Clinical Evidence*, and *Evidence-Based Nursing Journal* are a few examples.

FUTURE CHALLENGES

Facilitating research utilization in nursing practice is not an easy task, but neither is it an impossible dream. With rapidly advancing technology, we are now at the point where nurses at the bedside could carry a small device, no larger than a cellphone, which would allow them to access evidence at the bedside. The evidence is there, the technology is available. What is needed to make this happen?

The missing piece at the present time is knowledge. Nurses also need to be taught how to access the filtered evidence and how to use it to make good clinical decisions. It is not yet clear how to reach so many nurses, but once we find a way, the potential for improvement in clinical care is immense. Putting the evidence in useable form into the hands of nurses in practice creates a new world in which reliance on the tried and true is lessened and where expectations of nurses change drastically. This new era may be just around the corner.

CRITICAL THINKING QUESTIONS

1. What are the three kinds of research use?
2. Define evidence-informed practice.
3. How does the filtered literature differ from the unfiltered literature?
4. What are the stages of diffusion of an innovation?
5. Who are the stakeholders in evidence-informed practice?

WEB SITES

NurseONE: The Canadian Nurses Association portal: http://www.nurseone.ca
Registered Nurses Association of Ontario, Best Practice Guidelines: http://www.rnao.org/bestpractices/
Bandolier: Evidence-Based Thinking About Health Care: http://www.medicine.ox.ac.uk/bandolier
Sponsored by Oxford University, compiles information about evidence-informed health care—with humour.
The Cochrane Collaboration: http://www.cochrane.org

REFERENCES

Alcock, D., Carroll, G., & Goodman, M. (1990). Staff nurses' perceptions of factors influencing their role in research. *Canadian Journal of Nursing Research*, 22(4), 7–18.

Blizz-Holtz, J. (2007). Evidence-based practice: A primer for action. *Issues in Comprehensive Pediatric Nursing*, 30, 165–182.

Bock, L. (1990). From research to utilization: Bridging the gap. *Nursing Management*, 21(3), 50–51.

Brett, J. L. (1987). Use of nursing practice research findings. *Nursing Research*, 36(6), 344–349.

Carroll, D., Greenwood, R., Lynch, K., Sullivan, J., Ready, C., & Fitzmaurice, J. (1997). Barriers and facilitators to the utilization of nursing research. *Clinical Nurse Specialist*, 11(5), 207–212.

Chambers, C. (1989). Barriers to the dissemination and use of research in nursing practice. *NRIG Newsletter*, 11(2), 2–3.

Chapman, G., & Elstein, A. (2000). Cognitive processes and biases in medical decision making. In G. Chapman, & F. Sonnenberg (Eds.), *Decision making in health care: Theory, psychology, and applications.* Cambridge: Cambridge University Press.

Ciliska, D., DiCenso, A., & Guyatt, G. (2005). Summarizing the evidence through systematic reviews. In A. DiCenso, G. Guyatt, & D. Ciliska (Eds.), *Evidence-based nursing: A guide to clinical practice.* St. Louis, MO: Mosby.

DiCenso, A., Ciliska, D., Dobbins, M., & Guyatt, G. (2005). Moving from evidence to action using clinical practice guidelines. In A. DiCenso, G. Guyatt, & D. Ciliska (Eds.), *Evidence-based nursing: A guide to clinical practice.* St. Louis, MO: Mosby.

Dobbins, M., Ciliska, D., Estabrooks, C., & Hayward, S. (2005). Changing nursing practice in an organization. In A. DiCenso, G. Guyatt, & D. Ciliska (Eds.), *Evidence-based nursing: A guide to clinical practice* St. Louis, MO: Mosby.

Estabrooks, C. (1998). Will evidence-based nursing practice make practice perfect? *Canadian Journal of Nursing Research, 30*(1), 15–36.

Estabrooks, C. (1999). The conceptual structure of research utilization. *Research in Nursing & Health, 22*(3), 203–216.

Estabrooks, C., Thompson, D., Lovely, J., & Hofmeyer, A. (2006). A guide to knowledge translation theory. *The Journal of Continuing Education in the Health Professions, 26*, 25–36.

Funk, S. G., Champagne, M. T., Wiese, R. A., & Tornquist, E. M. (1991). Barriers: The barriers to research utilization scales. *Applied Nursing Research, 4*(1), 39–45.

Goodman, K. (2003). *Ethics and evidence-based medicine: Fallibility and responsibility in clinical science.* Cambridge: Cambridge University Press.

Gray, J. A. M. (1998). Evidence based policy making. In A. Haines, & A. Donald (Eds.), *Getting research findings into practice.* London: BMJ Books.

Haines, A., & Donald, A. (Eds.). (1998). *Getting research findings into practice.* London: BMJ Books.

Haughey, B. (1988). Utilizing research findings in nursing. *Clinical Nurse Specialist, 2*(4), 184.

Health Canada. (2004). *It's your health: Benefits and risks of hormone replacement therapy (Estrogen with and without Progestin).* Retrieved on March 26, 2008, from http://www.hc-sc.gc.ca/iyh-vsv/med/estrogen_e.html.

Horsley, J., Crane, J., & Bingle, J. (1978). Research utilization as an organizational process. *Journal of Nursing Administration, 8*(7), 4–6.

Kajermo, K., Nordstrom, G., Krusebrant, A., Bjorvell, H., & Nilsson-Kajermo, K. (1998). Barriers to and facilitators of research utilization, as perceived by a group of registered nurses in Sweden. *Journal of Advanced Nursing, 27*(4), 798–807.

Karkos, B., & Peters, K. (2006). A Magnet community hospital: Fewer barriers to nursing research utilization. *Journal of Nursing Administration, 36*(7), 377–382.

King, D., Barnard, K., & Hoehn, R. (1981). Disseminating the results of nursing research. *Nursing Outlook, 29*(3), 164–169.

Lander, J., Weltman, B., & So, S. (2006). EMLA and Amethocaine for reduction of children's pain associated with needle insertion. *Cochrane Library* (Issue 3).

LoBiondo-Wood, G., & Haber, J. (2006). *Nursing research: Methods and critical appraisal for evidence-based practice.* St. Louis, MO: Mosby.

O'Lynn, C., Luperell, S., Winters, C., Shreffler-Grant, J., Lee, H., & Hendrickx, L. (2009). Rural nurses' research use. *Online Journal of Rural Nursing and Health Care, 9*(1), 34–45.

Paterson, B. C., Thorne, S. E., & Canam, C. (2001). *Meta-study of qualitative health research: A practical guide to meta-analysis and meta-synthesis.* Thousand Oaks, CA: Sage Publications.

Pank, P., Rostron, W., & Stenhouse, M. (1984). Using research in nursing. *Nursing Times, 80*(11), 44–45.

Pravikoff, D., Tanner, A., & Pierce, S. (2005). Readiness of US nurses for evidence-based practice. *American Journal of Nursing, 105*(9), 40–50.

Profetto-McGrath, J., Smith, K., Hugo, K., Taylor, M., & El-Hajj, H. (2007). Clinical nurse specialists' use of evidence in practice: A pilot study. *Worldviews on Evidence-Based Nursing, 4*(2), 86–96.

Repko, L. (1990). Turn research reports into an assessment challenge. *RN, 53*(8), 56–61.

RNABC. (1993). *Nursing and research in clinical agencies: A.B.C. survey.* Vancouver: Author.

Rogers, E. M. (2003). *Diffusion of innovations* (5th ed.). New York: Free Press.

Toronto Public Health. (2009). Influenza immunization rates of healthcare workers in Toronto healthcare facilities. Retrieved on October 20, 2009, from http://www.toronto.ca/health/boh_reports.htm#003.

Tversky, A., & Kahneman, D. (1974). Judgment under uncertainty: Heuristics and biases. *Science, 185,* 1124–1131.

Tversky, A., & Kahneman, D. (1982). Availability: A heuristic for judging frequency and probability. In E. Kahneman, P. Slovic, & A. Tversky (Eds.), *Judgment under uncertainty: Heuristics and biases.* Cambridge: Cambridge University Press.

Wakefield, A., Murch, S., Anthony, A., Linnell, J., Casson, D., Malik, M., Berelowitz, M., Dhillon, A., Thomson, M., Harvey, P., Valentine, A., Davies, S., & Walker-Smith, J. (1998). Ileal-lymphoid-nodular hyperplasia, non-specific colitis, and pervasive developmental disorder in children. *The Lancet, 351,* 637–641.

Winters, C., Lee, H., Besel, C., Strand, A., Echeverri, R., Jorgensen, K., & Dea, J. (2007). Access to and use of research by rural nurses. *Rural Remote Health, 7*(3), 758.

10 Health Informatics and Canadian Nursing Practice

Kathryn J. Hannah and Margaret Ann Kennedy

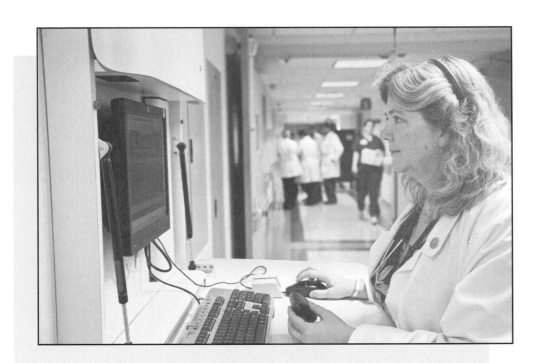

LEARNING OBJECTIVES

- To describe the factors that have led to the emergence of nursing informatics as a recognized specialty.
- To describe the scope of practice in nursing informatics and the competencies necessary to practise.
- To describe how standardized nursing languages can represent Health Information: Nursing Components in the health care system and why this is important for nursing.
- To explain how components of the e-Nursing Strategy are currently being implemented and identify future opportunities.
- To describe the various ways in which nurses can be active in nursing informatics communities.

Technology is providing unprecedented opportunities to document nursing practice, exchange information with diverse points of service, and facilitate access to information (such as pharmaceutical databases, laboratory values, and best-practice guidelines). The informatics revolution, identified by McBride (2005) and others, is shaping how nurses view health data and how they manage such data. Nurses, at the core of their work, are information and knowledge workers. Managing vast amounts of diverse information related to patient demographics and needs, diagnostic results, planned or ongoing treatment regimes, and coordinating community supports represents only a portion of the role performed by Canadian nurses on a daily basis. These activities are increasingly embedded in technology, and new considerations of this informatics revolution are facing nurses and challenging previous ways of doing and knowing.

Nursing has been at the very heart of this revolution. The management of health information through the use of electronic technologies has rapidly developed since the first computers were developed in the 1950s and 60s and continued to expand in clinical applications into the 1980s (Hannah, Ball, & Edwards, 2006, p. 28). The introduction of the computer for use at the organizational and individual levels, as well as its rapid evolution over a very few decades, has led to extensive computerization of basic operations in health care agencies and in management of clinical processes at the unit level. Current information management applications include patient scheduling and transfer, billing and financial management, diagnostic imaging, lab reporting, order entry applications, pharmacy, patient documentation systems, clinical support tools, and resource management applications. Many systems vendors offer sophisticated applications that integrate tools for all units in a health care facility or region. Many areas of the country are adopting such systems, having recognized the immense benefits of having health care information readily accessible to care providers regardless of location within or outside the health care facility.

In the midst of the range of technologies embedded in contemporary health care, however, Hannah (2005) notes that "the issues for nurses are no longer computers or management information systems, but rather information and information management. The computer and its associated software are merely tools to support nurses as they practice their profession" (p. 48). McBride (2005) observed that all aspects of nursing will be affected by the health information revolution as changes to professional practice continue to emerge from the penetration of technological advances in health care. It is imperative that nurses are actively engaged in developing systems that support professional practice and that they are attentive to the content of information systems rather than focusing primarily on the technology itself (Hannah, 2005).

THE EMERGENCE OF NURSING INFORMATICS

Concurrent with the explosive development of information technology in health care, several nurse leaders began to explore how nursing could use technology to support professional practice, and how nurses could respond to the demands of using such technology. This exploration culminated in the 1980s with the emergence of a new nursing specialty in information management. The field of nursing informatics (NI) has expanded rapidly since the term was initially coined by Dr. Marion Ball, an informatician and NI advocate. Ball presented her concept of the new specialty at the 1983 International Medical Informatics Association (IMIA) Conference in Amsterdam, which was only the third global conference on health informatics (Englebardt & Nelson, 2002). Emerging from medical informatics and health care informatics, NI is a specialty in its own right. The first text on NI was published in 1984 by Dr. Ball from the United States and Dr. Kathryn Hannah from Canada (Ball & Hannah, 1984). Since that time, the proliferation of academic and applied texts, printed and online journals, conferences and educational programs, all directed at preparing nurses to capitalize on applying technology to its optimal potential, has provided ample evidence of the progression of NI within Canada and internationally.

As a result of technological innovations, nurses have had to assume new responsibilities for patient care. Indeed, nurses' roles have evolved from monitoring patient response to treatment to understanding and working with the technological applications that have become an integral part of care. The evolution in nurses' roles has mirrored evolutions in the development and definitions of NI. Table 10.1 presents an overview of definitions, reflecting the progression of development and the scope of practice in NI, as examined by Staggers & Bagley Thompson (2002).

Staggers and Bagley Thompson further extended the breadth of their definition by suggesting that "the goal of nursing informatics is to improve the health of populations, communities, families, and individuals by optimizing information management and communication. This includes the use of information and technology in the direct provision of care, in establishing effective administrative systems, in managing and delivering educational experiences, in supporting lifelong learning, and in supporting nursing research" (2002, p. 260). Thus, the *effective identification, collection, representation, management, and communication* of nursing data lie at the core of all nursing activities regardless of practice setting, and it is this attention to nursing information management that is the central focus of NI.

TABLE 10.1	Definitions of Nursing Informatics		

FOCUS OF DEFINITION	DATE	AUTHOR	DEFINITION
Information technology	1984; 1994	Ball & Hannah; Hannah, Ball, & Edwards	"Any use of information technologies by nurses in relation to the care of their patients, the administration of health care facilities, or the educational preparation of individuals to practice the discipline is considered nursing informatics."
	1986	Saba & McCormick	"Systems that use computers to process nursing data into information to support all types of nursing activities."
	1989	Zeilstorff, Abraham, Werley, Saba, & Schwirian	Central role of technology
	1996	Saba & McCormick	"Use of technology and/or a computer system to collect, store, process, display, retrieve, and communicate timely data and information in and across health care facilities that administer nursing services and resources, manage the delivery of patient and nursing care, link research resources and findings to nursing practice, and apply educational resources to nursing education."
	1998	IMIA	"The integration of nursing, its information, and information management with information processing and communication technology, to support the health of people world wide."
	2000	Ball, Hannah, Newbold, & Douglas	"All aspects of nursing—clinical practice, administration, research and education— just as computing holds the power to integrate all four aspects."
	2001b	CNA	"The application of computer science and information science to nursing. NI promotes the generation, management and processing of relevant data in order to use information and develop knowledge that supports nursing in all practice domains."
Conceptual	1986	Schwirian	"Solid foundation of nursing informatics knowledge [that] should have focus, direction, and cumulative properties."
	1989	Graves & Corcoran	A combination of computer science, information science, and nursing science designed to assist in the management and processing of nursing data, information, and knowledge to support the practice of nursing and the delivery of nursing care
	1996	Turley	Development of an NI model that included cognitive science, information science, and computer science

Continued

TABLE 10.1	Definitions of Nursing Informatics—cont'd		
FOCUS OF DEFINITION	DATE	AUTHOR	DEFINITION
Role-centred	1992	American Nurses Association (ANA)	"Specialty that integrates nursing science, computer science, and information science in identifying, collecting, processing, and managing data and information to support nursing practice, administration, education, and research and to expand nursing knowledge. The purpose of nursing informatics is to analyze information requirements; design, implement and evaluate information systems and data structures that support nursing; and identify and apply computer technologies for nursing."
	1994	ANA	"Specialty that integrates nursing science, computer science, and information science in identifying, collecting, processing, and managing data and information to support nursing practice, administration, education, research, and expansion of nursing knowledge. It supports the practice of all nursing specialties, in all sites and settings, whether at the basic or advanced level. The practice includes the development of applications, tools, processes, and structures that assist nurses with the management of data in taking care of patients or in supporting their practice of nursing."
	2002	Staggers & Bagley Thompson	Nursing informatics is a specialty that integrates nursing science, computer science, and information science to manage and communicate data, information, and knowledge in nursing practice. Nursing informatics facilitates the integration of data, information, and knowledge to support patients, nurses, and other providers in their decision making in all roles and settings. This support is accomplished through the use of information structures, information processes, and information technology.

Source: Hannah, K.J., & Kennedy, M.A. (2009). Nursing informatics and Canadian nursing practice. In Potter, P.A., Perry, A.G., Ross-Kerr, J.C., & Wood, M.J. (Eds.). *Canadian fundamentals of nursing* (4th ed., pp. 235–36). Toronto: Elsevier Canada.

Most recently, the Nursing Informatics Special Interest Group of the International Medical Informatics Association (IMIA-NI) formally adopted a new nursing informatics definition at the General Assembly meetings in Helsinki on June 28, 2009.

Nursing Informatics science and practice integrates nursing, its information and knowledge and their management with information and communication technologies to promote the health of people, families and communities world wide (IMIA-NI, 2009).

This new IMIA-NI definition supports the direction taken by Staggers & Bagley Thompson to position the focus of NI firmly on the central and unique role of nursing.

As information management becomes increasingly important to all nursing practice settings, NI becomes less and less a specialty practice and a more integral tool or practice skill that contributes to the provision of safe, effective care (CNA, 2006a). This necessitates that, aside from practice-based competencies, nurses also develop and maintain competencies in NI. The Canadian Nurses Association (CNA) has specifically articulated the need for nurses to develop competencies in the use of technology and information management strategies and tools as a necessity for competent and effective care (CNA, 2000, 2001b, 2001, November, 2003, 2006a, 2006b). Numerous authors have devoted attention to the development of nursing informatics competencies for both novice and more advanced practitioners. Grobe (1989) was one of the first nurses to explore and provide recommendations on the specific range of competencies. Reporting on the conclusions of an IMIA-NI expert working group, Grobe documented a hierarchy of skills that would enable nurses to function effectively across each domain of nursing (practice, education, administration, and research), although levels of competencies were not linked to specific domains. Hebert (2000) also presented the initial recommendations for NI competencies. Staggers, Gassert, & Curran (2001) offer the most current summary of specific competencies for nurses in each practice domain and describe NI competencies as going "beyond computer literacy skills to the set of skills, knowledge, attitudes and perceptions nurses need" (p. 306). Staggers et al. developed a set of NI competencies, validated by an expert panel of nurses, for four levels of nurses involved in NI. Table 10.2 lists the specific skill sets considered essential for each category of nurse—beginning nurses, experienced nurses, informatics specialists, and informatics innovators.

Nurses wishing to perform a self-assessment on their NI skills can go to many Web sites to complete tools that will guide their development. One such site is located at http://www.nursing-informatics.com/niassess/index.html. This site was developed by Canadian educator June Kaminski (2007) and is designed around three levels of NI skills identified in Hebert's report (2000), each with specific competencies—user/technical competencies, modifiers/utility competencies, and innovator/leadership competencies. The site also features such tools as tutorials, self-tests, the PATCH test to evaluate attitudes, and a plan for development.

REPRESENTING NURSING DATA IN HEALTH CARE

There are several key stakeholders in the collection and dissemination of health information in Canada, and nurses should have a working knowledge of them. The Canadian government has made significant progress in promoting connectivity in Canada, establishing programs such as the Community Access Program, SchoolNet, and others (CNA, 2006b). As the result of the Wilk Task Force and its vision of a strong health information system in Canada, four health information groups were integrated in 1992 to create a single national health information authority—the Canadian Institute for Health Information (CIHI) (Hannah, 2005). CIHI is the national, independent, and not-for-profit body that

TABLE 10.2 Categories of Nursing Informatics Competencies

CATEGORIES	LEVEL 1: BEGINNING NURSE	LEVEL 2: EXPERIENCED NURSE	LEVEL 3: INFORMATICS SPECIALIST	LEVEL 4: INFORMATICS INNOVATOR
Computer Skills				
Administration	√	√	-	-
Communication	√	-	-	-
Data access	√	√	-	-
Decision support	√	-	-	-
Documentation	√	-	-	-
Education	√	√	-	-
Monitoring	√	√	-	-
Basic desktop software	√	√	√	-
Systems	√	√	√	-
Quality improvement	-	√	√	√
Research	-	√	-	-
CASE tools	-	-	√	-
Project management	-	-	√	-
Simulation	-	-	√	√
Informatics Knowledge				
Data	√	√	√	-
Impact	√	√	√	√
Privacy/security	√	√	-	-
Systems	√	√	√	-
Education	-	√	√	√
Research	-	√	-	-
Usability/ergonomics	-	-	√	-
Regulations	-	-	√	-
Informatics Skills				
Evaluation	-	√	√	√
Role	-	√	√	-
Analysis	-	-	√	√
Data structures	-	-	-	√
Design/development	-	-	√	√
Fiscal management	-	-	√	-
Implementation	-	-	√	-
Management	-	-	√	√
Privacy/security	-	-	√	-
Programming	-	-	√	-
Requirements	-	-	√	-
Systems maintenance	-	√	√	-
System selection	-	-	√	-
Testing	-	-	√	-
Research (funding)	-	-	-	√
Training	-	-	√	-
Education	-	-	-	√

Source: Staggers, N., Gassert, C., & Curran, C. (2001). Informatics competencies for nurses at four levels of practice. *Journal of Nursing Education, 40*(7), 307.

records and disseminates essential data and analysis on Canada's health system and the health of Canadians (CIHI, 2007). Although CIHI collects valuable health data, such as health care services and spending, health human resources, and population health, gaps still existed in the health information available to care providers and decision makers. The National Forum on Health recommended a pan-Canadian electronic health record (EHR) (Hannah, 2005). In response to recommendations, the federal government committed $500 million to the development of e-health, including the EHR, telehealth, and Internet-based health information (CNA, 2006b; Hannah, 2005). Canada Health Infoway was a key outcome of the federal/provincial/territorial partnership and was incorporated in 2001 (CNA, 2006b; Hannah, 2005). Infoway is the federally funded, independent, not-for-profit body whose primary focus is the development of a secure, integrated, and patient-centred electronic health record (CNA, 2006b; Hannah et al., 2005). Since 2004, Infoway has also targeted telehealth applications for development (CNA, 2006b).

Clearly, much has been accomplished in the drive to ensure that accessible health data exist for both care providers and decision makers. However, much work remains to be done. Nursing, as a professional practice, has long been observed to be disadvantaged by a lack of formal and tangible recognition in the health care system (Clark & Lang, 1992; Marck, 1994; Conrick & Foster, 1997; Colliere & Lawler, 1998; Clark, 1999; Norwood, 2001; CNA, 2000; Weyrauch, 2002; Hannah, Ball, & Edwards, 2006; Rutherford, 2008). Hannah et al. (2005) noted that nurses' contributions to health care were not recorded in institutional or national databases representing essential elements of care provision. As a consequence, they argued that nurses lack a position of political agency or authority from which to exert control over their own nursing practice and influence systemic health care decision making. Clark and Lang (1992, p. 109), in their seminal article on nursing visibility and representation, noted that "if we cannot name it, we cannot control it, finance it, teach it, research it, or put it into public policy." The stance forwarded by Clark and Lang (1992) and others (such as CNA, 2006a; Hannah, 2005; CNA, 2000; Hannah et al., 2005; Graves & Corcoran, 1989; Werley, 1988) argues that in order to give nursing visibility, a standardized language to reflect what nursing is and what nursing does is required. Clark (1999, p. 42) advocated for a standardized nursing language using the argument that "without a language to express our concepts we cannot know whether our understanding of their meaning is the same, so we cannot communicate them with any precision to other people."

Over the last two decades, numerous health reports and commissions have repeatedly articulated a specific need for better information to support health care decisions. Reports at provincial, territorial, and federal levels, including the Lalonde (1974), Kirby (2002), and Romanow (2002) reports, all recommend improved data collection to support effective and appropriate decision making (Hannah, 2005, 2007). In spite of the calls for improved health care data, nursing contributions to health care are *still* not included on patient discharge abstracts or in provincial or national data repositories (Hannah, 2005). CIHI records only nursing human resource data, and the pan-Canadian electronic health record (EHR) at the time of writing does not address recording nursing data in any standardized manner or in a way that makes nursing contributions evident (Hannah, 2005). This trend continues to ignore the contributions nurses make to health care and health outcomes and results in decisions about fiscal allocation being made without calculating the contributions of the largest sector of health care providers (Hannah, 2007). Clark's (1999, p. 42) observation that "nursing is invisible in health policy decisions, in descriptions of health care, in contracts and service specifications" continues to reflect current practices.

In Canada, the process of working toward capturing nursing data was initiated in the early 1990s by the Alberta Association of Registered Nurses (AARN) at a national conference to generate consensus on the Canadian Nursing Minimum Data Set (NMDS) (Giovannetti, Smith, & Broad, 1999). The CNA supported this initiative and held the conference in 1992, when discussions focused on the content of and issues concerning a Canadian NMDS (Giovannetti et al., 1999). The Canadian version of an NMDS is recognized as Health Information: Nursing Components (HI: NC) and enjoys consensus on patient status, nursing interventions, patient outcomes, nursing intensity, and nurse identifier (CNA, 2000; Hannah, 2005).

The Canadian Nurses Association describes HI: NC as the "most important pieces of data about the nursing care provided to the patient during a health care episode" (2000, p. 5); see Box 10.1. Enormous work in education and promotion has been done since the HI: NC were identified and achieved consensus. As Hannah (2005) notes, it is "essential in Canada that the nursing data elements constitute one component of a fully integrated health information system, e.g. the CIHI Discharge Abstract Database… or an EHR such as that being developed under the leadership of Infoway" (p. 49).

As Hannah (2005) noted, identifying the essential nursing data is really only the first step in representing nursing contributions. It is essential to have standardized data for trending, comparison, and analysis. Many specific languages and taxonomies have been

---

BOX 10.1	Definitions of Health Information: Nursing Components

- **Patient status** is broadly defined as a label for the set of indicators that reflect the phenomena for which nurses provide care, relative to the health status of patients (McGee, 1993). Although patient status is similar to nursing diagnosis, the term patient status was preferred because it represents a broader spectrum of health and illness. The common label "patient status" is inclusive of input from all disciplines. The summative statements referring to the phenomena for which nurses provide care (i.e., nursing diagnosis) are merely one aspect of patient status at a point in time, in the same way as medical diagnosis.
- **Nursing interventions** refer to purposeful and deliberate health-affecting interventions (direct and indirect), based on assessment of patient status, which are designed to bring about results which benefit patients (Alberta Association of Registered Nurses [AARN], 1994).
- **Patient outcome** is defined as "patients' status at a defined point(s) following health care [affecting] intervention" (Marek & Lang, 1993). It is influenced to varying degrees by the interventions of all care providers.
- **Nursing intensity** "refers to the amount and type of nursing resource used to [provide] care" (O'Brien-Pallas & Giovannetti, 1993).
- **Primary Nurse identifier** is a single unique lifetime identification number for each individual nurse. This identifier is independent of geographic location (province or territory), practice sector (e.g. acute care, community care, public health) or employer.

Source: Hannah, K.J. (2005). Health informatics and nursing in Canada. *Healthcare Information Management and Communications*, *XIX*(3), 49. Reprinted by permission of Healthcare Computing and Communications Canada, Inc.

created in attempts to present nursing data in standardized ways. The North American Nursing Diagnosis Association (NANDA), the Omaha Classification System, the Home Health Care Classification (HHCC), the Nursing Intervention Classification (NIC), and the Nursing Outcome Classification (NOC) have all attempted to quantify nursing into standardized formats according to the various foci of the taxonomy or classification system (Hannah et al., 2005).

In an effort to represent nursing in a standard unified way, the International Council of Nurses (ICN) approved a resolution at its 1989 conference in Seoul, Korea, to establish the International Classification for Nursing Practice (ICNP) (ICN, 2005). The scope of ICNP is what nurses do (interventions) to address specific needs (diagnoses) to achieve specific results (outcomes) (ICN, 2005). ICNP has evolved from its early stages as a vocabulary and classification with separate multi-axial classifications for Nursing Phenomena (diagnoses and outcomes), and Nursing Intervention (actions), to its current state of development as Version 1. Many nurses from countries around the world assisted in the evaluation of terms and coding structures and collaborated with ICN to promote changes in ICNP. Additionally, collaboration was necessary to translate ICNP® into the many languages now available to nurses.

Today, ICNP® is defined as a "unified nursing language system and a compositional terminology" (ICN, 2005, p. 21). ICNP® Version 1 was created using description logic and Web Ontology Language (OWL) in order to address the complexities of developing a fully functional and robust tool that could document nursing practice, eliminate redundancy between terms, and avoid hierarchical coding structures. Further, ICNP® Version 1 is unique from previous iterations in that the single seven-axis is used to create statements containing nursing diagnoses, nursing actions, or outcomes in nursing practice (see Figure 10.1). Also new to Version 1 is the inclusion of catalogues of terms. Catalogues, which are made up of subsets of diagnoses, actions, and outcomes specific to various practice areas or specialties, continue to be developed (ICN, 2005). ICNP® Version 2 was launched on July 2, 2009, at the ICN 24th Quadrennial Congress, held in Durban, South Africa (ICN, 2009). This new version reflects continued efforts to develop more terms, customized catalogues, and extensive collaboration opportunities with the ICNP® community.

ICNP® presents nurses with a tool that functions as a cross-mapping tool to accommodate existing vocabularies, assist in developing new vocabularies (compositional vocabulary), and identify relationships (reference terminology) (ICN, 2005, p. 19). This tool enables nurses to document their practice, regardless of geographical location, practice setting, or language, and allows for comparison of standardized data.

The seven axes supporting Version 1.0 include Focus, Judgement, Means, Action, Time, Location, and Client (see Table 10.3). Terms are situated within a hierarchical navigational construct and are used to create nursing diagnoses, nursing interventions, and nursing outcomes. Similar to previous iterations, both nursing diagnoses and nursing outcomes must contain a term from the Focus Axis and the Judgement Axis and may include terms from additional axes as needed to fully describe the phenomenon of attention. Nursing Interventions must include a term from the Action Axis and the Target Axis and may include additional terms from other axes as necessary.

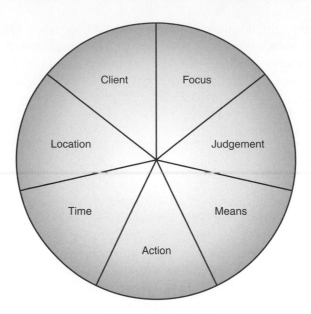

ICNP® 7 Axis Model

FIG 10.1 7 Axis model of ICNP Version 1.0. Source: International Council of Nurses (2005). International Classification for Nursing Practice, Version 1.0 (p. 29). Geneva: Author. Reproduced with permission of the International Council of Nurses.

In 2000, the Canadian Nurses Association developed a discussion paper supporting the ICNP®. Strong support from nurses led to the endorsement of ICNP® for use in representing nursing data in Canada (CNA, 2001b, 2003, 2006a). Nurses have further recognized the need for standards governing nursing data and have actively participated in the development of international nursing models and terminologies to support a standardized approach to nursing representation and communication.

A key example of standards upholding nursing data is the ISO 18104 Reference Terminology Model for Nursing and its subsequent adoption in Canada (Hannah, 2005, p. 50; Saba, Hovenga, Coenen, McCormick, & Bakken, 2003). The ISO Reference Terminology Model for Nursing sets forth the relationships between nursing concepts to ensure a consistent ontological representation between nursing reference terminologies and interface terminologies—essentially to support interoperability. In accordance with ISO practices, ISO 18104 was subjected to review in 2008–09 to ensure it is updated for continued relevance and guidance. Canada, through involvement in ISO, IHTSDO, and other nursing informatics associations, continues to contribute to this essential standard and to ensure that any revisions or additions represent Canadian nursing needs.

Thede & Sewell (2009) define an interface terminology as the terminology that clinicians would interact with in an electronic health management system, while a reference terminology is defined as the standardized terminology, embedded in a system's

TABLE 10.3	Definitions and Terms for 7-Axis Model in ICNP® Version 1.0

AXIS	DEFINITION	SAMPLE TERMS
Focus	The area of attention relevant to nursing	Elder abuse, Child Bearing, Arterial Ulcer, Fever
Judgement	Clinical opinion or determination related to the focus of nursing practice	High, Partial, Risk, Decreasing Level
Means	A manner or method of accomplishing an intervention	Wound Drainage Bag, Denture, Feeding Bottle, Cast, Nebulizer
Action	An intentional process applied to or performed by a patient	Assisting, Patient Advocating, Listening, Resuscitating
Time	The point, period, interval or duration of an occurrence	Always, Onset, Situation, Appointment, Afternoon
Location	Anatomical or spatial orientation of a diagnosis or intervention	Residential building, Anterior, Supine, Abdominal cavity, Finger, Intravenous route
Patient	Subject to which a diagnosis refers and who is the recipient of an intervention	Female-headed single family, Community, Elder, Infant

Source: Adapted from International Council of Nurses. (2005). International Classification for Nursing Practice®, Version 1.0 (pp. 29–30). Geneva, Switzerland: Author. Reproduced with permission.

BOX 10.2	Interface Terminology vs. Reference Terminology

- **Interface Terminology:** The terminology that clinicians would interact with in an electronic health management system (Thede & Sewell, 2009).
- **Reference Terminology:** The standardized terminology, embedded in a system's architecture, to which terms from an interface terminology may be mapped for communication with other systems (ISO TC 215, 2003).

architecture, to which terms from an interface terminology may be mapped for communication with other systems (ISO TC 215, 2003) (see Box 10.2).

Further, Canada Health Infoway, in consultation with various health care groups, adopted the **S**ystematized **No**menclature of **Med**icine-**C**linical **T**erms (SNOMED CT)® as the terminology for use in the pan-Canadian EHR. CNA and nurses on the various Infoway committees lobbied vigorously for parallel adoption of ICNP® without success. However, ongoing efforts by CNA and others did achieve the milestone invitation for ICNP® to work collaboratively with SNOMED to ensure that nursing data are accurately and effectively captured, and that terms are cross-mapped to provide comprehensive documentation. In March 2010, a joint announcement was issued by IHTSDO and ICN confirming the completion of a formal agreement to collaborate.

CNA continues to encourage nurses to apply ICNP® to support ongoing evaluation, not only to improve ICNP® itself, but also to determine how best to approach applying ICNP® to represent Canadian nursing data (CNA, 2001b, 2003). Research on ICNP® in Canada began with Lowen's (1999) examination of ICNP® Alpha Version in community-based nursing practice. In Lowen's research, ICNP® captured approximately two-thirds of the nursing data. Kennedy's (2005) research extended the Canadian application of ICNP® Beta 2 Version across multiple practice settings, including acute care, mental health, home-based care, and long-term care. ICNP® Beta 2 was effective in capturing the majority of nursing assessments and nursing actions across all practice domains, although nursing documentation was incomplete in a high percentage of nursing records (Kennedy, 2005). Nursing outcomes were conspicuously absent in the nursing documentation from every domain, and consequently, ICNP® could not be evaluated on outcomes measurement (Kennedy & Hannah, 2007; Kennedy, 2005). Doran's work (2004, 2006) in nursing-sensitive outcomes measurement has significant potential to contribute to ICNP® evolution and guide future research. With funding from Canada Health Infoway, the Canadian Nurses Association (CNA, 2007a, 2007b) is currently implementing the collection of nursing-sensitive patient outcomes using ICNP® in partnership with the provinces of Ontario, Manitoba, and Saskatchewan. ICNP® is an integral component to collect standardized, comparable nursing data from this project, which is titled Canadian Health Outcomes for Better Information and Care (C-HOBIC), and builds on the excellent work done in Ontario for the Health Outcomes for Better Information and Care (HOBIC) project (CNA, 2006a). The specific nursing-sensitive outcomes targeted for implementation in C-HOBIC include functional status, therapeutic self-care (or readiness for discharge), symptom management (pain, nausea, fatigue, dyspnea), and patient satisfaction (CNA, 2007b). Research related to the collection of data about nursing practice and outcomes, and the representation of that data, provides a rich research opportunity in Canada.

🔍 CANADIAN THEORY TO PRACTICE

The Canadian Health Outcomes for Better Information and Care (C-HOBIC) Project represents a key Canadian initiative linking nursing practice and decades of research on standardized nursing data (see Figure 10.2). C-HOBIC is a jointly funded initiative in partnership with the Canadian Nurses Association, Canada Health Infoway, and three Canadian provinces to include nursing-sensitive patient information in electronic health records (EHRs). Ontario, Prince Edward Island, and Saskatchewan were the initial provincial participants, and in May 2008, Manitoba joined the initiative.

C-HOBIC uses the International Classification for Nursing Practice (ICNP®) to enable collection and extraction of nursing data in secure jurisdictional EHRs, data repositories, or databases. C-HOBIC targets data on functional status, pain, fatigue, dyspnea, nausea, falls, and pressure ulcers and makes this data available to nurses for use in patient care across four sectors: acute care, complex continuing care, long-term care, and home care.

As a result of the work implemented in the C-HOBIC Project, Canada has contributed to the development of the ICNP® catalogue of terms by identifying new terms and recommending pre-coordination of terms to effectively capture the intent of the nursing item. The International Council of Nurses has welcomed the C-HOBIC Project as a leading example of standardized nursing data, and the C-HOBIC terms are being used by other countries, including Ireland.

The C-HOBIC Project promotes widespread, systematic use in Canada of standardized patient assessments and standardized related documentation. Based on the data captured by the C-HOBIC Project, nurses are able to retrieve feedback about patient outcomes by comparing patient assessments at different times.

This groundbreaking initiative offers numerous benefits, including the following:
1. Relevant information to support clinical practice
2. Improvements to patient care by fostering information access across care sectors
3. Opportunity to collect aggregated data that accurately reflect nursing activity

Updates on the C-HOBIC Project may be obtained through the Canadian Nurses Association.

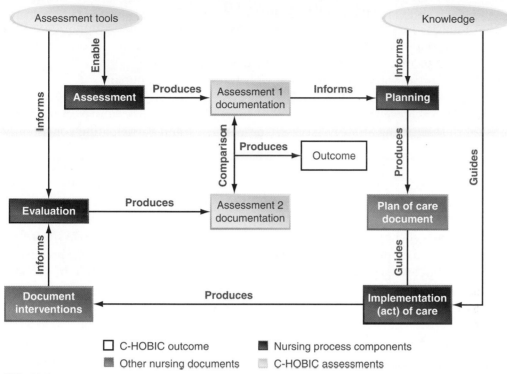

FIG 10.2 Relationship between C-HOBIC and the Nursing Process. Source: Hannah, K.J., White, P., Nagle, L., & Pringle, D. (2009). Standardizing nursing information in Canada for inclusion in electronic health records: C-HOBIC. *Journal of the American Medical Informatics Association, 16*, 524–530. Reproduced with permission of JAMIA.

E-NURSING

In 2006, CNA released the *E-Nursing Strategy for Canada* to guide the collaborative and coordinated development and integration of technology into Canadian nursing practice. With the ultimate goal of improving both nursing practice and outcomes for patients and clients, the strategy addresses both medium- and long-term goals. This strategy is intended to "fully integrate information and communication technologies (ICT) so that it becomes recognized as one of many tools used in practice—and within a few years, the 'e' part of the term will disappear" (CNA, 2006b, p. 3). Two working groups developed both the e-nursing and e-learning strategies that make up the comprehensive strategy for ICT and Canadian nursing practice. CNA (2006b, p. 4) identified seven key outcomes that were anticipated as a result of the e-Nursing Strategy. These are the seven outcomes:

1. Nurses will integrate ICT into their practice to achieve good patient outcomes.
2. Nurses will have the required information and knowledge to support their practice.

3. Human resources planning will be facilitated.
4. New models of nursing practice and health services delivery will be supported.
5. Nursing groups will be well connected.
6. ICT will improve the quality of nurses' work environments.
7. Canadian nurses will contribute to the global community of nursing.

In order to achieve the stated outcomes, CNA identified three fundamental directions for the e-Nursing Strategy. Access, Competencies, and Participation consistently emerged from the working groups and feedback from nurses across the country as critical paths to achieve success in fully integrating ICT in nursing practice. CNA identifies access to ICT as imperative if Canadian nurses are to realize the full benefits of technology in their practices. CNA notes that health care organizations have a responsibility to ensure that nurses have connectivity that will support professional practice—tools such as computers, mobile technology (e.g., laptops, PDAs, wireless technology), and resource databases/Internet resources (CNA, 2006b). As previously noted, CNA encourages nurses to develop competencies in the application of ICT and recommends that such competencies be part of both undergraduate and graduate-level nursing programs. Finally, CNA identified participation as including strategic partnerships with nurses in clinical practice, employers and administrators, federal/provincial/territorial ministries, nursing organizations (professional associations, regulatory bodies, educational groups, and unions), and educators and researchers (CNA, 2006b, p.12).

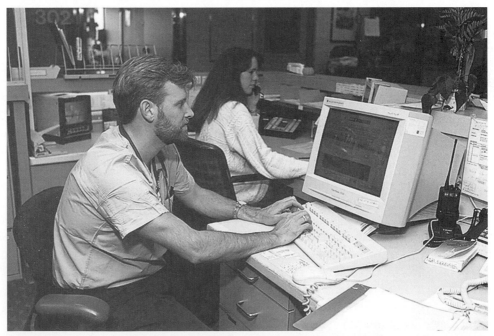

A nurse documenting patient care at a computer terminal.

A key component of the e-Nursing Strategy is the Canadian nurses' portal. The development of the portal was initially funded from a grant from the First Nations and Inuit Health Branch (FNIHB) of Health Canada (CNA, 2006b). The nursing portal, now known as NurseOne, enables nurses to register at http://www.nurseone.ca/index.php ?option=com_content&view=article&id=50&Itemid=67&lang=en, to create their own profile, and to customize their use of the site's tools and resources. NurseOne provides such services as Professional Links (resources with clinical or professional orientation), Professional Development (including resources for continuing competence, continuing education, and career development), Library (access to numerous educational resources), and NurseConnect (using the portal to create discussion groups among individual subscribers) (CNA, 2006c). Additional resources available to subscribers include conducting self-assessments, creating learning plans, and developing a professional online portfolio. Nurses also have the option of tracking current news and nursing information, receiving updates and alerts on items of interest, accessing educational opportunities, and searching for practice support on the NurseOne site. This valuable nursing tool will further develop over time and continue to support implementation of the e-Nursing Strategy.

REFLECTIVE THINKING

Consider the projected key outcomes of the e-Nursing Strategy launched by the Canadian Nurses Association:

1. Do you think the informatics competencies recommended by Staggers, Gassert, & Curran (2001) support the development of these key outcomes?
2. What additional factors might influence the development of competencies to support these outcomes?

CANADIAN E-NURSING SHOWCASE

As the CNA proceeds to implement the e-Nursing Strategy, many nurses are already engaged in projects that demonstrate innovations using technology to support practice and patient outcomes. These projects are as diverse as telehealth applications and researching change management to support technological innovations.

Examples of telehealth—the assessment, treatment, and monitoring of patients located at great or small distances from the health care providers who care for them—have grown rapidly since the 1990s. Telehealth is a global term that encompasses the various specialty applications, such as telemedicine, tele-education, and telenursing (or nursing telepractice). For instance, telemedicine reflects health services provided at a distance by physicians to support diagnostic information and consultation, while tele-education is the use of telehealth networks to support education of health care providers (CNA, 2000 November). The Canadian Nurses Association defines nursing telepractice as "a nursing-specific application of telehealth that includes all patient-centred forms of nursing practice and the provision of information, conferences, and courses for health care professionals occurring through, or facilitated by, the use of telecommunications or electronic means" (CNA, 2001a, p.1). The Canadian Nurses Association (2001a) also acknowledges the challenges associated with providing care to patients at a distance, and notes that "nurses engaged in telepractice are considered to be practising in the province/territory where they are located and currently registered, regardless of where the patient is located. As such, they must provide nursing telepractice services consistent with the *Code of Ethics for Registered Nurses*, professional practice standards, relevant legislation and practice guidelines of the province/territory in which they are registered and practising" (p. 2).

The first recorded example of a telehealth application occurred in the 1950s, with the first poison control centre at the Montreal General Hospital. This program served as a model for the rest of Canada and such projects were initiated in many large centres. Many universities have also implemented telehealth applications, such as the University of Ottawa, which assumed responsibility for providing health services to the Baffin Island population, and which is offering to patients in the far north a variety of health services involving nurses and physicians. Additionally, the University of Ottawa, School of Nursing has a tele-education partnership with two provinces in China involving the preparation of nurse clinicians. Likewise, the Faculty of Nursing at the University of Alberta is partnered with the Faculty of Nursing at the University of Ghana and is assisting in the development of a master's program in nursing in Ghana. Athabasca University offers nursing education programs online, and many other Canadian universities, from Dalhousie University on the east coast to the University of Victoria on the west coast, employ such communication technologies as WebCT, virtual classrooms, online lectures, and other e-learning applications to ensure students from off-site locations are able to access health education (CNA, 2006b).

Clinical examples of telehealth applications include the provincial tele-triage and health information call centre (Roberts, Tayler, MacCormack, & Barwich, 2007). In this example, nurses provide support to patients in the palliative care program by answering questions or linking patients to specialized palliative care nurses when appropriate. Telenursing enables patients to receive professional health care information and support 24 hours a day, 7 days a week, being accessible when most offices are closed and patients are at their most vulnerable. Another current clinical example involves the provision of cardiac rehabilitation services for patients in remote areas of Ontario. In this case, four sites, ranging between 100 and 385 kilometres from the primary program site, are able to offer patients access to lifestyle education and risk-factor modification through a telemedicine network. Additionally, a Web site provides access to procedures and tools, policies and forms, and best practices. Patients are also able to have access to professional counsellors, diagnostic testing, and medical specialists through the telemedicine network. Future plans include adapting this program to a culturally sensitive application for a remote First Nations community.

Other examples of e-nursing include the transition to computerized patient assessments at the Interior Health Authority in British Columbia (Kraft & Scott, 2007), and the cardiac program described by Kmill, Sherrington, and Third (2007). These initiatives shared a desire to improve patient access to care and ensure optimal outcomes despite remote geographical location from centres of care. Both programs necessitated significant attention to change management and standards of information management.

Challenges remain, and remote communities continue to be marginalized by a lack of access to health care. However, progress is being made and efforts are underway across the country by communities in partnership with Canada Health Infoway, and other professional bodies and funding agencies, to implement projects that serve to improve outcomes and support health care practice.

PRIVACY AND CONFIDENTIALITY IN A DIGITAL PRACTICE DOMAIN

A significant issue in nursing, regardless of the presence or absence of technology, relates to patient privacy and the security of patient information. Where computerized records are shared across jurisdictions, the protection of privacy and confidentiality becomes an even greater area of concern. The provincial Standards of Practice and national *Code of Ethics* govern nurses' actions in regard to the protection of patient information. Privacy legislation varies among provinces, and nurses should have a working knowledge of the relevant legislation, both provincially and nationally.

The federal government has two separate pieces of legislation regarding the privacy of personal information. These include the *Privacy Act* and the *Personal Information Protection and Electronic Documents Act* (Government of Canada, 2004). Each Act sets forth specific regulatory parameters in regard to personal information. In the *Privacy Act*, the regulation states, "8.(1) Personal information under the control of a government institution shall not, without the consent of the individual to whom it relates, be disclosed by the institution…" (Government of Canada, 1983, Section 8.1). The *Personal Information Protection and Electronic Documents Act* (PIPEDA) (Government of Canada, 2000) takes the *Privacy Act* one step further to address the specific risks associated with electronic data collection, storage, retrieval, and communication. PIPEDA addresses personal health information specifically and notes that personal health information, with respect to an individual, whether living or deceased, means

(a) information concerning the physical or mental health of the individual;
(b) information concerning any health service provided to the individual;
(c) information concerning the donation by the individual of any body part or any bodily substance of the individual or information derived from the testing or examination of a body part or bodily substance of the individual;
(d) information that is collected in the course of providing health services to the individual; or
(e) information that is collected incidentally to the provision of health services to the individual (Government of Canada, 2004, Section 1.2).

Further, PIPEDA stipulates that disclosure of personal information may be permitted only under the most stringent of conditions, such as law enforcement (Government of Canada, 2004, Division 1, Section 7.3).

Regardless of the practice setting or mode, nurses are professionally and ethically obliged to protect the personal information of all patients in their care. Knowledge of these two pieces of federal privacy legislation, in addition to provincial privacy legislation, can support nurses as they uphold the Standards of Practice and *Code of Ethics.*

NURSING INFORMATICS COMMUNITIES AND RESOURCES

Since the development of the World Wide Web in the early 1990s, the Internet has transformed communications around the world. In nursing, it facilitates the acquisition and exchange of knowledge. Norris (1999) has differentiated between Internet use in a "writerly context," in which the user is an active participant in the inquiry, and a "readerly context," which implies a more passive response. Internet access to nursing and health-related resources is immensely helpful to nurse clinicians, administrators, educators, and researchers studying particular topics. Web sites have been launched by organizations and individuals to provide information and assistance in relation to their mission or principal interests. Thus, information that previously might have taken nurses days or weeks to obtain can be accessed within minutes. Web sites may also contain information about the principal staff and divisions of an organization as well as listing names and telephone numbers of contacts for particular kinds of assistance, thereby providing valuable networking opportunities.

Today, nurses routinely use the Web for accessing up-to-date health information or to network with professional colleagues. The success of electronic discussion groups is perhaps one of the most exciting professional developments for nurses. In 2002, there were upward of 70 public discussion lists and many newsgroups, bulletin boards, and chat rooms for nurses on the World Wide Web. Today, the presence of "blogs" (an online commentary, generally hosted by an individual—or less commonly, by a group—with writers posting their comments on diverse or specific topics) has assumed prominence not only in informal communication, but also among professional groups. Mediblogopathy (http://mediblogopathy.blogspot.com/) is one such site that provides links to most other nursing blogs and provides opportunities for nurses to informally discuss professional information as well as pursue discussions that have a more educational flavour.

These forms of communication have assumed importance for nurses functioning in a variety of roles. The term "on-line nursing communities" was coined by Norris (1999, p .198) to refer to the various electronic communication resources for nurses. The important professional outcomes of the resources that she cites include networking and collegial support, nursing education, research and other scholarly activity, and political action (p. 199).

Nurses interested in joining a network or nursing informatics community will find several groups readily accessible through the Web. Although not every province has a nursing informatics special-interest group, the Canadian Nursing Informatics Association

(CNIA) (http://www.cnia.ca/intro.htm) has a Web site offering access to a variety of educational resources, informatics events, and networking opportunities. Links to existing provincial NI groups are available on the CNIA Web site. The International Medical Informatics Association—Nursing Informatics (IMIA-NI) (http://www.imiani.org/) is an international organization of significant value to nurses interested in NI. This group has multiple working groups and represents the interests of nurses internationally.

COACH, Canada's Health Informatics Association (http://www.coachorg.com/default.asp), is another group of interest to nurses and was formed in 1975 by several health professionals and vendors in the medical industry. COACH's 900 members include health care executives, physicians, nurses and allied health professionals, researchers and educators, CIOs, information managers, technical experts, consultants, and information technology vendors. Organizational members include health care service delivery organizations, government and nongovernment agencies, consulting firms, commercial providers of information and telecommunications technologies, and educational institutions. The Canadian Society of Telehealth (CST, http://www.cst-sct.org/en/index.php), was created in 1998. The CST was the first Canadian nonprofit health association devoted to telehealth. The society brought together the many key stakeholders involved and interested in furthering the development and implementation of telehealth practices, acts as a major resource for information and knowledge sharing, contributes to telehealth policy and standards development, and is the Canadian voice for telehealth both at home and internationally. As of April 1, 2010, COACH and the CST have merged under the COACH name.

Today, there are a multitude of online resources for nurses. Library catalogues of most universities and major university health centres are for the most part fully online, with access to full-text journal articles. Further, online lectures with leading experts are offered by many groups. The NurseOne site also incorporates many of these features to support nursing education and professional practice.

GLIMPSES INTO THE FUTURE

The Canadian Nurses Association released its vision for future nursing practice in its landmark document *Toward 2020: Visions for Nursing* (CNA, 2006d). This document highlights areas that will change as we progress toward 2020. Changes predicted in the report include the use of robots to perform mundane or repetitive tasks, changes in human resource management, and an education revolution in how nursing programs are structured.

It is difficult to predict with any certainty how technology will affect the professional practice of nursing, but as technology advances, nurses will respond to both challenges and opportunities. Saba (2001) has predicted that as the technology evolution continues, and with the continued integration of telephone, computer, and media technologies, "nursing will change from 'electronic care' to 'mobile care' using wireless technology tools." Further, nurses will "be linked to desktop computers via wireless communication." Already this is true of many health care settings, as agencies incorporate encrypted wireless technology to enhance point-of-care delivery and data collection.

Many technologies offer real and potential value to nursing. Anonson (2007) suggests that the iPod can be used to support both practice and education through podcasts and wireless mobility. Other examples of innovative applications include Healthphone—an international health software company that is using SMS or text messages on cellular phones to support smoking cessation and partnering with the Victorian Order of Nurses (VON) to provide a mobile wound management service. Further, the CNA e-Nursing Strategy (2006b, p. 47) notes that future nursing practice and education will include technologies such as rich media (or streaming video/audio), virtual reality/simulations, 3D virtual instructors, blogs, wikis (essentially highly interactive blogs), and mobile technology.

CONCLUSION

Although the nursing practice environment has evolved significantly with the integration of technology, the philosophy and goals of the professional discipline of nursing have remained constant. The patient-centred focus of the profession is as important as it always has been. It may even have assumed more importance as patients undergoing new and potentially frightening procedures for diagnosis or treatment require support and reassurance.

The vast array of informational resources that have been made accessible by computer technology will continue to benefit nurses and their patients. Enhancements to communications resources are occurring on an almost daily basis. Nurses will continue to advocate for patients in the midst of a health care environment that is laden with technology and continue to support the central goals of competent and caring nursing practice.

CRITICAL THINKING QUESTIONS

1. You are part of a multidisciplinary team at your local hospital or community centre, planning for a new health information system. What other disciplines are important to have as team members? Why? What specific competencies would you need to be an effective nursing representative? How will these competencies contribute to your participation?
2. You and your nursing team are examining ways to examine the outcomes of nursing care on your unit. The manager has required that a standardized nursing language must be used to perform the analysis. What are some of the issues you may confront with colleagues unfamiliar with such languages? How would you explain the necessity and value of standardized languages in nursing?

WEB SITES

NurseOne: http://www.nurseone.ca/
Canadian Nursing Informatics Association: http://cnia.ca/intro.htm
International Medical Informatics Association—Nursing Informatics (IMIA-NI):
    http://www.imiani.org/index.php
Canada Health Infoway: http://www.infoway-inforoute.ca/

REFERENCES

Alberta Association of Registered Nurses (AARN). (1994). *Client status, nursing intervention, and client outcome taxonomies: A background paper*. Edmonton: Author.

American Nurses Association (ANA). (1992). *Congress of nursing practice: Report on the designation of nursing informatics as a nursing specialty*. Washington, DC: American Nurses Association.

American Nurses Association (ANA). (1994). *The scope of practice for nursing informatics*. Washington, DC: Author.

Anonson, J. (2007). From Pens to Pentium: A review of tools used by registered nurses for the processing of client information. *Canadian Journal of Nursing Informatics*, 2(2), 20–29.

Ball, M. J., & Hannah, K. J. (1984). *Using computers in nursing*. Reston: Reston Publishing.

Ball, M. J., Hannah, K. J., Newbold, S. K., & Douglas, J. V. (Eds.), (2000). *Nursing informatics: Where caring and technology meet* (3rd ed.). New York: Springer.

Canadian Institute for Health Information (CIHI). (2007). Taking health information further. Retrieved on August 31, 2009, from http://secure.cihi.ca/cihiweb/dispPage.jsp?cw_page=profile_e.

Canadian Nurses Association (CNA). (2000). *Collecting data to reflect nursing impact: Discussion paper*. Ottawa: Author.

Canadian Nurses Association. (2000, November). Telehealth: Great potential or risky terrain? *Nursing Now*, 9. Retrieved on August 31, 2009, from http://www.cna-nurses.ca/CNA/documents/pdf/publications/Telehealth_November2000_e.pdf.

Canadian Nurses Association. (2001, November). *Position statement: Collecting data to reflect the impact of nursing practice*. Ottawa: Author.

Canadian Nurses Association. (2001a). The role of the nurse in telepractice. Ottawa: Author. Retrieved on August 31, 2009, from http://cna-aiic.ca/CNA/documents/pdf/publications/PS52_Role_Nurse_Telepractice_Nov_2001_e.pdf.

Canadian Nurses Association. (2001b). What is nursing informatics and why is it so important? *Nursing Now*, 11. Retrieved on August 31, 2009, from http://www.cna-nurses.ca/CNA/documents/pdf/publications/NursingInformaticsSept_2001_e.pdf.

Canadian Nurses Association. (2003). International classification for nursing practice: Documenting nursing care and client outcomes. *Nursing Now*, 14. Retrieved on August 31, 2009, from http://www.cna-nurses.ca/CNA/documents/pdf/publications/NN_IntlClassNrgPract_e.pdf.

Canadian Nurses Association. (2006a). Nursing information and knowledge management. Ottawa: Author. Retrieved on August 31, 2009, from http://cna-aiic.ca/CNA/documents/pdf/publications/PS87-Nursing-info-knowledge-e.pdf.

Canadian Nurses Association. (2006b). E-Nursing Strategy for Canada. Ottawa: Author. Retrieved on August 31, 2009, from http://www.cna-nurses.ca/CNA/documents/pdf/publications/E-Nursing-Strategy-2006-e.pdf.

Canadian Nurses Association. (2006c). NurseOne. Retrieved on September 5, 2009, from http://www.nurseone.ca/.

Canadian Nurses Association. (2006d). Toward 2020: Visions for nursing. Retrieved on September 5, 2009, from http://cna-aiic.ca/CNA/documents/pdf/publications/Toward-2020-e.pdf.

Canadian Nurses Association. (2007a). CNA moves forward on e-Nursing Strategy. *Canadian Nurse*, 103(5), 11.

Canadian Nurses Association. (2007b). Canadian health outcomes for better information and care. Retrieved on August 31, 2009, from http://www.cna-aiic.ca/c-hobic/.

Clark, D. J. (1999). A language for nursing. *Nursing Standard*, 13(31), 42.

Clark, J., & Lang, N. M. (1992). Nursing's next advance: An international classification system for nursing practice. *International Nursing Review*, 39(4), 109–112, 128.

Colliere, M., & Lawlor, J. (1998). Marie Francoise Colliere—nurse and ethnohistorian. A conversation about nursing and the invisibility of care. *Nursing Inquiry*, 5(3), 140–145.

Conrick, M., & Foster, J. (1997). Nurses: Invisible forever? *Contemporary Nurse, 6*(2), 92.

Doran, D. (2004). Enhancing continuity of care through outcomes measurement. *Canadian Journal of Nursing Research, 36*(2), 83–87.

Doran, D., Harrison, M., Laschinger, H., Hirdes, J., Rukholm, E., Sidani, S., McGillis Hall, L., Tourangeau, A., & Cranley, L. (2006). Relationship between nursing interventions and outcomes achievement in acute care settings. *Research in Nursing & Health, 29*(1), 61–70.

Englebardt, S., & Nelson, R. (2002). *Health care informatics: An interdisciplinary approach.* St. Louis, MO: Mosby.

Giovannetti, P., Smith, D., & Broad, E. (1999). Structuring and managing health information. In J. Hibberd, & D. Smith (Eds.), *Nursing management in Canada* (2nd ed.), (pp. 297–318). Toronto: W.B. Saunders.

Government of Canada. (1983). The Privacy Act. Bill C-21. Retrieved on August 31, 2009, from http://laws.justice.gc.ca/en/ShowFullDoc/cs/P-21///en.

Government of Canada. (2000). Personal Information Protection and Electronic Documents Act. BillC-6. Retrieved on August 31, 2009, from http://www.parl.gc.ca/PDF/36/2/parlbus/chambus/house/bills/government/C-6_4.pdf.

Government of Canada. (2004). Privacy legislation in Canada. Retrieved on August 31, 2009, from http://www.privcom.gc.ca/fs-fi/02_05_d_15_e.asp.

Graves, J. R., & Corcoran, S. (1989). The study of nursing informatics. *Image: Journal of Nursing Scholarship, 21*, 227–231.

Grobe, S. J. (1989). Nursing informatics competencies. *Methods of Information in Medicine, 28*(4), 267–269.

Hannah, K. J. (2005). Health informatics and nursing in Canada. *Healthcare Information Management and Communications, XIX*(3), 45–51.

Hannah, K. J. (2007). The state of nursing informatics in Canada. *Canadian Nurse, 103*(5), 18–22.

Hannah, K. J., Ball, M. J., & Edwards, M. J. A. (1994). *Introduction to nursing informatics.* New York: Springer-Verlag.

Hannah, K. J., Ball, M., & Edwards, M. (2006). *Introduction to nursing informatics* (3rd ed.). New York: Springer-Verlag.

Hannah, K. J., Hammell, N., & Nagle, L. M. (2005). Nursing informatics in Canada. In V. K. Saba, & K. A. McCormick (Eds.), *Essentials of nursing informatics* (4th ed.), (pp. 607–620). Philadelphia: McGraw-Hill.

Hannah, K. J., White, P., Nagle, L., & Pringle, D. (2009). Standardizing nursing information in Canada for inclusion in electronic health records: C-HOBIC. *Journal of the American Medical Informatics Association, 16*, 524–530.

Hebert, M. (2000). A national education strategy to develop nursing informatics competencies. *Canadian Journal of Nursing Leadership, 13*(2), 11–14.

International Council of Nurses. (2005). *International Classification for Nursing Practice®, Version 1.0.* Geneva: Author.

International Council of Nurses. (2009, June). ICNP® Bulletin No. 1. Retrieved on August 9, 2009, from http://www.icn.ch/icnpbulletin.htm.

International Medical Informatics Association Special Interest Group—Nursing Informatics (IMIA-NI). (2009). Definition of nursing informatics. *Retrieved on September, 5,* 2009, from http://www.imiani.org/index.php.

Kaminski, J. (2007). Nursing informatics competencies: A self assessment. Retrieved on August 31, 2009, from http://www.nursing-informatics.com/niassess/index.html.

Kennedy, M. A. (2005). *Packaging nursing as politically potent: A critical reflexive cultural studies approach to nursing informatics.* Adelaide, Australia: University of South Australia.

Kennedy, M. A., & Hannah, K. J. (2007). Representing nursing practice: Evaluating the effectiveness of a nursing classification system. *Canadian Journal of Nursing Research, 39*(7), 58–79.

Kirby, M. L. (2002). *Standing Senate Committee on Social Affairs, Science, and Technology. Final Report: The Health of Canadians—The Federal Role (Volume Six: Recommendations for Reform).* Ottawa: Queen's Printer. Retrieved on October 22, 2009, from http://www.parl.gc.ca/37/2/parlbus/commbus/senate/com-e/SOCI-E/rep-e/repoct02vol6-e.htm..

Kmill, C., Sherrington, L., & Third, G. (2007). Increasing access to cardiac rehabilitation through telemedicine technology. *Canadian Nurse*, *103*(5), 8–9.

Kraft, L., & Scott, P. (2007). Computerized patient assessments: A change in practice. *Canadian Nurse*, *103*(5), 28–31.

Lalonde, M. (1974). *A new perspective on the health of Canadians*. Ottawa: Queen's Printer.

Lowen, E. (1999). *The use of the International Classification for Nursing Practice® for capturing community-based nursing practice*. Winnipeg, Manitoba: University of Manitoba.

Marck, P. (1994). The problem with good nursing care…it is often invisible. *Alberta Association of Registered Nurses Newsletter*, *50*(5), 10–11.

Marek, K., & Lang, N. (1993). Nursing sensitive outcomes. In Canadian Nurses Association (Ed.), *Papers from the Nursing Minimum Data Set Conference* (pp. 100–120). Ottawa: Canadian Nurses Association.

McBride, A. B. (2005). Nursing and the informatics revolution. *Nursing Outlook*, *53*(4), 181–191.

McGee, M. (1993). Response to V. Saba's paper on Nursing Diagnostic Schemes. In Canadian Nurses Association (Ed.), *Papers from the Nursing Minimum Data Set Conference* (pp. 64–67). Ottawa: Canadian Nurses Association.

Norris, J. R. (1999). The Internet: Extending our capacity for scholarly inquiry in nursing. *Nursing Science Quarterly*, *12*, 197–201.

Norwood, S. (2001). NP education: The invisibility of advanced practice nurses in popular magazines. *Journal of the American Academy of Nurse Practitioners*, *13*(3), 129–134.

O'Brien-Pallas, L., & Giovannetti, P. (1993). Nursing intensity. In Canadian Nurses Association (Ed.), *Papers from the Nursing Minimum Data Set Conference* (pp. 68–76). Ottawa: Canadian Nurses Association.

Roberts, D., Tayler, C., MacCormack, D., & Barwich, D. (2007). Telenursing in hospice palliative care. *Canadian Nurse*, *103*(5), 24–27.

Romanow, R. J. (2002, November). *Building on values: The future of health care in Canada*. Ottawa: Queen's Printer.

Rutherford, M. (2008). Standardized nursing language: What does it mean for nursing practice? *OJIN: The Online Journal of Issues in Nursing*, *13*(1). Retrieved on August 31, 2009, from www.nursingworld. org/MainMenuCategories/ANAMarketplace/ANAPeriodicals/OJIN/TableofContents/vol132008/No1Jan08/ArticlePreviousTopic/StandardizedNursingLanguage.aspx.

Saba, V. K. (2001). Nursing informatics: Yesterday, today and tomorrow. *International Nursing Review*, *48*, 177–187.

Saba, V. K., Hovenga, E., Coenen, A., McCormick, K. M., & Bakken, S. (2003). Nursing language—Terminology models for nurses. *ISO Bulletin*, 16–18, (September).

Saba, V. K., & McCormick, K. A. (1986). *Essentials of computers for nurses*. Philadelphia: Lippincott.

Saba, V. K., & McCormick, K. A. (Eds.). (1996). *Essentials of computers for nurses*. New York: McGraw-Hill.

Schwirian, P. (1986). The NI pyramid: A model for research in nursing informatics. *Computers in Nursing*, *4*(3), 134–136.

Staggers, N., & Bagley Thompson, C. (2002). The evolution of definitions of nursing informatics: A critical analysis and revised definitions. *Journal of the American Medical Informatics Association*, *9*(3), 255–262.

Staggers, N., Gassert, C., & Curran, C. (2001). Informatics competencies for nurses at four levels of practice. *Journal of Nursing Education*, *40*(7), 303–316.

Thede, L. Q., & Sewell, J. (2009). *Informatics and nursing: Opportunities and challenges* (3rd. ed.). Philadelphia: Lippincott Williams & Wilkins.

Turley, J. P. (1996). Toward a model of nursing informatics. *Image: Journal of Nursing Scholarship*, *28*(1), 309–313.

Werley, H. H. (1988). Introduction to the nursing minimum data set and its development. In H. H. Werley, & N. M. Lang (Eds.), *Identification of the nursing minimum data set* (pp. 1–15). New York: Springer.

Weyrauch, B. (2002). President's message: DNA joins alliance to increase nursing's visibility. *Dermatology Nursing*, *14*(6), 356.

Zielstorff, R., Abraham, L., Werley, H., Saba, V. K., & Schwirian, P. (1989). Guidelines for adopting innovations in computer-based information systems for nursing. *Computers in Nursing*, *7*(5), 203–208.

PART 3

NURSING CARE DELIVERY

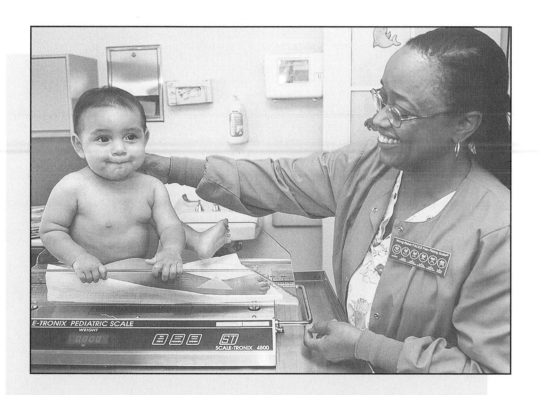

Primary Health Care: Challenges and Opportunities for the Nursing Profession

Linda Reutter and Linda Ogilvie

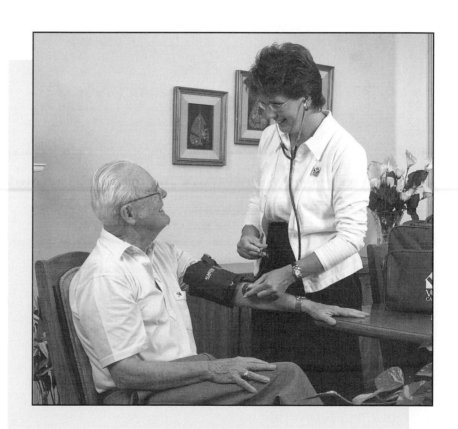

LEARNING OBJECTIVES

- To situate Primary Health Care (PHC) within international and historical contexts.
- To foster understanding of the five interrelated principles of PHC.
- To identify examples of current PHC initiatives in Canada.
- To highlight nursing involvement and potential nursing leadership in the evolution of PHC in Canada.
- To introduce the challenges and complexities of reorienting the Canadian health care system to meet PHC goals.

With the Alma-Ata Declaration of 1978, Primary Health Care (PHC) was introduced as "the key to attaining ... a level of health that will permit ... all peoples of the world by the year 2000 ... to lead a socially and economically productive life ... as part of development in the spirit of social justice" (World Health Organization [WHO], 1978a, p. 3). The goal of this international meeting was captured in the slogan "Health for All by the Year 2000." Primary Health Care was defined as

> *essential health care based on practical, scientifically sound and socially acceptable methods and technology made universally accessible to individuals and families in the community through their full participation and at a cost that the community and country can afford to maintain at every stage of their development in the spirit of self-reliance and self-determination. It forms an integral part both of the country's health system, of which it is the central function and main focus, and of the overall social and economic development of the community. It is the first level of contact of individuals, the family and community with the national health system bringing health care as close as possible to where people live and work, and constitutes the first element of a continuing health care process. (WHO, 1978a, pp. 3–4)*

From the beginning, PHC was conceptualized as a social justice model, although care was taken to articulate the autonomy of nations in operationalizing the concept. The nursing profession was envisioned as being key to attaining health for all (Mahler, 1985). Nurses around the world, including in Canada, embraced PHC as fundamental to nursing's role in enhancing health, and nurses have been actively involved in efforts to bring about PHC reform.

DECONSTRUCTING PRIMARY HEALTH CARE

PRINCIPLES OF PHC

Although the PHC concept remains ambiguous, there is general agreement that it is based on five principles (see Figure 11.1). Key to understanding the concept of PHC is the interrelatedness of these principles, including the importance of incorporating all principles in a health care approach.

Accessibility implies health care that is geographically, financially, and culturally accessible, and that is appropriate and acceptable to people (Canadian Nurses Association

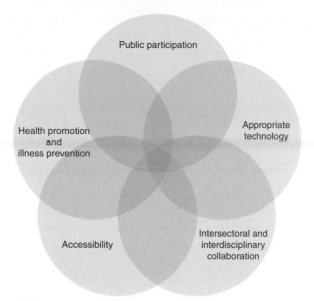

FIG 11.1 Principles of Primary Health Care

[CNA], 1988). In the spirit of the Health for All philosophy of reducing health inequities, some have suggested that the definition of accessibility be expanded beyond its conventional meaning of access to health care services to access to the prerequisites for health (WHO, 1997a) or determinants of health (Advisory Committee on Population Health [ACPH], 1994, 1996) that lie outside health care services (Reutter, 2000; Stewart, 2000).

Public participation refers to maximum individual and community involvement in the planning and operation of health care services (CNA, 1988). Consumer control, support by volunteers, mutual aid, partnership with lay helpers, and professional–client interactions are all compatible with the public participation principle (Stewart, 2000). Collaborative partnerships include partnerships at all levels—governmental, nongovernmental, corporate, and community.

The principle of **health promotion and illness prevention** reflects the concern that to date there has been greater emphasis on cure and treatment of illness than on prevention and health promotion. A broad view of health promotion as enabling control over determinants of health (WHO, Health and Welfare Canada, & the Canadian Public Health Association [CPHA], 1986) necessarily incorporates the principles of public participation and intersectoral collaboration, which are required to address health determinants outside the health sector. Six of the eight essential elements of PHC (WHO, 1978a) address prevention: health education, nutrition, sanitation, maternal and child health care, immunization, and prevention and control of endemic diseases.

Appropriate technology refers broadly to the appropriate use of all health care resources, such as funds, facilities, equipment, tools, and techniques (Stewart, 2000). It also includes the most effective use of personnel and evidence-informed interventions and strategies. This principle relates directly to issues of cost and sustainability.

Intersectoral and interdisciplinary collaboration is a crucial principle to achieving Health for All and is highly interrelated with the above principles. A focus on the broad determinants of health requires attention to areas outside the traditional health sectors, such as education, labour, employment, and social services. Addressing these determinants also requires collaboration among a range of disciplines.

The Declaration of Alma-Ata, when examined closely, was a radical document when it was published in 1978. It implied a need for far-reaching structural changes in how health services were delivered and changes in the skills needed by the health workers providing guidance and care (Ogilvie, 1993). In early WHO documents advocating the shift to PHC (1978a, 1978b), there appeared to be little appreciation of the difficulty of making structural changes in health systems, particularly in situations of scarce resources and obvious social inequities (Navarro, 1986). It should therefore be of no surprise that, while significant strides were being made, by the 1990s it was obvious that the goal of Health for All by the Year 2000 would not be met.

Several WHO publications provide analyses of reasons for not meeting the goal of Health for All 2000 (WHO, 1990, 1995, 1996, 1997b, 1998, 1999, 2000). The 2001 WHO report, *Health for All in the Twenty-first Century*, while continuing to reiterate the values of PHC, identified the following barriers to Health for All: lack of political commitment, slower than anticipated socioeconomic development, insufficient financial input for health, problems achieving intersectoral collaboration, the speed with which epidemiological and demographic changes are occurring, and the occurrence of natural and human-made disasters. Moreover, it was noted that poverty, the greatest determinant of health, had increased globally, with the worst population health status indicators in countries where per capita incomes are inadequate or where wide disparities in the distribution of resources are apparent (WHO, 2001). This finding underscores the problem of inequity and the need for increased emphasis on strategies based on the principle of social justice.

HEALTH EQUITY—A KEY COMPONENT OF HEALTH FOR ALL

Several international initiatives continue to acknowledge the significance of health equity as a key component of Health for All. The United Nations Millennium Development Goals, adopted in 2000, emphasize the essential elements of PHC articulated in 1978: poverty reduction; universal primary education; gender equality and empowerment of women; reducing child mortality; improving maternal health; combating HIV/AIDS, malaria, and other diseases; environmental sustainability and access to safe drinking water and sanitation; and global partnerships for development (United Nations, 2006). The WHO Commission on the Social Determinants of Health (WHO, 2008a) was established in 2005 to promote models and practices that will effectively address social determinants of health, thereby narrowing health inequalities to achieve Health for All. The Bangkok Charter for Health Promotion (WHO, 2005) emphasizes health as a fundamental human right and the responsibility of government, civil society, and the private sector. The 2008 World Health Report (WHO, 2008b) focused on PHC and recommended four sets of reforms: promotion of equity and social justice through universal coverage; people-centred health service delivery; enhanced focus on the health of communities through public policy reforms; and promotion of inclusive, participatory leadership styles. Recent Canadian health care documents give messages consistent with the social determinants of health focus advocated in WHO circles, and iterate a new commitment to PHC.

 REFLECTIVE THINKING

> How are the five principles of PHC reflected in your workplace? In what ways could they be more fully incorporated?

PRIMARY HEALTH CARE IN THE CANADIAN CONTEXT

HISTORICAL PERSPECTIVES

Prior to the 1978 Declaration of Alma-Ata, the federal and provincial governments in Canada had moved in a direction congruent with some of the main tenets of PHC. Universal health care insurance was introduced in 1966, and in 1977 greater responsibility for health-service development shifted to the provinces (Legowski & McKay, 2000). As well, the Lalonde Report (Lalonde, 1974) articulated the difference between health and health care and the need for intersectoral collaboration if the health status of the Canadian population was to improve in a significant way. The groundwork for building an accessible health care system oriented to prevention, health promotion, and intersectoral collaboration was in place.

From the beginning, health promotion in Canada focused on a behavioural perspective of health, which emphasized decreasing behavioural risk factors. Limited emphasis was given to the other health-field determinants identified in the Lalonde Report, such as environment or the social conditions influencing health. However, the 1980s ushered in the shift to a more social conceptualization of health, with the introduction of *Achieving Health for All: A Framework for Health Promotion* (Epp, 1986), which was Canada's blueprint for achieving Health for All. The report followed the *Canada Health Act*, which in 1984 entrenched the principles of accessibility, universality, portability, comprehensiveness, and public administration of hospital and medical services (Health Summit '99, 1999). The Epp Report identified the major challenges to health as reducing inequities, increasing prevention, and enhancing coping. Self-care, mutual aid, and healthy environments were viewed as the relevant health-promotion mechanisms. Fostering public participation, strengthening community services, and coordinating healthy public policy were suggested as implementation strategies. The Epp Report was congruent with the Ottawa Charter (WHO, Health and Welfare Canada, & CPHA, 1986). Together, the Ottawa Charter and the Epp Report reinforced four of the five principles of Primary Health Care. The political will required for transforming the Canadian health system to incorporate PHC principles appeared strong.

Political will for health promotion, however, began to dissipate in 1989. Concerns were raised about budgetary deficits. Health promotion was seen by some as too diffuse to guide specific actions. Evidence-informed practice, with quantitative data perceived as "best evidence," was perceived as most useful for informing policy. The social justice thrust of health promotion was not congruent with the "emerging political agendas of the late 1980s and 1990s, which generally criticized social programs as undermining individual initiative and unnecessarily draining the public purse" (Legowski & McKay, 2000, p. 26).

The population health paradigm, initiated by the Canadian Institute of Advanced Research (CIAR) in the 1990s, significantly influenced the direction of government health initiatives. This approach is characterized by a strong epidemiological research base, a focus on determinants of health, and a life-cycle approach (children and youth, early and middle adulthood, and later life). A framework to achieve population health, as outlined in *Strategies for Population Health* (ACPH, 1994), was adopted by the federal government to guide health policy (Pinder, 2007). The document identified nine determinants of health, which in 1996 were expanded to twelve: income and social status, social support networks, education, employment and working conditions, physical environments, biology and genetic endowment, personal health practices and coping skills, healthy child development, health services, gender, culture, and social environments. In line with the new emphasis on a population health approach, in 1995, the Health Promotion Directorate was replaced by the new Population Health Directorate (Pinder, 2007). Early on, there was considerable debate on the similarities and differences between population health and health promotion. In an effort to integrate these two approaches, Health Canada developed the *Population Health Promotion Model* (Hamilton & Bhatti, 1996), which clearly identified the contributions of each approach: the determinants of health that need to be addressed (population health) using five broad action strategies (health promotion).

An emphasis on deficit and debt reduction in the 1990s, with resultant cuts to health care spending, led to a renewed commitment to ensuring access to illness care services. The National Forum on Health (1997) highlighted public concerns about the impact of fiscal constraints on health care spending and reported a public perception that health care was deteriorating in Canada. The subsequent Romanow Commission (Commission on the Future of Health Care in Canada, 2002), however, suggested that there remained a strong public commitment to publicly funded health care.

The discourse on health reform in the past decade has shifted to PHC as a way to sustain our publicly funded health care system and to meet the increasing challenges of access to health services. Two provincial commissions—in Quebec (Quebec Commission on Health and Social Services, 2000) and Saskatchewan—emphasized the principles of PHC in their recommendations for a sustainable health care system. The Fyke Report (Saskatchewan Commission on Medicare, 2001) recommended the establishment of primary health teams comprising a range of health providers, primary health centres, and accessibility to primary services 24 hours a day, seven days a week ("24/7"). The Romanow Commission strongly supported PHC as a key element of health-system reform (CNA, 2003c). Although it is important to analyze critically how PHC is being conceptualized in these documents (i.e., as synonymous with primary medical care rather than encompassing the five essential principles outlined previously), nevertheless it is significant that provincial and federal documents and Web sites acknowledge the principles in varying ways. For example, the Health Canada Web site clearly articulates that PHC includes all services that contribute to health (e.g., income, housing, education, and environment) and that Primary Care, one element of PHC, focuses on health care services including health promotion, illness and injury prevention, and the diagnosis and treatment of illness and injury (Health Canada, 2006).

FEDERAL SUPPORT FOR PHC INITIATIVES

Tangible evidence of the renewed emphasis on PHC in the past decade is the significant government funding allocated to initiatives in PHC. In 1997, the federal government established the Health Transition Fund (HTF) in response to the National Forum on Health's recommendation to support innovation for a more integrated system of health care. The $150-million fund supported 141 projects and many sub-studies across Canada to test and evaluate innovative ways to deliver health care. Primary Health Care/ Primary Care (the terms are sometimes used interchangeably) was one of four priority areas in this initiative. These PHC projects addressed one or more principles of PHC. Examples included evaluating nursing practice models in PHC settings, improving the effectiveness of PHC through the collaboration of family physicians and nurse practitioners, strengthening multidisciplinary teams, evaluating community health centres, and advocating telehealth as appropriate technology (Health Canada, 2001).

Again, in September 2000, the first ministers identified PHC reform as a priority for the renewal of Canada's health care system. Accordingly, the Government of Canada established the $800 million Primary Health Care Transition Fund (PHCTF) to support the provinces and territories to improve the delivery of PHC over the next four years (the project was completed in 2006). The goals for the PHCTF were to increase the number of people who have access to primary health care organizations, which are accountable for a clearly defined set of comprehensive health services to a defined population; increase health promotion, disease and injury prevention, and the management of chronic diseases; expand 24/7 access to essential health services; ensure the most appropriate health care, provided by the most appropriate professional, which was thought to be achieved through multidisciplinary primary health care teams; and ensure that people's health care is coordinated and integrated with other health services (Health Council of Canada, 2005). The federal government also emphasized increasing access to PHC in rural Canada through its Innovations in Rural and Community Health initiative ($11 million) for health projects addressing accessibility and integration of health services in rural areas.

Assisted by federal funding, the provinces and territories pursued innovative approaches to PHC. Over half of British Columbia's allocation under the PHCTF was devoted to the Primary Care Demonstration Project, involving seven sites, that incorporates multidisciplinary teams, integrated primary care, and an alternative to fee-for-service payment to physicians. All of Alberta's $11-million allocation of the PHCTF was used to fund 27 projects under the umbrella Alberta Primary Health Care Project, including demonstration projects and evaluation of existing PHC models. The projects provided useful lessons about successes and challenges. A detailed description of projects and a synthesis of general trends and lessons learned are reported in the Health Canada document *Sharing the Learning: Health Transition Fund* (Mable & Marriott, 2002).

The PHCTF initiative set the stage for the directions proposed in the First Ministers' 2003 and 2004 health accords. The 2003 Health Accord identified the goal that, by 2011, 50% of Canadians would have 24/7 access to an appropriate health care provider, and that residents would routinely receive needed care from multidisciplinary PHC organizations or teams (Health Council of Canada, 2005). This target was reiterated in September 2004 in the Ten-Year Plan to Strengthen Health Care, at which time the First Ministers also established the Best Practices Network to facilitate information sharing and collaboration among jurisdictions. Overall, these health accords allocated more than $50 billion to health-sector reform (Villeneuve & MacDonald, 2006). The 2002 and 2003 First Ministers' health accords also made a commitment to reducing health disparities, which necessarily involves action on the social determinants of health (Health Disparities Task Group, 2004).

PROGRESS IN IMPLEMENTING PHC

The Health Council of Canada is analyzing the progress being made in moving toward a PHC system. Its background document on Primary Health Care (Health Council of Canada, 2005) outlines specific strategies being incorporated by each Canadian jurisdiction (see Box 11.1). The council points out that 24/7 access has been advanced primarily by expanding nursing roles in rural areas and providing telephone access to a nurse after hours. Because responsiveness to community needs is a key element of PHC, there is no "one size fits all" model. However, a key feature of PHC reform in Canada has been the use of multidisciplinary teams working in a variety of collaborative practice models—many involving nurse practitioners. Such teams are well positioned to focus on health promotion and the management of chronic illness, and to increase access and information sharing (Health Canada, 2006). The Health Council of Canada has recently produced excellent documents that identify the benefits of Primary Health Care teams, using examples of initiatives across Canada, particularly in the management of chronic diseases and in serving vulnerable populations (Health Council of Canada, 2009a, 2009b).

Why this emphasis on PHC? Armstrong and Armstrong (2001) provide a review of salient factors that may have led to the recent emphasis on PHC. A major factor relates to

---

BOX 11.1   Examples of Primary Health Care Strategies in Canada

- Developing nurse practitioner legislation and funding and implementing nurse practitioner initiatives
- Creating community health centres and shared care models
- Establishing telephone-based health information systems and electronic health records
- Promoting primary health care teams, family medicine groups, and family health centres
- Implementing "Healthy Living Strategies"

Source: Health Council of Canada. (2005). *Primary Health Care*. Toronto: Author.

the recognition of inadequacies in the current system of primary-care physician services, particularly the fee-for-service payment scheme, the inability to provide 24/7 coverage (often resulting in non-urgent emergency care), and the limited set of skills (diagnosis and treatment rather than health promotion and disease prevention) in which physicians are engaged. In addition, hospital downsizing and restructuring have resulted in more care being provided outside hospitals, with insufficient community facilities to cope with the demand. This problem is accentuated by a physician fee-for-service payment scheme that is a disincentive to providing adequate medical backup for families and health care providers (McWilliam & Sangster, 1994). As well, there are fewer physicians in family practice, and many do not take new patients, so that, by 2005, 14% of Canadians were without a family physician (Health Council of Canada, 2005), with the percentage of the population lacking family physicians in some jurisdictions continuing to increase. Lack of continuity of care between providers and institutions was also a concern (Health Canada, 2006). At the same time, new technologies have created possibilities for increased access to health services, such as better access to health advice through telephone advice lines, and information systems that allow for greater exchange of patient and provider information. The move to regionalization in most provinces may also have encouraged a more integrated system of health services, an important element of PHC (Rachlis & Kushner, 1997). Canada's strong history of intellectual refinement of the concepts of health and health promotion perhaps facilitated the incorporation of more health promotion and illness prevention in newer models of PHC. Finally, the consistent commitment and lobbying efforts of nursing associations (e.g., the CNA) for a health care system focused on principles of PHC and the conclusions of the Romanow Commission may have influenced the agenda.

🔍 CANADIAN RESEARCH FOCUS

Molzahn, A., Hibbert, M.P., Gaudet, D., Starzomski, R., Barrett, B., & Morgan, J. (2008). Managing chronic kidney disease in a nurse-run, physician-monitored clinic: The CanPREVENT experience. *Canadian Journal of Nursing Research, 40*(3), 96–112.

A qualitative design was used to explore the care provided to people with chronic kidney disease in nurse-run, physician-monitored clinics in five hospitals across Canada. Seven nurses, five physicians, and twenty-three patients participated in interviews to answer the following research questions: *What is the nature of the care provided by nurses and physicians? How do the nephrologists and nurses work together? How do patients, nurses, and physicians describe their experience with the clinic?* The following findings are particularly relevant to primary health care. Patient-centred care increased accessibility through home visiting, taking blood samples in the clinic, and flexibility in appointment scheduling. Nurses and physicians promoted health by responding to issues related to health practices (weight loss, smoking cessation), with an emphasis on health education. Beyond the collaborative relationships developed by nurses and physicians, nurses also facilitated a partnership model with patients and communication within a multidisciplinary team (e.g., social workers, physiotherapists, general practitioners). Overall, participants in the study reported satisfaction with the clinic. For example, patients reported weight loss, lower blood pressure, increased control of blood glucose, and enhanced feelings of well-being. Nurses and physicians described better outcomes for some of their patients. Nurses appreciated being able to work to a full scope of practice, demonstrating the primary health care principle of appropriate technology through better use of health personnel.

LINKING NURSING, PHC, AND THE CANADIAN CONTEXT

Given the congruence of the PHC principles with the key concepts underlying nursing practice, it should be no surprise that nurses quickly embraced the concept. The International Council of Nurses (ICN) pledged support for PHC, encouraging nurses worldwide to become involved in the planning and implementation of PHC in their own countries (WHO, 1978b). Nevertheless, Maglacas, the chief nurse of WHO, assessed nursing's response worldwide to PHC as "fragmented, sporadic, unplanned and uncoordinated, and [as involving] few, if any, other disciplines or sectors" (Maglacas, 1988, p. 67). The ICN reiterated support for PHC in a 1999 position statement (ICN, 2000).

MacPhail (1991, 1996) and Ogilvie and Reutter (2003), in past editions of this book, tracked the response of Canadian nurses to the challenge of PHC. Early on, nurse practitioner programs, focusing on primary care and nurses as substitutes for physicians, developed in Canada primarily to increase access to essential health services in underserved areas. Skills needed for primary medical care, as opposed to PHC, were emphasized in such programs. Graduates were employed primarily in northern health centres where consultation with physicians was available, using telephone or other technology, and in urban centres, often in clinics serving marginalized populations. All of the educational programs, except that at Dalhousie University, were phased out by the late 1980s, partly in recognition of the difficulty of adequately educating nurses through relatively short courses for the complexity of implementing PHC. Integrating knowledge, skills, and attitudes into baccalaureate education was perceived as more appropriate (MacPhail, 1996). More recently, the thrust has been toward master's level programs to prepare advanced practice nurses whose scope of practice encompasses extended clinical responsibilities and autonomy.

NURSING ASSOCIATION SUPPORT FOR PHC

The Canadian Nurses Association (CNA), along with provincial and territorial nursing associations, has provided leadership for nursing contributions to PHC in Canada. Rodger and Gallagher (2000) provide an excellent analysis of the paradigm shift in nursing thought and action in Canada from 1985 to 1998. They conclude that "the leadership role of the CNA in the move toward PHC from 1985 to 1998 is impressive" (p. 38). Numerous documents were produced, including position statements on health care reform (CNA, 1988), implementation strategies for specific target populations, and issues such as Aboriginal peoples and mental health (CNA, 1989a, 1991, 1992, 1994, 1995a), and policy statements (CNA, 1995b, 1995c). Briefs on needs for health care reform congruent with PHC principles were submitted to the Standing Committee of the House of Commons on Health and Welfare, Social Affairs, Seniors, and the Status of Women (CNA, 1989b); the Royal Commission on New Reproductive Technologies (CNA, 1990); and the National Forum on Health (CNA, 1996). Three nurses participated as members of the National Forum on Health.

The CNA has continued to support efforts to incorporate PHC in health reform. In 2001, the CNA Board of Directors identified PHC as a priority and designated a position of PHC corporate representative. More recently, a Primary Health Care consultant was employed until 2006. CNA strongly endorsed PHC in its presentations to the Commission on the Future of Health Care in Canada (the Romanow Commission) and the Standing Senate Committee on Social Affairs, Science and Technology (Kirby Commission) (CNA, 2005a) and developed documents and fact sheets in support of a public health system based on PHC principles (e.g., CNA, 2002b, 2003c, 2004). Moreover, CNA partnered in five different projects funded under the government PHCTF: the National Implementation of an Integrated Client Centred Approach to the Management of Arthritis, focusing on chronic disease management in a multidisciplinary community health setting; the Enhancing Interdisciplinary Collaboration in Primary Health Care Project to support effective collaboration among health care providers; the Canadian Collaborative Mental Health Initiative, aimed at improving collaboration between providers of mental health services; the Canadian Nurse Practitioner Initiative; and the Multidisciplinary Collaborative Primary Maternity Care Project (CNA, 2005a).

The CNA has actively advocated the role of nurse practitioners in a reformed PHC system. It has developed numerous documents and fact sheets related to cost-effectiveness (2002a), funding (2002c), and legislation, regulation, and education (2002d, 2003a). The revised position statement on the role of the nurse practitioner (CNA, 2003b) advocated the formalization of this role through appropriate advanced education, supportive legislation, and remuneration mechanisms. In 2005, the CIHI and CNA released *The Regulation and Supply of Nurse Practitioners* (CIHI & CNA, 2005), which outlined the status of regulation in the provinces and territories. The CNA led the PHCTF-funded Canadian Nurse Practitioner Initiative (CNPI) to facilitate sustained integration of the nurse practitioner role in the health system. This initiative resulted in several documents, including a competency framework, implementation and evaluation toolkit, and communication products for stakeholders (available through the CNA Web site). The role of the nurse practitioner in these documents is much broader in scope, and hence more in line with nursing's scope of practice, than earlier initiatives developed in response to the Boudreau Report (*Report of the Committee on Nurse Practitioners*, 1972). In addition to the leadership provided at CNA, all provincial and territorial nursing associations have encouraged nursing involvement in PHC, exemplified by their involvement on provincial or territorial government task forces for health system reform by 1993 (Rodger & Gallagher, 2000) and by updated position statements related to nursing and PHC in recent years (e.g., Association of Registered Nurses of Newfoundland and Labrador, 2004a, 2004b; College and Association of Registered Nurses of Alberta, 2005).

CANADIAN NURSING CONTRIBUTIONS TO PHC

In the previous edition of this text (Ogilvie & Reutter, 2003), we outlined numerous examples of Canadian nursing contributions to PHC compiled by Rodger and Gallagher (2000). They concluded that much of the nursing activity was related to health promotion and disease and injury prevention, with nurses participating in projects related to bicycle helmets, tobacco use, and myriad other health-related issues. The telephone health information systems, staffed by nurses (e.g., Health Link in Alberta), are exceptions as they are often the point of first contact for persons seeking information for specific health concerns. There are many other examples of nurses' involvement in projects that reflect the principles of PHC. The Registered Nurses' Association of Ontario (RNAO) has moved more explicitly in the direction of activity related to root causes and determinants of health than have other nursing associations. The RNAO is one of 11 Ontario member organizations of the Coalition for Primary Health Care, formed in 2000, that represents over one million consumers. In the media release announcing the formation of the coalition, a strong statement is made. "More than 25 reports have been written over the last 10 years or so calling for changes to Primary Health Care in Ontario. The time has come to end the report writing, and to take action." The RNAO has recently reiterated its stand on PHC by calling for funding for more nurse practitioner (NP)–led clinics and NP PHC positions, and for the removal of legislative and regulatory barriers to enable NPs with extended-care qualifications to practise to their full scope (RNAO, 2008). Before moving to a discussion of barriers to the implementation of PHC, including issues of particular interest to nurses, we will describe an interdisciplinary PHC project in more detail and introduce an interesting new initiative in Ontario. To obtain information on the diversity of initiatives being implemented in Canada, we recommend the excellent examples provided in the Health Council of Canada (2009a, 2009b) documents available on the council's Web site, and the videos available through the council's online library (see the Web site resources at the end of the chapter).

A PHC centre providing integrated services and built on the five principles of PHC is the North East Community Health Centre (NECHC) in Edmonton, Alberta. Established in 1999, the centre was planned using extensive community participation and consultation on what services should be provided, and incorporating the unique health needs of highly vulnerable, often marginalized, populations in the area. The NECHC provides both community health and emergency services. Access to services was enhanced by addressing language and cultural differences through employing multicultural health brokers, physician shortages through shared care models, and transportation barriers through partnerships with public transportation services. Maximum intersectoral and multidisciplinary collaboration is reflected in interdisciplinary teams made up of general practitioners, multicultural health brokers, social workers, dietitians, nurse practitioners, and others. Intersectoral collaboration with agencies such as Alberta Alcohol and Drug Abuse Commission, Alberta Mental Health Board, and others addresses the specific needs of the population served. A key feature of health promotion service delivery is the location of several public health services within the centre. Appropriate technology is reflected in the types of individuals employed, including nurse practitioners, and the availability of diagnostic services normally available only in tertiary centres (Gallagher, Relf, & McKim, 2003).

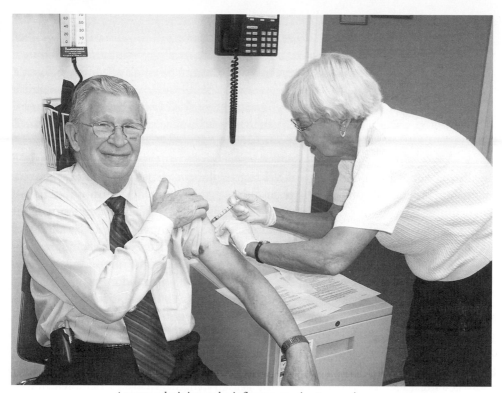

A nurse administers the influenza vaccine to a senior.

On August 30, 2007, the first nurse practitioner–led clinic opened in Sudbury with funding from the Ontario government (Registered Nurses' Association of Ontario, 2007). There are four nurse practitioners, support staff, and physician partners, with plans to employ a dietitian and a social worker in the future. In addition to the main clinic, there are two satellite sites in smaller communities. With nursing leadership, there may be greater potential for actualizing a population health focus more congruent with PHC principles than is currently the norm.

IMPLEMENTATION OF PHC: ISSUES AND CHALLENGES

Although there appears to be considerable movement toward PHC in Canada, several issues will need to be addressed if PHC is to be implemented in a manner that indeed provides Health for All. In its *Annual Report to Canadians*, the Health Council of Canada (2006) indicated that progress toward the 2003–2004 Health Accord goals "has been halting," with the biggest roadblock a reluctance of governments and health care leaders to set targets and be held accountable for progress. The council states, "At the current pace, key aspects of renewal that are fundamental to success—such as the shift to primary health care teams and electronic health records—won't be fully in place for many years" (p. 1). The council concluded that the focus of government action has been on access

BOX 11.2	Issues and Challenges in the Implementation of Primary Health Care

- Clarifying the concept of PHC
- Balancing accessibility to health determinants and to health care
- Ensuring individual and community participation
- Removing legislative barriers for health providers
- Implementing appropriate models of care

to health services (a response to public concerns) but believes that "renewal should set its sights on a higher destination: better health for Canadians [and proposes] a balanced journey along three pathways: quicker access to needed care, better quality of services, and a focus on determinants of population health outside the health care system" (p. 1). In Box 11.2, we present a summary of the challenges and issues discussed below.

CLARIFYING THE CONCEPT OF PHC

There is still considerable ambiguity about what is meant by PHC. This lack of agreement was reiterated by the National Primary Health Care Conference in Winnipeg in May 2004 (Health Council of Canada, 2005). Lack of consensus on terminology makes it difficult to report progress but, even more importantly, may limit the potential for PHC. Viewing PHC as synonymous with primary medical care (a person's first contact with the health care system during illness or injury) may have led to a focus on the accessibility principle, with the emphasis on 24/7 access. Moreover, this emphasis inadvertently may have been "facilitated" by legislation permitting nurses to engage in extended services that were previously the purview of physicians. Although such activities may indeed enhance nursing's complementary role within an interdisciplinary team, they also have the potential to erode nursing's main emphasis on health promotion. Politically, extending nursing roles in primary care through legislation may be much easier than integrating health-promotion activities into all facets of the health care system. Economic arguments oriented to short-term gains, under the guise of maintaining accessibility to illness care, may subvert real efforts at reform.

The integration of health promotion principles in a PHC system has been viewed as nursing's main contribution within an interdisciplinary, intersectoral team (Besner, 2006; Hills, Carroll, & Vollman, 2007). Although access to primary care is an important and necessary element of Primary Health Care, it is clearly not sufficient for attaining the total intent of PHC. Nurses, with a strong focus on health promotion and public participation, need to continue to advocate for the inclusion of all the principles of PHC, particularly health promotion, intersectoral collaboration, and public participation. Health reform, not merely increased accessibility to existing services provided in new ways, is required. PHC is a package of five interrelated principles and requires a fundamental change in funding structures and organization of health services if potential health gains for populations are to be achieved.

Nevertheless, it should be noted that there is room for greater accessibility to the whole range of health care services. A recent survey of the Canadian public's experience with the health care system found that timely access to quality health care by appropriate providers remains an issue for many Canadians (Health Council of Canada, 2008), an issue that perhaps is even more critical today. Over and above the current concerns about wait lists for a variety of primary care services, vulnerable populations, such as those living in poverty, cultural minorities, rural communities, and Aboriginal peoples, are particularly at risk for inaccessible health care (Hay, Varga-Toth, & Hines, 2006). For example, those on limited incomes may be unable to access counselling services, dental care, alternative therapies, chiropractic services, or physiotherapy (Stewart et al., 2005). Immigrant and Aboriginal populations may encounter linguistically inaccessible, culturally inappropriate, and culturally incomprehensible services. Hay et al. (2006) have identified innovative approaches currently being used across Canada to begin to increase access to health care for vulnerable populations, particularly rural and inner-city populations. The challenges faced by nurses in rural and remote areas have been identified by a group of Canadian nursing scholars (MacLeod et al., 2004).

BALANCING ACCESSIBILITY TO HEALTH DETERMINANTS AND ACCESSIBILITY TO HEALTH CARE

The Health Council of Canada (2005) suggests that a continuing challenge is the need to balance the current focus on accessibility to health care services with a greater emphasis on those determinants of health that lie outside the health care system. Accessibility must include access to the prerequisites and determinants of health, which can be achieved only through intersectoral collaboration. Although the documents advocating for PHC acknowledge the role of health determinants other than health care services, the implementation of this principle is less evident. Given that the underlying impetus for the PHC movement in 1978 was the observed health inequities brought about by social inequality, it is indeed noteworthy that social determinants, social inequality, and access to health (over and above access to health care) have received less attention from both nursing associations and government health departments. Advocacy, intersectoral collaboration, and political action become important nursing roles. The Health Council of Canada (2006) proposed that improving population health demands an "aggressive" and collaborative approach to reducing health inequalities with emphasis on children and Aboriginal groups. The council points out that the federal Healthy Living strategy targets in the areas of healthy eating, physical activity, and healthy weights do not address inequalities in health.

There have been at least three recent national initiatives focused on reducing health inequities through action on the social determinants of health. The Federal/Territorial/Provincial Advisory Committee on Population Health and Health Security in 2004 launched the Task Force on Reducing Health Disparities to document the extent of health disparities, the factors leading to disparities, and priority areas for their reduction (Health Disparities Task Group, 2004). In 2007, the Canadian Standing Senate

Committee on Social Affairs, Science, and Technology established the Subcommittee on Population Health to examine the impact of social determinants of health on disparities and inequities in health among population groups. The committee's final report, *A Healthy Productive Canada: A Determinant of Health Approach*, was recently released (Senate Subcommittee on Population Health, 2009). The *Report on the State of Public Health in Canada* (Public Health Agency of Canada, 2008), released by Canada's first chief public health officer also focused on health inequalities produced by social determinants of health. These documents emphasize that in order to achieve *Health for All* there is a need to ensure *Health in All Policies* or "healthy public policies," because the most significant influences on health lie outside the health care sector. The need to address social determinants of health to achieve *Health for All* is supported by many Canadian nurses and health scholars (e.g., Cohen & Reutter, 2007; Falk-Rafael, 2005; Raphael, 2009a, 2009b). Yet, despite this strong intellectual tradition in Canada that emphasizes a socio-environmental view of health and health determinants, a study of the involvement of federal and provincial and territorial ministries of health and health regions in addressing root causes of poverty revealed that health sectors only infrequently were involved in using political strategies to advocate for policies that would alter economic conditions that contribute to poverty (Williamson, 2001). More recently, Frankish (2007) reported limited support for addressing key nonmedical determinants of health (e.g., income and gender) among health regions in Canada.

Nurses and nursing associations at the provincial and national levels also need to expand their efforts to address the social determinants of health. Nurses are in a key position to advocate for policies that influence health: they work with people in all settings and observe first-hand how policies influence health; they are the largest group of health care providers, and they are organized into professional and labour organizations (Cohen & Reutter, 2007; Reutter & Williamson, 2000). In 2002, the CNA Board of Directors identified social justice as a priority issue, and the CNA has produced documents on the need to incorporate an understanding of social determinants in nursing practice (CNA, 2005b) and to utilize a social justice lens in CNA policies (CNA, 2006). Professional nursing organizations, however, generally have been slow to advocate for policies that address social determinants of health beyond health care (see Cohen & Reutter, 2007). Of the provincial associations, RNAO appears to be a leader in this area as demonstrated by its advocacy efforts directed to poverty reduction.

ENSURING INDIVIDUAL AND COMMUNITY PARTICIPATION

A third challenge in implementing PHC relates to the principle of ensuring individual and community participation. Overall, there has been increasing emphasis on citizen participation in program and policy development (Abelson & Lomas, 1996; Gauvin, Abelson, MacKinnon, & Watling, 2006; Kushner & Rachlis, 1998), as citizen participation is important in ensuring that programs and policies are relevant and effective. The concept of empowerment, which requires participation in defining problems and determining solutions, is the essence of health promotion. It is important, however, to consider the types of participation and the degree to which this participation is empowering. If participation is to be truly meaningful, people should be able to influence the configuration of services available and not just the ways in which already mandated services are to be delivered. Participation in the political process, through elections and public forums, provides civil society with a voice in decisions related to health and health care. As well, there is a need to ensure inclusivity for those who have traditionally had little voice in decision making (e.g., visible minorities, low-income people) by providing the supports needed to enable participation (Labonte & Edwards, 1995; Wharf Higgins, 1999). Nurses often work in organizations with established programs and little time or flexibility for creativity in stretching the boundaries. These organizations are embedded in government and other systems whereby options are limited by fiscal constraints. Participation, although a necessary and attractive principle of PHC, is in fact a slippery concept to actualize.

REMOVING LEGISLATIVE BARRIERS FOR HEALTH PROVIDERS

Another challenge that has received increased attention in recent years pertains to legislative barriers that prevent access to appropriate health care providers (AARN, 1998; Rachlis & Kushner, 1997). This challenge relates to the principle of appropriate technology. For example, in hospitals, physicians currently are the gatekeepers to nonphysician services. In the community, the public has always had direct access to public health nurses, but this is not the case with other health care providers. Without changes in how physician services are funded, it will be difficult to shift rules for entry into the system. It appears that the argument that a high-quality and sustainable health care system is possible through better use of existing or new human resources for health is receiving credence. New Health Professions acts (e.g., statutes revised in 2000 with amendments in force on March 1, 2002, in Alberta), enacted in some jurisdictions and in progress in others, allow increased scopes of practice for health care providers (Province of Alberta, 2000, 2005). These legislative changes open possibilities for advanced practice nurses in nurse practitioner and other roles. The boundaries among health care providers scopes of practice are more flexible. A current example is a pilot project in Alberta allowing a limited number of pharmacists with the requisite education to renew prescriptions or prescribe some medications for patients, provided that a diagnosis has already been established. Telehealth, through Internet health databases and information, computer transmission of images, and conversations and assessments across long distances, is revolutionizing the need for specialist services to be located with the patient. What services need to be where, with what provider, is a question that needs to be addressed.

The current labour shortage of health professionals, particularly family physicians and nurses, is a key challenge for health care systems, making health human resource planning of interest worldwide. Labour shortages are particularly acute in rural areas (Hay et al., 2006). The College of Family Physicians in Canada estimated that Canada was short 3,000 family physicians in 2002 and that number would double by 2010 unless new recruitment and retention strategies were implemented (Villeneuve & MacDonald,

2006). There is also a current and projected nursing shortage, due to the aging work-force and a high rate of absenteeism. The situation is compounded by the concern that all types of nurses—LPNs, RPNs, and RNs—are not working to their scope of practice (Villeneuve & MacDonald, 2006). The labour shortage may be an incentive for working in intra- and multidisciplinary teams, with each professional group working to its scope of practice. Caution must be exercised, however, to ensure that nurses use their health promotion expertise and do not merely take on a medical role. Already there is some evidence that nursing practice in both community health and acute-care facilities could reflect a stronger health-promotion focus (Besner, 2006; Browne & Tarlier, 2008). Obstacles to working to the full scope of practice were identified as heavy workloads, lack of resources, and unsupportive management.

IMPLEMENTING APPROPRIATE MODELS OF CARE: COMMUNITY HEALTH CENTRES

What model of health care will best serve the health needs of Canadians in the twenty-first century? The answer, of course, is that nobody knows for sure. Community health centres (CHCs) with salaried multidisciplinary teams; integration of curative, preventa-tive, and health-promotion programs; accessibility to the population being served; facili-tation of public participation; and creation of intersectoral links are viewed by many as the best options for a health care system truly oriented to PHC. CHCs in Canada gener-ally offer both primary health care and social programs and services, thereby addressing many social determinants of health (Hay et al., 2006). For example, the Calgary Urban Project Society (CUPS) offers a variety of services in inner-city Calgary, including multi-disciplinary staffed health clinics (e.g., prenatal and maternal–child clinics, chiropractic care, dentistry, shared-care mental health, eye care); counselling and advocacy; family resource centre (e.g., life skills and parenting programs, breakfast and hot lunch; basic needs services, referrals, socialization); community outreach (e.g., home visits, referrals, emergency transportation); educational and early intervention programs; and a housing registry (CUPS, 2005). Other excellent examples are the St. Joseph's Community Health Centre in St. John, New Brunswick, and the Great Slave Community Health Clinic in Yellowknife, Northwest Territories (Health Council of Canada, 2009b). The promise of CHCs is reflected in the establishment of the Canadian Alliance of Community Health Centre Associations (CACHCA), whose objective is to promote community health cen-tres as a cost-effective and successful method for delivering PHC.

THE WAY FORWARD

There are promising developments to move the PHC agenda forward. Nursing associa-tions have served nurses well in setting the guidelines for their potential involvement in such a system. At the political level, there seems to be openness to trying to do things differently. Funding for innovative projects and for research is available. The Canadian Health Services Research Fund (CHSRF) continues to see PHC as a cross-cutting theme in its funding initiatives, and the Institute for Health Services and Policy Research of CIHR (Canadian Institutes of Health Research) has identified primary health care reform as a key area for research under the strategic priority research area of Appropriate Care across the Continuum. There is at least one Canada Research Chair focused exclusively on Primary Health Care.

Substantial scholarly work in nursing exists to provide guidance, in Canada and elsewhere. Nursing textbooks and curricula emphasize PHC. The international journal *Primary Health Care Research and Development* is devoted to disseminating PHC research and practice. Nurses need to embrace the challenge and, perhaps most importantly, contribute to the research evidence that a system truly based on PHC principles can enhance the health of Canadians.

To meet the challenge of a reformed health system based on PHC principles, we believe that nursing education will need to concentrate on several key areas. First, nurses must be educated to work in community settings. The CNA envisions that in 2020, two-thirds of nurses will be employed in community settings, rather than in hospitals. They will be expected to play "active roles in health maintenance, case management, health education, and health advocacy" (Villeneuve & MacDonald, 2006, p. 80). Currently, many nursing programs concentrate students' clinical practice in hospital settings. As first-contact providers in PHC teams, nurses will require advanced assessment skills. Current curricula do provide basic physical assessment skills; this may need to be expanded in future to incorporate a broader focus on assessment of the influence of the social context on health situations (Besner, 2006), as this is where nurses will provide unique contributions to the PHC team. To better prepare nurses to work in multidisciplinary teams, interdisciplinary education will need to be strengthened. There are examples of initiatives in this area; however, this needs to be extended in a more systematic way. Finally, to realize the health promotion contribution of nursing, nurses will need a comprehensive understanding of the whole range of health determinants that influence individual health; moreover, they will require skills to work collaboratively with other sectors and disciplines to influence these determinants through strategies such as policy advocacy and community development. Nursing curricula must therefore provide a strong foundation in health promotion principles and strategies at the individual, community, and societal levels in a spirit of social justice. In many ways, a health-promotion focus in the broadest sense of the term is crucial to "reorienting health systems" to a PHC model (Hills et al., 2007).

CONCLUSION

In the past five to ten years in Canada, much effort and funding have been invested to develop a health system based on PHC principles. Some of the initiatives have been spurred on by the need to provide more accessible Health for All. It remains to be seen if these initiatives will become "permanent" aspects of our health system. Nurse academics, educators, administrators, and practitioners (in the widest sense) need to join forces with nursing associations, other health professionals, consumers, and other public sectors if a system based on PHC principles is to become a viable alternative to Canada's current health system, or perhaps more alarmingly, to a more privatized system with greater inequities than currently exist. Meeting the challenges addressed in this chapter will require risk and innovation by nurses and nursing associations as they work collaboratively with others to create a health care system that will meet the needs of Canadians in the twenty-first century.

CRITICAL THINKING QUESTIONS

1. How can the use of multidisciplinary teams facilitate a PHC approach to care?
2. What impact do you think the current human resource "crisis" will have on realizing a reformed health care system based on PHC principles?
3. What attitudes, knowledge, and skills do you think are most fundamental to nurses working within a PHC system?

WEB SITES

Health Council of Canada: http://www.healthcouncilcanada.ca
   This Web site provides excellent examples of primary health care initiatives both in document form and in online videos.
WHO Commission on Social Determinants of Health: http://www.who.int/social_determinants/thecom mission/finalreport/en/index.html
Senate Committee on Population Health: http://www.parl.gc.ca/40/2/parlbus/commbus/senate/com-e/ popu-e/rep-e/rephealth1jun09-e.pdf
WHO Report 2008 Primary Health Care: Now More Than Ever: http://www.who.int/whr/en/index.html

REFERENCES

Abelson, J., & Lomas, J. (1996). In search of informed input: A systematic approach to involving the public in community decision making. *Health Care Management FORUM, 9*(4), 48–52.

Advisory Committee on Population Health. (1994). *Strategies for population health: Investing in the health of Canadians.* Ottawa: Minister of Supply and Services Canada.

Advisory Committee on Population Health. (1996). *Report on the health of Canadians.* Ottawa: Minister of Supply and Services Canada.

Alberta Association of Registered Nurses. (1998). *Barriers to the implementation of Primary Health Care: A background paper.* Edmonton: Author. Retrieved on April 5, 2002, from http://www.nurses.ab.ca/ ARNDocs/primary.htm.

Armstrong, P., & Armstrong, H. (2001). *Primary Health Care reform: A discussion paper.* Ottawa: Canadian Health Coalition.

Association of Registered Nurses of Newfoundland and Labrador. (2004a). *Position statement: Primary Health Care.* St. John's: Author. Retrieved on August 30, 2007, from http://www.arnnl.nf.ca/PDF/ Position%20Statements/Primary_Health_Care.pdf.

Association of Registered Nurses of Newfoundland and Labrador. (2004b). *Position statement: Role of the registered nurse in Primary Health Care.* St. John's: Author. Retrieved on August 30, 2007, from http://www.arnnl.nf.ca/PDF/Position%20Statements/Role_of_Registered_Nurse_in_Primary_Health_ Care.pdf.

Besner, J. (2006). Optimizing nursing scope of practice within a primary health care context: Linking role accountabilities to health outcomes. *Primary Health Care Research and Development, 7,* 284–290.

Browne, A., & Tarlier, D. (2008). Examining the potential of nurse practitioners from a critical social justice perspective. *Nursing Inquiry*, *15*(2), 83–93.

Canadian Institute for Health Information and Canadian Nurses Association. (2005). *The regulation and supply of nurse practitioners in Canada*. Ottawa: CIHI.

Canadian Nurses Association. (1988). *Health for all Canadians: A call for health care reform*. Ottawa: Author.

Canadian Nurses Association. (1989a). *Health care reform for seniors*. Ottawa: Author.

Canadian Nurses Association. (1989b). *Submission to the Standing Committee of the House of Commons on Health and Welfare, Social Affairs, Seniors and the Status of Women: Select issues in health care delivery*. Ottawa: Author.

Canadian Nurses Association. (1990). *New reproductive technologies: Accessible, appropriate, participative*. Brief to the Royal Commission on New Reproductive Technologies. Ottawa: Author.

Canadian Nurses Association. (1991). *Mental health care reform*. Ottawa: Author.

Canadian Nurses Association. (1992). *Annual meeting minutes*. Ottawa: Author.

Canadian Nurses Association. (1994). *Comprehensive school health*. Ottawa: Author.

Canadian Nurses Association. (1995a). *Health in Canada: Perspectives on urban Aboriginal people*. Ottawa: Author.

Canadian Nurses Association. (1995b). *A framework for health care delivery*. Ottawa: Author.

Canadian Nurses Association. (1995c). *The role of the nurse in Primary Health Care*. Ottawa: Author. Retrieved on April 5, 2002, from http://www.cna-nurses.ca/_frames/advocacy/advocacyframe.htm.

Canadian Nurses Association. (1996). *Commitment required: Making the right changes to improve the health of Canadians*. Brief to the National Forum on Health. Ottawa: Author.

Canadian Nurses Association. (2002a). *Cost-effectiveness of the nurse practitioner role. Fact Sheet*. Ottawa: Author.

Canadian Nurses Association. (2002b). *Effective health care equals Primary Health Care. Fact Sheet*. Ottawa: Author.

Canadian Nurses Association. (2002c). *Funding the nurse practitioner role in Canada. Fact Sheet*. Ottawa: Author.

Canadian Nurses Association. (2002d). *Legislation and regulation of nurse practitioners in Canada. Fact Sheet*. Ottawa: Author.

Canadian Nurses Association. (2003a). *Legislation, regulation, and education of the nurse practitioner in Canada. Fact Sheet*. Ottawa: Author.

Canadian Nurses Association. (2003b). *Position statement. The nurse practitioner*. Ottawa: Author.

Canadian Nurses Association. (2003c). Primary Health Care: The time has come. *Nursing Now*, *16*, 1–4.

Canadian Nurses Association. (2004). *Building a strong, viable, publicly funded, not-for-profit health system*. Ottawa: Author.

Canadian Nurses Association. (2005a). *Primary Health Care: A summary of the issues. CNA Backgrounder*. Ottawa: Author.

Canadian Nurses Association. (2005b). *Social determinants of health and nursing: A summary of the issues. CNA Backgrounder*. Ottawa: Author.

Canadian Nurses Association. (2006). *Social justice … a means to an end, an end in itself*. Ottawa: Author.

Cohen, B., & Reutter, L. (2007). Developing public health nurses' role in addressing child and family poverty: A framework for action. *Journal of Advanced Nursing*, *60*, 96–107.

College and Association of Registered Nurses of Alberta. (2005). *Primary Health Care*. Edmonton: Author. Retrieved on August 30, 2007, from http://www.nurses.ab.ca/Carna-Admin/Uploads/Primary%20 Health%20Care.pdf.

Commission on the Future of Health Care in Canada. (2002). *Building on values: The future of health care in Canada. Commissioner Roy Romanow*. Ottawa: Author.

CUPS (Calgary Urban Project Society). (2005). *Programs*. Retrieved on August 3, 2007, from CUPS web site, www.cupshealthcentre.com/programs.htm.

Epp, J. (1986). *Achieving health for all: A framework for health promotion*. Ottawa: Health and Welfare Canada. Retrieved on April 5, 2002, from http://www.hc-sc.gc.ca/english/care/achieving_health.html.

Falk-Rafael, A. (2005). Speaking truth to power: Nursing's legacy and moral imperative. *Advances in Nursing Science, 28*(3), 212–223.

Frankish, J. (2007). *Intersectoral collaboration on non-medical determinants of health: The role of health regions in Canada*. Presentation at University of Alberta Centre for Health Promotion Lecture Series, April 2007.

Gallagher, S., Relf, M., & McKim, R. (2003). Integrated services in northeast Edmonton. *Canadian Nurse, 99*(7), 25–29.

Gauvin, R., Abelson, J., MacKinnon, M., & Watling, J. (2006). *A primer on public involvement*. Toronto: Health Council of Canada. Available at www.healthcouncilcanada.ca.

Hamilton, N., & Bhatti, T. (1996). *Population health promotion: An integrated model of population health and health promotion*. Ottawa: Health Promotion Development Division, Health Canada.

Hay, D., Varga-Toth, J., & Hines, E. (2006). *Frontline health care in Canada: Innovations in delivering services to vulnerable populations*. Research Report F/63. Family Network (CPRN). Toronto: Canadian Policy Research Networks.

Health Canada (2001). *Health Transition Fund*. Ottawa: Author. Retrieved on April 5, 2002, from http://www.hc-sc.ca/htf-fass.

Health Canada (2006). About Primary Health Care. *Health Care Systems*. Retrieved on July 31, 2007, from www.hc-sc.gc.ca/hcs-sss/prim/about-apropos/index_e.html.

Health Council of Canada. (2005). *Primary Health Care*. Toronto: Author.

Health Council of Canada. (2006). *Health care renewal in Canada. Executive Summary*. Retrieved from Health Council of Canada Web site, www.healthcouncilcanada.ca.

Health Council of Canada. (2008). *Fixing the foundation: An update on Primary Health Care and home care renewal in Canada*. Toronto: Health Council. Available at www.healthcouncilcanada.ca.

Health Council of Canada. (2009a). *Getting it right: Case studies of effective management of chronic disease using Primary Health Care teams*. Toronto: Health Council.

Health Council of Canada. (2009b). *Teams in action: Primary Health Care teams for Canadians*. Toronto: Health Council. Available at www.healthcouncilcanada.ca.

Health Disparities Task Group. (2004). *Reducing health disparities—Roles of the health sector: Discussion paper*. Prepared by the Health Disparities Task Group of the Federal/Provincial/Territorial Advisory Committee on Population Health and Health Security. Ottawa: Public Health Agency of Canada.

Health Summit '99. (1999). *Think about health: An Alberta framework for discussion*. Edmonton: Alberta Health.

Hills, M., Carroll, S., & Vollman, A. (2007). Health promotion and health professions in Canada: Toward a shared vision. In M. O'Neill, A. Pederson, S. Dupere, & I. Rootman (Eds.), *Health promotion in Canada* (2nd ed.), (pp. 330–346). Toronto: Canadian Scholars' Press.

International Council of Nurses. (2000). *Nurses and Primary Health Care*. Geneva: Author. Retrieved on July 13, 2007, from http://www.icn.ch/psprimarycare.htm.

Kushner, C., & Rachlis, M. (1998). Civic lessons: Strategies to increase consumer involvement. *Canada health action: Building on the legacy. Making decisions: Evidence and information* (Vol. 5), (pp. 303–347). Ste-Foy, PQ: Editions MultiModes. Commissioned paper by National Forum on Health.

Labonte, R., & Edwards, R. (1995). *Equity in action: Supporting the public in public policy*. Toronto: Centre for Health Promotion.

Lalonde, M. (1974). *A new perspective on the health of Canadians: A working paper*. Ottawa: Government of Canada.

Legowski, B., & McKay, L. (2000). *Health beyond health care: Twenty-five years of federal health policy development*. Discussion Paper No. H/04, October 2000. Ottawa: Canadian Policy Research Networks. Retrieved on April 4, 2002, from http//www.cprn.org/cprn.html.

Mable, A., & Marriott, J. (2002). *Sharing the learning: Health Transition Fund: Synthesis Series: Primary Health Care*. Ottawa: Health Canada.

MacLeod, M., Kulig, J., Stewart, N., Pitblado, R., Banks, K., D'Arcy, C., et al. (2004). *The nature of nursing practice in rural and remote Canada*. Retrieved on August 17, 2009, from http://www.chsrf.ca/final_research/ogc/pdf/macleod_final.pdf.

MacPhail, J. (1991). Primary Health Care: The means for reaching nursing's potential in achieving Health for All. In J. Kerr, & J. MacPhail (Eds.), *Canadian nursing: Issues and perspectives* (2nd ed.), (pp. 321–335). Toronto: Mosby.

MacPhail, J. (1996). Primary Health Care: The means for reaching nursing's potential in achieving Health for All. In J. Ross-Kerr, & J. MacPhail (Eds.), *Canadian nursing: Issues and perspectives* (3rd ed.), (pp. 390–406). Toronto: Mosby.

Maglacas, A. M. (1988). Health for all: Nursing's role. *Nursing Outlook, 36*(2), 66–71.

Mahler, H. (1985). *Nurses lead the way. WHO Features* (No. 97). Geneva: World Health Organization.

McWilliam, C. L., & Sangster, J. F. (1994). Managing patient discharge to home: The challenges of achieving quality of care. *Journal for Quality in Health Care, 6*, 147–161.

Molzahn, A., Hibbert, M. P., Gaudet, D., Starzomski, R., Barrett, B., & Morgan, J. (2008). Managing chronic kidney disease in a nurse-run, physician-monitored clinic: The CanPREVENT experience. *Canadian Journal of Nursing Research, 40*(3), 96–112.

National Forum on Health. (1997). *Canada health action: Building on the legacy*. Ottawa: Author.

Navarro, V. (1986). *Crisis, health, and medicine: A social critique*. New York: Tavistock Publications.

Ogilvie, L. (1993). *Nurses and Primary Health Care in Nepal*. Unpublished doctoral thesis. Edmonton: University of Alberta.

Ogilvie, L., & Reutter, L. (2003). Primary Health Care: Complexities and possibilities from a nursing perspective. In J. Ross-Kerr, & M. Wood (Eds.), *Canadian nursing: Issues and perspectives* (4th ed.), (pp. 441–465). Toronto: Elsevier.

Pinder, L. (2007). The federal role in health promotion. In M. O'Neill, A. Pederson, S. Dupere, & I. Rootman (Eds.), *Health promotion in Canada* (2nd ed.), (pp. 92–105). Toronto: Canadian Scholars' Press

Province of Alberta. (2000). *Health Professions Act*. Edmonton: Alberta Queen's Printer.

Province of Alberta. (2005). *Health Professions Act: Registered nurses profession regulation*. Edmonton: Alberta Queen's Printer.

Public Health Agency of Canada. (2008). *Report on the state of public health in Canada 2008: Addressing health inequalities*. Retrieved on June 30, 2009, from http://www.phac-aspc.gc.ca/publicat/2008/cpho-aspc/pdf/cpho-report-eng.pdf.

Quebec Commission on Health and Social Services. (2000). *Emerging solutions: Report and recommendations (Clair Commission)*. Quebec City: Health and Social Services. Retrieved on June 15, 2010, from http://www.publications.msss.gouv.qc.ca/acrobat/f/documentation/2001/01-109-010.pdf.

Rachlis, M., & Kushner, C. (1997). *Primary Health Care in Canada: A report for the Health Transition Fund, Health Canada*. Unpublished manuscript.

Raphael, D. (Ed.). (2009a). *Social determinants of health* (2nd ed.). Toronto: Canadian Scholars' Press.

Raphael, D. (2009b). Poverty, human development, and health in Canada: Research, practice, and advocacy dilemmas. *Canadian Journal of Nursing Research, 41*(2), 7–18.

Registered Nurses' Association of Ontario. (2007). *First nurse practitioner-led clinic opens doors in Sudbury*. Toronto: Author. Retrieved on August 30, 2007, from http://www.rnao.org/Page.asp?PageID=924&ContentID=2146.

Registered Nurses' Association of Ontario. (2008). Briefing note: Increasing access to Primary Health Care. Retrieved on July 12, 2009, from http://www.rnao.org/Page.asp?PageID=122&ContentID=2319&SiteNodeID=467.

Report of the Committee on Nurse Practitioners. (1972). Ottawa: Department of National Health and Welfare.

Reutter, L. (2000). Socioeconomic determinants of health. In M. J. Stewart (Ed.), *Community nursing: Promoting Canadians' health* (2nd ed.), (pp. 174–193). Toronto: W. B. Saunders.

Reutter, L., & Williamson, D. (2000). Advocating healthy public policy: Implications for baccalaureate nursing education. *Journal of Nursing Education, 39*, 21–26.

Rodger, G. L., & Gallagher, S. M. (2000). The move toward Primary Health Care in Canada: Community health nursing from 1985 to 2000. In M. J. Stewart (Ed.), *Community nursing: Promoting Canadians' health* (2nd ed.), (pp. 33–55). Toronto: W.B. Saunders.

Saskatchewan Commission on Medicare. (2001). *Caring for Medicare: Sustaining a quality system.* Regina: Author. Retrieved on April 5, 2002, from http://www.health.gov.sk.ca/info_center_pub_commission_on_medicare-bw.pdf.

Senate Subcommittee on Population Health. (2009). *A healthy, productive Canada: A determinant of health approach.* Standing Senate Committee on Social Affairs, Science and Technology. Final Report of the Subcommittee on Population Health. Retrieved on June 30, 2009, from http://www.parl.gc.ca/40/2/parlbus/commbus/senate/com-e/popu-e/rep-e/rephealth1jun09-e.pdf.

Stewart, M. J. (2000). Framework based on Primary Health Care principles. In M. J. Stewart (Ed.). *Community nursing: Promoting Canadians' health* (2nd ed.), (pp. 58–82). Toronto: W.B. Saunders.

Stewart, M. J., Reutter, L., Makwarimba, E., Rootman, I., Williamson, D., Raine, K., et al. (2005). Determinants of health service use by low-income people. *Canadian Journal of Nursing Research*, *37*(3), 104–131.

United Nations (2006). *The Millennium Development Goals Report.* New York: United Nations Department of Economic and Social Affairs.

Villeneuve, M., & MacDonald, J. (2006). *Toward 2020: Visions for nursing.* Ottawa: Canadian Nurses Association.

Wharf Higgins, J. (1999). Closer to home: The case for experiential participation in health reform. *Canadian Journal of Public Health*, *90*, 30–34.

Williamson, D. (2001). The role of the health sector in addressing poverty. *Canadian Journal of Public Health*, *92*, 178–183.

World Health Organization. (1978a). *Primary Health Care: Report of the international conference on Primary Health Care: Alma-Ata, USSR.* Geneva: Author.

World Health Organization. (1978b). *World Health Assembly Resolution 36:11.* Geneva: Author.

World Health Organization. (1990). *Achieving Health for All by the year 2000: Midway reports of countries' experiences.* Geneva: Author.

World Health Organization. (1995). *World Health Report: Bridging the gap.* Geneva: Author.

World Health Organization. (1996). *World Health Report: Fighting disease, fostering development.* Geneva: Author.

World Health Organization. (1997a). The Jakarta declaration on health promotion into the 21st century. (Online: http://www.dnttm.ro/arspms/jakarta.html)

World Health Organization. (1997b). *World Health Report: Conquering suffering, enriching humanity.* Geneva: Author.

World Health Organization. (1998). *World Health Report: Life in the twentieth century: A vision for all.* Geneva: Author.

World Health Organization. (1999). *World Health Report: Making a difference.* Geneva: Author.

World Health Organization. (2000). *World Health Report. Health Systems: Improving Performance.* Geneva: Author.

World Health Organization. (2001). *Health for all in the twenty-first century.* Geneva: Author.

World Health Organization. (2005). *Bangkok Charter for health promotion.* Geneva: Author.

World Health Organization. (2008a). *Closing the gap in a generation: Health equity through action on the social determinants of health. Commission on Social Determinants of Health. Final Report. Executive Summary.* Retrieved on March 13, 2009, from http://whqlibdoc.who.int/hq/2008/WHO_IER_CSDH_08.1_eng.pdf.

World Health Organization. (2008b). *World Health Report 2008: Primary Health Care—Now more than ever.* Retrieved on August 17, 2009, from http://www.who.int/whr/en/index.html.

World Health Organization. (1986). Health and Welfare Canada, & Canadian Public Health Association (1986). *Ottawa Charter for Health Promotion.* Ottawa: Canadian Public Health Association.

12 Quality of Care: From Quality Assurance and Improvement to Cultures of Patient Safety

Greta G. Cummings and Carol A. Wong

We gratefully acknowledge the assistance of Christy Raymond-Semeniuk in final preparation of this chapter.

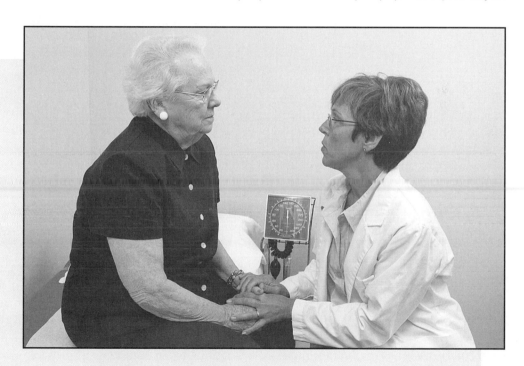

LEARNING OBJECTIVES

- To define the concept of quality assurance in health care.
- To review the historical development of quality assurance.
- To outline the limitations of quality assurance.
- To describe the key concepts of continuous quality improvement.
- To review the steps of continuous quality improvement processes.
- To outline the applicable tools used when examining and assessing outcomes related to quality improvement and assurance.
- To discuss the role of patient safety, nursing-sensitive outcomes, and best-practice guidelines in current quality improvement initiatives.
- To situate quality improvement and quality assurance in the current health care context.
- To describe possible future directions of quality improvement and quality assurance in Canadian nursing.

Increasing diversification and sophistication in the health care field have accompanied steady increases in national expenditures for health care. Meanwhile, public attitudes reflect parallel changes in social values about health: better informed health consumers are demanding increased accountability in health care. The activities of consumers' rights groups have attracted media attention and raised public awareness; health lobbyists have argued for environmental protection, health promotion, and provision of health care services that are accessible, effective, and appropriate. As a result, North American attitudes toward health care and health care providers have undergone a significant transition. This is reflected in the perception that health care is a right rather than a privilege, and the expectation that health care providers provide not just care, but quality care.

Historically, *quality assurance* in health care was defined as the self-regulating activities of various professions. In 2009, *quality improvement* (QI) in health care included actions designed to improve both processes and outcomes of care; specifically, actions aimed at increasing the value of services, improving responsiveness to those receiving care, and enhancing overall outcomes of care (Alexander & Hearld, 2009). Donabedian (2003) describes *quality assurance* as "all actions taken to establish, protect, promote, and improve the quality of health care" (p. xxiii).

The traditional view that only relevant health care providers could describe the nature of competent practice meant that physicians, nurses, and other professionals were not challenged about how they dealt with matters of professional misconduct. Today, the situation is very different. Although professional groups still have the privilege of autonomously conducting regulatory functions, there is more public scrutiny of the process. In many provinces, lay members of professional governing boards and their disciplinary committees are appointed by the government to represent the public interest in professional deliberations. The professional conduct of physicians, nurses, and other health care providers is a subject for public discussion and debate, something that was unheard of in the past. The media have constantly pressured professional groups for full and open disclosure of the results of disciplinary operations. In the past decade, several provincial governments have introduced omnibus legislation for the regulation of health providers that includes mandatory quality assurance/continuing competence programs and professional conduct hearings that are open to the public.

HISTORICAL DEVELOPMENTS IN QUALITY ASSURANCE

The assessment of nursing care quality has been an important and essential strategy for monitoring and stimulating excellence in nursing practice, administration, education, and research. The first documented study in health care and nursing, based on the use of standards, is attributed to Florence Nightingale, who in 1858 investigated the quality of care provided to military personnel (Nightingale, 1858). The development of standards for health care was formalized in the United States in 1918. The US standards were subsequently adopted in Canadian hospitals and applied to all disciplines and services. In 1952, the Joint Committee on Accreditation of Hospitals (JCAH) was formed, assuming responsibility for accrediting Canadian hospitals until 1958. At that time, the Canadian Council on Hospital Services Accreditation (CCHSA) was established to accredit health care agencies in Canada. Since then, the CCHSA has provided the external stimulus for quality assurance programs in nursing. Accreditation standards and requirements have been revised regularly and reflect increasingly strenuous monitoring. Beginning in the 1970s, the CCHSA standards required the presence of a quality assurance program in hospitals across Canada.

Over the following decade, considerable effort led to formal programs for assessing, monitoring, and improving care. Although quality assurance activities were visible in all disciplines, the primary focus was directed toward developing quality-monitoring programs in nursing, undoubtedly because nursing was the largest and most critically important service in health care agencies. Provincial professional associations in nursing also instituted quality assurance activities by developing guidelines for implementing quality assurance programs and nursing practice standards. Nursing consultants with quality assurance expertise were retained by professional associations to assist nursing service departments in provincial health care agencies in developing programs or ongoing quality assurance activities. Many hospitals established a quality assurance department within the division of nursing with responsibility for implementing and monitoring quality-related activities. Nursing expertise has also been important in developing standards at the past CCHSA Board of Directors, where the Canadian Nurses Association (CNA) was also represented. In 2008, CCHSA launched the Qmentum Accreditation Program and changed its name to Accreditation Canada. Although the name was changed, the approach and processes remain similar.

The common denominator of quality assurance programs has been standards. Donabedian (1980, 2003) proposed three levels for assessing quality: structure, process, and outcome. *Structural* standards or criteria focused on relationships among available human and material resources within a health care setting. Examples included the philosophy of the institution, resources and supplies, staffing patterns, and environmental characteristics. *Process* standards or criteria focused on nursing roles and activities to meet patient care goals. Examples of process standards were the nursing process, communication between nurses and patients, and nursing activities. *Outcome* standards or criteria were mainly patient oriented and described anticipated results of the care process. Outcomes generally referred to the results of health care delivery. It has been difficult to attribute outcomes to any one health care profession because a team effort is necessary to achieve results.

The major effort in quality assurance programs was directed at process levels of care because health care professional activities could be assessed and measured directly at this level. This assessment was concurrent or, more frequently, retrospective. If concurrent, nursing care was reviewed or measured as it was delivered; if retrospective, the review took place after care was provided. Concurrent methods have the potential for collecting more and better information and direct information from patients. Because information was gathered sooner, any necessary changes could be made quickly. Disadvantages included increased costs and possible disruption to nursing unit activities. Retrospective reviews were attractive because costs tended to be lower, with less disruption to the nursing unit because the review usually focused on the patient's record. However, it was not usually possible to collect information directly from the patient, and nurses responsible for chart data were not available to elaborate or answer questions that arose. Because both concurrent and retrospective reviews provided valuable and unique information about the process of care, many agencies implemented both types in their quality assurance programs.

The literature on quality assurance has been plentiful (Trussel & Strand, 1978; Ventura, Hageman, Slakter, & Fox, 1980; Giovannetti, Kerr, Bay, & Buchan, 1986), with descriptive publications covering the nature of quality; components of a quality assurance model or framework; categorizations of quality; rationale for developing quality assurance techniques and programs; and establishing, maintaining, and improving quality assurance programs. The research literature dealing with quality assessment has been limited, focusing primarily on instrument development with little attention to the type of testing that should be integral to the process. Most instruments demonstrated little more than face validity, raising questions about the value of results in quality assessment programs using inadequately tested instruments. This has also posed problems for the interpretation of research based on instruments purporting to measure the quality of nursing care.

LIMITATIONS OF QUALITY ASSURANCE PROGRAMS

Quality assurance programs have shown some significant limitations. A constant and major challenge facing executive officers of agencies is the cost-effectiveness of all programs, including quality assurance programs. As the number of professionals required for successful operation of quality-monitoring programs increased, so did costs associated with programs implemented by external consultants. Funds expended were considerable and, some suggest, disproportionate to the results achieved.

Another area of concern was whether those responsible for design and implementation were knowledgeable in research and quality assessment. Knowledge about the research literature was important, as was the ability to assess strengths and weaknesses of various approaches to quality that maximize the former and minimize the latter in programs selected for implementation. Many nurses responsible for in-service education were also given responsibility for managing quality assurance activities in health care agencies. Although this was an expedient way for agencies to implement quality monitoring, it assumed that those responsible had the time, interest, background, and expertise to function effectively in both spheres. Limited testing of instrument reliability and validity for monitoring quality was a major concern for nursing departments. Many instruments did not measure dimensions of quality consistently and therefore provided little value for judging performance within the institution based on the results obtained. Ventura et al. (1980) and Giovannetti et al. (1986) noted that measurements must be made carefully so that quality-monitoring processes yield reliable findings. Controlled conditions required that raters be carefully trained and monitored. This meant that certain nurses were designated as quality auditors and seconded to the program for a period of time. Although this system supported principles of good data collection, the process was seen as delegating the responsibility for quality care to a few individuals whose role was primarily inspection. Another limitation of quality assurance programs was the retrospective focus on achievement of standards. Considerable emphasis on quality-monitoring activities occurred after the fact when it was least possible to make necessary changes. Also, minimum standards of achievement were acceptable in determining whether criteria were met.

Perhaps the greatest limitation was the largely department-specific focus of quality assurance programs. This limited the resolution of interdisciplinary issues such as admission, transfer, discharge, consultation, and materials distribution, which have been resistant to change despite a variety of quality-monitoring techniques. These issues are not confined to individual departments; improvement in quality of care requires the concerted efforts of all disciplines and departments working together.

Finally, the foundation of quality assurance programs—achieving predetermined standards in the clinical setting—began to be seen as somewhat arbitrary. Administrators and program directors established the level to which each standard was to be achieved. Critical standards were expected to be achieved 100% of the time, while less critical standards, perhaps 80 to 90% of the time. For example, within nursing, random chart reviews were completed to determine how often nurses recorded their assessment of medication efficacy when analgesia were given as needed in the postoperative period. Eighty percent achievement was acceptable. Yet where was the evidence that achieving 80% on a particular standard was an appropriate goal? Was the goal even reasonable? In the world of quality assurance, a standard could be achieved to the desired level without any discussion as to its appropriateness. For example, anaesthetic and surgical procedures could be performed to standard 100% of the time, yet the particular surgical procedure might be performed too often or not often enough. In quality assurance chart reviews, questions of timing, frequency, or indication for the procedure were rarely asked. Perhaps the provider performing a procedure was not the most appropriate; it could have been completed more cost effectively by a health care provider from another discipline.

Although quality assurance had for several decades provided the focus for improving the care given to patients, a new approach to quality—using processes of continuous improvement rather than achieving predetermined standards—began to stir the corporate health care environment in the early 1990s. This approach to quality was initially known as total quality management (TQM); however, the lasting moniker is continuous quality improvement (CQI).

THE TRANSITION TO TQM/CQI

Total quality management is a "structured, systematic process for creating organization-wide participation in planning and implementing continuous improvement in quality" (Whetsell, 1990, p. 16). Its origins date back to the 1930s, when Dr. W. Edwards Deming, a graduate from Yale University and consultant in statistical studies, put forward his theory of continuous improvement to Western Electric Laboratories (later AT&T Bell Laboratories) and other US industries. He believed that problems with (and therefore opportunities to improve) quality were built into complex production processes and that defects in quality could rarely be attributed to the people involved with the process. Problems were generally caused not by poor motivation or effort but rather by job design. In his theory of continuous improvement, Deming (1986) advocated a strong and long-term commitment by management, including the need for clearly defined mission and vision statements. He believed quality should be the central focus of the organization and that emphasis needed to shift from inspection to prevention. Preventing defects and improving processes so that defects do not occur are the goals toward which all organizations should strive. Establishing long-term relationships with suppliers was more important than accepting the lowest bid. Deming believed that training and retraining of employees was critical to organizational success and that management's role was to coach employees. Finally, he believed that reducing variability in processes would ultimately lead to sustaining process improvements.

In the 1980s, both Canadian and American health care agencies began to face significant pressures, previously experienced in industry, to improve the quality of services while reducing steadily increasing costs. Quality assurance programs in hospitals were not providing the foundation on which to make the significant changes thought to be necessary. Further, the culture of quality, so much a part of the fabric of successful industries, was not identifiable in the health care industry. The successes that industries made in improving quality and reducing costs caught the attention of hospital managers. Could the quality improvement principles, proven to be successful in industry, have application in hospitals? Many were sceptical that any relationships could be found between manufacturing products and the highly complex, people-focused hospital milieu.

Donald Berwick (Berwick, Godfrey, & Roessner, 1990), professor of Pediatrics at Harvard Medical School and pediatrician with the Harvard Community Health Plan, disagreed with this view. Although steps taken in both Canada and the United States to control costs and improve health were unsuccessful, he believed that challenges facing industries over the previous two decades were no different than those facing health care. In 1987, he launched the National Demonstration Project on Quality Improvement in Health Care (NDP), an exploratory study designed to answer the question "Can the tools of modern quality improvement, with which industries have achieved breakthroughs in performance, improve health care?" This landmark study, described in *Curing Health Care* (Berwick et al.), documented the efforts of 21 health care organizations, paired with an equal number of industrial quality management experts, to use quality management principles to implement hospital-based pilot projects.

During the eight-month demonstration study, 17 hospitals completed projects that improved processes such as transport of critically ill neonates, use of portable X-ray machines, appointment waiting times, patient discharge, and hiring of nurses. At least 15 projects were considered successful, leading to several discoveries. These pioneer teams found that

- quality improvement methods and tools were applicable to health care;
- cross-functional teams were valuable in improving health care processes;
- data useful for quality improvement abounded; and
- poor quality correlated with high cost.

Involving physicians in the quality improvement process was difficult but essential, and quality transformation was dependent on leadership. This work was the first documented evidence that quality management principles initially implemented in industry could be applied to hospital processes. Many hospitals have continued to make profound changes, providing a model for successful implementation of a quality improvement philosophy in Canadian hospitals.

KEY CONCEPTS OF CONTINUOUS QUALITY IMPROVEMENT

A number of key concepts are central to the CQI approach and reflect a significant shift in thinking away from quality assurance. Successful implementation in industry and health care guided the development of these concepts (Walton, 1986; McLaughlin & Kaluzny, 1990; Thompson, 1991; Harrigan, 2000).

PROCESSES OF HEALTH CARE AND HEALTH CARE DELIVERY

Continuous quality improvement focuses on key processes rather than individual people. This approach is based on the premise that 85% of problems encountered in organizations result from cumbersome or poorly defined processes. Problems are attributable to staff performance only 15% of the time. Health care processes are complex and cross traditional departmental and disciplinary boundaries.

Most processes flow across the organization and between departments rather than up and down the hierarchy. Therefore, quality teams are made up of people who are most knowledgeable about the process. The team leader could be anyone in the organization who is knowledgeable about the process under review and who has demonstrated group leadership skills, knowledge of the quality improvement process, and skill in using quality tools. Only after a process is carefully analyzed to determine what it entails can changes be made to improve it. Staff are dedicated to providing high-quality care; it is the process itself that requires improvement.

CUSTOMER FOCUS

A customer is anyone who receives or is affected by a product or a process, and therefore patients, families, hospital visitors, hospital employees, physicians, volunteers, and suppliers are all viewed as customers of particular processes. In fact, service providers often have other service providers as their customers, and internal providers may also serve groups that are external to the organization. In this way, everyone within the organization is serving a customer and often is a customer.

CONTINUOUS MONITORING OF QUALITY

Meeting and exceeding the needs of patients and staff is a priority goal and involves not only an evaluation of current services but expectations and ideas for improvement. These expectations and requirements are data driven. Decisions are made based on fact, not opinions. Quality improvement tools and techniques are used by teams to create a systematic approach to problem analysis, resolution, and evaluation. The process of improvement adapted by the organization provides a consistent proactive approach to problem solving that is used by all teams. Approximately 50 to 70% of the time spent on a quality improvement process is focused on collecting and analyzing data. Team members frequently report that data analysis revealed information about root causes that differed from commonly held opinion.

Quality improvement is a continuous cycle of improving processes before errors are made or complaints are received. Doing the right thing right the first time and all the time is considered much more cost-effective than redoing work. Responsibility for improving processes rests with those directly involved in the process. CQI involves more than improving one process at a time or in one moment in time. It is an ongoing initiative for continuous improvement of all care processes and services within the organization. There is no point at which a final solution is achieved. The central tenet of CQI is that there is always room for further improvement.

EDUCATION AND LEARNING

Everyone in the organization is involved in continuous quality improvement. Working within the guidelines and boundaries established by managers, staff are empowered by receiving information, resources, and authority to improve work processes that will benefit patients and themselves. Problem resolution occurs at the lowest possible level of the organization, where staff have the greatest knowledge about potential causes and solutions. Staff education and training at all organizational levels are central to a motivated and contributing workforce. Education programs include an awareness of CQI principles, steps in quality improvement, use of quality improvement tools, just-in-time training, and teamwork skills.

LONG-TERM COMMITMENT

The process of cultural transformation is a long-term commitment that may take five to ten years in most hospitals. Even with a five-year implementation plan, results will depend on a variety of factors, including resources, dedication, organizational stability, organizational priority setting, and commitment by staff and physicians.

THE PROCESS OF CONTINUOUS QUALITY IMPROVEMENT

The following steps in the quality improvement process are generic and reflect a basic scientific approach:

1. Select and define a problem.
2. Organize a knowledgeable team.
3. Gather data to identify root causes of the problem.
4. Implement a plan of action based on the data analysis.
5. Continuously monitor results.

Two more formalized methods are now being widely used to standardize the process of improvement. Figure 12.1 shows the sequence of steps designed by Juran (1989), a student of Deming. This model conceptualizes the process as a journey having four phases: project definition and organization, a diagnostic journey, a remedial journey, and holding the gains.

A second commonly used model involves a nine-step method called FOCUS-PDCA (James, 1989, p. 33).

- **F**ind a process to improve.
- **O**rganize a team familiar with the process.
- **C**larify current knowledge of the process.
- **U**nderstand sources of variation.
- **S**elect the process improvement.
- **P**lan a change.
- **D**o carry out the change.
- **C**heck and observe the effects of the change.
- **A**ct, adapt, or modify the plan.

These two methods, and others less commonly used, are cyclical. As a process is improved, the cycle begins again, either to achieve a new level of performance or to

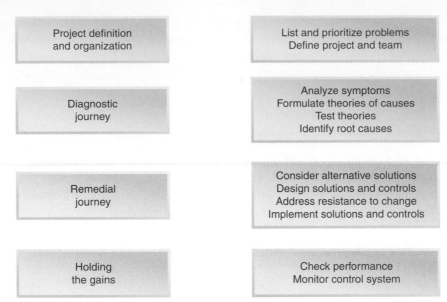

Project definition and organization	List and prioritize problems Define project and team
Diagnostic journey	Analyze symptoms Formulate theories of causes Test theories Identify root causes
Remedial journey	Consider alternative solutions Design solutions and controls Address resistance to change Implement solutions and controls
Holding the gains	Check performance Monitor control system

FIG 12.1 Steps in the Quality Improvement Process Source: Plsek, P.E., Onnias, A., & Early, J.F. (1988). *Quality improvement tools.* Wilton, CT: Juran Institute (p. 1).

address a new quality improvement opportunity. The goal is prevention, not detection, of errors through continuous improvement.

THE TOOLS OF QUALITY MANAGEMENT

Seven tools are used to identify and analyze work processes and to assess outcomes (Plsek, 1990). These quality tools and other techniques have gradually replaced routine auditing associated with quality assurance programs.

- A **flow chart** provides a pictorial representation of the steps in a process and how they relate to each other. For example, flow-charting the process of patient admission provides common understanding for team members and is usually enlightening.
- A **check sheet** is a form that shows the frequency of events and is particularly useful in showing patterns and translating opinions into facts. Recording the number of times equipment is unavailable or broken provides factual data.
- A **Pareto chart** uses data derived from a check sheet that shows the frequency of occurrence. Using data, the Pareto (or 20-80) rule, is applied, which states that 20% of issues account for 80% of occurrences. If a team is studying reasons for delay in patient transport to radiology, a check sheet will identify the factors contributing to delays and a Pareto chart will determine the specific factors that cause delays 80% of the time.

- A **cause-and-effect** (or **fish-bone**) **diagram** is used to record contributing causes of a problem—for example, methods, materials, people, or equipment. A check sheet and Pareto chart are then used to determine the "vital few" that require improvement.
- A **histogram** is a bar graph that displays the distribution of data within a category. If a team were studying the response time of the hospital's pharmacy to a narcotic order, this instrument would show the frequency with which the response time fell within a time interval.
- A **run chart** is used to display data over time, such as the length of time a nonemergent patient waits to see a nurse in the emergency department.
- A **scatter diagram** is used to plot two variables to determine whether a correlation exists. For example, the number of patient days per month could be plotted with the number of nursing hours, to see if staffing is efficient.

QUALITY IMPROVEMENT INDICATORS

Prior to 2008, the Canadian Council on Health Services Accreditation (CCHSA) had defined indicators as a measurement tool, screen, or flag to monitor, evaluate, and improve the quality of patient care, clinical services, support services, and organizational functions that affect patient outcomes (CCHSA, 1996). Currently, Accreditation Canada's Qmentum program has updated those standards and implemented more automated measurement tools (Accreditation Canada, 2009). Health care agencies are now monitoring quality indicators such as wait times for emergency care, cancer surgery, preoperative deaths, readmissions, and others.

The quality improvement movement occurred in times of recession and reform that necessitated deep cuts in health and social service spending with resultant major shifts in roles and functions of all health team members. The move of care from the acute setting to the community was also a factor influencing the continuing development of quality improvement programs. With regionalization of health care authorities from many independent hospital boards, the quality indicators being measured shifted from health care delivery indicators to include more general population health indicators. Accreditation Canada's Qmentum Program evaluates the three main categories of standards, which are system-wide areas, population-based aspects, and service excellence components of health care organizations. Overall, the Qmentum accreditation program "emphasizes health system performance, risk prevention planning, patient safety, performance measurement, and governance" (Accreditation Canada, 2009).

HEALTH REFORM

Health reform and the restructuring of health care delivery systems have had a significant impact on the ability of health care agencies to provide quality care in a consistent and seamless fashion (Hetherington, 1998; Cummings & Estabrooks, 2003). The 1990s were times of rapid and unprecedented change in health care. All structures, functions, roles, and expectations that defined delivery and consumption of health care services were challenged. Traditional hierarchical models were reconfigured, and functions historically organized by department (such as nursing, medicine, pharmacy, laboratory) were redefined.

Management literature is clear that structural changes alone will not lead to lasting organizational quality changes. Structural changes must be supported by modifications in roles, relationships, attitudes, and resource allocation. Concepts such as cross-functional teams, seamless organizations, clinical treatment teams, functional work groups, empowerment, coaching, and continuous quality improvement are central to the paradigm shift from traditional management processes to a system-wide quality improvement philosophy. Transformational leadership within health care can mitigate the external forces of change, leading to opportunities to improve organizations and services, and outcomes for patients (Cummings, Hayduk, & Estabrooks, 2005; Wong & Cummings, 2007).

In 1998, the International Study of Hospital Organization and Staffing on Patient Outcomes was launched in Canada, England, Scotland, Germany, and the United States to analyze the impact of the restructuring of health care on quality of care, availability of professional nurse staffing, and patient outcomes, including complication rates and mortality. Numerous reports have shown relationships between more hours of nurse staffing, a richer nurse skill mix, nurse education, and physician–nurse relationships and lower patient mortality (Aiken, Clarke, Sloane, Sochalski, & Silber, 2002; Estabrooks, Midodzi, Cummings, Ricker, & Giovannetti, 2005).

PATIENT SAFETY MOVEMENT

Another recent phenomenon in the international media is the focus on an epidemic of patient injury caused by health care (Wilson, 2001). The Royal College of Physicians and Surgeons (2007) define patient safety as the "reduction and mitigation of unsafe acts within the health care system, as well as the use of best practice, shown to lead to optimal patient outcomes." The Canadian Adverse Events Study (Baker et al., 2004) followed on the heels of the US Institute of Medicine's (IOM) report *To Err Is Human: Building a Safer Health System* (IOM, 2000) and the *Quality in Australian Health Care Study* (Wilson, 1995). In Canada, 1 in 13 adult patients admitted to acute-care hospitals in fiscal year 2000 experienced adverse events and sparked renewed interest in patient safety (Baker et al., 2004). A 7.5% incidence rate for adverse events, of which 36.9% were highly preventable, accounted for 1.1 million additional hospital days. Patient safety continues to be a major concern for health care consumers and providers while, at the same time, hospitals struggle with declining revenues and climbing costs.

In a follow-up to the *Err Is Human* report, the IOM pointed to the critical role nursing plays in providing safe care and identified health care management practices necessary to create a positive patient safety culture (IOM, 2004). Identified practices included creating and maintaining trust throughout the organization, deploying health care workers in adequate numbers, creating a culture of openness regarding reporting and prevention of errors, involving workers in decision making pertaining to work design and work flow, and actively managing the process of change (IOM, 2004). The report specifically targeted the salient role of strong nursing leadership to implement effective management practices that create "cultures of safety" (IOM, 2004, p. 253) and improve patient outcomes. The Canadian safety report also profiled the need for safer patient care environments and echoed the call for leadership to make the required changes (Baker et al., 2004). The IOM emphasized that quality of patient care is directly affected by the degree to which hospital nurses are active and empowered participants in decisions about their patients' plans of care and by the degree to which they have an active and central role in organizational decision making (IOM, 2004).

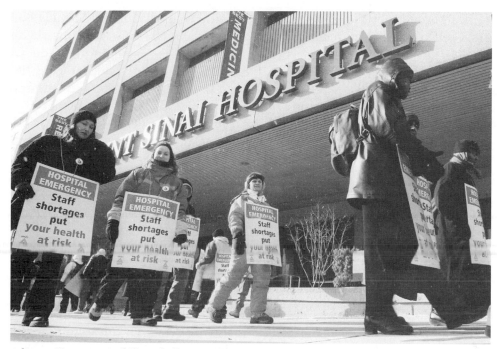

Advocacy is a responsibility of all nurses. Ontario nurses are shown here protesting against staff shortages that they fear will put patient health and safety at risk.

In 2002, the National Steering Committee on Patient Safety (NSCPS) reported 19 recommendations for a comprehensive and integrated national strategy to make patient safety a national priority for the Canadian health care system (NSCPS, 2002). One recommendation included the establishment of the Canadian Patient Safety Institute (CPSI) in 2005 with a mission to provide leadership on patient safety issues by advising governments, stakeholders, and the public on effective strategies, fostering information sharing, influencing culture change, supporting systems change, and collaborating with stakeholders in an ongoing dialogue on patient safety (NSCPS, 2002). In addition to producing original resources, CPSI provides peer-reviewed and annotated links to externally developed tools, articles and other resources and they link with key health care organizations and other groups involved in patient safety.

NURSING-SENSITIVE OUTCOMES AND BEST-PRACTICE GUIDELINES

The majority of care to patients in most health sectors is delivered by nurses, but very little information about the influence of nursing care is documented in administrative databases (Pringle & Doran, 2003). With the increasing imperative for professional and financial accountability in health care, we need health databases to include better information about the contributions of nurses. Recent efforts by professional and regulatory groups in both the United States and Canada have recommended health databases be expanded beyond mortality and morbidity (clinical complications) to include nurse-sensitive outcomes to measure the quality of nursing care. The American Nurses Association (2000) included patient satisfaction with pain management and patient education in the *Nursing Care Report Card for Acute Care*. The Ministry of Health and Long-Term Care of Ontario and its Expert Panel on Nursing and Health Outcomes recommended including functional status, symptom control, therapeutic self-care, pressure ulcers, and falls in Ontario administrative databases (Pringle & White, 2002). Outcomes sensitive to nursing are those that are relevant, based on nurses' domain and scope of practice, and for which empirical evidence links nursing inputs and interventions to the outcome (Doran, 2003).

In a feasibility study conducted with 890 patients from acute-care hospitals and long-term care facilities, Doran et al. (2006) demonstrated that the outcomes tools, functional status, symptom severity (pain, nausea, dyspnea, fatigue), and frequency and therapeutic self-care used were sensitive to change in patient condition, and that select nursing interventions were related to these outcomes. These findings suggest it is possible to collect data on nursing-sensitive patient outcomes in a reliable and valid way and to integrate this data collection into routine and daily nursing assessment and documentation. Inclusion of nursing-sensitive outcomes in health system monitoring is critical to effective evaluation of quality care but it is also important for nurses to understand how to use patient outcome results to assess and improve nursing interventions in daily nursing practice.

An associated domain of outcomes measurement is the use of evidence-informed best-practice guidelines as support to nurse decision making in the delivery of quality nursing care. Best-practice guidelines are systematically developed statements based on the best available evidence to assist clinician and patient decision making about appropriate health care for specific clinical circumstances (Field & Lohr, 1990). The implementation of evidence-informed or best practice should contribute to improved care outcomes. In Ontario, the Registered Nurses' Association of Ontario (RNAO) developed, pilot-implemented, evaluated, disseminated, and supported the uptake of nursing best-practice guidelines (BPGs) since 1999 (Virani & Grinspun, 2007). The BPG program is funded by the Ministry of Health and Long-Term Care of Ontario and to date more than 30 BPGs have been developed and utilized with reported evidence of improved clinical outcomes. Pilot-tested BPGs include those for asthma, breastfeeding, diabetic foot complications, delirium/dementia/depression, smoking cessation, and venous leg ulcers. RNAO attributes the success of the BPG program to four key fac-tors: intense grassroots engagement in BPG guideline development, dissemination, and uptake; comprehensive recommendations; government funding support; and strong staff leadership and expertise (Virani & Grinspun, 2007). The rationale behind the BPG project is that nurses are knowledge professionals whose practice must be based on the most valid and reliable evidence. This is essential to achieve best health and clinical out-comes for patients and positive organizational results. See the Canadian Research Focus box for an example of research that has evolved from the RNAO's work on BPGs and how BPGs can be examined to inform quality improvement processes.

REFLECTIVE THINKING

1. How is quality improvement and assurance actualized in my setting and how can I participate in ensuring the care provided to patients and their families fosters positive outcomes?
2. How do individual-level actions for improving patient care enhance the overall efforts of total quality management (TQM) and continuous quality improvement (CQI)?

CANADIAN RESEARCH FOCUS

Edwards, N., Davies, B., Ploeg, J., Virani, T., & Skelly, J. (2007). Implementing nursing best practice guidelines: Impact on patient referrals. *BMC Nursing*, *6*, 4.

Research into quality improvement and quality assurance reveals important findings that inform the science of implementation. One aspect worth studying is how best-practice guidelines are introduced to nurses and then actualized in the clinical setting. Edwards et al. (2007) studied the effects of an educational intervention aimed at increasing nurses' application of six RNAO Best Practice Guidelines (BPGs) using a prospective before and after design. The BPGs included in the study were related to asthma, breastfeeding, delirium/dementia/depression, venous leg ulcers, and diabetes. More specifi-cally, the researchers examined whether attempts to increase awareness and knowledge about the guidelines' referral recommendations led to more patient referrals to community resources. The results were mixed, as significant increases were seen in referral rates for three of the six BPGs. Numerous factors may have influenced the nurses' use of the BPG recommendations, resulting in a nonsignifi-cant increase in referral practices. Factors that may have decreased effectiveness of the educational intervention were the general versus specific nature of the BPGs, nurses' potentially limited knowledge of the health issue, and nurses' potential unfamiliarity with the available referral resources. From this study, the researchers suggested that having more specific BPGs inclusive of contextual application would possibly increase nurses' referral practices. Clear communication and documentation systems about referral processes may increase their use and promote overall continuity of patient care. Finally, nurses participating in this study gained more knowledge about BPGs and their role in referring patients to important community resources.

FUTURE DIRECTIONS ENSURING QUALITY OF CARE

Continuous quality improvement has established a foothold in the Canadian health care system along with establishing a presence internationally (Harrigan, 2000). Harrigan referred to the 1993 World Health Organization (WHO) standard that, by the year

2000, all member states would ensure continuous quality improvement in health care and appropriate development and use of health technologies. Since then, the WHO has launched global patient safety research funding and promotion of a conceptual framework for a cyclical, continuously improving approach to services management. Future WHO activities will include providing technical support for nation capacity building in countries involved in the promotion and implementation of quality improvement, and assistance to countries to monitor their own quality improvement development (WHO, 2008).

In the early 1990s, the CCHSA Survey Standards reflected a quality improvement focus and the consequent elimination of separate standards for departments providing patient care services. The standards focused on facility-wide integration of clinical and support processes across departmental boundaries and team functioning that is essential for effective and efficient implementation. Patient safety will continue as a priority for quality improvement efforts. Accreditation Canada and its Qmentum accreditation program is currently committed to playing a major role in improving patient safety through accreditation. The accreditation process is a way of identifying conditions of unsafe practice and supporting health care organizations to promote safe care. When Qmentum standards are met, the potential for adverse events occurring within health care and service organizations is reduced. Consequently, the Qmentum accreditation program has made patient safety an essential element, reinforcing that health service cannot be of high quality unless it is safe.

Nursing has directed and will continue to direct quality monitoring of nursing care, thus ensuring that professional standards are maintained for individual nurses. Quality-monitoring instruments, which have underpinned nursing quality assurance programs, continue to be used to monitor standards of nursing practice; however, the audit process is being replaced by new methodologies associated with a continuous quality improvement philosophy, the ongoing measurement of nursing-sensitive outcomes, and the implementation of nursing best-practice guidelines.

Many factors determine successful CQI, all of which must be addressed by leaders in the organization. The way forward through all the significant quality issues addressed in this chapter is to place patients and their needs at the centre. Then, by using the best available evidence to determine required care processes, measurement to inform and direct the processes, an organizational rather than an individualized approach, and the application of process-change management, we can ensure a culture of continuous quality improvement that actually results in improved outcomes. These improvements are based on a true cultural transformation, a well-developed quality strategy, ongoing educational programs available to all staff regardless of level in the organization, well-prepared team leaders, empowerment of front-line staff, and a quality improvement council charged with prioritizing quality issues, developing policy, and identifying a process for the identification of projects and teams.

The shift from quality assurance programs to a system-wide quality management philosophy has shown promising results in the pursuit of cost-effective, quality care. Nurses have been at the forefront in developing and monitoring standards of practice that have provided the foundation for the future. Efforts by the nursing profession to improve patient care and public accountability by refining and enhancing quality processes will continue to be instrumental in the ongoing redesign of health care. Quality improvement and patient safety cultures are interdisciplinary, interdependent approaches to managing our health care system for which comprehensive and integrated data need to be a driver. These data and commitment at all levels of the health care system will ensure a cyclical and continual improvement to quality of care regardless of internal and external challenges.

 REFLECTIVE THINKING

1. What might quality assurance and quality improvement within nursing look like in the future?
2. What working groups are in place to study and/or investigate issues related to quality improvement in Canada?

CRITICAL THINKING QUESTIONS

1. A nurse has been appointed to participate on a committee to reduce the number of families without access to adequate respite care in the community. What tools or processes should he or she suggest to help explore and improve the issue?
2. How does the concept of continuous quality improvement differ from quality assurance?
3. Why is it important for health care databases to include information about nursing interventions and nursing-sensitive outcomes?
4. What are some ways in which a nurse in any clinical setting can make patient safety improvement and reducing errors not just an organizational priority but a personal one in his or her everyday practice?
5. How can nurses demonstrate effective leadership related to quality improvement?

WEB SITES

Accreditation Canada: http://www.accreditation.ca/en/default.aspx
Accreditation Canada is an independent organization that is accredited by the International Society for Quality in Health Care (ISQua) and provides an external peer-review function for health care organizations. Accreditation Canada's new accreditation program is now called Qmentum.
Canadian Institute for Health Information: http://www.cihi.ca
The CIHI is an independent organization that provides data and information on the health status of Canadians and how the health care system is functioning overall. CIHI keeps track of data supplied by many health care partners ranging from government agencies to individual Canadians. National health indicators are also monitored by CIHI; they create an overall picture of the quality of health care in Canada. Examples of information published by CIHI include rate of falls in hospitalized patients, obesity statistics in Canada, and the number of adverse events that occur in acute-care settings.

Canadian Patient Safety Institute (CPSI): http://www.patientsafetyinstitute.ca/
> CPSI is an independent organization in Canada that partners with various health care stakeholders to promote safe patient care.

Corporate Nursing Quality Improvement Work Group: Ottawa Hospital: http://www.ottawahospital.on.ca/hp/dept/nursing/npp/wg/wg09-index-e.asp
> The Ottawa Hospital's Nursing QI group is one example of how institutions are fostering and monitoring quality health care.

International Society for Quality in Health Care (ISQua): http://www.isqua.org/
ISQua is an international organization that assists all levels of health care providers to achieve excellence in health care.

REFERENCES

Accreditation Canada. (2009). Qmentum accreditation program. Retrieved on September 24, 2009, from http://www.accreditation.ca/en/content.aspx?pageid=50.

Aiken, L. H., Clarke, S. P., Sloane, D. M., Sochalski, J., & Silber, J. H. (2002). Hospital nurse staffing and patient mortality, nurse burnout, and job dissatisfaction. *Journal of the American Medical Association, 288*(16), 1987–1993.

Alexander, J. A., & Hearld, L. R. (2009). Review: What can we learn from quality improvement research? A critical review of research methods. *Medical Care Research and Review, 66*, 235.

American Nurses Association. (2000). *Nurse staffing and patient outcomes in the inpatient hospital setting: Report.* Washington, DC: Author.

Baker, G. R., Norton, P. G., Flintoff, V., Balis, R., Brown, A., Cox, J., Etchells, E., Ghali, W. A., Hébert, P., Majumdar, S. R., O'Beirne, M., Palcios-Derflingher, L., Reid, R. J., Sheps, S., & Tamblyn, R. (2004). The Canadian Adverse Events study: The incidence of adverse events among hospital patients in Canada. *Canadian Medical Association Journal, 170*(10), 1678–1686.

Berwick, D., Godfrey, A. B., & Roessner, J. (1990). *Curing health care: New strategies for quality improvement.* San Francisco: Jossey-Bass.

Canadian Council on Health Services Accreditation (CCHSA). (1996). *Survey standards.* Ottawa: Author.

Canadian Council on Health Services Accreditation (CCHSA). (2008, January). Strengthening the accreditation program: An overview of the new program. Retrieved on January 20, 2008, from http://www.cchsa.ca.

Cummings, G., & Estabrooks, C. A. (2003). The effects of hospital restructuring that included layoffs on individual nurses who remained employed: A systematic review of impact. *International Journal of Sociology and Social Policy, 8/9*, 8–53.

Cummings, G. G., Hayduk, L., & Estabrooks, C. A. (2005). Mitigating the impact of hospital restructuring on nurses: The responsibility of emotionally intelligent leadership. *Nursing Research, 54*(1), 2–12.

Deming, W. E. (1986). *Out of crisis.* Cambridge, MA: MIT Press.

Donabedian, A. (1980). *Explorations in quality assessment and monitoring.* (Vol. 1). Ann Arbor, MI: Health Administration Press.

Donabedian, A. (2003). *An introduction to quality assurance in health care.* New York, NY: Oxford University Press.

Doran, D. (Ed.). (2003). *Nursing sensitive outcomes: The state of the science.* Boston, MA: Jones and Bartlett Publishers.

Doran, D. M., Harrison, M. B., Laschinger, H. S., Hirdes, J. P., Rukholm, E., Sidani, S., McGillis-Hall, L., & Tourangeau, A. (2006). Nursing-sensitive outcomes data collection in acute care and long-term care settings. *Nursing Research, 55*(2S), S75–S81.

Edwards, N., Davies, B., Ploeg, J., Virani, T., & Skelly, J. (2007). Implementing nursing best practice guidelines: Impact on patient referrals. *BMC Nursing, 6*, 4, [online article].

Estabrooks, C. A., Midodzi, W. K., Cummings, G. G., Ricker, K. L., & Giovannetti, P. (2005). Determining the impact of hospital nursing characteristics on 30-day mortality among patients in Alberta acute care hospitals. *Nursing Research, 54*(2), 74–84.

Field, M. J., & Lohr, K. N. (Eds.). (1990). *Guidelines for clinical practice: Directions for a new program*. Washington, DC: Institute of Medicine, National Academies Press.

Giovannetti, P., Kerr, J. C., Bay, K., & Buchan, J. (1986). *Measuring quality of nursing care: Analysis of reliability and validity of selected instruments—file report*. Edmonton: Faculty of Nursing: University of Alberta.

Harrigan, M. L. (2000). *Quest for quality in Canadian health care: Continuous quality improvement* (2nd ed.). Ottawa: Health Canada.

Hetherington, L. T. (1998). Evaluating quality management systems. *Journal of Nursing Care Quality*, *13*(2), 56–66.

Institute of Medicine (IOM). (2000). *To err is human: Building a safer health system*. Washington, DC: National Academies Press.

Institute of Medicine (IOM). (2004). *Keeping patients safe: Transforming the work environment of nurses*. Washington, DC: National Academies Press.

James, B. C. (1989). *Quality management of health care delivery*. Chicago: American Hospital Association.

Juran, J. M. (1989). *Juran on planning for quality*. New York: Free Press.

McLaughlin, C., & Kaluzny, A. (1990). Total quality management in health: Making it work. *Health Care Management Review*, *15*(3), 7–14.

National Steering Committee on Patient Safety (NSCPS). (2002). *Building a safer system: A national integrated strategy for improving patient safety in Canadian health care*. Ottawa: Author.

Nightingale, F. (1858). *Notes on matters affecting the health, efficiency and hospital administration of the British army*. London: Harrison & Sons.

Plsek, P. (1990). A primer on quality improvement tools. In D. Berwick, A. Godfrey, & J. Roessner (Eds.), *Curing health care* (pp. 177–220). San Francisco: Jossey-Bass.

Plsek, P. E., Onnias, A., & Early, J. F. (1988). *Quality improvement tools*. Wilton, CT: Juran Institute.

Pringle, D., & Doran, D. M. (2003). Patient outcomes as an accountability. In D. M. Doran (Ed.), *Nursing-sensitive outcomes: State of the science* (pp. 1–25). Sudbury, MA: Jones and Bartlett.

Pringle, D. M., & White, P. (2002). Nursing matters: The Nursing and Health Outcomes Project of the Ontario Ministry of Health and Long-Term Care. *Canadian Journal of Nursing Research*, *33*, 115–121.

Royal College of Physicians and Surgeons. (2007). *The Canadian patient safety dictionary*. Ottawa: Author.

Thompson, R. (1991). The six faces of quality. *Health Care Executive*, *6*(2), 26–27.

Trussel, P. M., & Strand, N. (1978). A comparison of concurrent and retrospective audits of the same clients. *Journal of Nursing Administration*, *8*(5), 33–38.

Ventura, M., Hageman, P. T., Slakter, M. J., & Fox, R. N. (1980). Interrater reliabilities for two measures of nursing care quality. *Research in Nursing and Health*, *3*(1), 25–32.

Virani, T., & Grinspun, D. (2007). Best practice guidelines—RNAO's Best Practice Guidelines Program: Progress report on a phenomenal journey. *Advances in Skin & Wound Care*, *20*(10), 528–535.

Walton, M. (1986). *The Deming management method*. New York: Dodd, Mead.

Whetsell, G. (1990). Total quality management. *Health Progress*, *71*(8), 16–19.

Wilson, R. (1995). The Quality in Australian Health Care Study. *Medical Journal of Australia*, *163*, 458–471.

Wilson, R. (2001). Quality improvement will require a major commitment. *Hospital Quarterly*, *4*(3), 20–24.

Wong, C., & Cummings, G. G. (2007). The relationship between nursing leadership and patient outcomes: A systematic review. *Journal of Nursing Management*, *15*, 508–521.

World Health Organization (WHO). (2008). *Management of quality care*. Retrieved on January 31, 2008, from http://www.who.int/management/quality/en.

13

The Practising Nurse and the Law

Lori L. Kerr

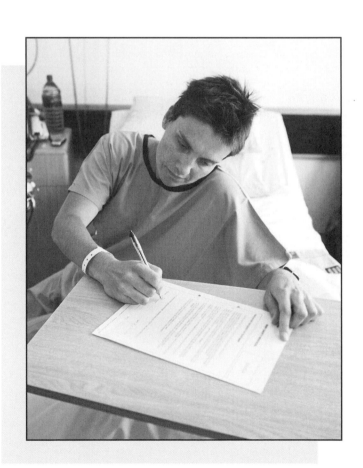

▌ LEARNING OBJECTIVES

- To introduce the common legal issues nurses may become involved in.
- To highlight the role of nurses as professionals and the obligations of self-regulation.
- To outline all the elements of a nursing negligence action.
- To appreciate the complexities required for a valid consent to health care treatment, informed consent, and capacity to consent for minors and dependent adults.
- To identify the legal obligation of nurses to keep treatment records.
- To understand the legal obligation to maintain privacy and confidentiality of patients.
- To understand that the legal aspects of nursing practice are not static and evolve with the development of nursing practice.

On a daily basis, nurses confront a myriad of factors that have a direct impact on their ability to make informed decisions regarding the quality of care they give. Legal challenges to nursing activities were once rare and posed little concern in the nursing profession. However, this situation has changed. The extension of the nurse's scope of practice, substantial improvements in salaries and working conditions for nurses, and a greater propensity for the public to seek damages for professional negligence are all reasons for nurses to be aware of the risks and responsibilities inherent in their practice. The potential benefit of understanding rights and responsibilities under the law, particularly as they apply to the health care field, is clear when one considers the close and continuing contact between patients and nurses in health care environments.

Nurses' responsibilities traditionally have been seen as falling largely in the area of comfort and less in the area of treatment procedures. However, the continuous transfer of functions from medicine to nursing and the exponential increase in knowledge and technology relating to health have had a far-reaching impact on nursing and nurses' roles. The expanded scope of practice in nursing from hospitals to home care, physicians' private offices and health clinics, and other facilities has been such that nurses have taken on the performance of procedures that entail considerable risk. The primary types of legal proceedings that may affect nurses' professional abilities throughout their careers include negligence actions, disciplinary proceedings, public inquiries, criminal charges, and employment arbitrations. Although each proceeding will differ, it is essential not only that nurses be knowledgeable and competent in the practice of their profession, but also that they are aware of and respect the legal rights of their patients. This chapter provides an overview of the law and the principal areas of nurses' involvement in the legal system. The information is not intended as a comprehensive treatment of the subject, but rather as a cursory review to introduce areas of concern, stimulate thinking about issues, and encourage further research.

PROFESSIONAL STATUS OF NURSES

Nurses have professional status in all provinces and territories in Canada that allows for exclusivity of practice, right of self-regulation, and the obligation to monitor and discipline its own membership. Nurses are governed in some provinces and territories by individual health profession legislation. However, other jurisdictions have moved to umbrella legislation for all health professionals. The common principle throughout each province is the designation by the legislation of a statutory body whose role is to register, monitor, and discipline nurses within the province or territory.

Each jurisdiction's nursing governing bodies are charged by legislation to provide and enforce standards of practice and a code of conduct as well as establish requirements for entry to practice. Even after nurses have met the qualifications and competencies required for registration, they have a continuing legal obligation to remain familiar with developments in the profession and to remain capable of performing tasks that the public would expect a competent nurse to perform. Additional to their regulatory functions, most nursing "associations" or "colleges" take on voluntary functions in the interest of promoting the nursing profession, except for a few jurisdictions whose legislation requires that the regulatory body and the voluntary functions remain separate (College of Nurses of Ontario and the Registered Nurses Association of Ontario).

When incidents occur that involve complaints against a nurse for failure to meet the standards of practice, for incompetence, or for incapacity, the governing body protects the public by investigating such complaints about members' practice. Investigations performed by the registrar, employer through mandatory reporting, or regulated health provider may arise as a result of complaints from patients, colleagues, or members of the public. Any professional conduct or discipline process must meet the requirements of the governing legislation. A hearing related to a complaint may be held when issues are of a serious nature and the allegations of professional misconduct or incompetence are supported by evidence. A hearing is similar to a court proceeding; each side will have opening and closing statements, examinations and cross-examinations, and testimony of expert witnesses. The board or committee hearing the complaint will be empowered by the governing legislation to issue a decision with the appropriate penalty, the most severe being revocation of registration.

Each regulatory body will set out the appeal process of decisions of the board or committee of the hearing. Following the appeal, a further appeal to the appropriate court may be available. Where available, the appeal court has the ability to confirm the decision, to substitute its own decision, or to send the issue back for a new hearing. Complaints of professional misconduct or incompetence may also result in a negligence lawsuit and criminal charges. As discussed below, negligence lawsuits are primarily about compensation for damages whereas the complaints of professional misconduct or incompetence are about registration and practice permits.

NEGLIGENCE

The majority of lawsuits against health care providers are in tort law. Torts can be intentional or unintentional. The bulk of lawsuits against health care providers are unintentional torts, which are based on complaints of negligence. These will be the focus of this discussion. However, it is important to be aware of intentional torts, which are acts that deliberately violate the rights of another. In the health care context, some examples of this include battery, false imprisonment, or detaining patients against their will, and libel and slander (defaming a patient's reputation).

ELEMENTS OF NEGLIGENCE

Patients place their trust in nurses on a daily basis and have a right to expect the best possible care based on a reasonable standard of skill and knowledge. Negligence in this context is commonly defined as treatment falling below the standard of care that a reasonable and prudent nurse would follow in particular health care circumstances. The concept of the provision of a reasonable standard of nursing care has been upheld by the courts in case law. As commented in *Crits v. Sylvester* [1956]:

> *Every medical practitioner must bring to his task a reasonable degree of skill and knowledge and must exercise a reasonable degree of care. He is bound to exercise that degree of care and skill which could reasonably be expected of a normal, prudent practitioner of the same experience and standing…. (p. 601)*

A claim of negligence will succeed if the essential elements can be demonstrated by a plaintiff. These include the following: (1) the defendant must owe the plaintiff a duty of care; (2) the duty of care was breached—i.e., the nurse must have been careless or negligent; (3) the breach must have caused the injury; (4) the breach of duty must result in damages; and (5) the defendant must not be able to raise any defence to the plaintiff's claim.

In order to establish that a duty of care of a nurse is owed to a patient, it must be demonstrated that there was a relationship between the patient and nurse. A duty of care is seldom disputed as "the extreme vulnerability and dependency of patients upon their nurses and the obvious capacity of nurses to cause harm to their patients by substandard care combine to create in the eyes of the law an unquestionable duty owed to each patient to provide appropriate care and professional skill" (Sneiderman, Irvine, & Osborne, 2003). Most often, this element will be satisfied by the reliance on records documenting the nurse's involvement with the patient's care.

The second element, breach of duty or standard of care, tends to provide the focus of debate when a nurse is sued. The care would not have to have been the best care or even the optimum care, but the standard of care a "reasonable and prudent nurse" would have provided in a particular situation. The evidence establishing the standard of a "reasonable and prudent nurse" is developed in a number of ways, including relevant statements in articles and books by nursing authors that document the acceptability of certain practices, nursing practice standards developed by national and provincial professional nursing associations, curriculum content in schools of nursing, and testimony by expert witnesses who are nurses. As well, the individual nurse's practice, educational background, and experience are scrutinized by the court. In one important case (*Dowey v. Rothwell* [1974]), a nurse who had worked in a physician's office in Alberta for 22 years was found negligent after the court learned that she had failed to take any continuing education courses since the year after her graduation, some 40 years before. Even if there is more than one recognized method of care, a nurse would not be negligent as long as the nurse provided care that was consistent with accepted practice.

The next element requires that a plaintiff must be able to link the breach of duty to the patient's injury. To establish this link, it must be demonstrated on the balance of probabilities that if the nurse had not been negligent, the injury would not have been suffered. This element is usually established through testimony of expert witnesses. This is illustrated in *MacDonald v. York County* [1972], in which a patient treated for a fractured dislocation of the ankle developed gangrene and was forced to undergo an amputation of his leg below the knee. The trial judge found that the nurses had been aware that the patient's condition was deteriorating over an 18-hour period but had failed to advise a physician, and found the hospital and nursing staff partially responsible for the injuries. On appeal, the nurses' negligence was found not to have caused any harm to the plaintiff as the physician had provided evidence that he would not have acted even if the appropriate standard of care had been met by the nurses.

Even if all the previous elements are present, the breach of duty must have resulted in damages to the plaintiff. Although health care providers, including nurses, tend to view actions involving negligence as negative to reputation and integrity, the purpose of the law pertaining to torts is to compensate the party who is injured through the actions of another. For example, in the case of *Strachan (Guardian ad litem of) v. Reynolds* [2004], a mother and child were entitled to recover damages against a nurse, as the nurse had failed to recognize signs and symptoms of developing uterine rupture, which caused the child's oxygen deprivation and subsequent brain injury. The issue here is not punishment, but rather to compensate the plaintiff for injury by moving responsibility for loss from the plaintiff to the defendant. If a patient is not able to demonstrate damages, there would be no basis for a civil action, notwithstanding a patient could still initiate discipline proceedings.

In some jurisdictions, there may be legislation that affords nurses protection from liability if the applicable legislation contains an appropriate statutory limitation of liability. This was the case in *Wowk v. Edmonton (Health Board)* (1994), in which the plaintiff suffered an injury as a result of an influenza shot given by the defendant community health nurse. The court found that the *Public Health Act* (Alberta) shielded the community health nurse from liability for any act done or omitted in good faith in performing the services, as negligence was not itself a lack of good faith.

REFLECTIVE THINKING

What is the legal differentiation between an error and negligence of a nurse in nursing practice?

CONSENT TO NURSING CARE

A fundamental human right, historically respected in law, is the right to be free from interference. Except in the case of emergencies and other extraordinary circumstances, consent must be obtained prior to the provision of health care treatment. In 1993, the Supreme Court of Canada confirmed this right in stating that

> [e]veryone has the right to decide what is to be done to one's own body. This includes the right to be free from medical treatment to which the individual does not consent. This concept of individual autonomy is fundamental to the common law…. (Ciarlariello v. Schacter, [1993], p. 135)

The tort of battery involves intentional touching of another person. There need not be any injury for the charge to be upheld by the courts. Because nursing practice involves much touching of patients, it is important that patient consent be obtained for any nursing procedures that involve touching. Thus, the aim here is to provide a cursory discussion of the fundamental requirements for a legal consent. The present discussion represents a brief summary only. More specific references should be consulted to obtain a deeper understanding of the issues.

Age, health, and mental status of patients, and circumstances surrounding the situation, often make it difficult for nurses to obtain informed consent. Nurses usually rely on the patient's verbal expression of consent to nursing-care activities. In the past, the majority of these activities have been considered low risk. However, with the steady expansion of the scope of nursing practice and the increase in independent nursing functions, many current nursing-care procedures are considered high risk. Thus, it is crucial that nurses understand all the fundamental requirements for a valid consent, as well as their role in documenting it. Health care workers who rely on implied consent in the absence of emergency or for high-risk procedures are exposing patients to unauthorized intrusion on their bodies and themselves to possible liability (Philpott, 1985). In *Canadian AIDS Society v. Ontario* (August 4, 1995), the court had to consider whether consent could have been implied by a blood donor to have his donated blood tested ten years after the fact. Thus, express consent is preferred even if implied consent may be valid.

Much of the law surrounding consent has been settled in case law or by the relevant legislation in the provinces. In an attempt to provide a degree of certainty, some provinces have enacted legislation that defines how and by whom consent can be given. For example, Ontario's *Health Care Consent Act* holds that valid consent relating to treatment must be informed and voluntary and must not be obtained by misrepresentation or fraud (*Health Care Consent Act*, 1996). In the absence of specific legislation within the nurse's jurisdiction, the law has recognized four basic requirements for consent to be valid: (1) it must relate to the treatment; (2) it must be informed; (3) it must be given voluntarily; and (4) the patient must have the capacity to consent to the proposed treatment. A brief explanation of each the four elements noted above will reveal the importance and complexity of this issue.

TREATMENT AND PROVIDER OF TREATMENT

Consent to care given must be specific to the proposed treatment or procedure. As noted in *Dixon v. Calgary Health Region* [2006], a patient sued after being treated with multiple intramuscular injections of Demerol, which the patient claimed caused weakness in his right leg, causing him to fall and injure his back. The court ruled that informed consent had been provided and that separate written consents were not required for each injection. Additionally, consideration should be taken if a patient consented to the performance of a procedure by a particular health care provider; this does not authorize substitution of another, less qualified, or different type of, health practitioner.

INFORMED OF THE NATURE AND RISKS OF TREATMENT

Generally, in all provinces for consent to be informed prior to commencing treatment, the patient must be provided with information concerning the nature of the treatment and its gravity, the expected benefits of the treatment, the material risks of the treatment and material side effects of the treatment, alternative courses of action, and potential consequences of not having the treatment. The patient should also have an opportunity to ask questions and receive responses to the questions. The courts have found that "material risk" is dependent on each situation. Not every conceivable risk or mere possibility needs to be disclosed but normally just those risks that may result in serious consequences. Through the *Health Care Consent Act* in s. 11(3), Ontario has set out the "reasonable person" as the standard used as a basis for determining how much information needs to be disclosed to a patient.

VOLUNTARY CONSENT

To be considered voluntary, consent must be freely given and must be obtained without undue influence or misrepresentation about the nature of the treatment. Even though each case depends on its facts, fundamentally patients have the full right to control their own medical treatment. The court will examine any pressure brought on a patient and determine whether it was sufficient to affect the decision making of that individual. In *Re T [1992]*, a minor who was 34 weeks pregnant refused to have a blood transfusion. Though the minor was not a Jehovah's Witness, her mother was a member of that faith. Upon the request of the minor's father, the court granted application to order the transfusion. On appeal, the court held that there was undue influence upon the minor by her mother and so upheld the decision to authorize the transfusion.

As well, it is important to remember that patients have a right to make their own health care decisions. A patient also has a right to withdraw consent to any procedure at any time before or during it. The Supreme Court of Canada confirmed that if there is any basis for the withdrawal of consent to a medical procedure even while it is underway, the procedure must be halted except if termination of the procedure either would be life-threatening or would cause serious problems for the patient (*Ciarlariello v. Schacter*, [1993], p. 135).

CAPACITY TO CONSENT

The patient must have the legal capacity to consent to treatment or substitute consent must be obtained from a person with legal standing to make the treatment decision. Capacity in this context refers to the individual's age and mental competence. Adults with disabilities and children are the two groups for whom questions of consent in health matters become a more complex issue. It can be difficult not only to identify the appropriate decision maker but also to determine the basis on which the decision is to be made. The limits on decision-making authority depend on a number of factors. For adults without capacity, most jurisdictions have enacted comprehensive legislation to deal with the substitute consent and the ability to create a legally valid personal or advance directive or to appoint a health care agent (Downie & Caulfield, 1999). In the absence of legislation, the courts are likely to apply many of the principles embodied in existing legislation (Morris, Ferguson, & Dykeman, 1999, p. 146).

In addition to the legislation for adults without capacity, health care providers should be aware of relevant legislation in their provinces that addresses age of consent for minors. Although parents are routinely consulted in regard to treatment, their decisions are not absolute. The courts have the jurisdiction to challenge a parent's decision if it is not deemed to be in the best interests of the child. Some jurisdictions have enacted legislation that creates an independent tribunal to review decisions not in the best interest of the child. For example, in Ontario, the Consent and Capacity Board is an independent body created by the provincial government of Ontario under the *Health Care Consent Act* that considers whether the substitute decision maker followed the principles for making substitute decisions.

A common situation occurs when, for example, in the opinion of health care providers, a blood transfusion is required but is refused by the parents for religious reasons. The courts will take into consideration age, intelligence, education, and previous experiences in determining whether a child can understand the nature and consequences of the proposed treatment and thus give consent. In the 1986 decision by the Alberta Court of Appeal, *C. (J.S.) v. Wren* [1986], a 16-year-old sought an abortion and obtained the consent of her doctor and the Therapeutic Abortion Committee, both of which were required at the time. Her parents attempted to stop the procedure and argued that their daughter was a minor and therefore could not give consent to the abortion. Although the court confirmed parental rights, it held that the evidence established that the daughter was a normal 16-year-old who had sufficient intelligence and understanding to make up her own mind. Thus, the court upheld the Committee's original order.

Along with physicians, nurses often face the issue of consent as they are often involved in asking patients to sign consent-to-treatment documents. The case of *B.H. (Next friend of) v. Alberta (Director of Child Welfare)* [2002] illustrates the complexity of this issue. In February 2002, a 16-year-old minor was diagnosed with acute myeloid leukemia, and based on her religious beliefs, she refused to consent to blood transfusions or the administration of blood products. The Alberta Director of Child Welfare made an application to the Provincial Court for an apprehension order and a medical treatment order. The court granted the orders that made the minor a ward of the state, and the essential treatment was administered. The decision was upheld by the Alberta Court of Appeal and leave to appeal to the Supreme Court of Canada was refused. Although this difficult issue has arisen before, it serves as a reminder of the complexities involved in obtaining a minor's consent.

CANADIAN RESEARCH FOCUS

Sklar, Ronald. (2007). *Starson v. Swayze*: The Supreme Court speaks out (not all that clearly) on the question of "capacity." *Canadian Journal of Psychiatry, 52*(6), 390–396.

The case of *Starson v. Swayze* put the issue of capacity to consent to treatment front and centre in Canada. The decision of the Supreme Court of Canada (SCC) focused on the interpretation of the "understanding" requirement for capacity in Ontario's *Health Care Consent Act*. The court looked at many factors, including the question of whether the patient's best interests are to be factored into the determination of a patient's capacity and subsequently the right of a capable patient to refuse treatment. In this 2007 article, the author discusses and analyses the SCC's decision, including its clinical and constitutional implications for Ontario and the rest of Canada.

NURSING DOCUMENTATION

Most health professionals have a legal obligation to maintain an account of the care and treatment to the minimum standard set out by legislation as well as standards set by the health professions governing body. The primary purpose of creating health records is to facilitate communication among health care providers in treating a patient. Health records reflect a contemporaneous account of the care and treatment of patients and are a vital part of communication among members of the health care team. Once created, the health record becomes a legal document. Documentation should be done in compliance with a number of legal requirements with respect to content, retention, and disclosure of the health record. Other sources that set out the frequency, quantity, and detail of documentation include provincial legislation, hospital bylaws, policies and procedures, standards of the professions, regulatory guidelines, and complexity and severity of the patient's health problems.

Courts have over time recognized that in many situations a written record may be more dependable than a witness's oral recollection of the events. The leading case with respect to admissibility of hospital records into evidence, including nurses' notes, is the Supreme Court of Canada case *Ares v. Venner* [1970]:

> *Hospital records, including nurses' notes made contemporaneously by someone having a personal knowledge of the matters then being recorded and under a duty to make the entry or record, should be received in evidence as prima facie proof of the facts stated therein. This should in no way preclude a party wishing to challenge the accuracy of the records or entries from doing so. (p. 626)*

Before this decision, nurses' notes were considered hearsay evidence and were not admissible in court. There are differences, however, among provinces as to whether various kinds of nursing records that form a part of the hospital record are admissible as evidence in court. Philpott (1985) notes that the *Canada Evidence Act* and the majority of provincial laws concerning evidence accept those parts of the record that are considered business records. However, there are variations in nursing records and whether any part or all of a record is consistent with the definition of "business records" is decided by the province involved.

In many cases, problems with nursing notes introduced as evidence in court have engendered criticism in court records of the proceedings. Frequent criticisms include failure to record events contemporaneously, gaps in recording, and recording of care by someone other than the nurse who provided the care. As illustrated in the case of *Kolesar v. Jefferies* (1974), the case involved the death of a patient who was found dead the morning after a spinal fusion operation. The chart was important in establishing liability as no nursing entries were made from 22.00 hours to 05.00, when the death was discovered. The lack of nursing notes enabled the court to infer no nursing care was provided during the time frame.

In general, it is difficult to verify that any care not recorded was actually provided. Cases often come to trial long after the events in question occurred. In these circumstances, it is difficult for principals to remember details of what happened. Thus, clear, accurate, and complete recording of events at the time of the event is essential as the contemporaneous record will generally be accepted over anyone's recollection of the events. The court in *Chancey v. McKinstry* [2000] demonstrated this principle by its reliance on the medical record. The case involved a patient who assaulted his wife after he had stopped taking lithium after 20 years of treatment for a bipolar disorder. The patient at trial alleged that his psychiatrist had told him to stop taking the lithium. The court accepted the psychiatrist's notes as demonstration that it was his standard practice not to interfere with patients' prescriptions.

The desired characteristics of nursing notes include many essential elements. The recording of information should be contemporaneous by the nurse who had first-hand knowledge of what was described in the record. It is considered very poor practice to record the actions of another health care provider, as the recording nurse would not have personal knowledge of the event and not be able to testify as to the truth of it. Therefore, record only what you performed, saw, and heard. It is important to record chronologically, frequently, and accurately in preparing a "factual, concise and totally objective" record of the events (Ross, 1973, pp. 102–103). These principles are exemplified in the case of *Meyer v. Gordon* [1981], which involved an infant who suffered a serious brain injury during birth. The trial was held five years after the incident and the nurse's sole evidence was her chart. The chart was found to be insufficient to demonstrate that she provided adequate care to the patient and she was found to be negligent.

Nevertheless, many believe that there is a good deal of unnecessary charting in which nurses are required to spend a great deal of time recording routine care. This is thought to be wasteful both in using the time of highly skilled nurses unnecessarily and the space and time required for storage and retrieval of the data. Thus, charting by exception is being used in many health care centres. This is a method by which routine care and normal procedures are documented in an abbreviated method and only unusual occurrences and exceptions are recorded by a narrative. Nevertheless, charting by exception should be used only when it is supported by standards and policies in place to ensure that consistency and commitment to documentation is maintained.

There may be failures or honest mistakes made in the documentation process. The best course of action is to strike out the incorrect information and fill in the correct information with the date and time corrected. Nurses may be considered negligent if information is erased, as the court must assume that important facts were hidden and the person or persons responsible for the act did so in self-interest. It is evident that dishonesty in matters pertaining to care will usually be discerned in court proceedings and will not reflect positively on the character, conduct, or professionalism of the nurse or nurses involved. Additionally, any falsification and destruction of nursing records by nurses most likely will result in criminal and disciplinary action taken by the employer as well as the regulatory body.

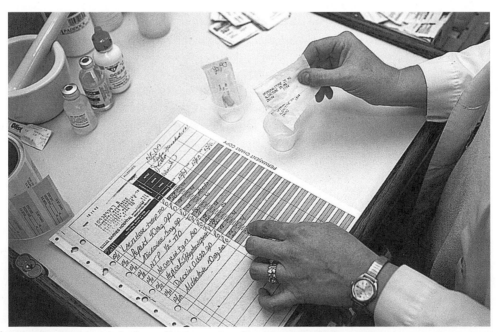

Nurse checking the label of a medication against the patient's medical administration record, to ensure accuracy.

ELECTRONIC HEALTH RECORDS

All the principles with respect to nursing documentation apply whether they are in paper or electronic format. The obligation for documenting is the same regardless of the form of charging. The guidelines and professional standards created by the regulating bodies support the notion that it is acceptable to maintain electronic records. The general requirements for electronic records are that

- they be secure from interference or unauthorized access,
- they can display and print each patient's record separately,
- they have automatic backup and recovery, and
- they maintain an audit trail.

Amendments to federal and provincial legislation were made to allow for computerized records. For example, *Ontario Regulation 965* requires that all orders for treatment shall be in "writing and shall be dated and authenticated by the physician, dentist or midwife giving the order" (Morris, Ferguson, & Dykeman, 1999, p. 89). Computer entries eliminate legibility problems, but the issues associated with the nature and quality of the recording remain.

Electronic health records (EHR) have enabled a highly efficient means of maintaining, storing, and retrieving patient health files. By their nature, EHRs permit easy transmission of patient information for those who have a legitimate purpose in accessing and using the record (Health Law Institute, 2005). Nevertheless, as EHRs contain personal health information of patients, significant concerns regarding privacy, confidentiality, and security are raised. Issues of patient confidentiality are important (as discussed below), and the parameters for maintaining confidentiality do not change with computerization. This issue is illustrated in an unreported Ontario case (Sanchez-Sweatman, 1997) in which a charge nurse was found to have breached confidentiality by using her access card to call up information on her nurse manager, who had been admitted to the hospital the previous day. It was determined that the nurse had inadvertently called up the chart on the screen and was initially dismissed for these actions. Although she was reinstated in this case, the fact that it is possible for many people to access computerized records underscores the need to ensure that systems are put in place that allow only those with the right to access patient records to do so.

▌ PRIVACY AND CONFIDENTIALITY

The right to privacy and the duty of confidentiality are related. However, they may be differentiated in that the duty of confidentiality is owed by a health care provider to a patient while the right to privacy is vested in the patient. The law specifies that "the duty of confidentiality is subject to disclosures required by the law; whereas the patient's constitutional right to privacy, as part of the supreme law of Canada, may affect the validity of laws" (Downie & Caulfield, 1999, p. 151). Statutes of the provinces that include laws addressing the patient's right to confidentiality in health records are usually included in hospitals' and health agencies' specific privacy legislation, although legislation that regulates nursing also contains provisions that reiterate the nurse's professional responsibility to maintain patient confidentiality. To fail in this responsibility is to be subject to allegations of professional misconduct.

The right of privacy is not explicitly protected in Canada, but the Supreme Court of Canada has established that privacy is a constitutionally protected right. Canadian courts have protected the right of privacy through sections 7 and 8 of the *Canadian Charter of Rights and Freedoms (Part 1 of the Constitution Act* [Canada]). This provides that "everyone has the right to life, liberty and security of the person and the right not to be deprived thereof except in accordance with the principles of fundamental justice and to freedom from unreasonable search and seizure." The Supreme Court has upheld the charter's provisions in both civil and criminal cases unless the infringement can be justified under section 1 of the Charter.

The modern health care system, with its rapid advances in technology, has created not only significant benefits to health, but also situations that have never arisen before in health and communications. There has been an erosion of the traditional ethical principles of confidentiality and the patient's right to privacy. Patients are in a vulnerable position. Their autonomy requires that they retain control over their health records, including the ability to access those records and control their disclosure. Federal and provincial governments have attempted to respond to the public's concern by putting in place comprehensive legislation that provides a clear framework governing rights of access and the collection, use, and disclosure of health information.

Today, privacy of personal information is a top priority of governments, as personal information gains more significance in the applications it can have in the public and private sectors. Health information is no exception because health records include such sensitive information as family health history, psychiatric conditions, and financial information. Processes to protect privacy are extremely important in order to protect such personal information from unauthorized access, collection, and disclosure. The difficulty in providing protection for personal information from access, collection, and disclosure must be balanced by the needs of health care providers who require the information to provide treatment to patients.

Currently, individual health records are protected through a patchwork of federal and provincial legislation and policies. The federal government's initiative, the *Personal Information Protection and Electronic Documents Act (PIPEDA),* endeavours to control the collection, use, or disclosure of most forms of personal information. The provisions of *PIPEDA* now well-established in Canadian law impacts interprovincial and international flows of personal information as well as personal health information in any province without supplemental legislation acceptable to the federal government. Manitoba, Alberta, Saskatchewan, and Ontario enacted dedicated health privacy statutes aimed specifically at substantially transforming their practices and policies relating to protection of privacy in health information. The provinces without stand-alone health privacy statutes are captured under *PIPEDA*/provincial private-sector or public-sector laws, depending on the location of the personal health information. The aim of the legislation is to establish minimum standards for the collection, use, disclosure, and safeguarding of the information. Other objectives of the legislation include providing patients with access to their health records; the ability to correct erroneous information, the ability to request an independent review to resolve complaints relating to the handling of health information, and the ability to obtain remedies for contraventions of the legislation. Generally, exceptions to the obligation to maintain include (1) patient consent (implied or express, depending on the application legislation) for disclosure of health information to persons; (2) statutory provisions for reporting certain diseases and child abuse to appropriate health and social services personnel; and (3) court orders, which are often used to obtain health records for the use of plaintiffs or defendants in trials. With regard to privacy, these legislative initiatives are a welcome start to standardizing the health sectors dealing with patients' personal information.

New technology has revolutionized the advancement and adoption of information and telecommunications technologies in the delivery of health care. Applications such as telehealth and the EHR continue to transform health care delivery in the information age by improving the accessibility, quality, and efficiency of health care. With the advancement of nursing practice using new technologies for sharing information and new ways of seeking treatment across jurisdictions, legal issues emerge. Some of the most prevalent issues are licensure, patient identification, privacy, and protection of personal and health information. Policies and legislation are emerging to deal with the legal issues. For example, British Columbia has enacted the *E-Health (Personal Health Information Access and Protection of Privacy) Act*. The legislation provides an EHR for every individual in the province and governs the collection, use, and disclosure of personal health information in government databases. As most jurisdictions continue to build their capacity to use the new information and telecommunication technologies, only the passage of time will demonstrate whether the new legislation achieves the balance required between access and protection for health providers and patients.

UNDERSTANDING THE LEGAL ASPECTS OF NURSING

It is evident that the professional nurse must have some knowledge of the law, legal processes, the judicial system, and patient rights. The increasing complexity of professional practice has been associated with increased risks in nursing procedures, and higher-risk procedures increase the potential for legal action. There have been many changes in the nurse's role over time, and the pace of development has accelerated in recent years. The establishment of the baccalaureate standard for entry to practice in the profession is likely to result in even more change in the direction of augmented responsibility and increased risks for the nurse. There is no substitute for maintaining a high level of competence in nursing practice, excellent communication with patients, and an awareness of the risks involved in performing various procedures.

The Canadian Nurses Protective Society (CNPS) was established by the Canadian Nurses Association in 1988 at the request of the provincial and territorial professional associations in nursing as a result of escalating costs of professional liability insurance. It is a nonprofit organization that offers liability insurance purchased by 10 of the 12 provincial and territorial associations on behalf of their members. It also offers advice about professional liability to nurses 24 hours a day all year round. Nurses may contact the CNPS if they have had personal involvement in or knowledge of any situation in which there are ethical or legal implications of concern by calling a toll-free number: 1-800-267-3390 or by e-mail at info@cnps.ca for nonconfidential matters only. The CNPS offers the opportunity to speak with a nurse-lawyer who will give advice immediately and provide assistance with the steps to be taken in documenting an unusual occurrence, in understanding legal processes that might be applicable, and in referring nurses to experienced legal counsel.

Nurses have an obligation to respect their professional and ethical guidelines that are respecting the law. In order to meet these obligations, nurses require extensive knowledge and skills for competent and ethically based practice. Now as never before, nurses engaged in practice need a fundamental understanding of the law and legal aspects of nursing. This chapter is not meant to be a comprehensive discussion of the issues nor should it be considered legal advice. It is meant to shed light on and raise awareness of some of the legal issues that nurses may face in their practice and encourage further thought and study on the topic.

CRITICAL THINKING QUESTIONS

1. Identify the principles of informed consent to health care treatment.
2. What elements constitute negligence in nursing practice?
3. What is the legal importance of documentation in legal proceedings in nursing practice?

WEB SITES

Canadian Nurses Protective Society: http://www.cnps.ca/
Canadian Nurses Association: http://www.cna-nurses.ca/

REFERENCES

Ares v. Venner, [1970] S.C.R. 608 at 626.
B.H. (Next friend of) v. Alberta (Director of Child Welfare) 2002 ABQB 371, 2002 ABCA 109, [2002] S.C.C.A. No. 196.
C. (J.S.) v. Wren, [1986] 76 A.R. 118 (Alta. C.A.).
Canadian AIDS Society v. Ontario, unreported August 4, 1995 (Ont. Gen. Div.).
Canadian Charter of Rights and Freedoms, Part 1 of the *Constitution Act, 1982,* being Sch. B of the *Canada Act,* 1982 (U.K.), 1982, c.11.
Chancey v. McKinstry, [2000] B.C.J. No. 2008 (S.C.).

Ciarlariello v. Schacter, [1993] 2 S.C.R. 119 at 135.

Crits v. Sylvester [1956] O.R. 132, 1 D.L.R. (2d) 502 (C.A.) affirmed 1956 CarswellOnt 84, [1956] S.C.R. 991, 5 D.L.R. (2d) 601.

Dixon v. Calgary Health Region, [2006] ABQB 235, 398 A.R. 199, 2006 CarswellAlta 378.

Dowey v. Rothwell, [1974] 5 W.W.R. 311, 49 D.L.R. (3d) 82 (Alta. S.C.).

Downie, J., & Caulfield, T. (1999). *Canadian health law and policy.* Toronto: Butterworths Canada.

E-Health (Personal Health Information Access and Protection of Privacy) Act, [SBC 2008] c. 38

Health Care Consent Act, 1996, S.O. 1996, c. 2. Sched. A.

Health Law Institute, University of Alberta. (April 2005). *Electronic Health Records and the Personal Information Protection and Electronic Documents Act.*

Kolesar v. Jeffries (1974), 9 O.R. (2d) 41, 59 D.L.R. (3d) 367 (H.C.).

MacDonald v. York County Hospital, [1972] 3 O.R. 469, 28 D.L.R. (3d), [1976] 2 S.C.R. 825.

Meyer v. Gordon [1981] B.C.J. NO. 524 (S.C.)(QL).

Morris, J. J., Ferguson, M., & Dykeman, M. (1999). *Canadian nurses and the law.* Toronto: Butterworths Canada.

Philpott, M. (1985). *Legal liability and the nursing process.* Toronto: W.B. Saunders.

Re T, [1992] All. E.R. 649 (C.A.).

Personal Information Protection and Electronic Documents Act (Canada), S.C. 2000, c. 5.

Ross, M. W. (1973). The nurse as an employee. In S. R. Good, & J. C. Kerr (Eds.), *Contemporary issues in Canadian law for nurses* (pp. 95–106). Toronto: Holt, Rinehart & Winston.

Sanchez-Sweatman, L. (1997, August). Nurses, computers and confidentiality. *The Canadian Nurse,* 93(7), 47-48.

Sklar, Ronald (2007). *Starson v. Swayze*: The Supreme Court speaks out (not all that clearly) on the question of "capacity." *Canadian Journal of Psychiatry,* 52(6), 390–396.

Sneiderman, B., Irvine, J. C., & Osborne, P. (2003). *Canadian medical law. An introduction for physicians, nurses and other health care professionals* (3rd ed.). Scarborough, ON: Carswell.

Straghan (Guardian ad litem of) v. Reynolds (2001), [2001] B.C.J. No 1110.

Wowk v. Edmonton (Health Board) (1994), 19 Alta L.R. (3d) 232.

Ethical Issues and Dilemmas in Nursing Practice

Marilynn J. Wood

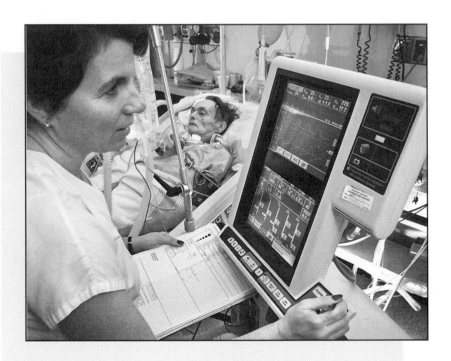

◾ LEARNING OBJECTIVES

- To understand the principles and concepts of ethics.
- To understand the rights of individuals relating to the principle of autonomy.
- To appreciate "do not resuscitate" orders as a case of advance directives.
- To understand advance directives as they pertain to health care ethics.
- To appreciate the unique case of the mentally ill.
- To interpret ethical dilemmas related to reproduction.
- To interpret issues related to allocation of health care resources.
- To understand the importance of codes of ethics in professional practice.

Closely related to the issues pertaining to legal aspects of nursing practice are issues and dilemmas concerning nursing ethics. Nurses have always been faced with ethical dilemmas and have had to make ethical decisions; however, the dilemmas are more complex today. Factors contributing to this complexity are the rapidly expanding body of knowledge about health and illness, and the development of new technologies to save or prolong human life. At the same time, changes in societal values have increased recognition of individual rights, freedoms, and responsibility for protecting those rights. Another influential factor is the availability of information—for example, the wealth of data available on the Internet, resulting in a better informed public that is more questioning and expects to be more involved in decisions about their own lives and health. In the past, Canadians have become familiar with cases such as those of Sue Rodriguez and Tracy Latimer, which have made "assisted suicide" and "euthanasia" household words. Because of the eradication of many diseases, increasing control over other diseases, and improved living standards, people are also living longer, a situation that creates new ethical questions regarding making decisions about prolonging life. The finite amount of available resources is another factor that raises questions about priorities in the health care system; when there are insufficient resources to meet all needs, complex decisions must be made about who will receive care and how funds will be spent.

Because of these interacting factors, nurses face many dilemmas. Who decides what is right for the individual or family involved? Is there always a right answer? Yeo, Moorhouse, and Dalziel (1996) define bioethics as "reasoned enquiry about the ethical dimension of interventions in the lives of human beings directed to or bearing on their good health, individually or collectively" (p. 4). Health care is one of the interventions in the lives of human beings. Nursing ethics is part of this broader picture and deals with how nurses ought to behave in given circumstances.

◾ PRINCIPLES AND CONCEPTS OF ETHICS

The field of ethics is a branch of the discipline of philosophy involving the study of social morality and includes reflection on society's norms and practices (Beauchamp & Walters, 2003). Morality is the concept of whether certain actions ought or ought not to be taken because of the effect they could have on other people. Children learn morality as they grow up in a family and community. The expectations of others as to appropriate behaviour are made clear in a series of standards. These standards deal with "doing good, avoiding harm, respecting others, keeping promises, and acting fairly" (Beauchamp & Walters, 2003, p. 1). The field of bioethics has arisen because of the dilemmas presented by advances in biology and medicine. Nursing ethics arise specifically from the need to examine the activities in the field of nursing and how they affect basic human rights of people in the care of nurses. Although ethical theory does not provide a formula for deciding what is right and proper behaviour, it does provide a context for examining a sub-discipline such as bioethics or nursing ethics. There is considerable discussion in the nursing literature about whether nursing ethics is a subset of bioethics or is a separate discipline (Norvedt, 1998; Scott, 2000; Beckstead & Beckstead, 2006; Holm, 2006). It is clear that the issues dealt with by nurses are unique to nursing and cannot be subsumed under another discipline. However, basic ethical theory can be applied to nursing ethics as well as to bioethics.

Knowledge of several types of ethical theory is needed for the study of bioethics because the literature on bioethics draws from methods and conclusions grounded in these theories. Without a theoretical base, discussion of ethical issues may be merely sharing of opinions. Moral philosophy is the area of philosophy concerned with theories of ethics, with how we ought to live our lives. Normative ethics is the approach from moral philosophy that encompasses nursing ethics. Normative ethics is concerned with providing a moral framework that can be used to work out what kinds of action are good and bad, right and wrong. There are three main traditions in normative ethics: virtue ethics, deontology, and consequentialism.

Virtue ethics stems from the work of Aristotle and focuses on the character of the person who is taking the action. Virtues are character traits that make one a good person who will take good actions. After many years of being ignored, virtue ethics is making a comeback in recent years. It has some advantages over the rule-based theories of ethics that have been more prominent. The main strength of virtue theory is that it gives a central role to character. Other ethical theories neglect this aspect of morality. Kantian ethics, for example, hold that it is important to act out of duty rather than inclination, that whether or not you want to do the right thing is irrelevant; all that matters is whether or not you do it.

The second tradition of normative ethics is deontology, which holds the belief that certain acts are intrinsically right or wrong. When we know this, we can set forth rules to follow to ensure ethical actions. Immanuel Kant is the foremost deontology theorist, and the ethical principles that have guided most health professions are based on his work.

Consequentialism is the theory that the moral status of an act is determined by its consequences. Consequentialism thus rejects both the virtue ethicist's view that the moral status of an act is determined by the moral character of the agent performing it, and the deontologist's view that the moral status of an act is determined by the type of act that it is. According to consequentialism, each of these factors is morally irrelevant. All that matters is what consequences an act leads to.

Although ethical theory does not provide a formula for making decisions as to whether certain behaviours are morally acceptable, the tradition of deontology provides principles that help us to take consistent positions on some issues. Three of these principles are particularly useful in nursing ethics. They are the principles of *respect for autonomy, beneficence,* and *justice.*

RESPECT FOR AUTONOMY

Respect for autonomy comes from the tradition of the importance of individual freedom and choice. Respect for autonomy is seen as intrinsically right. Being autonomous implies the freedom to decide and act. In bioethics, many issues stem from failure to respect autonomy or failure to recognize individuals' rights to hold their own views on issues and to make decisions based on their own perspectives. Issues of autonomy can range from whether a person has the right to refuse treatment to whether a person can decide to end his or her life. Codes of ethics for physicians and nurses all specifically address the principle of respect for autonomy. Problems arise when we try to interpret this principle when it conflicts with other principles, such as justice and beneficence. When can this principle be overridden? An example is the refusal of blood transfusions for religious reasons when it can be determined that the person may die without the treatment.

 REFLECTIVE THINKING

Consider a situation in which health care personnel determine that a child requires a blood transfusion. The parents of the child refuse this treatment on religious grounds. The hospital administration appeals to the judicial system to assume responsibility for the child and to authorize the treatment that may save the child's life. Identify the ethical principles that apply in this instance.

BENEFICENCE

Beneficence refers to the obligation to cause no harm to another person. In health care, it refers to the obligation of the health care providers to protect patients from harm and to promote their welfare. This principle is the foundation of nursing and medical ethics. Acts of beneficence are required by the fiduciary relationship between nurse and patient. Nurses know that the risks of harm must be weighed against the possible benefits for patients and that as nurses they have a duty to benefit others.

JUSTICE

Justice implies treatment that is fair, due, or owed. The principle of justice is based on the idea that everyone has certain rights. When these rights are met, justice has been served. The term "distributed justice" refers to a fair, equitable, and appropriate distribution in society as determined by norms of distribution. Usually, distributive justice applies to such matters as political rights and economic goods, but it can also apply to health care services. The *Canada Health Act* requires equal access to health care for all Canadians, which means that unequal access is an injustice.

The formal principle of justice has been interpreted in many ways for different situations and to accommodate a variety of philosophical perspectives. The following is a list of some of these interpretations:

- To each person an equal share
- To each person according to individual need
- To each person according to acquisition in a free market
- To each person according to individual effort
- To each person according to societal contribution
- To each person according to merit

Most societies use more than one of these principles of justice with the idea that different situations require different approaches (Beauchamp & Walters, 2003).

When conflicts arise among ethical principles, theorists have attempted to devise ways of determining which principle should prevail. Much of the discussion centres on the emergence of the idea that there are certain universal human rights. Historically, this notion arose out of the need to curtail the sovereign power of royalty, but rights have now become powerful principles to be considered in any relationship. There are both moral and legal rights, but moral rights are the subject of ethics, whereas legal rights belong to the judiciary.

Of most importance in health care are rights that stem from autonomy. Everyone agrees that liberty is a basic right for all people, but not complete liberty. Various moral principles have been designed to limit liberty in acceptable ways. The most common of these are the following:

- Harm: Liberty can be restricted to prevent harm to others.
- Paternalism: Liberty can be restricted to prevent harm to self.
- Legal moralism: Liberty can be restricted to prevent immoral behaviour.
- Offence: Liberty can be restricted to prevent offence to others.

These principles represent an attempt to deal with conflict over individual and societal rights to autonomy, and to balance liberty and other values. Of these four principles, the harm principle is generally accepted, but the other three generate much controversy. In health care the principle of paternalism is a major issue. Is there ever a situation that justifies limiting persons' autonomy "for their own good"? There are avid proponents of both sides of this issue.

The question of justice presents an ethical dilemma frequently described in the literature today because of inadequate staffing due to shortages in the nursing workforce, causing nurses to make difficult decisions about apportioning care when all needs cannot be met. A thorough knowledge of basic ethical concepts is necessary for nurses to be able to address the increasingly complex issues encountered daily in practice settings.

Although there is a tendency to consider only the dilemmas faced in acute-care settings, the issues are different but equally complex for practitioners in long-term care and home and community settings owing to increased longevity, early discharge from hospitals, and the use of technologies in the home that were previously limited to acute-care settings. Robillard et al. (1989) carried out one of the very few studies on the ethical issues in primary care, even though most health care is provided in primary care settings. Their study revealed that the issues are most frequently pragmatic, not dramatic, and are concerned with "patient self-determination, adequacy of care and professional responsibility, and distribution of resources" (p. 9). Thus, nurses practising in all types of health care settings need a knowledge base in ethical concepts and principles, as well as support and expert resources to assist them in ensuring that basic human rights are recognized and respected.

BASIC HUMAN RIGHTS RELATING TO THE PRINCIPLE OF AUTONOMY

Autonomy in health care means the right of the patient to accept or refuse treatment. This right is part of every professional code of ethics. However, when the consequence of respecting this right is the death of the patient, other values come into play for health care providers; in particular, respect for life itself. It is relatively easy for nurses to respect patients' decisions about treatment when these decisions agree with what the nurse believes to be the right decision.

The case of Nancy B. brought the issue of self-determination into prominent view in Canada (*Nancy B. v. Hôtel Dieu de Québec* [1992]). Nancy B. was a young woman with Guillain-Barré syndrome who was paralyzed and living on a respirator. She requested to be disconnected from the respirator. Her request created a moral dilemma for most of the nurses and physicians involved in her care. This case became a legal battle between lawyers for Nancy B. and the Hôtel-Dieu hospital in Quebec City. The major issue was whether this was a question of Nancy B.'s right to refuse treatment or a question of assisted suicide or homicide, both of which are illegal. The Superior Court of Quebec determined the issue to be an ethical one of the right to refuse treatment. This case clarified the right of Canadians to refuse treatment, even when that treatment is sustaining life.

Self-determination is not limited to life and death matters, but also involves making decisions about lifestyle. For example, individuals make decisions to continue with lifestyles and behaviour patterns that are known to be detrimental to their health and well-being, such as smoking, overeating, excessive drinking, refusing to wear seat belts, and engaging in unprotected sexual relations with people likely to be carriers of sexually transmitted infections. Although efforts to educate the public about the hazards of such habits are meeting with some success, many individuals still choose to do things that are harmful to their health. Politicians sometimes suggest that special charges for health care be levied on individuals whose medical conditions have been self-induced through poor health practices. This is an issue that will be debated many times in the future, as there is no easy solution.

INFORMED CONSENT

Because health care providers possess much knowledge about health and disease, the functioning of the human body, and various treatments for illnesses, knowledge that is not possessed by most members of the public, some difficult ethical issues are bound to arise. Lack of knowledge affects the ability of patients to make good decisions regarding their treatment, yet complete knowledge of all the issues may be impossible for the average patient to achieve, no matter how much information the nurse or physician imparts. What are the ethics governing this imbalance of knowledge?

In the past, health care providers were mainly concerned with doing good for the benefit of the patient, a situation fraught with beneficence and paternalism. Truth telling did not play a large role in professional practice. In fact, professionals were likely to decide that the truth would be harmful to the patient, and thus they would conceal facts they believed likely to cause distress. This attitude has changed, however, and in the present day, it is believed that patients have a right to know the truth. It is quite clear that patients need appropriate information to exercise their autonomy. Even though there may be a large knowledge gap between patients and health providers, the truth can be told in a way that is helpful to the patient. That means a communication in which the patient will understand what the health provider knows and believes to be true about the situation.

Occasionally, there may be differences of opinion between nurses and physicians about the meaning of being informed and whose responsibility it is to inform the individual or family. A confrontation may occur if information is withheld by a physician who believes this is in the best interest of the patient, and the nurse, who believes that the patient should be informed, is asked directly for such information.

The right to be informed has increased the need for obtaining informed consent before medical interventions are taken and before patients are asked to participate in research. Until the 1970s, there was no expectation or requirement for obtaining informed consent for participation in research, and people were sometimes exploited. There are many examples in the literature of unethical practices in research prior to that time. For example, in an experiment at the Allen Memorial Institute in Montreal in the late 1940s, patients were given mind-altering drugs, such as lysergic acid diethylamide (LSD), which had far-reaching effects on their mental health. These patients sought recompense in the mid-1980s.

THE RIGHT TO MAKE CHOICES IN RELATION TO DEATH

Dying and death give rise to many ethical issues and dilemmas. These issues revolve around one or more of the following events: (1) possible interventions by health care providers, such as resuscitation and passive euthanasia; (2) possible interventions by the family, health providers, or significant others, such as helping a terminally ill person to hasten death and end suffering; and (3) possible interventions by the afflicted person, such as suicide and claiming "a right to die."

The word "euthanasia" is derived from Greek and means good or pleasant death. Is death ever preferable to life? That question is difficult to answer, as there is always a context to be considered. Euthanasia is the putting to death, by painless method, of a terminally ill or severely debilitated person through the omission (intentionally withholding a lifesaving medical procedure or passive euthanasia) or the commission of an act (active euthanasia) (Duhaime, 2009). Passive euthanasia, or "letting someone die," may be performed by not initiating treatment or by stopping treatment, with or without the consent of the individual. These measures are still morally controversial and in fact may be difficult to distinguish from active euthanasia. For instance, disconnecting a respirator may be either active or passive euthanasia, depending on exactly what is meant by these terms. "Active euthanasia" generally means taking steps to bring about an individual's death with or without consent. Many people believe that intention makes a moral difference. For these people, passive euthanasia may be defined as action (or omission) that is intended for a purpose other than ending the life of the individual. Relieving unbearable pain, for instance, may be the primary intention. In this case, active euthanasia would involve taking an action that would hasten the person's death. This definition covers cases of assisted suicide as well, and in Canada, this action is illegal. Two sections of Canada's *Criminal Code (1985)* are relevant to this issue:

14. No person is entitled to consent to have death inflicted on him, and such consent does not affect the criminal responsibility of any person by whom death may be inflicted on the person by whom consent is given.

241. Everyone who counsels a person to commit suicide or aids or abets a person to commit suicide, whether suicide ensues or not, is guilty of an indictable offence and liable to imprisonment for a term not exceeding fourteen years.

The case of Sue Rodriguez (*Sue Rodriguez v. British Columbia* [1993]) is an example of the complexity of these issues. Rodriguez had been diagnosed with amyotrophic lateral sclerosis (ALS, or Lou Gehrig's disease). She asked to be assisted to die at such time as her condition might become unbearable to her. The Supreme Court of British Columbia dismissed her case, and the B.C. Court of Appeal and the Supreme Court of Canada concurred with this decision in 1993. In 1994, she died with the assistance of an anonymous physician, who administered a lethal injection. The physician's action was clearly illegal, as section 241b of the *Criminal Code (1985)* states that assisting someone to die is prohibited, as is intentional killing. Sue Rodriguez received much media and public support because she was seen as a mentally competent adult who had requested help to end her life. For many, this factor makes a significant difference.

The case of Tracy Latimer (*R. v. Latimer* [2001]), on the other hand, centres on a 12-year-old girl with cerebral palsy. Tracy was quadriplegic and unable to speak. How much Tracy understood about her own situation was unknown. She was in severe pain from muscle spasms and required several surgeries to alleviate the pain. She was being cared for by her family at home, and how long the family could continue this care was uncertain. Tracy's father, with the goal of ending her pain and suffering, arranged her death using carbon monoxide from an automobile. Tracy herself was unable to express any wishes in the matter.

The Rodriguez case raised questions about the limits on respecting an individual's autonomy. The Latimer case, by contrast, is unrelated to autonomy, since Tracy was incapable of requesting anything at all (Yeo, Moorhouse, & Dalziel, 1996). These cases raise many questions to which there are no easy answers. How does the concept of protecting human rights fit into euthanasia? Does a person ever have the right to die? Can one refuse lifesaving treatment? Is the lack of clear-cut policies and guidelines to help nurses and physicians in addressing such complex questions a reflection of there being no right or wrong answer? These are just a few of the difficult questions that arise from such ethical dilemmas.

DO NOT RESUSCITATE ORDERS

In recent years much has been written about the ethical dilemmas relating to "do not resuscitate (DNR) orders" (Blacksher & Christopher, 2002; Fins et al., 1999; Hamel, Guse, Hawranik, & Bond, 2002). If there are no written DNR orders and a patient arrests, is the nurse expected to "code" the patient? Who is, or should be, involved in making such a decision? Are there, or should there be, differences in DNR policy in community settings or long-term care institutions versus acute-care settings?

The development of guidelines for resuscitation has been encouraged through a joint effort of the Canadian Medical Association (CMA), the Canadian Nurses Association (CNA), the Canadian Hospital Association (CHA), and the Canadian Bar Association (CBA), which resulted in a "Joint Statement on Terminal Illness," published in *The Canadian Nurse* (CNA, CMA, & CHA, 1984). These guidelines were replaced by a new joint statement in 1994, which was still in effect in 2009. It is intended to be used in formulating institutional policy and procedure. Implementation of these guidelines would result in policy that assists with decisions regarding which situations, and which persons, require cardiopulmonary resuscitation (CPR). It encourages staff to assess the potential benefit from CPR for patients in their institution, so that persons who have rejected CPR, as well as those who would not benefit from it, are not given this treatment if a cardiac arrest occurs.

Although it is the physician's responsibility to write a DNR order and also convey the meaning of it to the nursing staff, there should be opportunity for nursing input into the development of such guidelines. Nurses are the ones who are most likely to see significant changes in a patient's condition that might require reconsideration of a DNR order. It should be noted that the Joint Statement makes it clear that a decision not to carry out CPR is not the same as withholding treatment and should not result in the withholding or withdrawing of any other treatment that might benefit or provide comfort to the patient (CNA, 1995).

The guidelines stress the importance of discussing the DNR order with the patient, guardian, and family, and also recording this in the patient's record; however, the literature raises questions about the extent to which patients are involved in such decisions.

Most DNR policies in hospitals pertain to terminally ill patients only. Godkin (1992) suggests that such policies be made known so that every individual understands that current policy requires CPR to be performed on all patients unless a DNR order is recorded on the chart. This would require that the issue be addressed, an undertaking that could reduce the dilemmas faced by families and staff regarding CPR, reduce costs of administering CPR that was not desired by the patient, and prevent the situation in which the patient is unable to participate in the decision by the time discussion is initiated.

Although autonomous decision making by the patient is highly valued by both nurses and physicians, research shows that frequently the patient is not involved in the decision when participation is possible. In a study of end-of-life care in hospital settings, researchers found that patients on a medical service were more likely to have DNR orders than those on a surgical service, and these were made earlier in the hospital stay for medicine than for surgery. In addition, although 22% of patients in the study had some form of advance directive on their chart, this had no impact on the frequency or timing of DNR orders (Morrell, Brown, Qi, Drabiak, & Helft, 2008). Since end-of-life decision making is taking place in intensive care units with more frequency, Westphal and McKee (2009) surveyed nurses and physicians in critical care units regarding their beliefs and practices about end-of-life care in the ICU. They found that nurses were more likely to ask if there was a living will and to read it. Only 53% of physicians read living wills; however, 90% of physicians consider the wishes in the living will when making recommendations to the family. Physicians are more likely to discuss DNR orders in the case where prognosis is extremely poor. The factors most likely to influence writing DNR orders are family dynamics and medical/legal concerns.

In the 1990s, Wilson (1993) found that 73% of 135 accredited health care facilities in Alberta had a written DNR policy. Most had been developed to optimize decision making and involve the patient in the process; however, these purposes had not been achieved in general. In-depth surveys of four of the facilities indicated that DNR policies were not commonly followed and that in almost one-third of all instances they were not implemented at all. Problems generally arose from late decision making that excluded the patient from end-of-life decisions. Hence, DNR policies seemed to have limited effect on practice.

ADVANCE DIRECTIVES

Advance directives are documentation of the preferences a person has for life-support procedures in the event that he or she becomes unable to communicate. Advance directives may take the form of an *instruction directive* or *living will*, which specifies what life-sustaining treatments the person would want instituted in a given situation, or a *proxy directive* or *power of attorney*, which designates who is to make health care decisions should the individual become unable. The legal status of these documents varies among provinces and territories, and therefore nurses must be familiar with the law in their own area.

The Joint Statement on Advance Directives by the Canadian Nurses Association, the Canadian Medical Association, and the Canadian Healthcare Association asserts as a principle the notion that all health care personnel must support the right of an individual patient to self-determination (CNA, 1994). It is intended to serve as a guide for the development of policies by health care institutions in areas that will support self-determination by the patient. It applies to all areas of care and treatment, including those that sustain life.

Advance directives can be portable and thus go with the patient from one facility to another, or from community to hospital. However, a DNR order must be written by a physician in each setting. Is this how things should be? It would be possible for an elderly person to receive CPR in a hospital emergency room even though an advance directive was in place requesting no CPR, if the ER physician has not yet written the order. This example highlights the challenges of the world we live in, where technologies that artificially prolong life are readily available. These technologies raise complex legal, ethical, and philosophical questions about the quality and dignity of life and individuals' rights to make their own decisions about health care. Decisions about health care have increasingly become moral decisions. Advance directives are necessary because medicine has the capacity to maintain survival in states that many health care providers find unacceptable (Payne & Thornlow, 2008).

A DNR order is the most specific case of an advance directive and is the most important because of the potential consequences that may be irreversible. Payne and Thornlow (2008) recommend careful guidelines be developed by organizations, including proper education of patient care staff. The minimum requirements for these guidelines would include the requirement for a physician's order, entered into the medical record and signed. A rationale, entered into the progress notes, must be consistent with accepted medical standards. Verbal DNR orders are not acceptable. Ideally, these directives are decided collaboratively by the physician, patient, and responsible family member and will address the following four kinds of treatments:

- CPR
- Level of medical interventions
- Treatment with antibiotics
- Administration of fluids and nutrition

The process of discussion and decision making regarding advance directives ensures that the individual's wishes are followed, provides guidance to health care providers regarding the individual's wishes in such circumstances, and also helps family members to make complex decisions (Flarey, 1991). When there are no advance directives, nurses face difficult situations when they find a patient in distress. One nurse described this dilemma as follows:

At that immediate time, when I was in the room and seeing him and not knowing this patient from anybody—ethically there was a part of me … that said to go ahead and run the code.

Because I didn't know this gentleman, … he could have been the most active 102-year-old gentleman I have ever met. But I didn't know him. But there was another part of me that said, 102 years old? My grandmother died at 102. I would have killed somebody who did that to my grandmother. (Varcoe et al., 2004, p. 320)

An advance directive in this case would have given the nurse some guidance in her decision.

THE UNIQUE CASE OF THE MENTALLY ILL

Many complex ethical questions derive from efforts to effect a change in deviant behaviour. In the case of the mentally ill, there may be a need to protect the public from violent or uncontrolled behaviour. This effort often affects the autonomy of the deviant individual. Bandman and Bandman (1978) stated the following:

Once a set of persons occupies a place within the circle of life, the problem of the right to live as persons arises. The limits to this right are found in the right a person has to be free to live well, without unjustified interferences of his or her freedom. Conversely, being free—and one can only be free if unmolested and free from unjustified harm, injury or threat of violence—is the presence of rules and norms for changing undesirable behavior. To induce changed behavior, reward and punishment are commonly used. (p. 4)

Although few people would argue about the need to control violence against others, what constitutes deviant behaviour is worthy of discussion. What establishes norms of standard behaviour? What authorizes people to try to change behaviour that does not meet these norms and under what conditions? Specific groups in society, such as prisoners, children, older persons, and the mentally ill, are particularly vulnerable to having their rights disregarded when professionals use behaviour modification methods.

Another societal concern about allowing the mentally ill to refuse treatment is that, if untreated, their condition will become chronic and they will become an economic burden on society. Peplau (1978) believed that releasing these patients into the community, which has been done in Canada and the United States for many years, is not as much a matter of their being a danger to society as their being a burden on others. In addition, they are in danger of being exploited by others ready to take advantage of the already disadvantaged. These words of Peplau continue to ring true well into the twenty-first century, as mentally ill people are frequently found living on the streets. Individuals who are treated in in-patient settings are likely to return to the streets after discharge unless stable housing is organized for them (Killaspy, Ritchie, Greer, & Robertson, 2004). Even with stable housing, mentally ill individuals encounter problems integrating into society. Drury (2003) describes a culturally based pattern of mutual avoidance between homeless mentally ill patients and caregivers that severely limits delivery of services to this population.

ETHICAL DILEMMAS RELATED TO REPRODUCTION

One of the major ethical issues pertaining to reproduction is abortion. Abortion continues to be a hot issue with strong arguments both for and against. Anti-abortionists claim that the personhood of the fetus is being denied, and that abortion is akin to murder. Pro-abortionists maintain that the woman's right to self-determination cannot be denied. They emphasize the burden imposed on society by an unwanted pregnancy and the possible outcomes for the welfare of the child in the future. Between the two extremes are those who support abortions in specific circumstances such as rape and incest. In the popular media, these two positions are known as pro-life and pro-choice.

The Supreme Court of Canada's decision, made in 1988, endorses women's rights to self-determination in relation to abortion. This has been challenged many times, but the challenges have not been supported. For example, Bill C-43, passed in 1990 by the House of Commons, would permit abortion only if a continued pregnancy would jeopardize the woman's physical or mental health, as diagnosed by one physician only. Physicians adamantly opposed this change because of the possibility of criminal charges against them and because they would be required to provide pre-abortion and post-abortion counselling. Bill C-43 was struck down, so the Supreme Court's decision still prevails. However, despite the legal acceptance of abortion, it remains an ethically contentious subject and one that creates extreme reactions. In many cases, health providers working in situations where abortions are performed have been in extreme danger from protesters.

The question of abortion may present problems for the individual nurse who is expected to participate in abortions within a health care agency. It is important that the nurse know the agency's policies about such participation before accepting a position. Health care agencies must have clearly defined policies that can be communicated to potential employees and referred to when situations arise that present an ethical dilemma to staff members. The nurse is responsible, legally and morally, for ensuring that patients' needs are met and that patients are not neglected because of differing values (Dickens, 2003; Jones & Chaloner, 2007).

Advancing technology has introduced other ethical issues relating to reproduction, with the introduction of cloning, stem cell research, and infertility treatment. These are not nursing issues per se, because they are basically medical procedures, but nurses are responsible for providing supportive care to patients who have chosen to undergo treatment for infertility or stem cell transplant as a treatment for cancer.

The rights to reproduce and have a family are considered basic human rights, and these apply to infertile couples as well as those who are able to reproduce. Recent medical advances have made possible many new reproductive possibilities in the realm of assisted reproduction. Although the basic right to reproduce is widely recognized, does this imply unlimited access to available technology for women who wish to have a child? Some say yes, because they believe that the right to form a family is a concept woven into the fabric of society. The issue, however, is to whom such technology should be provided and whether it should be publicly funded. This issue continues to be debated, and no solution is currently in place (Chan, 2006).

In recent times, headlines have reported women in their 60s who have carried pregnancies through in vitro fertilization. In these cases, the issue has been the age of the mother, and whether it is ethical to allow women to bear children when they may not live to see them grow up. Although these issues generate much public interest, there is not yet any public policy in Canada to limit the use of these treatments.

ALLOCATION OF HEALTH CARE RESOURCES

Ethical issues pertaining to allocation of health care resources may be encountered at several levels. At the government level, public policies are established that determine what type of health care can be provided. Nurses and other health care providers have a responsibility to exercise their prerogatives and communicate with legislators to influence these policies. For example, prior to a government's decision to require seat belt use by law, a considerable portion of the health care dollar was spent on people involved in automobile accidents.

The drastic budget cuts and changes to the health care system made by provinces during the 1990s created many ethical dilemmas for nurses. These issues have not been resolved and have carried over into the twenty-first century. Nurses are required to maintain patient safety in spite of layoffs, "bumping," and the delegation of nursing duties to lesser or unprepared health workers. Nurses find themselves working in unsafe environments with insufficient staff and inadequate staffing mixes, making safe patient care difficult. In some provinces, additional cuts to health care are once again occurring in response to the perceived recession. These will again cause migration of newly graduated nurses to other jurisdictions as jobs again become scarce and will create difficult situations for the nurses who are left to provide care with inadequate resources.

Policies that influence the use of health care resources are also established at the institutional level. Too often nurses have little influence on such policies, and they need to take action to influence decision making and priority setting. Decisions to develop programs are often made without adequate consideration of the implications for nursing practice; medical programs, such as heart transplantation and hip replacements, have enormous impact on the need for nursing care and can affect nurses' ability to respond to the demands placed on them. At the unit level, nurses have to delineate problems that result from new programs and provide data that will facilitate a reasoned decision, although values and emotions often enter into these decisions. Fortunately, nurses have become more vocal in expressing their concerns and in providing facts that can influence decision making, rather than merely responding to the decisions made by physicians and hospital administrators.

Is it ethically and morally right to support activities that may jeopardize the patient or result in unequal or unfair distribution of resources among different programs within a health care institution? Who decides the priorities in allocating resources, and what facts are considered?

With the increasing proportion of older people in Canada and other developed countries, the question of age may influence decisions. For example, a 99-year-old man had surgery for removal of an esophageal pouch that was making adequate nutrition impossible. He had been advised 17 years earlier not to have surgery because of his age, but the predictors of his life expectancy were inaccurate. Although he survived the surgery, it might have been easier at age 82. Many disadvantaged groups, such as the physically handicapped, the cognitively impaired, the poor, and ethnic minorities, are also exploited by such decisions and their rights are neglected.

Other factors that influence allocation of resources in health care legislation include consumer unrest and the patients' rights movement. Although nurses, individually and collectively, have become more involved in influencing public policy through lobbying and working effectively with consumers and care providers, their involvement needs to be increased. In addition to responding to particular issues, the professional organizations are working diligently to influence public policy about the allocation of health care resources.

Principles of just health care allocation have been offered by Chan (2006). It is understood that health care rationing or limiting the availability of potentially beneficial treatments is a necessity, both practical and moral. These principles can be very useful to policy makers who are responsible for the allocation of resources and who are subject to much pressure from special interest groups.

The first principle of resource allocation is that a basic level of health care must be provided for everyone. This requirement does not mean that everyone must have access to all potentially beneficial treatments or all the treatments that individuals request. Rather, it means if safe, ethical, and effective treatments are available, a caring society should provide them through the health care system.

The second principle is that treatment that is expected to be futile should not be provided. This principle ensures that limited resources are not wasted on nonbeneficial treatments. If, therefore, the effectiveness of a particular treatment cannot be proven, an individual cannot claim it as a right.

The third and last principle of just allocation is that allocation criteria for potentially beneficial treatments should be established in a public and democratic process. In this category, society must make decisions about what should be available for whom. This may result in a priority listing for costly procedures when there are limited resources available. In this case, treatments that provide significant benefits take priority over treatments that provide only marginal benefit; treatments that can benefit many take priority over treatments than can benefit only a few; and treatments that are less expensive take priority over treatments that are more expensive.

CODES OF ETHICS

A code of ethics is one of the characteristics of a profession. It is defined by the profession through the professional association and serves to inform members of that profession and society about the profession's expectations in ethical matters. For many years, physicians, upon graduating from medical school, have taken the Hippocratic Oath, which was derived from the time of Hippocrates. Although it provides some ethical direction, it also commits the physician to saving and prolonging life at any cost, which is one of the factors leading to difficulties between physicians and nurses today. For example, there is often a difference of opinion between these two professions about prolonging life. This difference has led to stressful interprofessional relationships because of the question of who should make the decision. Many physicians believe it is solely their responsibility, whereas many nurses believe the individual or family should be involved in making a decision that affects their lives.

Although some nurses have taken the Florence Nightingale pledge (which did not originate with Florence Nightingale but with Harper Hospital School of Nursing in Detroit), this pledge does not provide ethical direction for the issues and dilemmas encountered in practice. In 1955, the Canadian Nurses Association (CNA) adopted the code of ethics developed in 1953 by the International Council of Nurses (ICN) and replaced in 1973 by *The ICN Code for Nurses—Ethical Concepts Applied to Nursing*, which guided members in ethical decision making until the 1970s. At its 1978 annual meeting, the CNA made the development of a new national code a priority. A new code was approved in 1980, but revisions were deemed necessary soon after. An ad hoc committee appointed to make the revisions sought input from nurses across Canada and, after lengthy deliberations, published the *Code of Ethics for Nursing* in 1985 (CNA, 1985). Since that time, the code has been reviewed on an ongoing basis, with revisions published in 1991, 1997, 2002, and 2008. It is available on the CNA Web site, and feedback from nurses in practice is continuously sought. The latest version (2008, p. 1) has the following preamble:

> *The Canadian Nurses Association's* Code of Ethics for Registered Nurses *is a statement of the ethical values of nurses and of nurses' commitments to persons with health care needs and persons receiving care. It is intended for nurses in all contexts and domains of nursing practice and at all levels of decision-making. It is developed by nurses for nurses and can assist nurses in practising ethically and working through ethical challenges that arise in their practice with individuals, families, communities and public health systems.*
>
> *The societal context in which nurses work is constantly changing and can be a significant influence on their practice. The quality of the work environment in which nurses practise is also fundamental to their ability to practice ethically. The code of ethics is revised periodically … to ensure that it is attuned to the needs of nurses by reflecting changes in social values and conditions that affect the public, nurses and other health care providers, and the health care system. Periodic revisions also promote lively dialogue and create greater awareness of and engagement with ethical issues among nurses in Canada.*

The *Code of Ethics* sets out the specific values and ethical behaviour expected of registered nurses in Canada. It not only educates nurses about their ethical responsibilities, but also informs other health care providers and members of the public about the moral commitments expected of nurses. Codes of ethics not only provide guidance for individual nurses as to appropriate behaviour in practice, but also provide guidelines for health care institutions to assess policy for its appropriateness to professional nursing practice. In addition, professional organizations use the *Code of Ethics* extensively when reviewing cases in which nurses have been charged with malpractice.

The code is organized into two parts. The first part describes the core responsibilities central to ethical nursing practice. It is organized around seven values, or broad ideals. Each value is accompanied by responsibility statements that are intended to clarify its application in practice. These values are the following:

- Providing safe, compassionate, competent, and ethical care
- Promoting health and well-being
- Promoting and respecting informed decision making
- Preserving dignity
- Maintaining privacy and confidentiality
- Promoting justice
- Being accountable

The second part of the code outlines endeavours that nurses may undertake to address social inequities as part of ethical practice.

The values that make up the Canadian code stem from the heart of the professional nurse–patient relationship and illustrate what nurses believe to be important in that relationship. The Canadian *Code of Ethics* is considered by many to be the gold standard for nursing worldwide.

A tentative code of ethics for nurses in the United States, adopted by the American Nurses Association (ANA) in 1926, was revised a number of times over the years. The ANA code of ethics for professional nurses, adopted in 1950, was revised in 1960 to become the *Code for Professional Nurses*. After additional revision in 1976, the ANA adopted the *Code for Nurses with Interpretive Statements* (ANA, 1976; Flanagan, 1976). The latest revision to the ANA code was published in 2001, with interpretive statements.

Earlier codes of ethics, prescriptive in nature, were essentially rules to govern the personal and professional conduct of members of a profession; recent codes are more similar to guidelines for practice that provide a framework for nurses to make ethical decisions and fulfill their responsibilities to the public and the profession. Although codes of ethics may or may not be part of statutory regulations, in most provinces there is a statutory requirement within the act governing the nursing profession that mandates that nurses uphold ethical standards as defined by the nursing profession. This means that not only are individual nurses expected to uphold the precepts contained in codes of ethics, they are also obliged to hold colleagues accountable for adhering to them.

Because of the complexity of the ethical dilemmas that nurses confront today, they need more than a code of ethics. Rodney, Doane, Storch, and Varcoe (2006) studied ethical decision making among nurses through the use of focus groups in diverse practice settings. The findings suggest that currents within the moral climate of nurses' work significantly influence nurse's progress toward their moral horizon. Rather than prescribing a set of values for nurses and nursing students as in the past, values clarification strategies are being used increasingly both in nursing education programs and in continuing education programs for practising nurses.

CANADIAN RESEARCH FOCUS

Varcoe, C., Doane, G., Pauly, B., Rodney, P., Storch, L.J., Mahoney, K., McPherson, G., Brown, H., & Starzomski, R. (2004). Ethical practice in nursing: Working the in-betweens. *Journal of Advanced Nursing, 45*(3), 316–325.

   The purpose of this study was to explore the meaning of ethics from the perspective of nurses, and the enactment of ethical practice in nursing. This was a qualitative study conducted in four communities in Western Canada, in a variety of clinical settings. Through a series of focus groups, the nurses described ethics in their practice as both a way of being and a process of enactment in which they worked in-between their own values and those of the organizations in which they worked. They were caught in the middle between competing values and interests, and described a deep personal and professional struggle as they sought to "do good" while forces in the work setting constrained their ability to choose and act ethically. In doing this, they drew on a wide range of sources of moral knowledge. The major finding from this research was that nurses described ethical practice as relational and highly contextual. Conflict and tension characterized their enactment of practice in a context full of values that often contradicted their own.

 ## STRATEGIES FOR ADDRESSING ETHICAL DILEMMAS IN PRACTICE

The number and variety of ethical dilemmas that nurses encounter in practice have increased because of advancements in scientific knowledge and the development of technologies. Nurses and physicians often become embroiled in ethical dilemmas in which opinions differ, leading to decreased communication and failure to work together in the interests of patients. These results can be detrimental to patient care and to the mental health and well-being of nursing staff, particularly in intensive care units, where nurses and physicians may disagree on life and death decisions, on approaches to care, and on setting priorities. Even more troublesome is the fact that many nurses have difficulty dealing appropriately with ethical issues when they do arise. Over the last decade, according to Woods (2005), research in the field of nursing ethics reveals three phenomena that persist:

- "Many nurses feel concerned about the clinical dilemmas they face, but take no action, or are uncertain about what action to take, or feel that they are overruled by physicians, or cannot always overcome 'the barriers' and suffer some form of moral distress.
- "If they do take ethical action or advocate on behalf of their patients, nurses find themselves ostracized by other personnel and then seek covert or subversive ways to promote their own moral survival.
- "Newly graduated nurses do not assert themselves in the face of moral conflict, choosing instead to find ways to cope with their own moral distress, often by passive acceptance or compromise, sometimes at the expense of doing what they have been taught is the right thing to do." (p. 7)

Some health care agencies attempt to address ethical dilemmas through an ethics committee, which is called on an ad hoc basis to address dilemmas presented by health care providers. In some large teaching hospitals, an ethicist is employed to provide expert assistance and guidance. Most hospitals now have institutional ethics committees to provide assistance to professional staff and to set institutional guidelines for ethical practice. However, an ethics committee will not solve the problem of nurses who avoid confronting ethical problems.

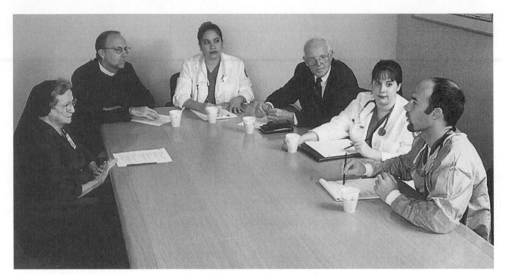

An ethics committee at work.

An attempt at a preventive strategy has been to improve the teaching of ethics in nursing education by ensuring that ethics is an official part of nursing curricula at the undergraduate and graduate levels and is taught by experts, not left to "chance" to be integrated into all teaching. Thompson and Thompson (1989) are advocates of this approach. They identify the goals of teaching ethics to students and health care providers as "to stimulate the moral imagination; recognize ethical issues; elicit a sense of moral obligation; develop analytical skills; and tolerate and reduce disagreements and ambiguity" (p. 86). They recommend using case studies, as do many textbooks on ethics; however, expert guidance should be provided during the process of analyzing the ethical issues and dilemmas presented. It is clear that giving students experience philosophizing on ethical issues is of value in preparing them for clinical practice (Penticuff & Walden, 2000). However, the best educational strategies have not been sufficient to enable new graduates to handle moral problems effectively (Woods, 2005).

Woods (2005) suggests some further changes to nursing ethics education. He believes an essential component is found in the use of appropriate role models in the clinical setting. The most effective way to do this is through the use of morally competent clinical preceptors who are prepared to carry out vigorous ethical discussions with students in the clinical setting. The subsequent validating of the students' knowledge and values from the classroom has the potential to create a whole new experience in which students "discover what they intuitively know alongside other nurses" (p.13). This type of educational strategy endeavours to give ethical idealism a sense of reality and thus bridges the gap between the classroom and the clinical setting.

Since many practising nurses who face ethical dilemmas every day have not had the benefit of this education, discussion of ethics should be included in workplace education and continuing education. After nurses have learned the theoretical foundation of ethics, ongoing ethics rounds can be organized for nurses and physicians. Ethics rounds are not intended to address issues encountered in the care of a specific patient, but to provide opportunities for open discussion of ethical issues when the professionals involved can consider various viewpoints and are not facing a specific ethical issue requiring an immediate decision.

This approach was developed by the John Dossitor Centre for Health Care Ethics at the University of Alberta. The project was originally the result of a collaborative effort to address ethical dilemmas and has equal representation from medicine, nursing, and philosophy through directors who plan and conduct bioethics rounds and are responsible for joint teaching in ethics for nursing and medical students. Such a collaborative approach facilitates addressing issues involving both professions, and decisions are reached that are in the best interests of the patients and the health care providers. This approach is based on the belief that collaboration in the delivery of health care is required to address complex ethical dilemmas; there are no right or wrong answers, but decisions must be made that will meet the needs of the consumers of health care.

CONCLUSION

This chapter has highlighted a few ethical issues and dilemmas; many more are addressed in books and journals for health care providers. The amount of literature on ethics has increased at a phenomenal rate in the past several decades, helping health care providers determine what action to take ethically in situations encountered in practice. Although there are no easy answers to ethical questions, health care providers must have resources available, in the literature and through consultation with ethicists, and they must use these resources in dealing with complex issues and dilemmas.

CRITICAL THINKING QUESTIONS

1. How does the abortion debate relate to current discussions about in vitro fertilization?
2. How can the CNA's *Code of Ethics* be of help to a nurse practising in a rural hospital who finds that staff in her agency have been cut to an unsafe level?
3. If reproduction is considered a basic human right, how would you deal with requests to make in vitro fertilization available on request to infertile couples?

REFERENCES

American Nurses Association. (1976). *Code for nurses with interpretive statements*. Kansas City, MO: Author.

American Nurses Association. (2001). *Code of ethics for nurses with interpretive statements*. Kansas City, MO: Author.

Bandman, E. L., & Bandman, B. (1978). *Bioethics and human rights*. Boston: Little, Brown.

Beauchamp, T. L., & Walters, L. (2003). *Contemporary issues in bioethics* (6th ed.). Belmont, CA: Thompson/Wadsworth.

Beckstead, J. W., & Beckstead, L. G. (2006). A multidimensional analysis of the epistemic origins of nursing theories, models and frameworks. *International Journal of Nursing Studies, 43*, 115–122.

Blacksher, E., & Christopher, M. (2002). On the road to reform: Advocacy and activism in end-of-life care. *Journal of Palliative Medicine, 5*, 13–22.

Canadian Nurses Association. (1985). *Code of ethics for nursing*. Ottawa: Author.

Canadian Nurses Association. (1994). *Joint statement on advance directives*. Ottawa: Author. Retrieved on May 9, 2002, from http://www.cna-nurses.ca/pages/ethics/ethicsframe.htm.

Canadian Nurses Association. (1995). *Joint statement on resuscitative interventions*. Ottawa: Author.

Canadian Nurses Association. (2008). *Code of ethics for registered nurses*, Centennial edition. Retrieved on October 5, 2009, from http://www.cna-aiic.ca/CNA/practice/ethics/code/default_e.aspx. Available in pdf format.

Canadian Nurses Association, Canadian Medical Association, & Canadian Hospital Association. (1984). Joint statement on terminal illness: A protocol for health professionals regarding resuscitative intervention for the terminally ill. *The Canadian Nurse, 80*(4), 24.

Chan, C. C. W. (2006). Infertility, assisted reproduction and rights. *Best Practice & Research Clinical Obstetrics and Gynaecology, 20*(3), 369–380.

Criminal Code, R.S. 1985, c. C-46, s. 241 (b).

Dickens, B. M. (2003). Legal duties to respect abortion choices. *Medicine & Law, 22*(4), 693–700.

Drury, L. (2003). Community care for people who are homeless and mentally ill. *Journal of Health Care for the Poor and Underserved, 14*(2), 194–207.

Duhaime, L. (2009). *Legal resources: Criminal law*. Retrieved on October 5, 2009, from http://www.duhaime.org/Legal Resources/CriminalLaw/LawArticle-100. Last updated January 21, 2009.

Fins, J. J., Miller, F. G., Acres, C. A., Bacchetta, M. D., Huzzard, L. L., & Rapkin, B. D. (1999). End-of-life decision-making in the hospital: Current practice and future prospects. *Journal of Pain and Symptom Management, 17*, 6–15.

Flanagan, L. (1976). *One strong voice: The story of the American Nurses Association*. Kansas City, MO: American Nurses Association.

Flarey, D. (1991). Advanced directives: In search of self-determination. *Journal of Nursing Administration, 21*(11), 16–22.

Godkin, M. D. (1992). *Cardiopulmonary resuscitation: Knowledge, attitudes and opinions of older adults in acute care and long-term care settings*. Unpublished master's thesis. Edmonton: University of Alberta Faculty of Nursing.

Hamel, C. F., Guse, L. W., Hawranik, P. G., & Bond, J. B. (2002). Advance directives and community-dwelling older adults. *Western Journal of Nursing Research, 24*, 143–158.

Holm, S. (2006). What should other healthcare professions learn from nursing ethics. *Nursing Philosophy, 93*, 165–174.

International Council of Nurses. (1973). *ICN code for nurses—Ethical concepts applied to nursing*. Geneva: International Council of Nurses.

Jones, K., & Chaloner, C. (2007). Ethics of abortion: The arguments for and against. *Nursing Standard, 21*(37), 45–48.

Killaspy, H., Ritchie, C. W., Greer, E., & Robertson, M. (2004). Treating the homeless mentally ill: Does a designated inpatient facility improve outcome? *Journal of Mental Health, 13*(6), 593–599.

Morrell, E. D., Brown, B. P., Qi, R., Drabiak, K., & Helft, P. R. (2008). The do-not-resuscitate order: Associations with advance directives, physician specialty and documentation of discussion 15 years after the Patient Self-Determination Act. *Journal of Medical Ethics*, *34*(9), 642–647.

Nancy B. v. Hôtel-Dieu de Québec, [1992], 86 D.L.R. (4th) 385 (Quebec Superior Court).

Norvedt, P. (1998). Sensitive judgement: An inquiry into the foundations of nursing ethics. *Nursing Ethics*, *5*(5), 385–392.

Payne, J. K., & Thornlow, D. K. (2008). Clinical perspectives on portable do-not-resuscitate orders. *Journal of Gerontological Nursing*, *34*(10), 11–16.

Penticuff, J. H., & Walden, M. (2000). Influence of practice environment and nurse characteristics on perinatal nurses' responses to ethical dilemmas. *Nursing Research*, *49*(2), 64–72.

Peplau, H. E. (1978). The right to change behaviour: Rights of the mentally ill. In E. L. Bandman, & B. Bandman (Eds.), *Bioethics and human rights* (pp. 207–212). Boston: Little, Brown.

R. v. Latimer, [2001] S.C.C. 1. File No.: 26980. Retrieved on March 26, 2002, from http://www.lexicongraphics.com/scdla/latimer_scc.html.

Robillard, H. M., High, D. M., Sebastian, J. G., Pisaneschi, J. I., Perritt, L. J., & Mahler, D. M. (1989). Ethical issues in primary care: A survey of practitioners' perceptions. *Journal of Community Health*, *14*(1), 9–17.

Rodney, P., Doane, G. H., Storch, J., & Varcoe, C. (2006). Workplaces: Toward a safer moral climate. *Canadian Nurse*, *102*(8), 24–27.

Scott, P. A. (2000). Emotion, moral perception and nursing practice. *Nursing Philosophy*, *1*, 123–133.

Sue Rodriguez v. British Columbia (Attorney General), [1993] S.C.R. 519.

Thompson, J. E., & Thompson, H. O. (1989). Teaching ethics to nursing students. *Nursing Outlook*, *37*(2), 84–88.

Varcoe, C., Doane, G., Pauly, B., Rodney, P., Storch, L. J., Mahoney, K., McPherson, G., Brown, H., & Starzomski, R. (2004). Ethical practice in nursing: Working the in betweens. *Journal of Advanced Nursing*, *45*(3), 316–325.

Westphal, D. M., & McKee, S. A. (2009). End-of-life decision making in the intensive care unit: Physician and nurse perspectives. *American Journal of Medical Quality*, *24*(3), 222–228.

Wilson, D. M. (1993). *The influences for do-not-resuscitate policies and end-of-life treatment or non-treatment decision.* Unpublished doctoral dissertation. Edmonton, AB: University of Alberta.

Woods, M. (2005). Nursing ethics education: Are we really delivering the good(s)? *Nursing Ethics*, *12*(1), 1–18.

Yeo, M., Moorhouse, A., & Dalziel, J. (1996). *Concepts and cases in nursing ethics.* Peterborough, ON: Broadview Press.

15 Shortage or Oversupply? The Nursing Workforce Pendulum

Eleanor Ross and Leslie J. Roberts

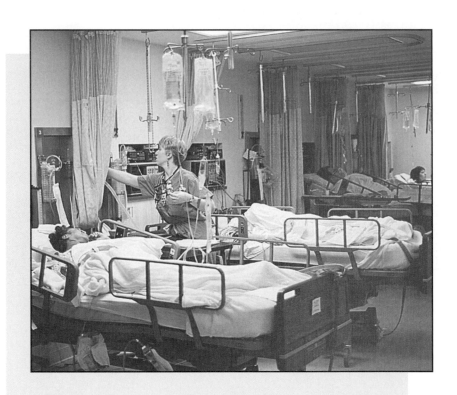

▌▐ LEARNING OBJECTIVES

- To examine trends in numbers and employment of registered nurses (RNs) in Canada.
- To discuss the trends in demand for RNs.
- To discuss issues in the supply of RNs.
- To examine the imbalances between demand and supply of RNs.
- To discuss the challenges facing the nursing profession.
- To identify implications of the shortage of nurses for health care of the future.
- To make recommendations for change.

The beginning of the twenty-first century has seen the health care system, in Canada and globally, continue to change and evolve under continuing cost-containment pressures, new technologies, and shifting health care demands. Within this changing environment, nurses continue to play a major role in delivering health services and to be recognized as invaluable to the health of individuals in Canada and globally (Oulton, 2006). Studies have documented trends in shortages of RNs (Buerhaus, Donelan, Ulrich, Noreman, & Dittus, 2005; Buerhaus, Auerbach, & Staiger, 2007; Buerhaus, Donelan, DesRoches, & Dittus, 2007). The importance of recruiting and retaining nurses has been studied and recommendations have been outlined (Buchan, 2002a, 2002b; Canadian Nurses Association [CNA], 2006; Oulton, 2006). Governments recognize that nursing manpower shortages have serious, negative repercussions on the availability of, access to, and scope of health services—precisely those attributes of the Canadian health system on which we pride ourselves. One of the most challenging tasks for nursing, hospital administrators, governments, and society is to ensure that enough nurses are available to provide care now and in the future.

Among the G8 countries, there were 5.3 regulated nurses for each physician in Canada and 5.5 regulated nurses for each physician in the United Kingdom (CIHI, 2008, p. 1). In addition, Canada had the second-highest number of regulated nurses and midwives per 10,000 population, with 101 to the United Kingdom's 128 (CIHI, 2008, p. 2). In comparison to the United Kingdom, Canada lags well behind the UK in the numbers of regulated nurses* per population.

Many studies in Canada and internationally (Aiken et al., 2001; Buchan, 2002a, 2002b; Upenieks, 2003; CNA, 2006; Oulton, 2006; Stordeur & D'Hoore, 2006) have indicated that autonomy, authority, workplace environment, and quality of work environment, including access to continuing professional development, need to be addressed in order to attract and retain nurses in the profession. This chapter describes trends in the employment of nurses, the demand for nursing services, the supply of nurses, supply imbalances, challenges facing the profession, governments, administration, and recommendations for change. The discussion is based on available data, with the recognition that certain data have limitations due to a variance in definitions over time and among sources of data collection.

---

* Definition: *Regulated nurses* includes all registered nurses, licensed practical nurses (registered practical nurses), and registered psychiatric nurses in Canada (CIHI, 2008).

TRENDS IN EMPLOYMENT OF NURSES

In 2007, registered nurses (RNs) continued to form the largest occupational group in Canada. In the past, the RN workforce increased rapidly from 1961 to 1981: an increase of 33% from 1961 to 1971, and 68% from 1971 to 1981 (Ross, 2003).

Figure 15.1 indicates that the average annual growth rate of the RN workforce was approximately 3.3% between 1980 and 1993. This growth curve flattens between 1993 and 2002, reflecting a period of fiscal restraint. This resulted in an average annual decline during this period of approximately -0.2%. Between 2002 and 2008, the annual growth rate returned to approximately 2.2% (CIHI, 2009). If the fiscal restraint period had not occurred and the annual growth rate of 3.3% had been maintained through this 27-year period, the number of RNs would have reached nearly 370,000, approximately 100,000 more RNs than we have today. The unanswered question is "Would this supply of nurses have met the current demand?"

Table 15.1 presents human resource data for 1995 to 2007 for selected occupations. The number of RNs has increased 18.1% (42,025) during this period. The number of licensed practical nurses (LPNs) decreased by -3.6% (2,937), which reflects a decrease of -21.7% (17,574) between 1995 and 2004 and an increase of 9.9% (14,637) between 2004 and 2007. The total percentage of regulated nurses (RNs and LPNs) decreased by 1.03% (3,248) between 1995 and 2004, while the percentage of increase for pharmacists

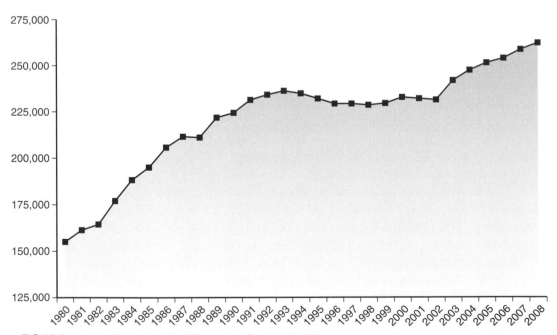

FIG 15.1 Registered Nursing Workforce, Canada, 1980 to 2008.
Source: Canadian Institute for Health Information. (2009). *Regulated Nurses: Canadian Trends 2004–2008* (Ottawa: CIHI, 2009), p. 6. Retrieved on January 14, 2010, from http://secure.cihi.ca/cihiweb/products/regulated_nurses_2004_2008_en.pdf.

| TABLE 15.1 | Nurses and Other Selected Health Care Occupations in the Canadian Labour Force |

	1995	2004	% CHANGE 1995–2004	2007	% CHANGE 1995–2007
Registered Nurses	232,249	246,575	6.2	274,274	18.1
Licensed Practical Nurses	81,017	63,443	−21.7	78,080	−3.6
Registered Psychiatric Nurses*	5,861	5,121	−12.6	5230	−10.8
Total Registered Nurses	313,300	352,354	25%		
Pharmacists	22,197	28,538	28.6		
Physiotherapists	12,551	15,607	24.3		
Nurse Practitioners	725	878	21.1	1,395	92.4

*Registered Psychiatric Nurses are in the four western provinces only.
Sources: CIHI. (2006b). *Health Personnel Trends in Canada, 1995 to 2004.* Retrieved on December 4, 2007, from http://secu re.cihi.ca/cihiweb/dispPage.jsp?cw_page=pub_e; CIHI. (2007c). *Highlights from the Regulated Nursing Workforce in Canada, 2006.* Retrieved on December 16, 2007, from http://secure.cihi.ca/cihiweb/dispPage.jsp?cw_page=pub_e; CIHI. (2008). *Regulated Nurses: Trends 2003–2007* (Ottawa: CIHI). Retrieved on August 21, 2009, from http://secure.cihi.ca/cihiweb/products/nursing_report_2003_to_2007_e.pdf.

and physiotherapists was significantly greater. However, between 1995 and 2007 the percentage increase of regulated nurses was 12.4% (39,088).

Between 1995 and 2007, the number of nurse practitioners increased by 92.4%. They are now licensed in every province in Canada and represented 3.2% of the nursing workforce in 2007 (CIHI, 2008). Nurse practitioners are employed in a variety of positions in the community and hospitals and are one example of new and evolving roles for RNs (see Table 15.1).

Table 15.2 indicates that there has been an overall increase in RNs of 17% between 1994 and 2007, including a small decrease between 1994 and 1997 with a continuing upward trend by 2007. During the same period, the number of full-time positions increased by 13.4%, and the part-time and casual positions increased by 17.9%. The average age of RNs has continued to increase and was 46.2 in 2007.

PLACES OF WORK

HOSPITALS

In 1994, 66.4% of all nurses worked in hospitals (Ross, 2003). This was a decrease from a high of 79.5% in 1971 (Meltz and Marzetti, 1988). As shown in Table 15.3, by 2007, the percentage of nurses working in hospitals had decreased to 62.3%, even though there was an increase in the numbers of nurses working in hospitals of 11.3% between 2002 and 2007. In addition, increasing numbers of nurses were employed in rehabilitation and convalescent centres.

COMMUNITY HEALTH AGENCIES

Community agencies, which include community health agencies, public health, home care and nursing stations, reported having a 17.9% increase in nurses overall. Nursing stations are frequently located in First Nations areas, where the population is growing dramatically. It is questionable whether the health care needs in this area will be addressed by a small increase in supply.

NURSING HOME/LTC

Nursing home/long-term care (LTC) facilities have significantly improved the number of RNs employed. However, the number of facilities is also increasing with the aging boomer generation.

OTHER PLACES OF WORK

The number of RNs employed in occupational health agencies, physicians' offices, educational institutes, and government, or who are self-employed, increased slightly during this period. However, the decline in the numbers of nurses in the occupational health and private agencies is of note.

| TABLE 15.2 | Registered Nurses in Canada 1994–2007: Average Age, Number, and Percentage of Nurses Working Full-Time and Part-Time |

	1994	1997	2000	2007	% CHANGE 1994–2007
Registered Nurses (total working)	234,393	229,813	232,412	274,274	17
Registered Nurses per 10,000 pop.	80.3	76.3	75.4	78.2	–2.1
Average Age	41.4	42.4	43.3	45.1	
Status: Full-time	128,796 (54.9%)	118,083 (51.5%)	127,472 (54.8%)	146,052 (56.6%)	13.4% (numbers) 1.7(%)
Status: Part-time (including casual)	92,570 (41.3%)	107,935 (47%)	95,032 (40.8%)	109,126 (42.3%)	17.9 (numbers) 1 (%)

Source: CIHI. (2007g). *Workforce Trends of Registered Nurses in Canada, 2006.* Retrieved on December 2, 2007, from http://secure.cihi.ca/cihiweb/dispPage.jsp?cw_page=pub_e; CIHI. (2005). *Workforce Trends of Registered Nurses in Canada, 2004.* Retrieved on January 15, 2008, from http://secure.cihi.ca/cihiweb/dispPage.jsp?cw_page=pub_e; CIHI. (2008). *Regulated Nurses: Trends 2003–2007* (Ottawa: CIHI). Retrieved on August 21, 2009, from http://secure.cihi.ca/cihiweb/products/nursing_report_2003_to_2007_e.pdf.

| TABLE 15.3 | Where Nurses Work in Canada, 2007 |

	2002	% TOTAL	2007	% TOTAL	% CHANGE
Hospitals	144,292	62.5	160,653	62.3	11.3
Community Health	30,544	13.2	36,024	14	17.9
Nursing Home/LTC Facility	24,372	10.6	27,111	10.5	11.2
Other	28,728	12.4	32,078	12.4	11.7
Not Stated	3,021	1.3	2,086	0.8	–30.9
Total	**232,959**		**259,959**		

CIHI. (2007g). *Workforce Trends of Registered Nurses in Canada, 2006.* Retrieved on December 2, 2007, from http://secure.cihi.ca/cihiweb/dispPage.jsp?cw_page=pub_e; CIHI. (2008). *Regulated Nurses: Trends 2003–2007* (Ottawa: CIHI). Retrieved on August 21, 2009, from http://secure.cihi.ca/cihiweb/products/nursing_report_2003_to_2007_e.pdf.

AREAS OF RESPONSIBILITY

Table 15.4 identifies the areas of responsibility where nurses are employed in Canada. An increase of 13.4% of RNs between 2002 and 2007 worked in direct care, with increases in all the specialization roles except for community health, home care, and oncology. However, public health and telehealth were reported for the first time in 2006, causing a reduction in the numbers in the community health sector. The modest increment in the number of nurse educators is of concern as there is an increasing demand for student

TABLE 15.4	RNs Employed in Nursing by Area of Responsibility, 2006				
	2002	%	2007	%	% CHANGE 2002–07
Direct Care	198,323	85.9	224,964	89	13.4
Medicine/Surgery	37,885	16.4	43,258	17.1	14.2
Psychiatry/Mental Health	11,321	4.9	13,255	5.2	17.1
Pediatrics	5,113	2.2	6,973	2.8	36.4
Maternity/Newborn	12,167	5.3	14,192	5.6	16.6
Geriatrics/Long-Term Care*	20,386	8.8	26,044	10.3	27.8
Critical Care*	16,537	7.2	18,604	7.4	12.5
Community Health	12,302	5.3	11,251	4.5	−8.5
Ambulatory Care	6,452	2.8	8,172	3.2	26.7
Home Care	9,255	4.0	7,316	2.9	−20.6
Occupational Health	2,616	1.1	3,020	1.2	15.4
OR/Recovery Room	9,507	4.1	12,056	4.8	26.8
Emergency Room	11,440	5.0	16,015	6.3	40
Several Clinical Areas	16,114	7.0	9,801	3.9	−39.1
Oncology	3,474	1.5	3,129	1.2	−9.9
Rehabilitation	3,128	1.4	3,888	1.5	24.3
Public Health			5,824	2.3	
Telehealth**			935	0.4	
Other Direct Care***	20,626	8.9	21,231	8.4	2.9
Administration	13,009		17,022	6.7	30.9
Education	9,644	4.2	8,607	3.5	−10.7
Teaching—Students	4,092	1.8	4,496	1.8	9.9
Teaching—Employees	1,546	0.7	852	0.3	−44.9
Teaching—Patients/Clients	1,676	0.7	643	0.3	−61.7
Other Education***	2,330	1.0	2,820	1.1	21.0
Research	2,301	1.0	1,878	0.8	−18.4
Nursing Research Only	1,189	0.5	910	0.4	23.5
Other Research	1,112	0.5	1,025	0.4	−7.8
Total	230,957		252,732	100	9.4

*Critical Care and Geriatric Long Term Care not submitted for Manitoba. Included in "Other Direct Care" for 2002.

**New Brunswick, Quebec, Alberta, and the Northwest Territories submitted information to CIHI for RNs in telehealth.

***Changes in Quebec forms for 2002 led to major changes in categories of Other Direct Care, Nursing Service, and Other Education

Source: CIHI. (2003b). *Workforce Trends of Registered Nurses in Canada, 2002.* Retrieved on January 5, 2008, from http://secure.cihi.ca/cihiweb/dispPage.jsp?cw_page=pub_e; CIHI. (2007g). *Workforce Trends of Registered Nurses in Canada, 2006.* Retrieved on December 2, 2007, from http://secure.cihi.ca/cihiweb/dispPage.jsp?cw_page=pub_e; CIHI. (2008). *Regulated Nurses: Trends 2003–2007* (Ottawa: CIHI). Retrieved on August 21, 2009, from http://secure.cihi.ca/cihiweb/products/nursing_report_2003_to_2007_e.pdf.

space, the educators are overwhelmed with their workload, and this group has one of the highest average ages, with significant numbers retiring in the near future (Bartfay & Howse, 2007).

Note: It is difficult to compare the numbers in Table 15.4 with those in 15.3 because of the way data was captured by CIHI.

The younger nurses and new graduates are a very mobile group with relatively high new registration and exit rates. CIHI (2008) states that the most likely reason for the high exit rates is the high rate of inter-jurisdictional mobility between provinces and territories, with Ontario, British Columbia, and Alberta gaining the most and Saskatchewan and the territories losing over 30% of this group. In 2007, there were 6,839 Canadian RNs working outside of their jurisdiction of registration, including the United States (53%), Canada (36.4%), and other foreign destinations (10.6%) (CIHI, 2008).

Exit rates of new RN entrants are very difficult to determine. However, CIHI has suggested that for new entrants in 2003, 18.7% of the under-35 group, 19.1% of the 35-to-49 age group, and 39.5% of the 50 and over age group have left the profession. Data for the international nurses group are higher (CIHI, 2008). There are many reasons for this mobility, such as marriage, pregnancy, and moving, but poor quality of work life and high stress levels have not been addressed and remain a major factor for nurses leaving the workforce.

The urban–rural distribution of the workforce is a major challenge for the health care sector in each province and territory. In 2007, 87.8% of the RN workforce worked in urban areas of Canada, ranging from highs of 98.4% in the Yukon and 93.9% in Ontario to lows of 57.1% in the Northwest Territories and Nunavut and 67.9% in Newfoundland and Labrador (CIHI, 2008, p. 39). Since many of these nurses are in the 50 and over age group, there is concern as to how health care will be provided in the rural and remote areas of Canada in the future.

"Of the RNs employed in Canada who reported their location of graduation in 2007, 92.1% (235,636) graduated from a nursing program in Canada and 7.9% (20,319) graduated from an international nursing program. Since 2003, the proportion of internationally educated graduates in the Canadian RN workforce remained between 7% and 8%" (CIHI, 2008, p. 37). International nurses are making a significant contribution to our supply of nursing graduates, but it is a stable number and significantly more than the number of Canadian nurses who have retained their registration here but work elsewhere.

In summary, the number of nurses working in hospitals has continued to increase although the number as a percentage of the total working RNs has continued to decrease since 1994. This decline is a result of increases in the community and other new and emerging roles. The numbers of nurses have continued to increase in rehabilitation and convalescent centres, nursing homes, and long-term care facilities. In community health agencies during this period, there was an overall increase of 17.9% (Fig. 15.3). Nurses working in community health centres and public health have increased by 15.9% since 2002.

Numbers are reflected differently in tables due to the way the data has been captured and reported by CIHI.

TRENDS IN DEMAND

The review of where nurses work and the actual numbers of RNs employed illustrates the increasing demand factors for nursing knowledge and skills. The trends have been identified nationally and internationally as shorter hospital stays; more complex diseases, resulting in increased acuity of care; a shift from hospital to ambulatory, home, and community care; new infectious and re-emerging diseases; an aging population; globalization; and a growing private sector (Oulton, 2006). In general, all the specialization roles of nurses in hospitals have increased except for a decrease in the number of RNs employed teaching employees and patients.

The factors driving the increasing need for RN knowledge and skills (see Box 15.1) include (1) the increase in specialization of nurse employment in hospitals and in the community; (2) the reduction in bed-to-RN ratio because of the increasing acuity and complexity of patients; (3) the variation in the number of aides, orderlies, and personal service workers; (4) the continuing number of nurses working part-time; and (5) the new and emerging RN roles, such as nurse practitioner, telehealth, and self-employment.

INCREASING SPECIALIZATION

The first factor relates to the continuous increase in the number of RNs in Canada other than a slight reduction between 1994 and 1997 (see Figure 15.1). The trend of increasing numbers of RNs working in hospitals, but a decreasing percentage of the total working RNs, is supported by studies indicating that there is an increasing acuity and workload in hospitals. Hospital beds have been reduced and many patients have a shorter length of stay. The use of new technologies allows procedures and major surgeries to be done on an outpatient basis and care to be delivered in the community.

Of interest, a review of LPN statistics indicates that there has been an increase in numbers from 2002 to 2006 of 7,177. In particular, LPNs have increased in mental health work by over 200% and rehabilitation and convalescent care by over 185% but have had a decrease in general hospitals by 7.9%) (CIHI, 2003a, 2007f).

In the 1980s, the increasing use of RNs instead of LPNs was explained by the fact that hospitalized patients were sicker and required more care than in years past; in reality, RNs were paid a relatively low wage and were very adaptable. RNs could perform a wide range of other functions from clerical jobs to therapists, could substitute for physicians under some circumstances, and could assume hospital management roles after regular

BOX 15.1	Factors Driving the Demand for Nursing Knowledge

- Increasing specialization
- Reduction in bed-to-RN ratio
- Variation in number and type of support workers available
- Fluctuation in part-time employment
- New and evolving RN roles

work hours. Nurses required little supervision and took responsibility for a wide range of duties. By 1993, however, nurses' salaries in Canada had increased because of pay equity legislation and negotiated salary increases. In 2006, salaries across Canada varied but have since increased (Canadian Federation of Nurses Unions [CFNU], 2007). During the 1990s, hospitals began downsizing and a number of layoffs occurred with decentralization, regionalization, and strategic alliances. Initial research about the downsizing of nursing resources indicated a decrease of 11% in paid hours between 1994–95 and 1996–97 (McGillis Hall, Pink, Johnson, & Schraa, 2000a, 2000b). Layoffs included middle-management nurses, staff nurses, and licensed practical nurses. In 2008, the discussions continued about the nursing shortage but also included the significant amount of overtime and absenteeism occurring in the nursing workforce.

In 2006, it is important to note the decrease in the number of RNs employed teaching employees and patients. When hospitals are in their cost-cutting mode, it is often nurses working in these areas who are considered expendable, with little regard for quality of care for patients and the stressors in the work environment for nurses.

REDUCTION IN BED-TO-RN RATIO

The second factor in the increase of employed RNs was the trend of reduction in the bed-to-RN ratio. Over the years, there have been increasing numbers of RNs per bed (Meltz & Marzetti, 1988). Between 1999–2000 and 2004–05, there was a decrease of almost 10,000 beds (7.8%) (CIHI, 2007b). RNs working in hospitals increased by 8.8% during the same period (CIHI, 2005). This trend appears to be due to the increased acuity and complexity of patient care in hospitals, a change that required more RNs around the clock. Inpatient hospitalizations in Canada decreased from 1995–96 to 2006–07 by 13.4% (3.2M to 2.6M) (CIHI, 2007d, 2007e). Interestingly, during the 1995 to 2007 period, the average length of hospital stay (ALOS) had remained at 7.2 and 7.3 days respectively (CIHI, 2007d, 2007e). However, a 30.6% increase in the day surgery visits is observed with over 1.3 million day surgery visits in 1995–96 compared with almost 1.8 million visits in 2005–06 (CIHI, 2007e). New technologies such as laser surgery have influenced where and how procedures are done.

The research evidence supports the importance of sufficient, well-qualified RNs in relation to patient outcomes and cost-effectiveness (McGillis Hall & O'Brien-Pallas, 2000; West, Barron, & Reeves, 2005; Hall et al., 2006; Hugonnet, Chevrolet, & Pittet, 2007; Stone et al., 2007; Stordeur & D'Hoore, 2006; Tourangeau et al., 2007; Aiken, Clarke, Sloane, Lake, & Cheney, 2008; Armstrong, Laschinger, & Wong, 2009).

VARIATION IN NUMBER AND TYPE OF SUPPORT WORKERS

The third factor was the variation in the number of assistants, aides, and orderlies (Meltz & Marzetti, 1988). In 1971, the number of RNs (104,635) was slightly smaller than the total number of supervisors, assistants, aides, and orderlies (112,775). By 1986, however, the number of RNs (221,980) was almost double that of the other three groups (136,635). RNs increased from 21.3% to 32.7% of the total employees in hospitals,

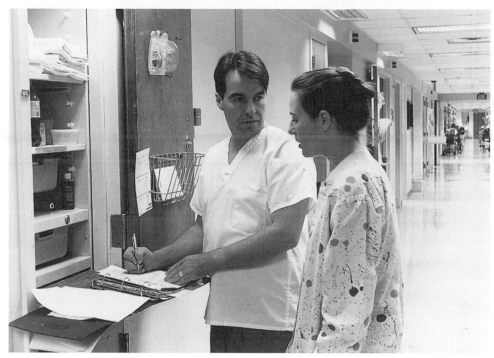

With increasing specialization in the health care field, some nurses may delegate specific elements of patient care to a personal support worker.

whereas assistants, aides, and orderlies decreased from 20.3% to 11.87% (Meltz & Marzetti, 1988). Data about orderlies, assistants, and aides are no longer captured.

Discussions about an implementation of a nurse extender, or a "generic worker," and the use of auxiliary staff to support the registered nurse began in the 1990s (McGillis Hall, 1997, 1998a, 1998b). In particular, discussions began about reducing the inappropriate utilization of nurses (Aiken, 1990; Miller, 1992). Although there has been much discussion about new models of care such as total patient care and patient-focused care, it is difficult to find evidence of much change in where and how services are delivered. Data about the aide or personal service worker are not captured in the available reports. Only the regulated professions are tracked and documented. It is uncertain how much the system and hospitals have changed in delivering care in hospitals. LPNs had been reduced in acute-care settings, but recent data indicate they have increased in certain areas such as palliative care (CIHI, 2003a, 2007f). Whether the assistive or generic worker (formerly aides and orderlies) who had been purported to assist and support RNs in the delivery of care is playing the support role is unclear.

FLUCTUATION IN PART-TIME EMPLOYMENT

The fourth factor in the increase of employed RNs was the increase in the proportion working part-time. Almost half of the RNs in Canada were working part-time by 1985 (Meltz & Marzetti, 1988), an increase from 27% of RNs working part-time in 1971.

This trend has continued (see Table 15.2). In 1994, 54.9% were working full-time; in 1997, that percentage dropped to 51.5%. A slight reversal occurred in 2000, with 54.8% working full-time and 56.3% in 2006. Nursing associations and governments in Canada have focused on increasing the numbers of full-time positions in the last 5 to 10 years; however, not much movement has occurred. Undoubtedly, a change in the number of hours worked by almost 100,000 nurses could substantially affect the number of full-time equivalent nurses. However, very few studies clarify whether the majority of RNs continue to work part-time and casually by choice because of the workplace issues and/ or work–life balance. As full-time positions have opened up, RNs do apply for them. In 2006, approximately 3,000 nurses were looking for work at the time of registration. Almost 4% were not employed and not seeking work (CIHI 2007g).

NEW AND EVOLVING RN ROLES

The fifth factor relates to the number of new RN roles in the health care system. Nurse practitioners are employed in a variety of positions in hospitals and the community in primary, secondary, and tertiary settings, as an example of these new and evolving roles for RNs. Also, new telehealth networks and telephone advice and information centres (Goodwin, 2007) require the knowledge and skills of RNs. Governments and the media discussed the nurse practitioner role as a cost-effective way of delivering health care in Canada and internationally (Ketefian, Redman, Hanucharurnkul, Masterson, & Neves, 2001). The new emerging RN roles continue to be discussed and implemented as seen by the recent statistics.

TRENDS IN SUPPLY

The supply of RNs in Canada comes from recent graduates from colleges and university programs; immigrants from other countries who have had nursing education; and former RNs returning to the workforce. In 1986, 87.5% of the employed RNs had graduated from Canadian schools of nursing; 9.1% had graduated from schools in other countries. In 2006, 92.1% (231,140) had graduated from a nursing program in Canada and 7.9% (19,836) were internationally educated. The percentage of graduates educated internationally has varied from 7 to 8% since 2003 (CIHI, 2006b). Enrolment in nursing programs in Canada and the United States fluctuated in the 1980s and 90s (Aiken & Mullinix, 1987). Interest in nursing as a career declined for a number of reasons, including increased career opportunities for women, rigid and capped salary structures for staff nurses, layoffs during the 1990s, and lack of economic return for degrees in nursing. The decrease in numbers of students enrolling was also due to the changes in education of RNs in Canada and a declining number of 18-year-olds and fewer young adults entering the workforce.

In Canada, nursing schools have increased their enrolment since discussions about an acute shortage began in the 1990s. In 2006, 6,559 candidates wrote the Canadian Registered Nurse Examination; 87% were educated in Canada and 13% were educated internationally. Over the last seven years, first-time exam writers have fluctuated between a low of 4,737 in 2000 and a high of 10,992 in 2004. The majority of both Canadian and international RN candidates continue to be female (93% and 88%, respectively) (CNA, 2007). Although 8,379 students graduated from Entry-To-Practice (ETP) programs in 2006, compared with 5,642 in 2001, a 48.5% increase (CNA & CASN, 2007), studies have indicated that 12,000 graduates per year, or an increase of 4,000 new graduates, are needed to address the projected nursing shortage (CNA & CASN, 2007). The number of graduates from ETP programs in 2006 was similar to the 1985 to 1993 numbers; however, the Canadian population has grown from 25.3 million in 1986 to 31.6 million in 2006, an increase of 24.9% (CNA & CASN, 2007).

Some hospitals have focused on unemployed nurses or nurses who had left the profession as a potential resource for employment as the shortages became more pronounced. However, a review of unemployment and employment data does not support this as a major source of RNs. Over 93% of RNs registered were working in 2006 (CNA & CASN, 2007; CNO, 2008).

A total of 6839 RNs with Canadian registration lived or worked outside of Canada in 2007. Of these, 53% were employed in the United States (CIHI, 2008). The reasons that nurses work in the United States are uncertain but full-time work and educational opportunities have been cited. In 2007 in Ontario alone, of the 93,941 registrants there were 3,457 RNs (3.7%) working in the United States, 4,959 (4.6%) working in non-nursing jobs, and 7,574 (7%) not working (CNO, 2008).

A study measuring the retention of RNs in Canada between 2000 and 2004 found that RNs aged 60 to 75 had a slightly higher exit rate from the system than RNs aged 25 to 34, and RNs with casual employment had an exit rate of approximately twice that of RNs with full-time or part-time employment (CIHI, 2006c; CIHI, 2008, p. 23).

SUPPLY–DEMAND IMBALANCES

The actual imbalance between supply and demand is complex. The supply of RNs varied in numbers of graduates over the years and into the twenty-first century. Meanwhile, the demands have continued to expand and increase over this same period. Imbalances in a labour market can occur through unfilled vacancies or unemployment and underemployment (Meltz & Marzetti, 1988). Vacancies indicate an inability to recruit people or to retain them in a particular position. Although vacancy rates had been reported in some areas across Canada in the 1980s, the rates had varied tremendously. Meltz and Marzetti found that critical care and long-term care consistently had high vacancy rates, and vacancy rates for chronic care, psychiatric care, and active teaching hospitals were also well above the provincial average. By 1993, the vacancy rate was virtually zero because of the funding cutbacks and downsizing that occurred in the 1990s. Recent data do not reveal vacancy rates. Individual workplaces have such data, but no central registry could be found. Nurse researchers have begun to analyze vacancy statistics and recommend a standard methodology that would better quantify vacancy rates and therefore provide a more accurate assessment of nurse utilization and shortage (Fisher, Baumann, & Blythe, 2007).

UNEMPLOYMENT

A low unemployment rate can indicate a shortage; a high rate can indicate a potential supply source of RNs. The Statistics Canada Labour Force Survey in 2006 indicates that the unemployment rate for health occupations was 1.2%, whereas the rate for all occupations was 6.3%, the lowest for 30 years (CIHI, 2006c). Canada has consistently low rates of unemployment for nurses that are 50% or less of general labour force unemployment rates. The CIHI data also suggest that unemployed nurses do not form a large untapped pool of workers. Between 2003 and 2007, the proportion of RNs who were employed in nursing remained the same at 93.4% (CIHI, 2007e) and increased to 94% by 2007. In 2007, 3% of RNs licensed in Canada were not employed and only 1.8% of these were seeking employment; 2% were employed in other than nursing and 21.7% (451) were seeking employment (CIHI, 2008). Of the 2,773 licensed RNs who were seeking employment as an RN in 2006, 87.8% were 30 years of age or older and 12.2% were under 30 years of age (CIHI, 2007e).

OVERTIME AND ABSENTEEISM

Nevertheless, there are four increasing areas of concern. The amount of overtime worked by nurses, nursing absenteeism, nursing turnover, and the aging nursing population are all worrisome (CNA, 2006). Research has shown that Canadian nurses have the highest rates of overtime and absenteeism. The rate of overtime equalled 10,000 full-time equivalents in 2005. "Nearly 10,000 full-time positions were taken up with absenteeism in 2005—a rate 58% higher than the average Canadian full-time worker" (CNA, 2006). Thus, the rate of overtime is equivalent to the absenteeism rate. Nurses have had the highest or second-highest rate of absenteeism of all workers in Canada over the past 15 years (CNA, 2006). Work-related injury and disability is high among nurses in Canada and globally (CIHI, 2006a). In Canada, research is determining factors contributing to healthy workplaces (Baumann et al., 2001; O'Brien-Pallas et al., 2004; Stone & Gershon, 2006; Stone et al., 2007; Hall, Doran, & Pink, 2008). Early conclusions indicate that the complexity and acuity of a nurse's work likely contribute to injuries and sick time (Shamian et al., 2001). Sufficient staffing might reduce workload and stress on the RN but also would improve patient care outcomes and the efficiency and cost-effectiveness of the health system (Donnelly, Yarbrough, & Jaffe, 1989; Aiken, Clarke, & Sloane, 2002; Aiken, Clarke, Sloane, Sochalski, & Silbur, 2002; Bower & McCullough, 2004; Tourangeau et al., 2007; Aiken et al., 2008; Armstrong et al., 2009).

TURNOVER

Turnover is a major challenge for health human resource planning in nursing. It has been considered an indicator of nurse dissatisfaction. Factors that have been identified as contributing to turnover are heavy workload, work stress, schedules, and staff burnout. Retention has been an area of study and recommendations over the past 20 years (Laschinger, Wong, & Greco, 2006; Leners, Wilson, Connor, & Fenton, 2006;

O'Brien-Pallas, Griffin, et al., 2006; Zeytinoglu et al., 2006; Pendry, 2007). Modifying the work environment by having participative management, career development, and continuing education opportunities has been recommended (Wittmann-Price & Kuplen, 2003; Wilson, 2005; O'Brien-Pallas, Duffield, & Hayes, 2006). A review of data does not support that much change has taken place across Canada. Some units in some institutions may have successfully implemented strategies to attract and retain nurses but they are not well documented. The authors perceive that teaching hospitals have attempted most of the changes. A new accreditation program, Qmentum Workforce, was introduced by Accreditation Canada, which includes Worklife as one of the six required organizational practices in patient safety (2008).

AGING AND RETIREMENT

Another growing concern is the aging of the profession and the large number of RNs who will retire in the next ten years. The average age of nurses in Canada is rising (see Table 15.2). The RNs providing direct care are the youngest group (average 44.5 years), while those in education are the oldest (average 48.1 years). In the age group of 40 years and older, the proportion of nurse educators exceeds that of the total RN workforce (CNA & CASN, 2007; CIHI, 2007g). A large group of nurse educators will be retiring over the next ten years. The numbers of nurse educators must be maintained in order to educate the nurses of the future (Bartfay & Howse, 2007).

In summary, the supply–demand imbalance is complex. These data emphasize the need to consider supply more broadly than new graduates. The retention of RNs, addressing the quality of the workplace environment, and increasing full-time positions are all important factors that must be addressed.

🔊 REFLECTIVE THINKING

With all the published research related to workplace environment, why has so little change taken place in the acute-care facilities, where the majority of registered nurses still work?

▌ CHALLENGES FACING THE PROFESSION

Major challenges continue to face the profession of nursing (see Box 15.2). Our health care system depends overwhelmingly on the work of women. Four out of five workers in health-related occupations are women; four out of ten workers overall are women (Ryten, 1988). In 2005, the Labour Force Survey of Statistics Canada reported that the percentage of women employed in all other industries varied from 5 to 6% in trades, transportation, and equipment to 70% in sales and service (CIHI, 2006b).

In 1985, only 57% of employed female graduate nurses worked full-time; 43% worked part-time (Meltz & Marzetti, 1988). This trend continues today. The most recent

BOX 15.2	Challenges Facing the Nursing Profession

- Full-time versus part-time employment
- Female versus male work patterns
- Reorganized health care systems that are slow to recognize and support RNs' need for additional knowledge and skills
- New structures that are slow to empower and value RNs
- Continued lack of coordinated recruitment and retention strategies
- Continued lack of structural changes to address working conditions and quality of work–life balance in nursing

statistics indicate that only 54.8% of employed female nurses worked full-time (CIHI, 2007g). The proportion of the general Canadian workforce working full-time (82%) and part-time (18%) has remained stable over the past decade. In comparison, more members of the health care workforce worked part-time (24%) and a higher proportion of nurses worked part-time (43%) in 2006. Part-time work is more prevalent in the mainly female occupations such as nursing and the younger female physicians (CIHI, 2006b).

Work patterns have continued to vary between men and women and among different health care occupations. For example, in 1985, 88% of male pharmacists and 70% of female pharmacists worked full-time, but 82% of female physicians worked full-time, and 57% of registered nurses worked full-time (Ryten, 1988). However, by 1995, 58% of those graduating in pharmacy were women with an increase to 77% by 2004. Likely, this will lead to a change in pharmacists' work patterns. Between 2000 and 2004, the number of female physicians increased by 14% while their male counterparts increased by only 0.6% (CIHI, 2006b). A 2001 report by the College of Physicians of Canada indicated that female physicians worked 21% fewer hours than male physicians. The difference in work hours between men and women was lowest at ages 25 to 29 and was the most notable between the ages of 35 and 44. Male physicians reached their peak work hours at ages 40 to 44 and females slightly later at 55 to 59 (CIHI, 2007a). This would indicate that female physicians reduce their workload to the greatest extent during their childbearing and early parenting years. It is very likely that if the same survey were repeated for nurses very similar results would have been determined. Health occupations have the highest percentage of employed women, averaging around 80%. Work–life balance is the most important factor for many women who work part-time (CIHI, 2007a). A higher proportion of women are pursuing higher education but are choosing different work patterns than men after entering the workforce. The profession of nursing has been in the forefront of these trends (CIHI, 2006b).

During the past 25 years, women have entered traditionally male occupations, such as medicine, veterinary medicine, and engineering; however, men have not entered traditionally female occupations, such as nursing, at the same rate. In the past ten years, more women than men have graduated from universities. Women have made great strides in pursuing higher education, but their participation has benefited fields of study that are not predominantly female (Ryten, 1988). A review of the Canadian labour market in general identifies two additional trends between 1980 and 2000: women increased their earnings (10.8%) and full-time employment (0.2%) while men lost earnings (-6.4%) and full-time employment (−3.8%) (Statistics Canada, 2005).

A key characteristic of the Canadian labour market in the 1980s and the 1990s is the continually increasing demand for well-educated and skilled workers. This trend reflects changes both in the occupational "mix" of employment toward business services in areas of professional, scientific, and technical services industries, and in the administrative and support, waste management, and remediation service industries. The computer and telecommunications (CT) sector, which combines "high-tech manufacturing and service activities, grew particularly fast in the 1990s" (Statistics Canada, 2005, p. 91). This trend in the general labour market is also evident in the health care industry, in hospitals, and in the nursing profession. Nevertheless, the health care system and hospitals have been slow to recognize and support RNs' need for additional skills and knowledge (Presho, 2006).

The 1990s witnessed a more turbulent, chaotic, and challenging economic and health care environment. Reorganization and decentralization were key principles in the many institutional changes. Program management, case management, and patient focus were the trends. Although many studies have highlighted that the nursing issues are related to lack of recognition, lack of professionalism, and lack of authority for responsibility, these new management structures have not necessarily addressed the empowerment of nurses or the need for the nurse to be a professional knowledge worker. Organizational and technological support for their work, however, remains as low as it has been in past decades (Bower & McCullough, 2004). In some structures, the lack of a chief executive nurse, who articulates a vision for nursing and excellent patient care, can be seen as a continuum of the devaluing of nurses' work (Health Canada, 2001).

In the new millennium, nurses face several challenges. First, the continued need for restructuring of health care systems, which will enhance the nurses' value, knowledge, and roles. These new ways of delivering care should enhance the work–life balance and create more efficient and effective work patterns (Bower & McCullough, 2004; Duxbury & Higgins, 2005). Second, there needs to be a continued focus on implementing recommendations for recruitment and retention (Wittman-Price & Kuplen, 2003; Wilson, 2005; Duffield, O'Brien-Pallas, Aitken, Roche, & Merrick, 2006) that will deal with the aging nursing population as well as the younger generations (Gifford, Zammuto, & Goodman, 2002; Andrews, Manthorope, & Watson, 2005; Carroll, 2005; Widger et al., 2007). Higher efficiency and productivity is required as we move toward the era of a reduction in birthrates, resulting in a decrease in the population (Statistics Canada, 2007). Nursing leadership is facing the challenges by "managing fiscal restraints while addressing current healthcare issues" such as "increasing service demands, integration of services and wait time strategies" (Vandevelde-Coke, 2007).

A review of the data in 2007 indicated that nurses have not been leaving the profession as is often suggested but were actually working and attempting to make changes in the system. The profession of nursing has become more vocal. Illegal strikes occurred in the 1980s and 1990s. Although there was much anger and unrest among nurses, causing salaries to improve, systemic change that would empower nurses has not resulted.

The aging of RNs is a major concern. On the other hand, some RNs, like the general population, might choose to continue working. Strategies to assist and encourage nurses to continue working need to be considered (O'Brien-Pallas et al., 2004; Hart, 2007). Every study since the 1980s in Canada and globally has recommended structural changes that would address unsatisfactory working conditions and quality of work life in nursing. However, these recommended changes have not been adopted by the health care system.

CANADIAN RESEARCH FOCUS

McGillis Hall, L., Doran, D., & Pink, L. (2008). Outcomes of interventions to improve hospital nursing work environments. *Journal of Nursing Administration, 38*(1), 40–46.

Patient outcomes and nursing effectiveness have been seen to be influenced by nursing work environments. This quasi-experimental study involved 16 unit managers, 1,137 patients, and 296 observations from registered nurses over time. Baseline measures were taken and interventions were designed according to the needs of the individual units and implemented with three- and six-month follow-up data collections. The findings demonstrated that unit characteristics can affect nurse and patient outcomes. Patient-to-nurse ratio was one of the most consistent unit characteristics to have a harmful effect on nurse outcomes, with high patient-to-nurse ratios negatively affecting nurses' perceptions of work and the work environment. A high ratio also had a negative effect on unit-based nursing leadership, and on nurses' job stress. It is evident from this study that change interventions can have a positive effect on nurses' perceptions of their work and the work environment. Also, a higher proportion of RNs was linked to patients achieving a higher level of independence related to activities of daily living.

RECOMMENDATIONS FOR CHANGE

A review of trends in the employment of nurses, the supply of and demand for nurses, and supply imbalances indicates that Canada has not had a real "shortage" of RNs if the numbers only are considered. However, with the number of part-time RNs remaining at over 40% of the total RNs working and the high rate of absenteeism, there is a shortage. The increasing number of aging nurses is a concern. The number of new graduates has increased a small percentage but not in sufficient numbers (CNA & CASN, 2007). The level of "surplus" would appear to be very little since over 93% of RNs have continued to reregister each year. In 1989, there were specialties, hospitals, and other nursing areas in Canada that had high vacancy rates; in 1993, there were no vacancies and an undetermined level of unemployment; in 2006, the data were not captured, but waiting times for certain procedures or care related to the nursing shortage remained in the news (see Box 15.3).

Because health care is a provincial matter in Canada, the provincial governments, in planning for health care, should have a coordinated human resources strategy to address the imbalances in supply and demand for RNs. Many organizations and reports (CNA, 2006; Oulton, 2006) have highlighted the human resources issues in health care and provided guidelines for human resources planning. In October 2000, Canada and the provincial governments developed a plan that addresses human resources planning in nursing over the long term (Health Canada, 2001, p. 16). The need for an ongoing

BOX 15.3	Recommendations for Change in Nursing

The "myth" of a nursing shortage is complex and requires a multifaceted approach to resolve the issue. Nursing leaders know that increasing the number of nurses alone will not be a solution. The "nursing shortage" has been acknowledged as a complex phenomenon requiring a comprehensive and collaborative approach to address the various issues. The need for government officials, hospital administrators, and nurses to collaborate has been identified.

coordinated human resources plan for health care based on the health needs of Canadians cannot be overemphasized.

Governments have a responsibility to review and update legislation that will enact structural changes to give nurses the authority to participate in decision making. This legislation is needed to ensure that nurses' participation in decision making occurs not simply by virtue of invitation, as it is at present in most provinces. Administrators of health care delivery organizations need to retain the nurses they have and preserve RNs' time for direct care of patients and families (Andrews, Manthorope, & Watson, 2005). Staffing affects quality and cost of patient care (Gifford, Zammuto, & Goodman, 2002; Lang, Hodge, Olson, Romano, & Kravitz, 2004). Organizations should design and implement innovative, cost-effective staffing methods that include job restructuring, use of support personnel, flexible scheduling plans, and labour-saving technology (Aiken & Mullinix, 1987; Donnelly, Yarbrough, & Jaffe, 1989; Glandon, Colbert, & Thomasma, 1989; Bower & McCullough, 2004). Also, administrators should consider nursing as a revenue centre rather than a cost centre and thus begin to value and recognize nursing's contribution to the organization (Johnson, 1989; Jones, 1990). Management must continue to introduce incentives to encourage experienced nurses to remain in clinical care. Wage structures and benefit packages that recognize experience and advanced education continue to be needed.

Although many new management models emerged in the 1990s, the health care system continues to be a hierarchical and bureaucratically managed system. As a result of the rapidity of the changes within the government's cost-cutting initiatives, many agencies have downsized not only in numbers of beds but in numbers of nurses. Meanwhile, these agencies and units are continuing to deliver care in the same traditional way of the past 30 years. The need for innovation, creativity, and entrepreneurial acts has never been greater. The need to maximize every nurse's skill and knowledge is paramount. Technology and delivery models must be used and designed to best use the RN's knowledge (Bower & McCullough, 2004). Every unit or agency likely requires a different system of delivering care based on the needs of a specific population of patients.

Nurses also have a part to play in addressing some of the issues. Each nurse must value and recognize the importance of nursing care and be able to articulate that value. Nurses should realize the strength of nursing; it includes many different groups, organizations, and specialties. External groups have suggested that a major problem in nursing is a lack of unity or a unified voice. However, this may be a "blame the victim" phenomenon similar to those seen in other women's issues. Such comments by government and administrators maintain the status quo; they need not do anything about the nursing problems since they are "nursing's problem." Therefore, systemic and legislative changes that would deal with quality of work-life and workplace issues are not addressed. Nurses should take pride in their differences and recognize that some among their number perceive the "shortage" issue to be a result of work-life balance and workplace problems common to nurses everywhere. Nursing has started to become more politically aware. Legislation and policies that direct how decisions are made and who makes them need to be fully appreciated by all nurses.

CONCLUSION

Data have shown that although Canada has not had a shortage of numbers of RNs, there is now a real possibility of a future shortage looming, the size and nature of which has been predicted by some recent reports. However, there are a number of problems related to working conditions that have been identified and solutions recommended but that are slow to be implemented. Retention of nurses along with recruitment is critical to address the ongoing nursing workforce pendulum. The problems continue to include lack of respect, limited autonomy and authority in clinical situations, lack of technological and management support, lack of educational opportunities, and an inability to participate in management decisions about resource allocation, which affects support services and staffing. The demand for nursing skills and knowledge continues and new and expanded roles for nurses are being implemented. Collaboration among government, administrators, and nurses continues to be a priority in order to deal adequately and comprehensively with the various quality-of-work-life issues facing nurses in Canada today.

CRITICAL THINKING QUESTIONS

1. Is the shortage of nurses caused by demand or supply factors?
2. Is there a "real" shortage of RNs?
3. What do you see as the most pressing issue for governments, nursing associations, administrators, and nurses to address?
4. What role might you play in dealing with the imbalance and challenges facing the profession of nursing?

WEB SITES

CANSIM: Statistics Canada's Key Socioeconomic Database: http://cansim2.statcan.ca/

Canadian Institute for Health Information (CIHI): http://secure.cihi.ca/cihiweb/dispPage.jsp?cw_page= home_e

Canadian Nurses Association of Canada: Publications & Resources: http://www.cna-aiic.ca/CNA/resources/ default_e.aspx

Nursing Education Program of Saskatchewan (NEPS) Reports: http://www.usask.ca/nursing/programs/ neps/reports.php

REFERENCES

Aiken, L. (1990). Charting the future of hospital nursing. *Image*, *22*(2), 72–78.

Aiken, L., & Mullinix, C. (1987). Special report: The nurse shortage—myth or reality? *New England Journal of Medicine*, *317*(10), 641–646.

Aiken, L. H., Clarke, S. P., & Sloane, D. M. (2002). Hospital staffing, organization, and quality of care: Cross-national findings. *Nursing Outlook*, *50*(5), 187–194.

Aiken, L. H., Clarke, S. P., Sloane, D. M., Lake, E. T., & Cheney, T. (2008). Effects of hospital care on patient mortality and outcomes. *Journal of Nursing Administration*, *38*(5), 223–229.

Aiken, L. H., Clarke, S. P., Sloane, D. M., Sochalski, J. A., Busse, R., Clarke, H., Giovanetti, P., Hunt, J., Rafferty, A. M., & Shamian, J. (2001). Nurses' reports on hospital care in five countries. *Health Affairs*, *20*(3), 43–53.

Aiken, L. H., Clarke, S. P., Sloane, D. M., Sochalski, J. A., & Silbur, J. H. (2002). Hospital nurse staffing and patient mortality, nurse burnout, and job satisfaction. *Journal of the American Medical Association*, *288*(16), 1987–1993.

Andrews, J., Manthorpe, M. A., & Watson, R. (2005). Employment transitions for older nurses: A qualitative study. *Nursing and Health Care Management and Policy*, *51*(3), 298–306.

Armstrong, K., Laschinger, H., & Wong, C. (2009). Workplace empowerment and magnet hospital characteristics as predictors of patient safety climate. *Journal of Nursing Care Quality*, *24*(1), 55–62.

Bartfay, W. J., & Howse, E. (2007). Who will teach the nurses of the future? *Canadian Nurse*, *103*(7), 24–27.

Baumann, A., O'Brien-Pallas, L., Armstrong-Stassen, M., Blythe, J., Bourbonnais, R., Cameron, S., et al. (2001). *Commitment and care: The benefits of a healthy workplace for nurses, their patients and the system*. Ottawa: Canadian Health Services Research Foundation.

Bower, F. L., & McCullough, C. (2004). Nurse shortage or nursing shortage: Have we missed the real problem? *Nursing Economics*, *22*(4), 200–203.

Buchan, J. (2002a). Global nursing shortages. *British Medical Journal*, *321*, 751–752.

Buchan, J. (2002b). Nursing shortages and evidence-based interventions: A case study from Scotland. *International Nursing Review*, *49*(4), 209–218.

Buerhaus, P. I., Auerbach, D. I., & Staiger, D. O. (2007). Recent trends in the registered nurse labor market in the U.S.: Short-run swings on top of long-term trends. *Nursing Economics*, *25*(2), 59–66.

Buerhaus, P. I., Donelan, B. T., DesRoches, C., & Dittus, R. (2007). Trends in the experiences of hospital-employed, registered nurses: Results from three national surveys. *Nursing Economics*, *25*(2), 69–79.

Buerhaus, P. I., Donelan, B. T., Ulrich, B. T., Norman, L., & Dittus, R. (2005). Is the shortage getting better or worse? From two recent national surveys of RNs. *Nursing Economics*, *23*(2), 61–71, 96.

Canadian Federation Nurses Union (CFNU). (2007). *CFNU Contract Comparison Document*. Nurses' Union Affiliated of CFNU and other unions representing nurses, researched and prepared by The Manitoba Nurses' Union, updated March 2007.

Canadian Institute for Health Information. (2003a). Workforce trends of licensed practical nurses in Canada, 2002. Retrieved on January 10, 2008, from http://secure.cihi.ca/cihiweb/dispPage.jsp?cw_page=pub_e.

Canadian Institute for Health Information. (2003b). Workforce trends of registered nurses in Canada, 2002. Retrieved on January 5, 2008, from http://secure.cihi.ca/cihiweb/dispPage.jsp?cw_page=pub_e.

Canadian Institute for Health Information. (2005). Workforce trends of registered nurses in Canada, 2004. Retrieved on January 15, 2008, from http://secure.cihi.ca/cihiweb/dispPage.jsp?cw_page=pub_e.

Canadian Institute for Health Information. (2006a). Findings from the 2005 National Health Survey of the Work & Health of Nurses. Co-published by Health Canada. Retrieved on December 5, 2007, from http://secure.cihi.ca/cihiweb/dispPage.jsp?cw_page=pub_e.

Canadian Institute for Health Information. (2006b). Health personnel trends in Canada, 1995 to 2004. Retrieved on December 4, 2007, from http://secure.cihi.ca/cihiweb/dispPage.jsp?cw_page=pub_e.

Canadian Institute for Health Information. (2006c). Measuring the retention of registered nurses in Canada: A study of 2000–2004 registration data. Source: Canadian Regulated Nursing Professions Database. Retrieved on January 7, 2008, from http://secure.cihi.ca/cihiweb/dispPage.jsp?cw_page=pub_e.

Canadian Institute for Health Information. (2007). *Registered Nursing Personnel Databases, Registered Nurses Database.* Retrieved September 11, 2009, from http://secure.cihi.ca/cihiweb/dispPage.jsp?cw_page=hhrdata_nursing_e.

Canadian Institute for Health Information. (2007a). Canada's health care providers, 2007. Retrieved on January 4, 2008, from http://secure.cihi.ca/cihiweb/dispPage.jsp?cw_page=pub_e.

Canadian Institute for Health Information. (2007b). Canadian MIS Database (CMDB), hospital financial performance indicators, 1999–2000 to 2004–2005 and Preliminary 2005–2006. Number of hospitals & number of hospital beds by province, territory and Canada. Retrieved on January 14, 2008, from http://secure.cihi.ca/cihiweb/dispPage.jsp?cw_page=statistics_a_z_e.

Canadian Institute for Health Information. (2007c). Highlights from the regulated nursing workforce in Canada, 2006. Retrieved on December 16, 2007, from http://secure.cihi.ca/cihiweb/dispPage.jsp?cw_page=pub_e.

Canadian Institute for Health Information. (2007d). Highlights of 2006–2007 inpatient hospitalizations and emergency department visits. Retrieved on December 16, 2007, from http://secure.cihi.ca/cihiweb/dispPage.jsp?cw_page=pub_e.

Canadian Institute for Health Information. (2007e). Trends in acute inpatient hospitalizations and day surgery visits in Canada, 1995–1996 to 2005–2006. Retrieved on December 16, 2008, from http://secure.cihi.ca/cihiweb/dispPage.jsp?cw_page=pub_e.

Canadian Institute for Health Information. (2007f). Workforce trends of licensed practical nurses in Canada, 2006. Retrieved on January 20, 2008, from http://secure.cihi.ca/cihiweb/dispPage.jsp?cw_page=pub_e.

Canadian Institute for Health Information. (2007g). Workforce trends of registered nurses in Canada, 2006. Retrieved on December 2, 2007, from http://secure.cihi.ca/cihiweb/dispPage.jsp?cw_page=pub_e.

Canadian Institute for Health Information. (2008). *Regulated Nurses: Trends 2003– 2007.* Ottawa: CIHI. Retrieved on August 21, 2009, from http://secure.cihi.ca/cihiweb/products/nursing_report_2003_to_2007_e.pdf.

Canadian Institute for Health Information. (2009). *Regulated nurses: Canadian trends, 2004 to 2008.* Ottawa: CIHI. Retrieved on January 14, 2010, from http://secure.cihi.ca/cihiweb/products/regulated_nurses_2004_2008_en.pdf.

Canadian Nurses Association. (2006). Toward 2020: Visions for nursing. Retrieved on November 14, 2007, from http://www.cna.aiic.ca/CNA/resources.

Canadian Nurses Association. (2007). Canadian Registered Nurse Examination (CRNE), statistics on CRNE writers for calendar year 2006. Retrieved on January 10, 2008, from http://www.cna.aiic.ca/CNA/resources.

Canadian Nurses Association and Canadian Association of Schools of Nursing. (2007). Nursing education in Canada statistics 2005–2006. Retrieved on January 10, 2008, from http://www.cna.aiic.ca/CNA/resources.

Carroll, T. L. (2005). Stressful life events among new nurses: Implications for retaining new graduates. *Nursing Administration, 29*(3), 292–296.

College of Nurses of Ontario. (2008). Membership statistics report 2007. Retrieved on January 12, 2008, from http://www.cno.org/docs/general/43069_stats_MemberStats2007-final.pdf.

Donnelly, L. J., Yarbrough, D., & Jaffe, H. (1989). Organizational management systems decrease nursing costs. *Nursing Management, 20*(7), 20–21.

Duffield, C., O'Brien-Pallas, L., Aitken, L., Roche, M., & Merrick, E. T. (2006). Recruitment of nurses working outside nursing. *Journal of Nursing Administration, 36*(2), 58–62.

Duxbury, L., & Higgins, C. (2005). Report Four: Who is at risk? Predictors of work–life conflict. Retrieved on January 25, 2008, from http://www.phac-aspc.gc.ca/publicat/work-travail/report4/index.html.

Fisher, A., Baumann, A., & Blythe, J. (2007). The effects of organizational flexibility on nurse utilization and vacancy statistics in Ontario hospitals. *Canadian Journal of Nursing Leadership (CJNL), 20*(4), 48–64.

Gifford, B. D., Zammuto, R. F., & Goodman, E. A. (2002). The relationship between hospital unit culture and nurses' quality of work life. *Journal of Healthcare Management*, *47*(1), 13–25.

Glandon, G. L., Colbert, K. W., & Thomasma, M. (1989). Nursing delivery models and RN mix: Cost implications. *Nursing Management*, *20*(5), 30–33.

Goodwin, S. (2007). Telephone nursing: An emerging practice area. *Canadian Journal of Nursing Leadership (CJNL)*, *20*(4), 38–46.

Hall, L. M., Doran, D., & Pink, L. (2008). Outcomes of interventions to improve hospital nursing work environments. *Journal of Nursing Administration*, *38*(1), 40–46.

Hall, L. M., Doran, D., Pink, L., LaLonde, M., Murphy, G. T., O'Brien-Pallas, L., Laschinger, H. K., Torangeau, A., Besner, J., White, D., Tregunno, D., Thomson, D., Peterson, J., Seto, L., & Akeroyd, J. (2006). Decision making for nurse staffing: Canadian perspectives. *Policy, Politics, & Nursing Practice*, *7*(4), 261–269.

Hart, K. A. (2007). The aging workforce: Implications for health organizations. *Nursing Economics*, *25*(2), 101–192.

Health Canada. (2001). *Healthy nurses: Healthy workplaces.* Proceedings of the 2000 National Stakeholder Consultation Meeting. The Office of Nursing Policy. Ottawa: Author.

Hugonnet, S., Chevrolet, J. C., & Pittet, D. (2007). The effect of workload on infection risk in critically ill patients. *Critical Care Medicine*, *35*(1), 296–298.

Johnson, M. (1989). Perspectives on costing nursing. *Nursing Administration Quarterly*, *14*(1), 65–71.

Jones, C. B. (1990). Staff nurse turnover costs: Part II measurements and results. *Journal of Nursing Administration*, *20*(5), 27–32.

Ketefian, S., Redman, R. W., Hanucharurnkul, S., Masterson, A., & Neves, E. P. (2001). The development of advanced practice roles: Implications in the international nursing community. *International Nursing Review*, *48*(3), 152–163.

Lang, T. A., Hodge, M., Olson, V., Romano, P. S., & Kravitz, R. L. (2004). Nurse–patient ratios: A systematic review on the effects of nurse staffing on patient, nurse employee, and hospital outcomes. *Journal of Nursing Administration*, *34*(7/8), 326–337.

Laschinger, H. K. S., Wong, C. A., & Greco, P. (2006). The impact of staff nurse empowerment on person-job fit and work engagement/burnout. *Nursing Administration Quarterly*, *30*(4), 358–367.

Leners, D. W., Wilson, V. W., Connor, P., & Fenton, J. (2006). Mentorship: Increasing retention probabilities. *Journal of Nursing Management*, *14*, 652–654.

McGillis Hall, L. (1997). Staff mix models: Complementary or substitution roles for nurses. *Nursing Administration Quarterly*, *21*(2), 31–39.

McGillis Hall, L. (1998a, January/February). The use of unregulated workers in Toronto hospitals. *Canadian Journal of Nursing Administration*, 8–30.

McGillis Hall, L. (1998b). Policy implications when changing staff mix. *Nursing Economics*, *16*(6), 291–297, 312.

McGillis Hall, L., Doran, D., & Pink, L. (2008). Outcomes of interventions to improve hospital nursing work environments. *Journal of Nursing Administration*, *38*(1), 40–46.

McGillis Hall, L., & O'Brien-Pallas, L. (2000). Redesigning nursing work in long term care environments. *Nursing Economics*, *18*(2), 79–87.

McGillis Hall, L., Pink, G., Johnson, L. M., & Schraa, E. G. (2000a). Developing a nursing practice atlas. Part 1: Methodological approaches to ensure data consistency. *Journal of Nursing Administration*, *30*(7/8), 364–372.

McGillis Hall, L., Pink, G., Johnson, L. M., & Schraa, E. G. (2000b). Developing a nursing practice atlas. Part 2: Variation in use of nursing and financial resources. *Journal of Nursing Administration*, *30*(9), 440–448.

Meltz, N., & Marzetti, J. (1988). *The shortage of registered nurses: An analysis in a labour market context.* Toronto: Registered Nurses Association of Ontario.

Miller, J. (1992). Use of unlicensed assistive personnel in acute care settings. *Journal of Nursing Administration*, *22*(12), 12–13.

O'Brien-Pallas, L., Duffield, C., & Hayes, L. (2006). Do we really understand how to retain nurses? *Journal of Nursing Management, 14,* 262–270.

O'Brien-Pallas, L., Griffin, P., Shamian, J., Buchan, J., Duffield, C., Hughes, F., Laschinger, H. K. S., North, N., & Stone, P. W. (2006). The impact of nurse turnover on patient, nurse and system outcomes: A pilot study and focus for a multicenter international study. *Policy, Politics & Nursing Practice, 7,* 169–179.

O'Brien-Pallas, L., Shamian, J., Thomson, D., Alksnis, C., Kerr, M., & Bruce, S. (2004). Work-related disability in Canadian nurses. *Journal of Nursing Scholarship, 36*(4), 352–357.

Oulton, J. A. (2006). The global nursing shortage: Overview of issues and actions. *Policy, Politics & Nursing Practice, 7*(3), 34S–39S.

Pendry, P. S. (2007). Moral distress: Recognizing it to retain nurses. *Nursing Economics, 25*(4), 217–221.

Presho, M. (2006). Earning and learning. Recruitment and retention in post registration nurse education. *Nurse Education Today, 26,* 511–518.

Qmentum. (2008). Accreditation Canada. Retrieved on June 24, 2010, from http://www.accreditation.ca/accred itationprograms/qmentum/required-organizational_practices/.

Ross, E. (2003). From shortage to oversupply: The workforce pendulum. In J. C. Ross-Kerr, & M. J. Wood (Eds.), *Canadian Nursing* (4th ed.) (pp. 229–243). Toronto: Elsevier Science Canada.

Ryten, E. (1988, June). *Women as deliverers of health care. Unpublished speech presented at the Canadian Association of University Schools of Nursing Annual Conference.* Windsor, Ontario: University of Windsor.

Shamian, J., O'Brien-Pallas, L., Kerr, M., Koehoorn, M., Thomson, D., & Alksnis, C. (2001). *Effects of job strain, hospital organizational factors and individual characteristics on work-related disability among nurses.* Toronto: Workplace Safety and Insurance Board.

Statistics Canada. (2005). Labour markets, business activity, and population growth and mobility in Canadian CMAs. Retrieved on January 27, 2008, from http://cansim2.statcan.ca/cgi.

Statistics Canada. (2007). Labour force projections for Canada, 2006–2031. Retrieved on January 27, 2008, from http://cansim2.statcan.ca/cgi.

Stone, P. W., & Gershon, R. R. (2006). Nurse work environment and occupational safety in intensive care units. *Policy, Politics & Nursing Practice, 7*(4), 240–247.

Stone, P. W., Mooney-Kane, C., Larson, E. L., Horan, T., Glance, L. G., Zwaziger, J., & Dick, A. W. (2007). Nurse working conditions and patient safety outcomes. *Medical Care, 45*(6), 571–578.

Stordeur, S., & D'Hoore, W. (2006). Organizational configuration of hospitals succeeding in attracting and retaining nurses. *Journal of Advanced Nursing, 57*(1), 45–58.

Tourangeau, A. E., Doran, D. M., McGillis Hall, L., O'Brien-Pallas, L., Pringle, D., Tu, J. V., & Cranley, L. A. (2007). Impact of hospital nursing care on 30-day mortality for acute medical patients. *Journal of Advanced Nursing, 57*(1), 32–44.

Upenieks, V. (2003). Recruitment and retention strategies: A magnet hospital prevention model. *Nursing Economics, 21*(1), 7–13, 23.

Vandevelde-Coke, S. (2007). Interview with Susan Vandevelde-Coke. *Canadian Journal of Nursing Leadership, 20*(4). Retrieved on January 23, 2008, from http://www.longwoods.com.libaccess.lib. mcmaster.ca/product.

West, E., Barron, D. N., & Reeves, R. (2005). Overcoming the barriers to patient-centred care: Time, tools and training. *Journal of Clinical Nursing, 14*(4), 435–443.

Widger, K., Pye, C., Cranley, L., Wilson-Keates, B., Squires, M., & Tourangeau, A. (2007). Generational differences in acute care nurses. *Canadian Journal of Nursing Leadership, 20*(1), 49–61.

Wilson, A. A. (2005). Impact of management development on nurse retention. *Nursing Administration Quarterly, 29*(2), 137–145.

Wittmann-Price, R., & Kuplen, C. (2003). A recruitment and retention program that works! *Nursing Economics, 21*(1), 35–38.

Zeytinoglu, I. U., Denton, M., Davies, S., Baumann, A., Blythe, J., & Boos, L. (2006). Retaining nurses in their employing hospitals and in the profession: Effects of job preference, unpaid overtime, importance of earnings and stress. *Health Policy, 79*(1), 57–72.

16 Political Awareness in Nursing

Janet C. Ross-Kerr

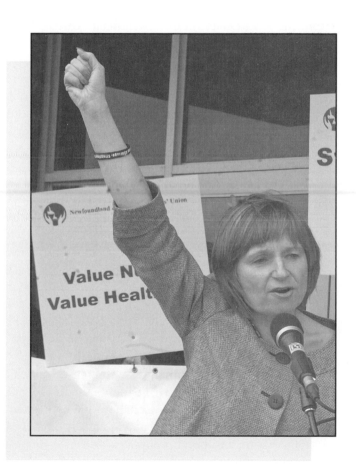

LEARNING OBJECTIVES

- To appreciate the importance of developing political awareness in professional practice.
- To understand the fundamentals of political action.
- To highlight the importance of interpersonal communication in meeting professional goals.
- To explain the importance of developing a base of support to achieve goals.
- To recognize the importance of developing strategies to achieve professional goals.
- To identify the benefits of enhanced political awareness.

Health care is "big business," and each of the health professions has an important stake in it. As the largest of the health professions, nursing must be unreservedly involved in the debate over the future of health care in Canada. Since the enactment of legislation establishing a national health insurance system for hospital and medical care, the philosophical basis of the system has been open to question. Historically, the proportion of private and public expenditures for health has remained relatively stable. Of health expenditures in 2007, 70% were funded from public sources, while 30% were funded from private sources (OECD, 2009). There has been a slight trend in the past five years toward higher private expenditures, accounted for by higher expenditures for pharmaceuticals. The public–private debate continues as more conservative elements of society argue for a system based entirely in the private sector, while those with more liberal leanings push either for maintaining the status quo or for increasing the proportion of costs funded through the public sector.

The fact that physicians have continued to be the sole gatekeepers to the health care system has led to continuing problems for those who wish access to the system, and to higher costs than would be incurred if nonphysician health care providers were used more effectively. Nurses in particular have historically been underused, despite the fact that a number of Canadian studies have demonstrated the effectiveness of services provided by nurses (Chambers, Bruce-Lockhart, Black, Sampson, & Burke, 1977; Hoey, McCallum, & LePage, 1982; Ramsay, McKenzie, & Fish, 1982). A study of 47,000 Ontario patients by the Institute of Clinical Evaluative Services provided evidence linking nursing knowledge to lower mortality rates (Canadian Nurses Association, 2002). Another study suggested that higher nurse staffing and a richer skill mix, particularly of registered nurses, resulted in improved patient outcomes (Lankshear, Sheldon, & Maynard, 2005). A review for the Cochrane Collaboration concluded that nurses in primary care settings could provide health care that was equally effective to that of physicians (Laurant et al., 2004). Compensation for physicians on a fee-for-service basis (versus salary or contract) is considered to be an important factor in the underutilization of nurses.

Since 10.1% of the gross domestic product was attributed to health expenditures in Canada in 2007 (OECD, 2009), any public-sector activity that involves substantial expenditure of tax dollars engenders considerable debate and competition among providers of the service. This is obvious in health care, where the various professions compete to increase their "share of the pie." Physicians have been extraordinarily successful in increasing income earned for services provided. Physicians' incomes have risen considerably over the past half century, attesting to the success they have had in the political arena. Nurses, through their unions and professional organizations, have demonstrated a growing ability to argue for proportionately greater compensation for their services. Significant gains have thus been made in the past 20 years.

The fact that nursing continues to be a sex-segregated profession must be considered a factor in its status, prestige, and ability to argue for appropriate funding for the professional services provided. Increased awareness of the need for respect for women's rights has occurred gradually over the past century, and important gains have been made in the past three decades. The parallel rise of the women's movement and unionism in nursing, which began in the 1960s, has been a significant development. Members of the profession challenge the status quo assiduously and assertively, striving for higher salaries and better working conditions. Nurses have gradually gained understanding of the processes and skills involved in influencing others, becoming more powerful and exercising more control over the factors that influence their working lives.

Although nurses are commonly thought of as political novices, there are many examples over time of situations in which nurses have engaged in political action and done so successfully. In the early history of Canadian nursing, Jeanne Mance could be considered a political activist par excellence, as she raised and sustained support for her hospital and for the colony in New France. Florence Nightingale's accomplishments as well are legendary, and the success of her nurses in ministering to sick and wounded soldiers in the Crimea brought the potential contributions of well prepared nurses who were women to the top of the public agenda. Nightingale's skill as a researcher was impressive, and her interpretation of the statistics she collected led to important and lasting changes in the organization of the health service of the British Army (Nightingale, 1858). She demonstrated the positive effect of sanitation and nutrition on the health of soldiers; her principles now apply to health care in the general population. There were important offshoots from her work for the British people—and indeed for people in other nations—as the principles that Nightingale championed were carried far afield.

Nurses in Canada argued strongly between 1900 and 1922 for legislation encompassing registration for nurses. The provincial campaigns were successful—every province had such legislation by 1922, when Ontario passed its first regulatory act for the nursing profession. More recent political activity by nurses has also been successful. The lobbying carried out by the Canadian Nurses Association (CNA) for the *Canada Health Act* of 1984 resulted in an amendment to the act after it was tabled in Parliament that permitted federal funding for "health practitioners." This legislation also made it possible for a provincial health plan to fund services of nurses or other health providers on a direct reimbursement basis, as the services of physicians and dental surgeons had been financed since the *Medical Care Act* of 1968 was passed. The fact that no province has yet implemented the health practitioner clause speaks to the lobbying power of physicians to maintain the medical profession's traditional and very expensive form of remuneration.

As primarily public-sector employees, nurses find themselves within highly hierarchical and bureaucratized structures in health organizations. In order to achieve their goals, they must lobby at a number of levels within organizations. Because health is a provincial responsibility at the level of the organized profession, nurses must approach provincial government legislators with their ideas for change, as it is this level of government that is responsible for public health expenditures. At the national level, the CNA interacts with the federal government in relation to national issues affecting health. Within each health agency, nurses must approach management with their ideas for systemic change. As most health agencies are unionized, the process for doing so at the agency level is normally outlined clearly.

There have been many other examples of nurses' involvement in lobbying for important public health measures. Some examples include campaigns by nurses to improve safety in the home, to encourage governments to enact seat-belt legislation, and to promote the use of bicycle helmets. A glance at the Web sites of the various provincial and territorial nurses' associations gives an indication of the breadth and depth of a multitude of issues being addressed today by organized nursing in Canada. A notable example of a unique Internet resource developed by the Registered Nurses' Association of Ontario is designed to develop nurses' counselling skills to assist individuals to stop smoking (RNAO, 2007). There have also been numerous examples of activism by nursing students. When the province-wide baccalaureate Nursing Education Program of Saskatchewan was developed in the 1990s (College of Nursing, University of Saskatchewan, 2009), the provincial government attempted to put a diploma exit in place. However, it was thwarted by nursing students protesting at the legislature in Regina, suitcases in hand, threatening to leave the province if the proposal went ahead. In September 2009, Alberta nursing students held a rally at the legislature in Edmonton to protest drastic provincial cuts in health care spending that would eliminate a large part of the nursing workforce, thus forcing new graduates to leave the province (McLean, 2009).

THE IMPORTANCE OF DEVELOPING POLITICAL AWARENESS

The term "politics" is used in many different ways. For some it may stimulate images of smoke-filled rooms, devious dealings, or power in the hands of a few. For others, the images have a different and more generic meaning. Among the earliest philosophers who attempted to understand the relationship between politics and people were Aristotle and Plato. Plato discussed the development of political leaders in some depth in *The Republic*, describing the qualities of leadership. For Aristotle, individuals were charged with the responsibility to support the common good through the domain of philosophy he called politics.

Politics can be viewed as the art of influencing another person. In practical terms, political activity means influencing for the purpose of allocating scarce resources wisely. In health care, recognition of the limits to growth of care and treatment has been a reality for some time. High-technology health care is expensive, and decisions may have to be made in some cases about health care priorities. Limits on the need to use certain technologies in the most effective and efficient way is increasingly meaning that not everyone can receive expensive care and treatment. Certain individuals will be responsible for deciding how to allocate the available resources, while others will have a political responsibility to provide the rationale for allocating resources in one way or another. Nurses have a responsibility to evaluate decisions that are made to allocate those resources and argue for just decisions for the care of their patients.

Many nurses recognize the importance of developing political skills, realizing that these are as important on the nursing unit as elsewhere. There tends to be more awareness of the importance of political factors in the development of policy than in patient-care environments. Where service is the primary activity, the politics of patient care may be less visible, but they are important and essential to good care. Nevertheless, there can be no better reason for enhancing the political skills of nurses than to improve the care of patients (see Box 16.1).

Nurses as a group have sometimes expressed a sense of powerlessness. Some nurses believe that nursing is low in the health care hierarchy when it comes to power and influence. These nurses adopt an indifferent approach, believing that expressing their views will not be useful because they will not be heard. A nurse who adopts such an attitude will not be able to argue for the needs of patients. These negative attitudes are based on false assumptions about society and a lack of understanding of the history of successful lobbying by the nursing profession. Fortunately, more nurses are taking an active interest in political activity and in learning how to influence others. Although professional groups have always recognized the value of lobbying for their objectives and using political skills to advantage, they are now attempting to educate members about developing political skills to enhance success in achieving goals.

Nurses have to work very hard at establishing and maintaining a power base, just as other professional groups devote considerable time, money, and energy toward a similar goal. There is strength in numbers, and that is an important factor where nursing is concerned because nurses are the largest group of health care professionals. Nurses have been striving to improve their educational level so that they will be on a par educationally with other members of the health team. The educational level is rising relatively rapidly, and 31.5% of registered nurses in 2005 held a baccalaureate degree (CNA, 2006). In addition, nurses have struggled with an image of subservience, partially because of gender-stereotyping of the profession. The proportion of the profession that is female

---

BOX 16.1   Why Should Registered Nurses Take Action?

- Nurses have a very high level of credibility with the public.
- Nurses bring a unique perspective and knowledge to health policy issues.
- Nurses are successful advocates!

Source: RNAO. (2006). *Framework for political action. Taking action!* (p. 3). Toronto. ON. Author. Retrieved on March 27, 2008, from http://www.rnao.org/Storage/18/1224_Framework_for_Political_Action_-_Sec_1.pdf.

was 94.2% in 2007 (Canadian Institute for Health Information, 2007). The medical profession, on the other hand, has historically been male dominated, but this is rapidly changing. In some medical schools, more than 50% of the students are women. The gender-stereotype in nursing is deeper, and men are not yet entering the nursing profession in rapidly increasing numbers—certainly not at the rate women are entering traditionally male-dominated professions. Nevertheless, changes are occurring because of the women's movement, increased recognition of human rights, and increased acknowledgement of nursing's contribution to health care. These factors bode well for nursing in the future, as arguments for restructuring and policy change within the health care system are likely to engender considerable interest and support.

 REFLECTIVE THINKING

1. From your perspective, reflect on how nurses can make a difference in the health care system through political action.
2. Highlight some of the most important contemporary health care issues and identify strategies involving political action to address these.

CREATING POLITICAL AWARENESS: UNDERSTANDING THE FUNDAMENTALS OF POLITICAL ACTION

Nurses can greatly enhance the achievement of their goals by learning how to work within the formal and informal systems in the workplace. Although it is essential to understand both, comprehending the informal structures and processes of an organization is a more difficult and less defined task than understanding formal ones. There is no substitute for understanding how an organization works or for thinking carefully about the nature and scope of problems and how they might be solved.

Although many nurses do not see themselves as able to take on political action in circumstances in which they would like to achieve a particular goal, those who do venture forth, if somewhat timidly at first, are often amazed by the fact that elected officials are often eager to hear what they have to say and show respect for their ideas. The fact of the matter is that the ordinary nurse is capable of communicating ideas effectively and being a highly positive asset in a campaign to achieve health care goals. Nurses are among the most highly educated of professional and occupational groups and have training in working with people and expressing ideas. Thus, they tend to be highly effective communicators and command respect from others for their knowledge.

It is also important to develop good communication skills in order to work effectively with others to understand both their roles and functions and the problems they face. Those wielding substantial power within the organization should be identified as key individuals, and the development of working relationships with these people is essential. Informal groups and social contacts within the organization may also be important, and although they may be organized around activities unrelated to the organization, they may represent networks for exchange of information and political activity.

Nurses must be risk takers, as no gains will be made if action is not taken. Timing is essential to achieving a goal. It is necessary to understand all sides of the question to develop a more effective strategy, and negotiation and compromise may be required in the final solution. A high degree of communication skill is required. The example provided by Cathy Crowe, a Toronto community health nurse, often referred to respectfully as a "street nurse," is instructive (Keung, 2009). Crowe has advocated for vulnerable populations for more than two decades and is clearly a highly skilled political activist and tireless worker whose objective is to improve conditions for homeless people in Toronto.

CANADIAN RESEARCH FOCUS

Hardill, K. (2006). From the Grey Nuns to the streets: A critical history of outreach nursing in Canada. *Public Health Nursing, 24*(1), 91–97.

The origins of outreach nursing in Canada can be found in the work of Marguerite d'Youville, who founded the Grey Nuns in 1737. Other examples of social activism for health cited as background include Florence Nightingale in the United Kingdom in the nineteenth century, Lillian Wald in the United States in the twentieth century, and Lady Ishbel Aberdeen in Canada who founded the Victorian Order of Nurses, also in the twentieth century. This unique work examines the origins of "street nursing" in Vancouver, Toronto, and Montreal and in doing so addresses a topic that has received little attention in the literature. Written by a nurse with a strong background in outreach nursing, this work underscores the need for political advocacy for vulnerable populations, and in particular those who are homeless and living in poverty. Indeed, a convincing case is made for political advocacy on behalf of the less fortunate and powerless in Canadian society.

A political action and advocacy guide prepared by the professional nursing association in Alberta (AARN, 2004) offers assistance in political action to individuals or groups of nurses, covering techniques such as individual communications and campaigns using letters, fax, and e-mail messages. There are also sections that address face-to-face meetings and telephone conversations with elected officials as well as dealing with the media. As it is important to have sufficient background when one is engaged in political activity with the goal of achieving a particular outcome, it is wise to gain as much information as possible in order to enhance the success of the effort. Another resource prepared by the Canadian Nurses Association (1997) focuses on lobbying the federal government and gives some suggestions for organizing a campaign to achieve particular goals at the national level.

INTERPERSONAL COMMUNICATION

The most important factor in the political arena is effective interpersonal communication. Because politics involves influencing others, effective relationships are essential. It is impossible to influence others if interpersonal activity is not positive and dynamic. As noted above, communication is the fundamental skill in political action, as all of the other techniques build on it. By communicating effectively with others, goals may be

enhanced and attained. Joining with others in pursuit of common goals is a very effective technique and is also recognized as an effective political strategy. It is important to
work cooperatively and willingly with others in pursuing collective goals. Approaching
others with respect and understanding increases the possibility that political activity will
be enhanced and more effective.

Although communication is important on every level, its fundamental tenets remain
the same. Attention has recently focused on networking, or joining together with others to achieve common goals. This can be accomplished in many ways. Networking is
an important political strategy, and it may be personally rewarding. Nursing curricula
usually contain courses designed to enhance interpersonal effectiveness. Because nurses
are in close contact with patients, preparation in the area of interpersonal communication is essential to good patient care. This is a subject that is emphasized in baccalaureate
degree programs.

The advent of the Internet as a vehicle for communication in the twenty-first century is revolutionizing communication around the world. In the sphere of politics,
legislators who ignore the power of the Internet for communicating with their constituents do so at their peril! In health care generally, people are turning to Web-
based health resources for assistance in understanding their health issues. With a
strong background in communication, nurses are well placed to assume important
roles in developing and maintaining e-health and telehealth-based resources. Nursing
informatics is an important and growing area, and the Canadian Nursing Informatics Association has been active in developing standards and competencies expected
of registered nurses (see Chapter 10). The NurseOne portal (CNA, 2009) launched
by the CNA provides Web-based access to learning resources for registered nurses.
This Web resource includes new health information of various kinds, public health
concerns and alerts, news bulletins, and professional responses to health issues. The
public home page includes login access for registered nurses for a broader range of
information.

DEVELOPING A BASE OF SUPPORT

Consolidating and developing a base of support often takes considerable skill and
time. Credibility must be established, and the desire to work in the best interests
of the organization and its goals must be demonstrated. In professional associations, this means working with the public interest in mind. It is important to demonstrate that clear and careful thought preceded the development of a campaign
for support on a particular issue, as this may be a powerful factor in convincing
potential allies that the issue is worth supporting. As noted previously, there is
power in numbers, and nursing has a great advantage in this respect. The campaign
is more likely to be successful if many people are committed to working toward
the goal. Although nurses have not always recognized the strength in their numbers, they have been successful in the past in mobilizing group support on crucial
issues. Many nursing organizations now recognize this potent force and are using
its power to advantage.

THE PURSUIT OF GOALS

Effective political strategy is a labour-intensive process that requires clear thinking and the ability to recognize factors, processes, and actors of importance. Identifying an issue or problem is crucial (see Box 16.2). Its relative importance must be measured against that of other issues or problems that arise. Action cannot be taken in all matters, so it is wise to choose one's issues. There is always some cost in pursuing a problem to its conclusion in the political sphere, and the possible negative consequences must be weighed against the positive benefits that may result. One must consider carefully the possible benefits and downsides of taking action on an issue to determine in advance, as much as possible, whether it is worth it.

Analysis is essential to determine whether pursuing the issue is reasonable. Once a decision has been made to pursue a particular goal, additional analysis determines what other resources might be helpful.

Because every issue is different, a plan of action must be outlined for the benefit of all those involved in the campaign. It is important to determine how the issue will be dealt with, both formally and informally. It is possible that many avenues will need to be taken to argue for or against the issue of concern. These need to be outlined at the outset and revised as necessary. One person alone may be able to make the case for change, or it may be necessary for an entire organization to be involved. This was the case when the Alberta Association of Registered Nurses (AARN) lobbied for the passage of a new act governing nursing in Alberta incorporating mandatory registration. The entire membership was asked to send letters of support to members of the Legislative Assembly and the Cabinet. Ultimately, the fact that so many of the AARN members got involved influenced the legislators to decide to move forward with the act.

Bowman (1985) refers to professional strategies, public strategies, and procedural strategies as categories that can be considered when plans are being developed to pursue an issue. A contemporary issue of interest across the country is the legalization of midwifery in Canada. Although midwifery developed from its roots in nursing, and currently the vast majority of midwives are nurses, midwives have, through extensive lobbying, been able to convince legislators and the general public that a separate and independent profession is in the public interest. Legislation to legalize midwifery has been passed in several provinces, and an infrastructure is emerging to support the regulation of the profession and the development of educational programs to prepare midwives.

BOX 16.2   How Can Registered Nurses Become Involved?

- Talk to your neighbours and co-workers about a health policy issue.
- Respond to a call for action from your provincial professional association.
- Write to your member of parliament or legislative assembly member about a health policy issue that is important to you.
- Lend your expertise and voice as an RN to a community issue.
- Run for office.
- Call your professional association and colleagues and ask for assistance.

Source: Adapted from RNAO. (2006). *Framework for political action: Taking action!* (p. 3). Toronto, ON: RNAO. Retrieved on March 27, 2008, from http://www.rnao.org/Storage/18/1224_Framework_for_Political_Action_-_Sec_1.pdf.

BENEFITS OF ENHANCED POLITICAL AWARENESS

Much can be gained by developing a cadre of politically skilled professional nurses. Dr. Ginette Lemire Rodger (1993), CNA president from 2000 to 2002, has asserted that "our challenge is to exercise our power and influence and use the political process to help bring about a major change in the delivery of nursing services to the society" (p. 25). There are important public implications for such activity, at both the individual and collective levels. The priorities of patient care are subject to politics at all levels. Nurses spend more time with patients than any other group of health care providers and are in an excellent position to understand, appreciate, and argue for consideration of their needs and concerns. Nurses must also continue to work for optimum conditions in the workplace because the quality of nursing care will be enhanced through the pursuit of this goal. Collaboration between nurses and other health care providers can do much to enhance nurses' effectiveness. Most important of all, understanding the political process and recognizing political strategy is a decisive first step in developing the ability to influence others.

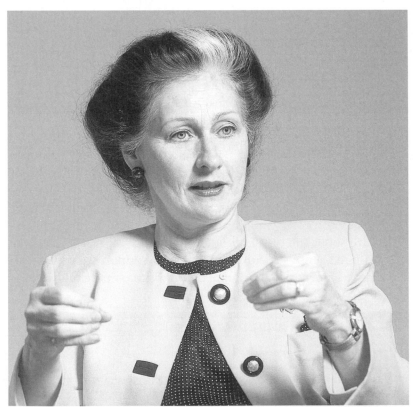

Dr. Ginette Lemire Rodger, president of the Canadian Nurses Association 2000–2002, encourages nurses to "use the political process to help bring about a major change in the delivery of nursing services."

CRITICAL THINKING QUESTIONS

1. Discuss the relevance of health care expenditures for the nursing profession.
2. What are some of the major issues for nurses in times of economic depression?
3. How can nurses advocate on behalf of their patients?
4. Identify some benefits of enhanced political activity by nurses.

WEB SITES

Canadian Nurses Association: http://www.cna-nurses.ca
Canadian Nurses Association NurseOne Portal: http://www.nurseone.ca/

REFERENCES

Alberta Association of Registered Nurses. (2004). *Turn up the heat! Political action and advocacy guide.* Edmonton: AARN. Retrieved on March 27, 2008, from http://www.nurses.ab.ca/pdf/Advocacy Guidefinal.pdf.

Bowman, R. A. (1985). Recognizing, developing, and pursuing an issue. In D. J. Mason, & S. W. Talbott (Eds.), *Political action handbook for nurses* (pp. 196–204). Menlo Park, CA: Addison-Wesley.

Canadian Institute for Health Information. (2007). *Workforce profile of registered nurses in Canada. 2007.* Retrieved on September 27, 2009, from http://secure.cihi.ca/cihiweb/dispPage.jsp?cw_page=statistics_results_topic_nurses_e&cw_topic=Health%20Human%20Resources&cw_subtopic=Nurses.

Canadian Nurses Association (CNA). (1997). *Getting started: A political action guide for Canada's registered nurses.* Ottawa: Author.

Canadian Nurses Association. (2002). Press release: Canadian study provides evidence linking nursing knowledge to lower mortality rates. Ottawa: Author.

Canadian Nurses Association. (2006). *2005 workforce profile of registered nurses in Canada.* Ottawa: CNA. Retrieved on March 27, 2008, from http://www.cna-nurses.ca/CNA/documents/pdf/publications/work force-profile-2005-e.pdf.

Canadian Nurses Association. (2009). *NurseOne portal, public home page.* Retrieved on April 29, 2010, from http://www.nurseone.ca.

Chambers, L. W., Bruce-Lockhart, P., Black, D. P., Sampson, E., & Burke, M. (1977). A controlled trial of the impact of the family practice nurse on volume, quality, and cost of rural health service. *Medical Care, 15*(12), 971–981.

College of Nursing, University of Saskatchewan. (2009). *History of the College of Nursing.* Retrieved on September 29, 2009, from http://www.usask.ca/nursing/college/history.php.

Hoey, J. R., McCallum, H. P., & LePage, E. M. (1982). Expanding the nurse's role to improve preventive service in an outpatient clinic. *Canadian Medical Association Journal, 127*(1), 27–28.

Keung, N. (2009). *Cathy Crowe: Toronto's street nurse.* Retrieved on September 29, 2009, from http://www.streetlevelconsulting.ca/biographies/Cathy_Crowe.htm.

Lankshear, A., Sheldon, T. A., & Maynard, A. B. (2005). Nurse staffing and healthcare outcomes: A systematic review of the international research evidence. *Advances in Nursing Science, 28*(2), 163–174.

Laurant, M., Reeves, D., Hermens, R., Braspenning, J., Grol, R., & Sibbald, B. (2004). Substitution of doctors by nurses in primary care (Review). *Cochrane Database of Systematic Reviews* (Issue 4), Art. No. CD00127/14651858.CD00127.pub2.

McLean, A. (2009). Generations of nurses will be lost to Alberta, students say. *Edmonton Journal,* September 25, 2009. Retrieved on September 29, 2009, from http://www.edmontonjournal.com/news/Alberta+nursing+students+protest+cuts/2028802/story.html#.

Nightingale, F. (1858). *Notes on matters affecting the health, efficiency and hospital administration of the British Army*. London: Harrison & Sons.

Organisation for Economic Co-operation and Development. (2009). *OECD Health Data 2009*. Retrieved on September 29, 2009, from http://stats.oecd.org/Index.aspx?DatasetCode=HEALTH.

Ramsay, J. A., McKenzie, J. K., & Fish, D. G. (1982). Physicians and nurse practitioners: Do they provide equivalent health care? *American Journal of Public Health*, *72*(1), 55–57.

Registered Nurses Association of Ontario. (2006). *Framework for political action: Taking action!* Toronto: RNAO. Retrieved on March 27, 2008, from http://www.rnao.org/Storage/18/1224_Framework_for_Political_Action_-_Sec_1.pdf.

Registered Nurses Association of Ontario. (2007). *Website that encourages nurses to counsel smokers is the first in Canada*. Toronto: RNAO. Retrieved on March 27, 2008, from http://www.rnao.org/Page.asp?PageID=122&ContentID=2016&SiteNodeID=382&BL_ExpandID=.

Rodger, G. L. (1993). Nurses and the political process. *AARN Newsletter*, *49*(2), 24–25.

17 Emergence of Nursing Unions as a Social Force in Canada

Janet C. Ross-Kerr

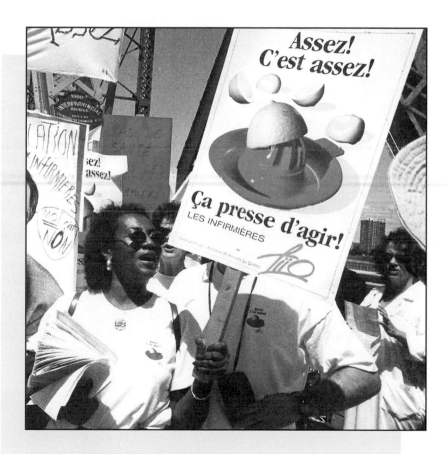

Quebec nurses' union representative Regine Laurent walks from Hull, Quebec, to Ottawa on the interprovincial bridge in July of 1999, while carrying 200 job demand slips. Striking nurses threatened to accept jobs in the Ottawa area if the Quebec government didn't give in to their demands.

◼ LEARNING OBJECTIVES

- To outline the legal case that served as a catalyst to the development of nursing unions in each jurisdiction in Canada.
- To describe the establishment, membership, and role of the Canadian Federation of Nurses' Unions.
- To highlight the gradual evolution of nursing unions in each jurisdiction of Canada.
- To understand the variation between jurisdictions in the membership of the bargaining unit.
- To discuss the looming nursing shortage and efforts to avert this situation.
- To highlight the nature of professional responsibility clauses in union contracts.
- To explore the issue of loss of the right to strike and its impact in particular jurisdictions.
- To discuss the outcomes from a public perspective of collective bargaining in nursing.
- To differentiate between the roles of professional associations and unions.
- To identify factors influencing cooperation and conflict in labour relations.

In the century following Florence Nightingale's championing of nursing as a legitimate and respectable profession for laywomen, it was never expected that nurses would engage in strike action. Indeed, it is unlikely that the rise of powerful and independent nursing unions could have been foreseen even at the midpoint of the twentieth century. However, the change in the gender balance of the profession, with the entrance of men in greater numbers, and the growing militancy among nurses who believe that their skills and the essential nature of their services have been undervalued and overlooked are but two factors in the new climate of confrontation and compromise over salaries and working conditions that characterizes the employment environment today. The power of unions in general, however, has been challenged by some provincial governments, and it would appear that unions, including nursing unions, have felt the impact of these threats to their hard-earned power base. Although the vast majority of staff nurses are covered by union contracts, there are groups of nurses who are not represented by unions. Nurses in private practice, private duty nurses, many groups of management nurses, and others in specialized sectors of practice may not be covered by union contracts. Some nurses may choose not to belong to a union, and in settings where nurses are unionized, nurses have the right to "opt out" of the union. However, under the Rand formula (Dion, 2009) applied in most areas, these nurses still have to pay membership dues.

Although there is considerable variation among provinces in approach and achievement, the thrust in nursing unions has been increasingly directed to consolidating membership, withstanding the threats to structural integrity, and maintaining the right to negotiate collective agreements on behalf of members. The impact of a worldwide climate of economic constraint and downsizing both in the mid-1990s and again in the late 2000s led to drastic and almost overnight downsizing of the health care system in each case. Widespread public-sector salary reductions in most provinces during each downturn have created an environment in which all unions struggle to preserve their mandates. These issues underscore the fact that economic conditions tend to be cyclical and exert a strong effect on nursing and health care.

THE RISE OF NURSING UNIONS

THE CATALYST FOR DEVELOPMENT OF NURSING UNIONS IN CANADA

In Canada, as well as in other countries, professional nursing associations played key roles in the development of nursing unions. However, in 1973 everything changed in Canada because of the decision made in a Saskatchewan case that was appealed to the Supreme Court of Canada. At issue was a dispute between the Service Employees International Union and the Saskatchewan Registered Nurses' Association (SRNA) over the SRNA's application for certification as a bargaining agent. The union charged that the SRNA should not be permitted to act as a trade union because its Board of Directors included nursing managers. The Court ruled in favour of the union and radically altered labour relations in nursing in Canada in little more than a decade. Because the rules governing the structure of the SRNA allowed for the election of nursing managers to its governing body, the association was presumed to have an inherent bias or conflict of interest that precluded participation in collective bargaining. Thus the way was paved for establishing new organizations across the country to assume the collective bargaining function of the professional associations.

STANCE OF THE CANADIAN NURSES ASSOCIATION

The Canadian Nurses Association (CNA) approved the principle of collective bargaining for nurses in the 1940s and affirmed that the bargaining agent at the provincial and territorial level should be the professional nursing association. The passage of the *Labour Relations Act* at the national level in 1944 giving federal employees collective bargaining rights was probably instrumental in the CNA decision to support collective bargaining among its member associations. The CNA was also on record as supporting a no-strike policy, a stand that became controversial two decades later and was repealed.

THE RNABC CERTIFIED AS FIRST BARGAINING AGENT IN CANADA

Nurses were concerned about possible management domination from the boards of directors of provincial associations after the 1944 decision (Rowsell, 1982). Because there was no formal collective bargaining at that time, the provincial associations struggled with the issues. Shortly after that, member organizations informed the CNA that it was not legally possible for them to act as bargaining agents. The first breakthrough in provincial labour legislation appeared in 1946, when the Registered Nurses Association of British Columbia (RNABC) became the first provincial association to apply successfully for certification as a bargaining agent under a labour relations act, beginning a movement that eventually involved all provinces.

THE "PERSONNEL POLICIES" APPROACH

Although they were not permitted to be formally involved in collective bargaining, the other nine provincial associations became engaged in promoting the social and economic welfare of their memberships in a less formal and proactive manner. It became customary in most provinces to publish annual personnel policies giving recommendations on salaries and working conditions. The associations then discussed the recommendations with employers or hospital associations. Although employers and employees had agreed on them, the personnel policies were not binding and often not implemented, leading to disillusionment with the process and its results. The failure to make progress using the personnel policy approach led to a search for a more effective approach to influence salary and wage decisions.

PROVINCIAL PROFESSIONAL ASSOCIATIONS ATTEMPT TO "TAKE UP THE TORCH"

During the expansionist decade of the 1960s, the majority of the provincial professional associations became more assertive in applying for the right to bargain collectively for the large groups of nurses employed in health care agencies. A number of factors were important in setting the stage for this new phase of development in nursing organizations. The economy was finally booming after a slow recovery through the postwar period and workers were making gains in financial status. The Royal Commission on the Status of Women in Canada (1967–70) drew attention to the need for equal opportunity for women in society and for removing inequities in a system that inadequately remunerated women. The new optimism in society brought what in the past had seemed impossible into the realm of the possible.

Because provincial professional nursing associations in all provinces except British Columbia could not be certified under provincial labour laws in the early 1960s, the associations established an important role for themselves by teaching staff nurses in hospitals and community health agencies about collective bargaining and helping them organize staff nurses' associations. Except in PEI, these organizations became the bargaining units that were eventually certified under the various labour acts. By the time of the Supreme Court decision that led to the separation of professional associations and unions, nurses had gained some experience and expertise in collective bargaining. As of 1987, the process was complete and the dual structure was in place in all provinces.

CHANGES IN ROLES OF PROVINCIAL PROFESSIONAL ASSOCIATIONS FOLLOWING SEPARATION

There were many advantages to the new organizational structure. Because professional nursing associations were no longer responsible for collective bargaining, they no longer protected their economic interests in public statements on health care issues and thus became more credible. Annual membership fees to professional associations no longer supported collective bargaining. Because collective bargaining is labour intensive and involves extensive time commitments from a bargaining team, and the involvement of labour relations consultants, lawyers, and others, it is an expensive process. Management involvement in professional associations and the fact that members' fees supported collective bargaining had always been sensitive issues. Complaints about the associations' strong thrust in the bargaining arena had come from groups of nurses not covered by union contracts. Creating separate unions addressed these complaints. Professional associations were able to focus on serving the public interest through self-regulatory functions, improving standards of nursing education and practice, promoting nursing research, and interacting with government and other health care professions as the official voice of the profession. However, it was also difficult for many nurses to understand that the professional association now stood truly apart from the bargaining function and could no longer intervene at difficult times to support a union stance in the face of a strike.

ESTABLISHMENT OF THE CANADIAN FEDERATION OF NURSES' UNIONS

Parallel to the development of provincial nursing unions as separate bargaining units, efforts were directed at establishing a national voice for unionized nurses. By the late 1960s, provincial labour relations staff began meeting under the aegis of the CNA Committee on Socio-Economic Welfare. With the controversial implementation of wage and price controls by the federal government and a code of ethics by the CNA, unionized nurses were convinced of the need for a more formal national structure to support their interests. In 1977, a labour relations service department was established under the auspices of the CNA to disseminate information on collective bargaining and to provide educational assistance to members. This was followed in 1981 by the establishment of an independent body, the National Federation of Nurses' Unions (NFNU) to represent unionized Canadian nurses in both watchdog and lobbying activities. The name of the organization was later changed to the Canadian Federation of Nurses' Unions (CFNU), and member unions include all provincial nursing unions except those in Quebec. By 2008, membership stood at 132,000 (CFNU, 2008). Since the responsibility for health care lies in each jurisdiction, the CFNU does not engage directly in collective bargaining. The role of this national body is to serve as a resource, providing member unions with assistance on the issues, strategies, and tactics, and representing unionized nurses to the national media and federal government.

REFLECTIVE THINKING

Reflect on the development of a nursing union in one jurisdiction and explain the current issues relative to its ongoing work.

THE ORGANIZATIONS: ESTABLISHMENT AND CONSOLIDATION

The development of separate and unique organizations for collective bargaining occurred within a relatively short time after the Supreme Court decision in 1973. Only 14 years elapsed between the inception of the first such organization, the Saskatchewan Union of Nurses, and the last, the PEI Nurses' Union, in 1987. The 1990s were characterized by cutbacks and health care restructuring, and nursing unions struggled to maintain what they had gained in the previous decade. This was a time of relative labour peace as the unions did not make big demands of employers as they fought to maintain staff positions. As the economic climate improved in the late 1990s, unions demanded higher wages, improved workloads, less overtime, and improved working environments (Archibald, 2004). Although the SARS crisis of 2003 impelled a period of consensus, labour strife was soon to follow as the economy went into overdrive. Although union demands were loud and clear, governments were less than willing to grant concessions, fearing that the long-term costs would be too high (Archibald, 2004). With the sudden economic downturn in 2008, unions had to do a "quick turn-around" and focus on nursing positions at risk when provinces began to slash their health care budgets as a result of declining revenues.

BRITISH COLUMBIA

Even though the RNABC was the first to be legally recognized as an official bargaining agent for nurses, at first it operated on the basis of annually approved personnel policies used as a basis for bargaining with hospital boards. Although this process was also used in other provinces, the difference was the legal recognition of the RNABC as bargaining agent. Dissatisfaction had arisen with the personnel policies route in all provinces. In 1959, many disputes went to conciliation, and strike votes were taken in a number of health care agencies. This led to the first province-wide collective bargaining for nurses in British Columbia in that year. The approach was successful and was used until 1974, when the RNABC disassociated the collective bargaining program from other association activity. This was a response to the Supreme Court decision and was likely an attempt to determine whether anything other than total separation was possible.

The BC Nurses' Union (BCNU) was formed in 1981 as an independent organization encompassing what had been the Labour Relations Division of the RNABC. Although the British Columbia government approved legislation in 1974 that gave government employees the right to bargain collectively and the right to strike, a decade later, new legislation revoked the right to strike for those designated as essential employees, including some nurses. Despite strong protests, the government stood firm. A nurses' strike in May to June 1989 provided an interesting example of the lack of solidarity between the BCNU members and leaders when the membership repudiated the memorandum of agreement approved by its leaders. An agreement was reached eventually, but the startling anger of the membership with their union leaders was evident.

In late 1989, under new leadership, structural changes led to a more cohesive organization, and subsequently the BCNU and the remaining two provincial unions representing health care workers—the Hospital Employees Union and the Health Sciences Association, negotiated a landmark employment security agreement. This tripartite agreement between the union, employer, and government was in effect until March 31, 1996, and ensured that should their present positions be abolished, nurses belonging to the union would be re-employed in similar positions in appropriate locales. Including retraining arrangements and early retirement packages, this agreement represented the successful amalgamation of independent unions in the pursuit of common goals. In September 1993, unionized nurses moved to a 36-hour work week, retaining the same salary agreements.

In the aftermath of the restructuring of the health care system that took place in the last half of the 1990s, BC nurses became disillusioned with their wages and benefits, which had not kept pace with those in other provinces. A bitter dispute between BCNU and the Health Employers Association of British Columbia (HEABC) occurred in the spring and summer of 2001. The government passed legislation imposing a contract that represented the final HEABC offer. Despite the imposition of the contract and the fact that it was $57 million less than one approved in Alberta months earlier, nurses achieved a 23.5% wage increase, the highest in British Columbia in more than a decade (BCNU, 2001). However, the legislation came back to haunt the BC government in 2007 when sections of it were declared unconstitutional by the Supreme Court of Canada (BCNU, 2007).

ALBERTA

Supported by the Alberta Association of Registered Nurses (AARN), nurses in Alberta became concerned about their social and economic status and held organizational meetings during the early 1960s. Working to help nurses in hospitals develop staff nurses' associations for bargaining, amendments made to the *Registered Nurses' Act* in 1965 allowed the AARN to act as the bargaining agent for the nurses. The AARN, like the RNABC, made bylaw changes in 1974 to create a unit for collective bargaining that would function separately from the rest of the association. However, nurses in Alberta decided to create a separate and autonomous structure for collective bargaining, and in 1977, the United Nurses of Alberta (UNA) was formed to act in this capacity. Shortly thereafter, the first nurses' strike occurred, involving seven hospitals and 2,000 nurses. Government intervened with a back-to-work order and a tribunal to rule on the items in dispute.

Subsequently, two nurses' strikes occurred in Alberta, one in 1980 and another in 1982. In 1983, the Alberta government enacted legislation that made it illegal for hospital nurses to strike. However, in January 1988, Alberta nurses defied the *Labour Act* and went out on an 18-day illegal strike. In 1992, the Supreme Court of Canada ruled against the appeal of criminal contempt convictions by the UNA. Thus, the substantial monetary penalties imposed on the union further to the 1988 strike were allowed to stand.

As in many other provinces, Alberta nurses became much more politically astute and assertive. Following the 1988 nurses' strike, two contracts were negotiated, each resulting in much less friction than in previous negotiations. However, billion-dollar health care cutbacks over the period from 1993 to 1997 and 5% wage rollbacks for public-sector workers, including nurses, led to layoffs of thousands of nurses, and a number of hospitals closed as 17 new regional health authorities (RHAs) were created to manage health services. These RHAs replaced boards of trustees of institutions and public health agencies, in effect becoming superboards. In 1997, the Staff Nurses Association of Alberta, representing a large group of nurses including those working at the University of Alberta Hospitals, amalgamated with the UNA (UNA, 1997). In 2001, the lucrative contract achieved by the UNA provided a bargaining chip for other Canadian union negotiations. With a collective agreement in force from 2007 to 2010, the UNA initially concentrated on workplace issues and the serious shortage of nurses in the province, focusing on criticisms of the provincial government for failing to address the nursing shortage (UNA, 2008). However, the impact of the worldwide economic depression beginning in late 2008 on resource revenues led the provincial government to initiate restructuring, creating one provincial health authority to replace the regional boards in 2008. In 2009, drastic cuts to health care were announced. Once again, nursing positions were on the line and the UNA's focus returned to trying to maintain nursing positions.

SASKATCHEWAN

In Saskatchewan, the SRNA became involved in collective bargaining prior to 1973 in response to demands from members in nongovernmental positions. Government-employed nurses represented by unions achieved significant improvement in salaries throughout the 1960s, whereas SRNA members who had no bargaining agent before 1968 did not. By 1972, collective agreements between the SRNA and the Saskatchewan Hospital Association encompassed about half of Saskatchewan hospitals (Botterill-Conroy, 1980). As previously noted, the amendment to the *Trade Union Act* that resulted from the question of the legality of the SRNA's role as bargaining agent for the nurses was ratified by the Supreme Court's 1973 decision. The Saskatchewan Union of Nurses (SUN) was created after the decision was made, and it orchestrated a walkout in 1974, followed by a strike in 1976.

Health care reform translated into regionalization in Saskatchewan with the appointment of regional health boards and the closing of a number of small acute-care hospitals. SUN refocused its efforts to argue for a "wellness model" consistent with the changes. Since many nurses had to relocate, the union directed its attention to labour adjustment strategies to protect nurses from the impact of the sweeping changes in the health care system. Strikes occurred in Saskatchewan in 1988 and 1999, the latter dispute resulting in the inclusion of a professional responsibility clause, giving nurses a mechanism to deal with patient care issues (Saskatchewan Union of Nurses, 2008).

Since then, successive contracts have been ratified by members, and attention has focused on the nursing shortage and retention and recruitment of nurses. SUN reached a four-year agreement with the Saskatchewan Association of Health Organizations (SAHO) in 2008 that resulted in substantial salary increases.

MANITOBA

Although nurses in Manitoba asked the Manitoba Association of Registered Nurses (MARN) to represent them in collective bargaining as early as 1953, the MARN did not become formally involved until 1969. To fill the void, the Winnipeg Civic Registered Nurses' Association was organized in 1965 to serve as an alternative to the provincial employee union, the Federation of Civil Employees. Even though the MARN became involved in bargaining, some ambivalence continued within the association because the *Labour Relations Act* clearly specified that unions must operate separately from management. Thus, the MARN followed the precedents set in Alberta and British Columbia, separating the organization from its collective bargaining sector so that the latter could function at arm's length from the rest of the association. As in the other provinces, this was a short-term solution to the problem, and in 1975, an independent organization, the Manitoba Organization of Nurses Association (MONA), was established (Botterill-Conroy, 1980), later becoming the Manitoba Nurses' Union (MNU). After a month-long strike in 1991, the MNU emerged more cohesive than previously: members were satisfied with an agreement that included joint trusteeship of pension plans, a professional responsibility clause, and differential salary increases for RNs and LPNs.

A successful "yellow ribbon" campaign in 1995 protesting emergency department closures attracted community support, and the government scaled back its wholesale closure efforts. Layoffs and out-migration affected the MNU tremendously as in other provinces. For those who remained in the system, working conditions were difficult at best (MNU, 2001). Manitoba nurses celebrated the agreement reached on March 8, 2008, after an arduous collective bargaining process (MNU, 2008).

ONTARIO

Events took a different course in Ontario, beginning in 1961 with the creation of a quasi-governmental body, the College of Nurses of Ontario, to assume the regulatory functions of registration and professional conduct. Collective bargaining rights were not achieved easily in Ontario as nurses tried unsuccessfully from 1958 until 1965 to gain legal recognition of bargaining. Even so, after 1965 bargaining had to be done individually, agency by agency. Not until 1973 did the Ontario Hospital Association (OHA) approve centralized bargaining by nurses for monetary issues only (Botterill-Conroy, 1980).

Although the RNAO had assumed the bargaining function for many years, the Ontario Nurses Association (ONA) separated from the RNAO in 1975, following the well-established trend in the rest of the country, but bargaining at the provincial level did not begin until 1979. Legislation passed in 1965 prevented nurses in hospitals and nursing homes from striking. However, it did not apply to community health nurses.

In 1989, the ONA was instrumental in obtaining an amendment to the *Public Hospital Act* to include an elected staff nurse on the Fiscal Advisory Committee. This was followed in 1991 by a contractual agreement that included ten incremental steps recognizing nurses with lengthy service records, expert clinical skills, and mentorship functions. Since then the ONA has focused on professional issues such as staff shortages, replacement of registered nurses with less-qualified personnel, unsafe working conditions, need for primary health reform, and strengthening Medicare (ONA, 2001, 2008). The organization announced ratification of a new three-year contract, expiring in 2011 (ONA, 2008).

QUEBEC

In Quebec, nurses were given legislative approval for collective bargaining in 1946 under the *Quebec Nurses' Act*. However, the Association of Nurses of the Province of Quebec did not develop a bargaining program. The reasons for this are unclear. However, after the enactment of the omnibus legislation that applied to a number of professional groups and the development of the Professional Code in Chapter 43 of the legislation applying to nursing, registration in the province became mandatory.

The Order of Nurses of the Province of Quebec (ONQ/OIIQ) was disqualified as the bargaining agent, not because of management domination, but because the right of free association guaranteed by the Quebec Labour Code was precluded by the mandatory membership provisions of the act. Therefore, nurses sought other representation in the socioeconomic domain. Several unions were formed—l'Alliance des Infirmières et Infirmiers du Québec, la Fédération des Syndicats Professionnels d'Infirmières du Québec (FSPIIQ), and in 1967, the United Nurses of Montreal (UNM). L'Alliance and FSPIIQ bargained separately for staff nurses and management nurses, whereas the UNM represented all nurses, including management nurses. This changed in 1970 when the UNM split into separate staff and management organizations—United Nurses Inc. (UNInc.) and United Management Nurses Inc. (UMNInc.).

In 1972, many public services were affected by a strike of the Quebec Federation of Labour that involved nurses who were members of l'Alliance. These nurses were ordered to return to work when the Quebec National Assembly passed legislation to end the interruption in public services. In 1975, UNInc. joined the Corps des Organismes Professionnels de la Santé (COPS) for the purpose of bargaining. Representing the vast majority of unionized nurses in Quebec, the organization also included among its members the FSPIIQ and many other groups in the health professions (Botterill-Conroy, 1980).

Three nursing unions merged in December 1987 to form La Fédération des infirmières et infirmiers du Québec (FIIQ). This move resulted in greater union strength in bargaining for salary increases for nurses in Quebec, traditionally among the lowest-paid nurses in Canada. The illegal walkout of members of the new organization in 1989, and the subsequent standoff between the nurses and the premier and his government in the midst of an election campaign, led to a seven-day strike that unified nurses and gained them considerable public support for their cause (FIIQ, 2001). The nurses' gains in this confrontation were impressive, and their public image was improved. Other groups of nurses have joined the federation, known since 2006 as the Fédération Interprofessionelle de la santé du Québec (FIQ), strengthening its ranks, so that it now represents some 47,500 members (FIQ, n.d.).

Over the years, Quebec has seen a substantial change in the way health care is delivered. The Centres Locaux de Services Communautaires (CLSCs), community health centres, serve as the means for the delivery of health and social services based in the community. Quebec has thus been in the forefront of the movement to establish community health centres in Canada. Attributable to the efforts of the FIIQ, collective bargaining rights were extended to these areas as nurses formerly based in hospitals moved out to these centres. A bitter dispute between the FIIQ and the employer group with which it bargains occurred in 1999 and was followed by a 23-day strike, in the aftermath of which financial penalties were imposed on the union. A new collective agreement was signed in 2000. As in other provinces, negotiations continue relative to collective agreements, and issues such as staff shortages and difficult working conditions (FIIQ, 2008). To their chagrin, nurses in Quebec had to work under a government decree rather than a collective agreement when the government halted negotiations and imposed the decree in May, 2006, with an expiry date of March, 2010. The organization of 58,000 members continued to fight privatization in its negotiations and had no contract as of the date of publications of this book. In the meantime, it has achieved higher salaries for nurse clinicians (FIIQ, 2008). However, the economic downturn is affecting nursing positions across the country and diverts the focus to the status quo and downsizing.

NEW BRUNSWICK

In the 1960s, nurses in New Brunswick became concerned about their socioeconomic status and disenchanted with the procedure for determining salaries. Originally, the New Brunswick Association of Registered Nurses (NBARN) provided recommendations on salaries and working conditions to the government on an annual basis. The first gain made to win more power was the NBARN's Social and Economic Welfare Committee's acquisition of standing committee status in 1967. After acquiring this status, the committee began helping nurses in health care agencies to organize staff associations throughout the province. In 1968, the NBARN Provincial Collective Bargaining Council was established as a separate entity from the NBARN.

The first serious collective bargaining in New Brunswick began in 1969, when employers agreed to negotiate with the NBARN Provincial Collective Bargaining Council. When a stalemate occurred in the negotiations, the majority of New Brunswick nurses resigned. These resignations were withdrawn when the employer group agreed to go back to the bargaining table to negotiate in a fair and equitable manner. An agreement was signed by both parties soon after. In the same year, provisions of the *Public Service Labour Relations Act* gave nurses in the public sector the right to bargain collectively. The right was extended to the private sector two years later through the *Industrial Relations Act*. The NBARN Provincial Collective Bargaining Council disassociated itself from the NBARN by becoming the New Brunswick Nurses' Provincial Collective Bargaining Council. The

New Brunswick Civil Service Nurses' Provincial Collective Bargaining Council was also established because public- and private-sector bargaining were separated legislatively. The two organizations merged in 1978 to become the New Brunswick Nurses' Union (NBNU) (Botterill-Conroy, 1980).

In 1991, the provincial government imposed a wage freeze and rescinded a previously agreed-to salary adjustment for nurses. The NBNU threatened to strike and then reached a settlement with the provincial government. In 1994, nurses were able to prevent the government from removing "nursing" from job qualifications (McGee, 1994). More recently, the NBNU has been working to alleviate staff shortages and pressing for the hiring of nurse practitioners (NBNU, 2008). In the post-2008 economic climate, in concert with other provincial and territorial organizations, the focus is on retaining the nursing workforce.

NOVA SCOTIA

In 1966, the Registered Nurses' Association of Nova Scotia (RNANS) (now known as the College of Registered Nurses of Nova Scotia) organized the Committee on Social and Economic Welfare to press for wage increases and improved working conditions. In 1968, RNANS was prepared to act as a bargaining agent for nurses employed in agencies, but did so only after they were able to change their legislative mandate. The RNANS then sought to assist nurses in health care agencies seek certification as bargaining agents under the *Trade Union Act,* the first being granted in 1969. Collective bargaining took place first under the aegis of the RNANS, and later under an independent organization, the Staff Nurses' Association of Nova Scotia. This organization was the forerunner of the Nova Scotia Nurses' Union (NSNU), which was organized in 1976.

In 1971, a brief strike at Amherst Hospital resulted in an agreement. Longer strikes took place at two institutions in 1972, and in 1975, nurses in 15 institutions withdrew their services because of a bargaining impasse. At that time, bargaining still primarily occurred at the local level but in 1978 began to take place collectively. By the next year, most agencies were involved in the process (Botterill-Conroy, 1980).

In 2001, the collective bargaining process undertaken between the NSNU and the Province of Nova Scotia was particularly difficult. Although a tentative agreement was reached on May 26, 2001 (Government of Nova Scotia, 2001), the offer was rejected by the membership. The Nova Scotia government introduced Bill 68, the *Health Care Continuation (2001) Act*, on June 14. The draconian measures incorporated in the proposed legislation stirred further anger and resentment in the NSNU because the legislation proposed suspending the right of employees to strike until March 31, 2004, and giving cabinet the power to impose a collective agreement if agreement could not be reached through bargaining. The NSNU received a strike mandate from its membership on June 29. In the meantime, a parallel union, the Nova Scotia Government Employees Union (NSGEU), began a legal strike on June 27, and its members were joined by nurses. The government rushed legislation to end the strike through the processes of approval and proclaimed it immediately.

When the NSNU and other unions threatened to submit their resignations en masse, the government retreated from its original position, and on July 5, all parties agreed to invoke a final-offer selection process to settle the outstanding contract issues. The agreement provided that the legislation would not apply to nurses, that the final report of the selector should be issued in just over a month, and that a three-year collective agreement would be developed. In this final-offer selection process, Susan M. Ashley, the arbitrator, selected the NSNU's position rather than that of the government, representing a considerable setback for the government in the dispute ("A final-offer selection," 2001). Currently an agreement has been reached for acute-care and long-term care sectors for a contract to be in place retroactively from 2006 until 2009 (Nova Scotia Nurses' Union, 2008).

PRINCE EDWARD ISLAND

Collective bargaining rights for nurses were included in the amended *PEI Nurses' Act* in 1972 because nurses had been excluded from the *PEI Labour Act*. Thus, the Provincial Collective Bargaining Committee of the Association of Nurses of Prince Edward Island (ANPEI) held legal responsibility for collective bargaining for nurses in the province. The first collective agreement was not negotiated until 1974 because the government and the ANPEI did not agree on the regulations to implement the act. Although nurses in PEI did not have the right to strike, a standoff between the nurses and the government was resolved when the government agreed to a compromise after the nurses threatened to resign.

For a time, it seemed that Prince Edward Island might be the only province that would not establish a separate organization for collective bargaining. But in 1987, the *PEI Nurses' Act* was amended to remove responsibility for collective bargaining from the ANPEI, and the *Labour Act* amended to ensure that nurses would not be excluded from its provisions. The PEI Nurses' Union was thus established.

As a result of health care reform in the 1990s, nurses in PEI faced similar problems over staff shortages and difficult working conditions to nurses in other provinces. Nurses are currently working under a much-disputed contract achieved long after the previous contract had expired through binding arbitration. This contract expires March 31, 2011 (Prince Edward Island Nurses' Union, 2009).

NEWFOUNDLAND

The Association of Registered Nurses of Newfoundland (ARNN) annually prepared recommendations for nurses' salaries and submitted them as part of a brief to the cabinet until 1970, when the process was deemed a failure and was discontinued. The ARNN, designated as the bargaining agent for civil service nurses and those employed by nongovernmental agencies, then bargained directly with government for the former and with the Newfoundland Hospital Association for the latter. The process, voluntary at first, became mandatory, and the first collective agreement was concluded in 1970. The passage of the *Public Service Act* in 1972 provided legal recognition of collective bargaining rights for nurses and other health care providers; it reflected the spirit and intent of the 1973 Supreme Court decision and precluded the ARNN from involvement in collective bargaining. The Newfoundland Nurses' Union (NNU) formed in 1974 to take responsibility for collective bargaining.

Because the Newfoundland economy was severely affected by recession, nurses were subjected to a wage freeze between 1991 and 1994 and saw the government withdraw its share of contributions to their pension plan. The severe retrenchment during the 1990s meant that job losses and lack of salary increments and benefits were the norm in Newfoundland, as elsewhere. In April 1999, nurses went on strike and were legislated back to work with an imposed contract. Members of the Newfoundland and Labrador Nurses' Union (NLNU) were very unhappy and subsequently engaged in a vigorous lobbying campaign. This endeavour succeeded, and in August 2000, the government reclassified nurses so that they received salary increases.

Subsequently. several contracts were negotiated in the presence of tremendous unrest across the country due to the shortage of nurses and inadequate resources for health care. Currently, nurses are covered by a contract in force from January 2007 to June 2008. However in late 2007, the provincial government agreed to reopen contract negotiations early at the request of the NLNU because of the crisis caused by staff shortages in the health care system (NLNU, 2008).

NORTHWEST TERRITORIES (NWT), NUNAVUT, YUKON TERRITORY (YT)

Nurses in these jurisdictions of Canada are mainly employees of the federal government and are represented in the Northwest Territories and Nunavut and in Yukon Territory by employees' unions that are members of the Public Service Alliance of Canada (PSAC). These organizations work very closely with the professional nursing associations in these jurisdictions as recruitment and retention of nurses are ongoing issues of concern.

UNION OR MANAGEMENT: WHERE TO DRAW THE LINE

It is difficult to describe the bargaining unit because of uncertainty about the appropriate classification of some supervisory positions. The dilemma is most prevalent at the level of first-line managers, and there are differences of opinion among the provinces as to whether certain employees can be included in the bargaining unit. In some areas, the "hiring and firing" standard has been used, and managers who perform these functions are disqualified. In other instances, management has redefined functions to ensure that first-line managers are not included in the bargaining unit. This redefinition has often occurred in provinces where the union has the right to strike as employers may see a need for expert assistance on the front lines in the event of a strike. (See Box 17.1.)

Many nurses do not wish to be removed from the bargaining unit because they will no longer have the security of a contract. However, after the retrenchment of the early 1990s, the "contract" clearly did not carry the same assurances and security as in the past. There is little protection for management nurses in comparison to those covered by the collective agreement. Only the province of Quebec has a union for nurse managers that actively

BOX 17.1	The Challenge: How to Avert a Nursing Shortage

The challenge for the provinces and territories is to integrate, recruit, and retain nurses in the face of a predicted national nursing shortage that could reach 78,000 by 2011 and 113,000 by 2016 (CNA, 2002). There are two ways to do this, and they are linked: (1) increase the number of nursing graduates in Canada by 12,000 annually, and (2) improve the quality of professional practice environments. As a result of the dramatic cuts to health care funding in the mid-1990s and the elimination of thousands of nursing positions, nurses became casual workers as full-time positions became increasingly hard to secure, especially for new graduates. The layoffs created an artificial surplus of nurses at a time when the nursing profession was projecting a growing shortage of RNs within 15 years. Concurrently, funding for seats in nursing programs was cut. In the early 1990s, the output level of nursing graduates in the country was close to 10,000. By the year 2000, that number had dipped below 5,000. Many Canadian nursing graduates were attracted by the promise of more supportive work environments and attractive salary packages in the United States, and others opted out of the profession altogether. The recognition of the looming crisis in staffing nursing positions led to increased recruitment efforts, and in 2006, the number of graduating nurses rose to 8,379 (CNA, 2007).

As work environments became more stressful, absenteeism rose. According to Statistics Canada, the average nursing professional is off sick 15.4 days a year, while the national average for other categories of workers is just 6.7 days.

There have been some increases in federal funding for health care and employer budgets in this decade, but there is still room for improvement. Provincial governments have had to recognize and address recruitment and retention of nurses. The Canadian Nurses Association (CNA) believes empowering nurses to make decisions about their workplace can go a long way in helping avert a nursing shortage. The cost-cutting measures of the mid-1990s resulted in overworked, stressed nurses working in less than adequate conditions. The quality of work environments and levels of patient care suffered as a result. An increased involvement of nurses in decision making about their work environment and a greater sense of control over that environment lead to improved work flow. In the past few years, research has provided evidence of the link between increased RN hours on a unit and higher patient survival rates.

As CNA past president Dr. Ginette Lemire Rodger has stated: "What is good for patients is inevitably good for nursing, and what is good for nursing is good for patients."

Source: *Globe and Mail*, "National Nursing Week" supplement, May 6, 2002, N7.

represents them. In other provinces, nurses in administrative positions are at the mercy of their employers for salaries and benefits. Perhaps more important, they are also vulnerable in the area of job tenure. This was particularly evident throughout the 1990s when all middle-management positions were endangered as organizations strove for the greater financial efficiency of "flat" structures. Employers are aware of the potential power of the nursing department, the largest and most costly sector of activity in any hospital. All these factors operative in the health setting effectively muzzle nursing administrators, who are in a unique position to evaluate the operational effectiveness of the system.

PROFESSIONAL RESPONSIBILITY CLAUSES

The climate of the setting in which nurses are expected to function has become a focus of concern for unions, and the advent of professional responsibility clauses as part of collective agreements is tangible evidence of this trend. Emphasis on salaries and wages continues, but working conditions for nurses have become a high priority in negotiations.

One consequence of the deep cuts to health-system funding has been staff shortages, as fewer nurses have been expected to carry heavier and heavier patient loads as well as work countless overtime hours.

Nurses are deeply concerned about the quality and safety of the care they can provide in particular health care settings. Structuring the collective agreement to allow nurses to negotiate with the employer about certain resources that may be necessary to provide safe care is an integral part of the collective bargaining process. Examples of difficulty in providing adequate care can be documented in waivers (disclaimer-of-responsibility forms) and diaries. These records provide data to support concerns discussed at meetings with management on professional responsibility committees.

IMPACT OF LOSS OF THE RIGHT TO STRIKE

The denial of the right of a particular professional group to strike is unusual and represents legislative interference with freedom to engage in the usual processes associated with collective bargaining (Anderson & Anderson, 1982). Ontario nurses lost the right to strike when the *Hospital Disputes Arbitration Act* of 1965 was passed. The right to strike was denied to nurses employed in hospitals in Alberta in 1983 after a period of acrimonious labour relations among Alberta nurses, the provincial government, and the Alberta Hospital Association. Three legal nurses' strikes between 1977 and 1982 motivated the Alberta government to enact legislation that denied hospital nurses and some other workers the right to strike because their services were deemed essential. This legislation imposed severe penalties on those who defied the law. As noted above, severe penalties under this legislation were imposed on the UNA as a result of an illegal strike in 1988. Quebec nurses also suffered penalties after their 23-day illegal strike in 1999. It is possible that events in Alberta convinced the government of British Columbia that legislation to prevent nurses' strikes was necessary. Prince Edward Island nurses also do not have the right to strike; in several other provinces, the right of nurses to strike is severely limited by conditions that must be satisfied during a strike.

A question that is often asked is whether the presence or absence of freedom to strike compromises a union's position at the bargaining table. In Ontario, nurses in hospitals and nursing homes have not had the right to strike for three decades, but salary levels appear to have been comparable with those in other provinces. Indeed, until Alberta nurses asserted themselves in the wake of a booming economy in the late 1970s and early 1980s, Ontario nurses had the highest salaries in Canada. Since then, Ontario, Alberta, and British Columbia nurses have been very close in their salary levels, with minor shifts in position with contract settlements. Unions provide a day-to-day evaluation of working conditions and issues that may be of concern to the professional nurse employee. Without the vigilance and concerted efforts provided by elected and paid union officials, it may be that nurses would not have made as much progress as they have in achieving gains in both salaries and reasonable and equitable working conditions.

REFLECTIVE THINKING

Explore the use of the strike "weapon" in nursing, and discuss how you might respond if you were asked to go on strike to support a union position further to the breakdown of collective bargaining in your agency.

PUBLIC IMPACT OF COLLECTIVE BARGAINING IN NURSING

It is difficult to determine the effect of the collective bargaining movement in nursing on public perceptions of nurses. Stereotypical images of nurses as passive and unassertive have been undermined, particularly in provinces where nursing unions have been militant, and relations with employer groups and governments have been acrimonious. However, public response to nurses' strikes has varied. In Alberta in 1977, public sympathy was against the nurses; however, in 1979 there was a virtual outpouring of sympathy for their bargaining position, and the public as well as members of other unions joined the picket lines, resulting in a large salary settlement. When Alberta's nurses went on strike again in 1982, there was little public support. In 1988, the Alberta public was reasonably supportive of the nurses during their illegal strike. Except for the substantial fines levied against the union, few repercussions against nurses resulted from this illegal walkout.

There have been some notable and successful efforts by a number of provincial governments to restrict the activities and processes that unions can use to exert pressure on their employers in the collective bargaining process. The fact that public protest has not usually persuaded these governments to reconsider their proposed course of action relative to passing the legislation suggests a lack of public support for the unions and their activities.

Nurses represent the largest group of health care providers in the labour force, and even small increases in their salaries affect the total budget of a health care agency significantly. Thus, employers may often attempt to keep nurses' salaries at a minimum level to effect cost savings and to balance budgets. Although collective bargaining rights for nurses did not appear to change the goals of employer negotiating groups, it gave the process of negotiation a higher profile and gave nurses more power.

Having fought hard for and achieved the right to bargain collectively with their employers, it is unlikely that nurses will ever again be remunerated so inadequately for their services as in the past. The "tables have turned" since nurses' salaries showed higher proportionate increases to other comparably prepared professionals. In the 1990s, the severe impact of the worldwide economic recession and decreasing tax revenues on publicly funded health and social services left federal and provincial governments hard pressed to find short-term and long-term solutions to benefit the consumer.

Although nurses were the clear targets of cost-cutting throughout the 1990s and have paid with their jobs (and in some cases, their careers), they recovered from this assault and gained strength in numbers once again. The labour strife of 1999 to 2002 attests to the fact that the nurses' unions will struggle hard to regain lost salary increases and benefits, to improve working conditions, and indeed, to maintain the respect for which they have had to fight so persistently over such a long period of time. The recession of 2008–2009 again raised the spectre of retrenchment along with salary freezes and job losses in some areas.

CHARACTERISTICS OF PROFESSIONAL ASSOCIATIONS AND UNIONS

Professional associations and unions have many common goals, including promoting the welfare of members and improving their working conditions. Since professional associations include many who are not members of nursing unions and whose economic interests are not served directly by unions, they continue to play an important role in advising and assisting. Most nurses in management are included in this group, as Quebec is the only province where a union for nurse managers exists.

Professional associations are also interested in ensuring that salaries and benefits for staff nurses continue at sufficiently high levels to maintain the status of the profession and to encourage prospective candidates to enter nursing. Professional associations and unions in nursing share a concern for professional ethics, although it is the provincial association that is responsible for ensuring that the standard of professional conduct reflected in the code of ethics is practised. Professional maturity has been observed during the past decade in the attention given to developing and approving a code of ethics at the national level. Before the first CNA *Code of Ethics* was approved and published in 1981, most provincial professional associations accepted the standard established by the International Council of Nurses (ICN) code published in 1953. Subsequent revisions to the CNA *Code of Ethics* in 1985, 1991, 1997, 2002, and 2008 have ensured that its provisions remain current (CNA, 2008).

Despite their common interests, professional organizations and unions are also different in many ways. The service ideal that is deeply embedded in the professional consciousness is reflected in legislation that regulates registration and professional conduct of registered nurses. Monitoring professional conduct is the responsibility of the professional association in every province and territory except Ontario, where the College of Nurses of Ontario, a separate, quasi-autonomous body partially funded by government, is responsible for regulatory functions. Thus, the focus of professional associations on the health and safety of recipients of nursing services is in the public interest. Standards of practice that support the public right to safe and competent care are of paramount importance. Unions are not legally bound to protect the public interest. They focus almost exclusively on the socioeconomic needs of members.

Unions are concerned with the development of legally binding agreements that regulate staff nurses' salaries, working conditions, and other negotiable benefits. Although concerned about appropriate salary levels and good working conditions, professional associations are not responsible for developing these agreements and therefore are not active in this area. In fact, professional associations must avoid involvement in the collective bargaining process because any interference may be viewed negatively by sectors of the membership and result in controversy and conflict. In times of labour unrest, many professional associations have been pressured by both union members and management nurses to take a position on issues on the negotiating table. These situations are difficult for professional associations, and any action must be based on maintaining appropriate standards of nursing care and serving the public interest.

The mandate of professional associations is also aimed at improving and maintaining standards of nursing education in provinces where the authority for doing so is vested with the professional association. Although there has been union support for educational standards, professional advancement, and improvements in programs, this area is clearly not in their mandate. For unions, the principle of seniority is normally the basis for approaches to advancement and other workforce decisions.

Finally, professional associations tend to value autonomy and independent action on the basis of individual evaluation and judgement. An individual approach to solving problems is contradictory to the approach taken by unions to achieve goals in collective bargaining. Individual needs are supplanted by those of the majority when pressing for contract demands, and the egalitarian view prevails: what is good for the average member is good for all members. Professional associations attempt to respond to the needs of various sectors of the membership and take public stands that will enhance standards of care and address the needs of different categories of members. Unions must negotiate agreements that incorporate all the items agreed to by unions and management; therefore, the needs of the "average" member prevail.

CANADIAN RESEARCH FOCUS

Hamelin-Brabant, L., Lavoie-Tremblay, M., Lefrançois, L., & Viens, C. (2007). Engaging health care workers in improving their work environment. *Journal of Nursing Management, 15*(3), 313–320.

In this study of nurses and other staff on a nursing unit, the authors attempted to determine the perceptions of these individuals involved in a project to reorganize care and work to create a more optimal work environment. Using a participatory approach, the authors established through interviews the perceptions of the subjects on the legitimacy of change; commitment, indifference, and resistance; day-to-day concrete changes as signs of hope; and the elements of the success of the participatory approach. The conclusion was drawn that the management team's support and leadership and the participatory approach were important in ensuring the success of the project. Since the work environment is a crucial factor in job satisfaction, the results of the study may be useful to those interested or engaged in the area of labour relations in nursing.

FACTORS INFLUENCING COOPERATION AND CONFLICT

A new genre of nursing organization since 1973, unions have introduced a range of new inter- and intra-organizational challenges. The development of leadership and of organizational culture and norms takes time, as both are evolutionary processes. Nurses have had to learn about the collective bargaining process and how to use collective power to advantage. Professional nursing associations, dating formally from 1910 and informally for many years before that, have had a much longer history than nursing unions. The maturity that characterizes the relationship between professional associations and unions is extremely important, as it will define the nature of the interactions between them. The initial growth period of unions has been characterized by positive and negative relationships between these organizations. Because unions were organizational newcomers in a relative sense, the independence and determined challenges from them may have come as a surprise to professional associations that had not expected to be at odds over issues with their counterpart union groups.

There is considerable controversy about whether it is possible for professional associations and unions to coexist in areas in which their objectives are sufficiently dissimilar to engender conflict. However, it is believed that predominantly professional values encourage good relationships and cooperation, whereas the reverse may lead to conflict between the organizations.

In Quebec, where there are many large nurses' unions, the Ordre des Infirmières et Infirmiers du Québec (OIIQ) took an unusual step more than two decades ago when it issued a public statement that the professional association would not endorse the use of strike tactics if patient care were jeopardized:

> Governed by its mandate to ensure the protection of the public, the Bureau of the Ordre declares it is against withdrawal of services in the health field. This is the position it has taken following its study, having considered the different components of the context of the organization of health services, those of labour relations and the harm suffered by the population. (OIIQ, 1982, p. 14)

At the same time, the OIIQ suggested to the Comité Permanente du Travail et de la Main-d'Oeuvre de l'Assemblé Nationale du Québec that a new approach to collective bargaining was needed, recommending compulsory arbitration that would require participation by professionals and consumers. Very few professional associations in nursing or in other professions have taken a similar stand, undoubtedly because of the likelihood of a negative interpretation by a large section of the membership. That OIIQ took this stand was impressive, possibly due in part to the strength of Quebec's mandatory registration legislation in nursing, empowering the OIIQ to vigorously monitor standards of nursing practice in the province.

The potential or actual use of the strike as a weapon may also be a source of conflict between professional organizations and unions. Historically, nurses have been ambivalent about the use of the strike. The no-strike policy adopted in 1946 by the CNA was rescinded in 1972 after nurses across the country were organizing and gaining the right to engage in collective bargaining (Mussallem, 1977). Although it may have been difficult for many of them, nurses were prepared to go on strike if labour negotiations did not produce the necessary outcomes. Whether it is ethical for members of a profession to strike has been debated at length aside from whether nurses have the legal right to strike. In any case, the latter is deemed to be "severely limited" by the public welfare concern. Hardingham (1999) debated the issues from both ethical and legal standpoints for nurses being asked by unions to go out on an illegal strike. She noted that "just as low pay is correlated with low self-esteem and low status, low status is linked to the lack of quality nursing care" (p. 17) and concluded that the ethical argument remained paramount. The CNA has now declared as a standard of ethical practice that "nurses planning to take job action or practising in environments where job action occurs take steps to safeguard the health and safety of people during the course of the job action" (CNA, 2008, A7).

There remain widely divergent views on how nurses should respond to conditions that they view as deleterious to patients as well as to their own health and well-being. Although conflict remains difficult to address, nursing unions have matured and developed over four decades in Canada to the point where they are able to develop action plans that drive home their views while holding the needs of patients and nurses at the forefront.

CRITICAL THINKING QUESTIONS

1. Explain why nurses found it necessary to develop programs to bargain collectively for their salaries, wages, and benefits within the various jurisdictions of Canada.
2. What impact has the loss of the right to strike had in jurisdictions where this has been mandated by provincial governments?
3. Explain the respective mandates of professional associations and unions.

WEB SITES

Canadian Federation of Nursing Unions: http://www.nursesunions.ca/
British Columbia Nurses' Union (BCNU): http://www.bcnu.org/
United Nurses of Alberta (UNA): http://www.una.ab.ca/
Saskatchewan Union of Nurses (SUN): http://www.sun-nurses.sk.ca/
Manitoba Nurses' Union (MNU): http://www.nursesunion.mb.ca/
Ontario Nurses' Association (ONA): http://www.ona.org/
Fédération Interprofessionelle de la santé du Québec: http://www.fiqsante.qc.ca/
New Brunswick Nurses Union (NBNU): http://www.nbnu-siinb.nb.ca/index.html
Nova Scotia Nurses' Union (NSNU): http://www.nsnu.ns.ca/
Prince Edward Island Nurses' Union (PEINU): http://www.peinu.com/
Newfoundland and Labrador Nurses' Union (NLNU): http://www.nlnu.nf.ca/
Public Service Alliance of Canada: http://www.psac.com/home-e.shtml

REFERENCES

Anderson, J., & Anderson, M. (Eds.). (1982). *Union-management relations in Canada.* Toronto: Addison-Wesley.

Archibald, T. (2004). Collective bargaining by nurses in Canadian health care: Assessing recent trends and emerging claims. *Health Law Journal, 11,* 77–198.

Botterill Conroy, M. D. (1980). *Labour relations, collective bargaining and nursing.* Edmonton: Unpublished manuscript, University of Alberta, Division of Health Services Administration and Community Medicine.

British Columbia Nurses' Union (BCNU). (2001). *Bargaining 2001, latest news—August 2001.* Retrieved on March 28, 2001, from http://www.bcnu.org/Latest_%20News_%20August.htm.

British Columbia Nurses' Union (BCNU). (2007). *Supreme Court strikes down Bill 29 provisions in landmark ruling: News Release.* Retrieved on March 8, 2008, from http://bcfed.org/files/Bill29jointB_backgrounder.pdf.

Canadian Federation of Nurses' Unions (CFNU). (2008). *History.* Retrieved on March 8, 2008, from http://www.nursesunions.ca/content.php?doc=44.

Canadian Nurses Association (CNA). (2002). *The nursing shortage—The nursing workforce.* Retrieved on March 11, 2008, from http://www.cna-aiic.ca/CNA/issues/hhr/default_e.aspx.

Canadian Nurses Association (CNA). (2007). *Nursing Education in Canada Statistics.* Ottawa: Author. Retrieved on March 8, 2008, from http://www.cna-nurses.ca/CNA/documents/pdf/publications/Nursing_Education_Statistics_2005_2006_e.pdf.

Canadian Nurses Association (CNA). (2008). *Code of ethics for registered nurses.* Ottawa: Author. Retrieved on October 10, 2009, from http://www.cna-nurses.ca/CNA/documents/pdf/publications/Code_of_Ethics_2008_e.pdf.

Dion, G. (2009). Rand formula. *The Canadian Encyclopedia, Law.* Historica-Dominion. Retrieved on October 2, 2009, from http://www.thecanadianencyclopedia.com/index.cfm?PgNm=TCE&Params=A1ARTA0006672.

Fédération des Infirmières et Infirmiers du Québec (FIIQ). (2001). *Notre histoire.* Retrieved on March 28, 2002, from http://www.fiiq.qc.ca/histoire.htm.

Fédération des Infirmières et Infirmiers du Québec (FIIQ). (2008). *Collective Agreement: A decree in lieu of a collective bargaining agreement.* Retrieved on March 10, 2008, from http://translate.google.com/translate?hl=en&sl=fr&u=http://www.fiqsante.qc.ca/&sa=X&oi=translate&resnum=1&ct=result&prev=/search%3Fq%3DFederation%2Bdes%2BInfirmiers%2Bet%2BInfirmieres%2Bdu%2BQuebec%26hl%3Den%26rls%3Dcom.microsoft:en-us:IE-SearchBox%26rlz%3DI1I7SUNA.

Fédération Interprofessionnelle de la santé du Québec (FIQ). (n.d.). *Historique de la FIQ, 2006.* Retrieved on October 10, 2009, from http://www.fiqsante.qc.ca.

A final offer selection in relation to the wage rates for registered nurses, licensed practical nurses, and other health care employees employed by the employer. (2001). Susan M. Ashley, Halifax. Retrieved on October 19, 2009, from http://action.web.ca/home/nsgeu/attach/fosdecision.pdf.

Government of Nova Scotia, Finance Department. (2001). *Selector's decision issued in health care labour dispute.* Retrieved on March 11, 2008, from http://www.gov.ns.ca/finance/news/release.asp?id=20010813004.

Hamelin-Brabant, L., Lavoie-Tremblay, M., Lefrançois, L., & Viens, C. (2007). Engaging health care workers in improving their work environment. *Journal of Nursing Management, 15*(3), 313–320.

Hardingham, L. (1999). Disobeying laws and rules. *Alberta RN, 55*(6), 16–17.

Manitoba Nurses' Union (MNU). (2001). *Standing up for the front lines of health care.* Retrieved on March 28, 2002, from http://www. nursesunion.mb.ca.

Manitoba Nurses' Union (MNU). (2008). *Bargaining '08: Highlights of settlement.* Retrieved on March 10, 2008, from http://www.nursesunion.mb.ca/march_10.htm.

McGee, A. H. (1994). *The strength of one: A history of the New Brunswick Nurses Union.* Fredericton: New Brunswick Nurses Union. Retrieved on March 11, 2008, from http://www.nbnu-siinb.nb.ca/documents/historyeng.pdf.

Mussallem, H. K. (1977). *Nurses and political action: Issues in Canadian nursing.* Toronto: Prentice-Hall.

New Brunswick Nurses' Union (NBNU). (2008). *NBNU in the news.* Retrieved on March 10, 2008, from http://www.nbnu-siinb.nb.ca/inthenews_archive.html.

Newfoundland and Labrador Nurses' Union (NLNU). (2008). *Government agrees to commence bargaining early.* Retrieved on March 11, 2008, from http://www.nlnu.nf.ca/publications/EarlyReturnNov2707.pdf.

Nova Scotia Nurses' Union (NSNU). (2008). *Acute and long term care agreements ratified February 29, 2008.* Retrieved on March 11, 2008, from http://www.nsnu.ns.ca.

Ontario Nurses' Association (ONA). (2001). *Annual report, 2000–2001.* Toronto: Author.

Ontario Nurses' Association (ONA). (2008). *ONA releases details of tentative settlement for 50,000 hospital RNs.* Retrieved on March 10, 2008, from http://www.ona.org/20080222HospSettlementDetailsRelease.

Ordre des infirmières et infirmiers du Québec (OIIQ). (1982). *Labour relations and withdrawal of services within the health sector.* Brief presented at the meeting of the Comité Permanente du Travail et de la Main-d'Oeuvre de l'Assemblé Nationale du Québec. Quebec: Author.

Prince Edward Island Nurses' Union. (2009). *President's message.* Retrieved on May 2, 2010, from http://www.peinu.com/presidents_message.html.

Rowsell, G. (1982). Bargaining: A means of conflict resolution. *International Nursing Review, 29*(5), 141–145.

Saskatchewan Union of Nurses (SUN). (2008). *History: 2006: A year in review.* Retrieved on March 10, 2008, at http://www.sun-nurses.sk.ca/history.php.

United Nurses of Alberta (UNA). (1997). *UNA history.* Retrieved on March 28, 2002, from http://www.una.ab.ca/documents/history/1997.html.

United Nurses of Alberta (UNA). (2008). *Conservative promises on the nursing shortage: Too little, too late say nurses.* Retrieved on March 9, 2008, from http://www.una.ab.ca/news/archive/nursing%20shortage.

PART 4

EDUCATING NURSES FOR THE FUTURE

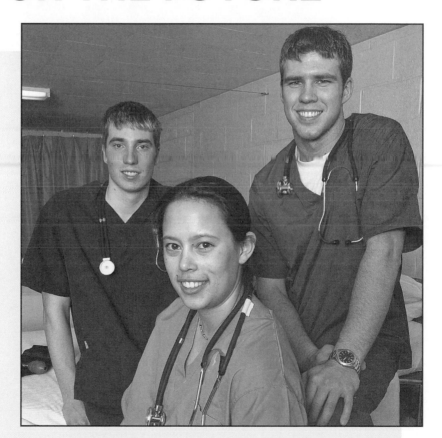

18 The Origins and Development of Nursing Education in Canada

Pauline Paul and Janet C. Ross-Kerr

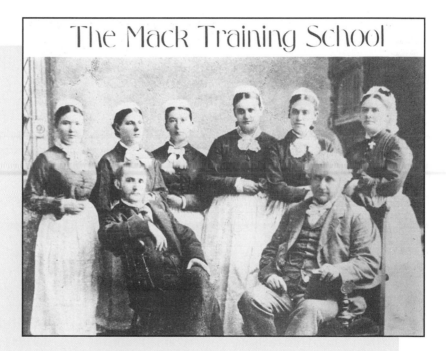

The first nurses to graduate in Canada are shown with their instructors from the Mack Training School in St. Catharines, Ontario, circa 1874.

LEARNING OBJECTIVES

- To recognize when women and nurses first had access to higher education.
- To acquire an understanding of the preparation of nurses prior to Nightingale.
- To understand the influence of the Nightingale model of nursing education.
- To describe the inception of the first hospital schools of nursing in Canada.
- To recognize how a number of reports demonstrated the need for better standards in nursing education.
- To understand the movement to establish two-year schools of nursing and identify how it played out in various provinces.
- To describe the emergence of university schools of nursing.
- To highlight the evolution of university nursing education in the 1920s and 1930s.
- To explain how university nursing education evolved between 1940 and 1950.
- To identify how the first two basic nursing baccalaureate degree programs in Canada emerged.

WOMEN AND HIGHER EDUCATION

In the late 1700s in the United States, a crusade began to allow women to gain entry into institutions of higher education, and feminist writer Mary Wollstonecraft presented an articulate case for the schooling of women (1787, 1792). However, it was not until 1837 that women began to slowly enter higher education in the United States. In Canada in 1862, Mount Allison University, in New Brunswick, was the first university to admit women and the first of the British Empire to confer a degree on a woman, when in 1875, Grace Annie Lockhart obtained a Bachelor of Science degree (Tunis, 1966; Mount Allison University, 2008).

Teaching was among the first professions to accept large numbers of women, and in the western United States, seminaries and normal schools for women were founded, where Jackel (1985) noted that "the need for fees fully as much as frontier egalitarianism dictated that these state-funded land-grant institutions would be coeducational from the outset" (p. 3). Although the more tradition-bound eastern states did not move as quickly, in 1887, philanthropist Grace Hoadley Dodge (1856–1914) founded the New York College for the Training of Teachers, which became Teachers College in 1892 and later a school of Columbia University (*Encyclopedia Britannica Online*, 2008). In 1899, Teachers College established a course in nursing, the first time in the world that nursing was a university subject area. Considering the concern Hoadley Dodge had for working women, and that normal schools in general were the first to welcome large numbers of women, it is not surprising that the first department of nursing in a university was at Teachers College. Teachers College rapidly became the beacon of university education in North America. In 1906, Mary Adelaide Nutting, a Quebec-born American nursing leader, became the director of its program at Columbia University and the first professor of nursing in the world. Columbia played a significant role in educating countless American and Canadian nursing leaders who shaped nursing education throughout the twentieth century.

However, during the twentieth century, most nurses did not study in universities but rather in hospital schools (and later in colleges) where nursing diplomas could be obtained. It is thus important to consider first how hospital nursing schools became the norm in the first half of the twentieth century in Canada.

EARLY PREPARATION FOR NURSING PRACTICE

Although nurses had some preparation for practice in the early days of the profession, it was largely informal. Observation, passing knowledge from one person to another, and on-the-job training were the principal forms of educational preparation for nurses in the seventeenth, eighteenth, and nineteenth centuries. Members of religious nursing orders like the Augustinians, who arrived at Quebec in 1639, received their preparation within their order, which had dedicated itself to the care of the sick. For several centuries, women who joined religious orders were taught the skills of nursing by experienced members of the sisterhood. Lay women rarely received this type of education. Among these exceptions were Jeanne Mance and later Florence Nightingale. Jeanne Mance, the founder of Hôtel-Dieu of Montreal and co-founder of the city, was the first lay nurse of New France, and she had designed her own course of nursing study, travelling to several centres in France to learn care methods before emigrating to New France in 1641. Similarly, Nightingale sought nursing knowledge at the Institution for Nursing Deaconesses at Kaiserswerth in Germany and with the Sisters of St. Vincent de Paul in Paris. The genius of Nightingale was to transform what she had seen into a school of nursing that brought the birth of modern nursing education.

THE NIGHTINGALE MODEL

In 1852, Florence Nightingale eloquently put the question "Why have women passion, intellect and moral activity—these three—and a place in society where no one of the three can be exercised?" (1929, p. 396). In a way, Nightingale answered her question in 1860, by founding the first school of nursing in conjunction with St. Thomas's Hospital in London. Evidently this development was needed in Western society, for the idea swept the world, and many hospital nursing schools were established throughout Europe and America. However, the first hospital schools of North America lacked an important aspect of the original Nightingale school, namely financial autonomy. The term "the historical accident," coined by Esther Lucile Brown (1948, p. 164), referred to the failure to apply the fundamental philosophy of the Nightingale model to the new schools of North America. In many of these schools, the concept of autonomy was lost in the financial administration of the enterprise. Such schools became completely dependent on the financial stability of the hospital with which they were associated, and policies were dictated by a board of trustees. The educational orientation was forgotten as the new schools-cum-service ministered to the needs of the sick. Thus, little attention was given to opportunities for instruction in the classroom or during clinical experience, and educational preparation was considered secondary to the needs of the hospital nursing service.

Certain principles of the first Nightingale school were present in new schools: women who were as well prepared in nursing as possible were placed in charge of the schools, courses were spread over a period of two or three years, and incidental instruction was accompanied by extended periods of practice. It was an apprenticeship system that lacked the master craftsman. In North America, off-duty students attended one or two hours of lectures that were given each week by a physician or the superintendent of nurses. Those who could attend related the information to those who could not because they were assigned to care duties.

One of the first schools in North America to advocate the principles of Florence Nightingale was the Bellevue Training School for Nurses, which was established in New York in 1873 by Sister Helen Bowden, an Anglican sister who had been educated at University College Hospital in England. Many Canadian women went to the United States to study during this period, and some, including Isabel Hampton Robb, Mary Adelaide Nutting, and Isabel Maitland Stewart, later became leaders in American nursing. Undoubtedly as a result of their influence, close contact was maintained between nurses in Canada and the United States through professional nursing organizations.

THE FIRST CANADIAN HOSPITAL SCHOOLS OF NURSING

The first hospital diploma school in Canada, the Mack Training School for Nurses in St. Catharines, Ontario, was initiated on June 10, 1874, by Dr. Theophilus Mack, an Irish-born physician who was convinced that "the prejudice held by many sick people against going into public hospitals could best be overcome by building up a profession of trained lay nurses" (Gibbon & Mathewson, 1947, p. 144). Healey (1990) notes that the date of the inception of the school "so closely parallels the start of Bellevue that in later years there will be those who seek to prove it was the first on the Continent to incorporate Nightingale's ideas" (pp. 31–32). Healey (1990) also indicates that "Dr. Mack is credited with having the idea [for the establishment of the school] as early as 1864" (p. 43). Constraints were again imposed, as "nursing was considered an undesirable vocation for a refined lady, the only acceptable profession being teaching" (Healey, 1990, p. 44).

Admission standards were "plain English education, good character, and Christian motives" (*St. Catharines Annual Report*; cited in Healey [1990]). The philosophy of the school is reflected in a statement concerning instruction:

> *Every possible opportunity is seized to impart instruction of a practical nature in the art of nursing, while teachings will be given in Chemistry, Sanitary Science, Popular Physiology and Anatomy, hygiene and all such branches of the healing art as a nurse ought to be familiar with. . . . The vocation of nursing goes hand in hand with that of physician and surgeon, and are absolutely indispensable one to the other. Incompetency on the part of a nurse renders nugatory*

the best effects of the doctor in the critical moments and has frequently resulted in loss of life. All the most brilliant achievements of modern surgery are dependent to a great extent upon careful and intelligent nursing.. . . The skilled nurse, by minutely watching the temperature, conditions of skin, pulse, respirations, the various functions of all the organs and reporting faithfully to the attending physician, must increase the chances of recovery twofold. (Healey, 1990, pp. 45–46)

The School for Nurses associated with the Toronto General Hospital was established in 1881; seventeen students enrolled, but eight resigned or were dismissed (Gibbon & Mathewson, 1947). When Mary Agnes Snively, a former schoolteacher from St. Catharines who had graduated from the Bellevue Hospital Training School of New York, was appointed superintendent of the school in 1884, there were no systems for work or study, no written orders, no history records, and no systems for obtaining ward supplies. The living conditions were distressing. The school was gradually reorganized and the modern plan developed (Gibbon & Mathewson, 1947). Snively worked hard to improve the educational component of the program as it developed and made it one of the most successful schools of nursing in the country (Kirkwood, 2005). Snively is also remembered for the roles she played in the International Council of Nurses (ICN) and the Canadian National Association of Trained Nurses (later the Canadian Nurses Association [CNA]).

At the Montreal General Hospital, which was founded in 1822, early interest in establishing a school of nursing led to the Committee of Management's correspondence in 1874 to secure assistance in developing "a system of trained hospital nurses such as approved of in England" (MacDermot, 1940, p. 17). Correspondence that ensued with Florence Nightingale and her brother-in-law Henry Bonham Carter, the president of the Nightingale Fund, dealt primarily with plans for the new hospital building that had been promised by the Committee of Management. Miss Machin, a Quebec native who had been nursing at the Nightingale Home in London, set out for Montreal with four Nightingale nurses, but the mission failed. The difficulties that arose during Machin's tenure at the hospital included a high staff turnover rate, and "there is reason to believe there was 'a lack of adaptability on the part of Miss Machin whose uncompromising purpose was to apply Nightingale principles of nursing care at whatever cost and without much thought for diplomacy'" (Redpath; cited in Baly, 1986, p. 146). The problems she encountered and her failure to accomplish her initial objective—establishing a training school for nurses—led to her perception of failure in her mission, and she returned to England in 1878. Baly (1986) notes that the Council of the Nightingale Fund did not make much of their efforts in Montreal or elsewhere because Cook (Nightingale's biographer) had given Montreal only a passing reference, and Carter clearly thought that the entire issue should be forgotten. Baly (1986) has taken issue with "nursing historians" who "have claimed that Nightingale missioners took reformed nursing to both Canada and Australia and have made much out of little evidence" (p. 147).

The School for Nurses at the Montreal General Hospital was finally initiated in 1890, under the direction of Nora Livingston, who was born the daughter of English parents in Sault Ste. Marie, Michigan, raised in Como, Quebec, and educated at the New York Hospital's Training School for Nurses (MacDermot, 1940). When she arrived in Montreal, she found deplorable conditions that she undertook to improve immediately to

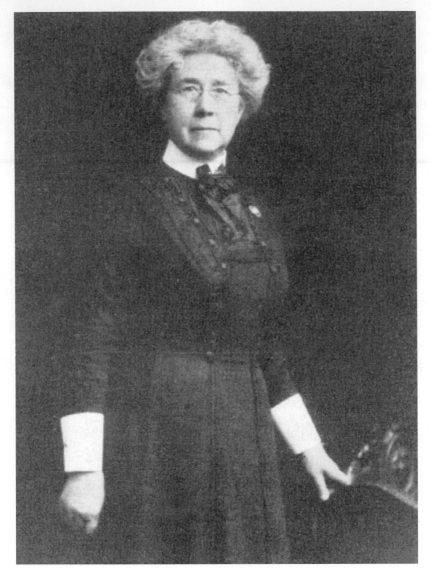

Mary Agnes Snively, superintendent of the School for Nurses at Toronto General Hospital and first president of the National Association of Trained Nurses (later the CNA).

ensure that the hospital and its nurses were soon held in high regard: "By reorganizing the work, gradually encouraging the appointment of nurses to positions of responsibility, and establishing specific duties, Livingston helped to define the proper functions of a nurse" (Cohen, 2000).

The popularity of the school increased rapidly. Livingston reported 169 applications in the first year, 80 of which were accepted on probation. Of the 80 students accepted,

42 proved satisfactory, four resigned, and two were dismissed (Gibbon & Mathewson, 1947). Recollections of Livingston's abilities are positive:

> *What an extraordinary amount of tact and gumption this remarkable woman possessed. Not only had she to change the incredible conditions of nursing but above all she had to change the attitudes of the administrators, men animated by good intentions but more accustomed to conducting the affairs of business than those of a hospital. (Desjardins, 1971, p. 103)*

The nursing education program gradually took shape, and one of the early graduates recalls: "Thinking of those days so long ago, I think I hear Miss Livingston say—'Nurse—the patient—always the patient first!' I think that spirit still lives within these old walls" (Gibbon & Mathewson, 1947, p. 149).

The move to establish hospital schools of nursing swept the country. The Winnipeg General Hospital initiated the first Training School for Nurses in the west in 1887. In the Maritime provinces, the Saint John General Hospital in Saint John and the Victoria Public Hospital in Fredericton opened training schools for nurses in 1887, and the Victoria General in Halifax and the Prince Edward Island Hospital in Charlottetown followed suit in 1890. In Vancouver, the General Hospital began an educational program in 1891, and a school was initiated at Medicine Hat in Alberta in 1894. By 1930, there were approximately 330 schools of nursing in Canada (CNA, 1968).

REFLECTIVE THINKING

Discuss the role of the hospital diploma schools of nursing in the evolution of nursing education in Canada.

RECOGNIZING THE NEED FOR IMPROVEMENT IN STANDARDS

Because hospitals were staffed primarily by students in the late nineteenth and early twentieth centuries, there were few opportunities for securing a staff position after graduation. Graduates who practised their profession usually did so as private-duty nurses in the homes of the sick. Therefore, one of nurses' first struggles after the hospital-based system of nursing education was established involved replacing students with graduate nurses as the primary providers of nursing care. Mabel Holt (1936) writes of an "experiment" in a Montreal hospital in which a nursing unit was totally staffed with graduate nurses and justified the endeavour as follows:

> *There are, however, other and even more important benefits . . . which have come about as a direct result of this new policy. Instead of adding to the output of graduate nurses during these difficult years by increasing the enrolment of our school of nursing, we have created employment for those who otherwise would have been obliged to enter an overcrowded and highly competitive field. (p. 10)*

The significance of the 1910 Flexner Report on medical education and its impact on nursing education have been noted by Allemang (1974). Funded by the Carnegie Foundation, the Flexner Report was commissioned because of concern for the quality of medical practice and medical education and the concomitant inability of the American Medical Association and the Council on Medical Education to achieve reforms. As a result of the Flexner Report, the character of medical education changed quickly; the proprietary schools that operated for profit were closed, and standards in medical education began to rise as the universities assumed major responsibility for the support and direction of the enterprise. According to Allemang (1974): "The Flexner report on medical education provided a model for the new approach to nursing reforms" (pp. 115–116). Thus, the call for improved standards of nursing education became more intense as the twentieth century progressed.

Increased awareness of deficiencies resulted in a number of surveys of nursing education in Canada and the United States. In 1923, the Goldmark Report, commissioned by the Rockefeller Foundation to investigate conditions in schools of nursing in the United States, described appalling conditions. The report advocated more attention for the educational preparation of nurses, more stringent admission requirements for nursing schools, and provision of federal grants to assist schools in raising their educational standards. In Burgess (1928) and the Committee on the Grading of Nursing Schools (1934), reports of a joint committee of several professional nursing associations and professional organizations of related health fields on the grading of schools of nursing restated the shortcomings of the system.

In Canada, similar unrest about hospital schools of nursing also surfaced in the 1920s. In 1927, a joint committee of the Canadian Medical Association (CMA) and the CNA was organized to study the problems. The committee appointed Dr. George Weir, of the Department of Education at the University of British Columbia, to conduct a survey to address these matters. The study documented the problems and drew attention to the changes needed to improve standards of education and service. The fact that small hospitals had established schools of nursing was a concern because students' education could be compromised as a result of the lack of variety in clinical experience in small institutions. The survey indicated that, in operating programs, schools associated with hospitals with fewer than 75 beds were more concerned with the financial needs of the hospital than with the educational needs of nursing students (CNA, 1968; Gibbon & Mathewson, 1947; Weir, 1932). The health of students was also a concern raised in the Weir report. It was common for schools to require students to work as many as 78 hours per week with just one half-day off duty. Overtime was also common, and students were not given time off to compensate for this. The gruelling hours had a consequent impact on the health of many students, and some did not complete their programs as a result. Classroom instruction was likewise lacking in planning and generally inadequate, with too few and ill-prepared instructors.

Suspicion about the general motives of hospitals in offering educational programs led to the recommendation that authority and responsibility for schools of nursing be vested within the general provincial system of education. "The development of training schools for nurses primarily as educational institutions functioning as an integral part of the general educational system of the province and financed on the same principle as are normal schools, should be made an immediate objective" (Weir, 1932, p. 116). This recommendation was repeated many times in the years before the basic diploma nursing education program began to move within the purview of the general postsecondary system of education.

The recommendations of the Weir report led the Canadian Nurses Association to organize a national curriculum committee with a mandate to develop a curriculum model (Letourneau, 1975, p. 6). The standard curriculum guide, published in 1936, was intended to serve as an interim measure that would help schools of nursing during their transfer to provincial educational systems (CNA, 1936).

THE DEMONSTRATION SCHOOL

The minimal progress through the next decade led the CNA to secure Red Cross funding for a demonstration school that would ascertain the feasibility of preparing a nurse in less than three years. The school, known simply as the Demonstration School, was established in 1948 in conjunction with the Metropolitan Hospital in Windsor, Ontario. Red Cross funding enabled the Demonstration School to be financially independent from the hospital. The experiment continued until 1952, when the Demonstration School reverted to its former status of financial dependence on the hospital. An extensive evaluation, conducted by a joint committee (chaired by A.R. Lord) of the CNA and the Canadian Education Association (CEA), indicated that the venture was a success; it was possible to prepare a nurse for practice in two years.

The conclusion is inescapable. When the school has complete control of students, nurses can be trained at least as satisfactorily in two years as in three, and under better conditions, but the training must be paid for in money instead of in services. Few students can afford substantial fees nor can the hospital pass on such additional costs to the "paying patient." Some new source of revenue is the only solution. (Lord, 1952, p. 54)

THE CENTRALIZED TEACHING PROGRAM

In Saskatchewan there was increasing concern about the lack of foundational courses in basic sciences for nursing students in diploma programs and the general shortage of suitably qualified faculty. The Saskatchewan Registered Nurses' Association (SRNA) sought and secured financial support from the W.K. Kellogg Foundation to centralize teaching of basic sciences for all schools of nursing in the Saskatoon and Regina areas. The program provided for

a duly authorized sixteen weeks' program of instruction in the basic sciences for nursing students. It is an integral part of the curriculum plan of the hospital school of nursing provided apart from the hospital school at a designated centre permitting centralization of effort and resources not immediately available in the local setting of the participating schools. (Schmitt, 1957, p. 6)

Although considerable effort was directed to organizing this effort and it was declared a success, it was not considered a panacea for the ills of basic nursing education. Although many areas of the country decided not to offer basic science instruction on a regional basis, this endeavour provided a solution to some problems and issues in basic diploma nursing education.

ACCREDITATION

The CNA next directed attention to the quality of instruction in schools of nursing. A pilot project under the direction of Executive Director Helen K. Mussallem was designed to determine whether schools were ready for a national voluntary accreditation program. The findings were somewhat disappointing; only 16% of schools met the criteria for accreditation. It was also determined that little progress had been made in improving the quality of schools since Dr. Weir had made his report public some 30 years before. Dr. Mussallem thus recommended that the CNA embark on a school improvement program rather than an accreditation program designed to lead to accreditation in the future (Mussallem, 1960). The CNA took this course of action, and accreditation was not seriously discussed again until the late 1970s. At that time, because of the associated costs, accreditation was not considered for diploma schools in the absence of an organization willing to provide the necessary funds.

THE ROYAL COMMISSION ON HEALTH SERVICES

In its brief to the Royal Commission on Health Services, the CNA favoured "introducing diploma schools of nursing into the post-high school system of the country" (Mussallem, 1964, p. 137). The Royal Commission on Health Services, known as the Hall Commission, surveyed the entire range of health services (including nursing), reporting in 1964 and recommending that schools of nursing function independently from hospitals and offer programs shorter than three years in length:

> The Commission believes this to be the right approach. The educational system for nursing should be organized and financed like other forms of professional education . . . not only [so] that we shall obtain equally, if not better, qualified personnel in shorter time, but that a substantial part of hospitalized patient-care will no longer depend, as it does now, upon apprentices. (Government of Canada, 1964, pp. 64–69)

A certain momentum created by the increased pace of change after the release of the Hall Commission Report may have led to the CNA's plan to press for change. Mussallem (1964) declared:

> Whether nursing education should be placed within the general educational system can no longer be considered a point of debate. It is possible and it can be done. . . . The Canadian Nurses' Association, in cooperation with its provincial counterparts, should take steps to implement the plan present in the study . . . leading to the inclusion of all nursing education within the general educational system of each province. (pp. 183–185)

THE MOVEMENT TO ESTABLISH TWO-YEAR SCHOOLS

QUEBEC

In Quebec the Royal Commission of Inquiry on Education, also known as the Parent Commission, reported in 1966 and argued against initiating one or two two-year schools as suggested by the Association of Nurses of the Province of Quebec (ANPQ), but a total transfer of programs to the general system of education. The commission contended that nursing recommendations were totally consistent with findings in other fields. Campbell (1971) has commented about the impact of the Parent Commission's report: "It would be difficult to name any royal commission in the history of Canadian education whose judgements more profoundly altered the structure and process of the entire educational system of a province and with greater speed" (p. 54).

In 1967, three programs were selected for transfer to the Collèges d'Enseignement Général et Professionnel (CEGEP) to serve as pilot projects; seventeen were selected in 1968, and others after that. "In 1972, the last Schools of Nursing attached to hospitals closed, ending three-quarters of a century of history. Now a network of 40 nursing options exists throughout 'la belle province'" (ANPQ, 1972, p. 1). With the two English-language CEGEPs that already had diploma programs, the number of programs was 42. Also, "a distinctively unique characteristic of education offered in a CEGEP is that it is tuition free for all full-time students" (Letourneau, 1975, p. 77). Thus, as nursing schools became part of the community college system in Quebec, nursing students began receiving the same educational benefits as students studying in other professions and vocations.

ONTARIO

The Nightingale School of Nursing in Toronto, established in 1960, was financed by the Ontario Hospital Services Commission. Situated near New Mount Sinai Hospital where nursing clinical experience was obtained, the school was administered by an independent board of directors. The Quo Vadis School of Nursing was established in 1964 under the auspices of the Catholic Hospital Conference of Ontario with a mandate to attract mature students. Financial support was provided by the Ontario Hospital Services Commission, and the school was administered by an independent board of directors (McLean, 1964).

The School of Nursing established at Ryerson Polytechnical Institute in Toronto in 1964 had the distinction of being the first nursing diploma program in Canada to be initiated in an educational institution (Letourneau, 1975). The efforts of the Registered Nurses' Association of Ontario (RNAO) were influential in instigating this effort. Similar programs were developed in colleges across the country. Although Ryerson's program was initially structured as a three-year program, it was later converted to a two-year program. Dr. Moyra Allen of McGill University and Professor Mary Reidy of the University of Montreal evaluated this program after five years and confirmed its soundness. The findings "point to the potential value of preparing a nurse in a college-level institution within the general system of education" (Allen & Reidy, 1971, p. 262).

In 1967, 20 colleges of applied arts and technology (CAATs) were created in the province by order of the Ontario government. In 1969, Humber College was the first of these institutions to develop a nursing program. Ontario moved ahead on another front before it began to develop schools of nursing within the CAAT system on a large scale, namely by developing freestanding schools of nursing called "regional schools" apart from the general education system. There were no regional schools in 1965, but "by the end of 1967 there were eight, and ten more . . . expected within the next five years" (Murray, 1970, p. 132).

The government also decided, in spite of the reservations expressed by the College of Nurses of Ontario, to move to "two plus one" programs, initially in a "ten-year plan leading to a gradual shortening and regionalization of schools of nursing" (Letourneau, 1975, p. 144). This change occurred rapidly, but it was a passing phenomenon as the move to establish two-year schools under the aegis of the CAATs received overwhelming support, and "in 1972, policies with regard to free room and board were altered, the year of internship was discontinued, and nursing students were required to pay tuition fees" (Letourneau, 1975, p. 145). By 1973, 56 schools had been absorbed by 23 CAATs.

WESTERN CANADA

Saskatchewan was the first Canadian province to consider implementing two-year diploma nursing schools. The Regina Grey Nuns Hospital School of Nursing received permission from the Saskatchewan Registered Nurses' Association (SRNA) to develop a two-year diploma program in nursing on an experimental basis, leading to the establishment of two-year diploma programs in Saskatoon and Regina in 1967. Letourneau (1975) cites the difficulties that occurred because "Saskatchewan had forged ahead in legislating change without having an educational system fully established to absorb programs" (p. 25). To avoid the development of isolated institutions that would be for nursing only, the SRNA (1966) insisted "that diploma nursing for nurses be established in post-secondary institutions for higher education" (p. 1). In Saskatchewan, "the trend was not for hospital schools of nursing to transmute to an educational institution, but rather to gradually phase out by ceasing to admit students" (Letourneau, 1975, p. 27). The two new two-year programs in Saskatchewan were developed at the Kelsey Institute in Saskatoon and at Wascana Institute in Regina.

In British Columbia, the first diploma nursing program to be established within the general educational system was a jointly planned venture of the British Columbia Institute of Technology (BCIT) and the Registered Nurses Association of British Columbia (RNABC) in 1967. The RNABC's (1967) position was well known:

Nursing can no longer be taught by apprenticeship methods; yet the students are part of the hospital service personnel. . . . We believe that the method of financing nursing education partly through hospital operating costs and partly through service rendered by students is no longer an adequate or desirable one. (p. 20)

Funding for this program was obtained through an agreement between the federal and provincial governments for vocational-technical education. During the development of the program, the RNABC successfully lobbied for changes in existing legislation to allow for development of new and innovative models of diploma nursing programs. Thus, community colleges throughout the province were able to develop nursing programs, and in 1965, Vancouver City College in Langara and Selkirk College in Castlegar initiated theirs. By 1974, four programs had been developed, and several others were in the planning stages, although four hospital diploma programs still remained in operation.

In Alberta, the transfer of diploma programs to the community colleges was a slow process. Mount Royal College in Calgary was the first college in the province to develop a diploma nursing program in 1967. Others included Red Deer College and the College St. Jean (merged with Grant MacEwan Community College in 1972) in 1968, Lethbridge Community College in 1969, Medicine Hat College in 1970, and Grant MacEwan Community College in 1972. Although seven hospitals had phased out their schools, six were still in operation in the province in 1974 (Letourneau, 1975). A report prepared by Dr. G.R. Fast in 1971 had recommended the transfer of remaining diploma programs to the Alberta college system, but lack of consultation and discussion prior to its release led to the shelving of the report. The last hospital schools of nursing did not close their doors until the 1990s.

The first and only college diploma program established in Manitoba in the 1970s was at Red River Community College (in 1970), as a result of "action on the part of the Departments of Health and Education and the adjoining cooperative efforts of the MARN" (Letourneau, 1975, p. 253). The Manitoba Association of Registered Nurses (MARN) was influential in establishing the program because it supported the inclusion of diploma nursing programs in the general system of education and the shortening of their duration to two years (MARN, 1968). Some diploma programs have been phased out in Manitoba, but Red River College continues to offer a diploma program in nursing.

THE ATLANTIC PROVINCES

By the end of 1974, there had been some activity in the Atlantic provinces in relation to the movement that was sweeping other parts of the country, but activity was limited. A study conducted by Katherine MacLaggan of nursing education in New Brunswick resulted in a recommendation that the general educational system be vested with responsibility for diploma nursing education (MacLaggan, 1965). According to Letourneau (1975), "Conflicting forces have rendered impossible the actual transfer of hospital programs to the system of education" (p. 275). In 1971, the Abbis Report recommended that four independent schools be established similar to a pilot program at the Saint John School of Nursing, which had been converted to a two-year program but financed through health dollars from the Department of Health (Study Committee on Nursing Education, 1971). Controversy over recommendations on registration and standards also contained in the document led the New Brunswick Association of Registered Nurses (NBARN) (1971) to say that it was "gravely alarmed at the import of these recommendations and quite surprised that they appear in the Report. . . . [We] earnestly recommend that they be rejected" (p. 23).

Because there was no authority for establishing community colleges in New Brunswick until 1974, transfer of diploma nursing programs to the system of general education across the province was not possible. Thus, four independent schools and one hospital school were established in Bathurst, Edmundston, Moncton, and Saint John (Letourneau, 1975). These programs were autonomous in all respects except finance. However, as Letourneau observed: "Trends point to an eventual orderly transfer of independent programs to the provincial system of education, but first the community college system must develop sufficiently to absorb these programs" (p. 290).

The Registered Nurses' Association of Nova Scotia (RNANS) had a leading role in pressing for changes in the system of nursing education in that province. The RNANS's appointment of a curriculum council to determine each school's plan for change may have hastened and facilitated self-study by the schools so that "seven hospital schools of nursing were authorized, in the period extending from 1969 to 1970, to begin a two-year program or to effect a change in this direction" (Letourneau, 1975, p. 293). As with nurses across the country, in 1969 nurses in Nova Scotia had to stop an attempt to remove the regulatory powers vested in their association. Like New Brunswick, Nova Scotia also faced the problem of having a community college system that needed to develop to accommodate the new programs.

The Association of Nurses of Prince Edward Island (ANPEI) requested that the three existing hospital schools of nursing in its province be phased out and replaced by one program to make the best use of staff and facilities and to provide the best possible education for students (Letourneau, 1975). The organization also sponsored a study that assessed the climate and readiness for change in the diploma nursing education system, reaching the conclusion that it was not the right time for major change (Rowe, 1967). In 1968, the ANPEI again pressed for change in the system, and this time the government responded by providing authority for developing one independent "two plus one" program for the province, replacing the three hospital schools (Letourneau, 1975). Efforts in 1974 to link the school with a community college, Holland College, were unsuccessful.

Letourneau (1975) has stated: "The transfer of hospital schools of nursing to the system of education is, as in other Atlantic provinces, non-existent in Newfoundland" (p. 308). Four hospital schools of nursing continued to exist there, although the Association of Registered Nurses of Newfoundland (ARNN) tried to encourage change. Arpin, a consultant hired by the ARNN to help formulate goals, recommended that "the three schools of nursing in St. John's develop their curriculum plans so that the theory and experience essential for meeting the school objectives is included in the first two years of the program" (1972, p. 1). By 1973, the three schools in St. John's had established "two plus one" programs and the Corner Brook program had reduced its length to two years.

EMERGENCE OF UNIVERSITY SCHOOLS OF NURSING

In view of the firm establishment and acceptance of the hospital-based educational system, the difficulty that the university-based system encountered in establishing its credibility in the eyes of patients, the public, and even nurses is easily understood. Bonin (1976) commented: "So deeply time-honoured became this system of nursing education that it became difficult to imagine nursing, like other professions, as belonging to a university setting for the education of its practitioners" (pp. xii–xiii).

University education for nurses was the subject of an address by Dr. Malcolm T. MacEachern to the British Columbia Hospitals Association in July 1919, after the May 26 Board of Governors' decision to approve the Senate's recommendation that a department of nursing be established at the University of British Columbia (Street, 1973). The founding of the department, a precedent in the history of Canadian nursing, occurred four years after the 1915 establishment of the university, largely through the efforts of Dr. MacEachern, the progressive medical superintendent of the Vancouver General Hospital. Universities were founded in the west as early as the second decade of the twentieth century, when agricultural and technical education were receiving attention from the federal government. The utilitarian philosophical orientation of the new western universities explains the location of the first school of nursing in the west—British Columbia.

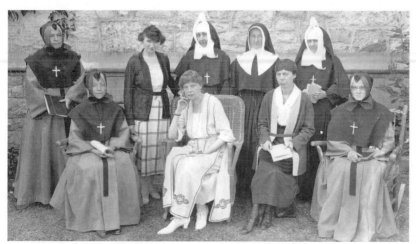

Ethel Johns, director of UBC's Department of Nursing, the first university degree nursing program in Canada, with her students in the summer of 1922.

THE DEPARTMENT OF NURSING AT THE UNIVERSITY OF BRITISH COLUMBIA

When the decision was made to establish the University of British Columbia's Department of Nursing, the source of funding for the school was reviewed:

The Board was advised that the Department would not involve any additional expense to the University. The minutes of this meeting do not add a fact of which the Board was aware: that the Vancouver General Hospital would pay the full salary of its director of nursing, who would also take charge of the University's Department of Nursing. (Street, 1973, pp. 118–119)

In subsequent communication to the Senate to inform members of the disposition of the recommendation, it was "emphasized that the action was taken on the understanding that the establishment of this Department would not involve any additional expense to the University" (Street, 1973, pp. 118–119). Under the terms of such a favourable arrangement, where the operating costs of the new department were to be borne by the hospital, the university was undoubtedly more easily persuaded by the persistent Dr. MacEachern that the entry of nursing into the academic world of the university was both possible and desirable.

The appointment of Ethel Johns as director of the new department was fortuitous; she was energetic, articulate, and of independent spirit. These qualities would be an asset, because in the beginning the way would not be easy for the first university school of nursing in the country. Street (1973) alludes to the "precarious early years" (p. 115) of the new program. In an address to a joint session of the British Columbia Hospitals Association and the Canadian Public Health Association in Vancouver in June 1920, Johns had an opportunity to appeal for positive attitudes, which had prevailed among physicians, toward the new development in nursing education:

To those who are in opposition or are in doubt, one last word, if there are any of such here: Will you not listen to the appeal of those upon whose shoulders you yourselves lay such heavy burdens? You see so many faults, so many blunders in our nursing service. So do we; they are not hidden from us. You cannot imagine why things should not run more smoothly, but we can; we know it is because of insufficient teaching and supervision. You do not realize how complex your own profession has become. How can we expect you to realize how difficult it is for us, with few of your educational advantages, to keep up with the advance shown in medicine? (Street, 1973, p. 132)

The degree program thus established was based on the prevailing U.S. model and "became the Canadian prototype of the pattern which came to be known as the non-integrated degree nursing course, or the 2+2+1 or 1+3+1 course, in which the university assumed no responsibility for the two or three years of nursing preparation in a hospital school of nursing" (Bonin, 1976, p. 7). The new program gradually became established. After the program was approved for its fifth year, there was a request from the Library Committee

for a grant of two hundred fifty dollars with which to purchase books for the Department of Nursing. But the Board had a long memory. After some discussion, it was decided to direct the attention of the Library Committee to the undertaking of the Hospital authorities that the University would not be asked to assume any financial responsibility in respect to the Department of Nursing. It was decided that a sum not to exceed one hundred dollars should be granted for books. (Street, 1973, p. 127)

THE IMPACT OF RED CROSS FUNDING

After World War I, the Canadian Red Cross Society participated in the formation of the League of Red Cross Societies and the planning of an international program for peace-time activity in public health. "It was decided that there should be a great worldwide public health organization to help bring up the standards of physical and mental fitness of the world . . . the promotion of health, the prevention of disease and the mitigation of suffering throughout the world" (Gibbon & Mathewson, 1947, p. 342).

In Canada, the Red Cross Society first directed its efforts to providing funds for the provision of facilities for postgraduate instruction in public health nursing "by sub-sidizing special courses for three years at the Universities of Toronto, McGill, British Columbia, Alberta, and Dalhousie" (Gibbon & Mathewson, 1947, p. 342). The financial incentive provided by these grants contributed to the creation of departments for the study of nursing at four of the institutions and encouraged the extension of what had been initiated the previous year at the University of British Columbia:

> In April 1920 the University of British Columbia accepted a proposal from the Provincial branch of the Canadian Red Cross Society to the effect that a Red Cross Chair of Public Health be established. For a period of three years from date of acceptance by the University, the Red Cross Society would pay five thousand dollars toward the salary of the professor. The expec-tation was that "the cause of Public Health, which everywhere is being regarded as of great importance, will be materially advanced throughout British Columbia." The Senate approved the proposal. (Street, 1973, p. 128)

The Red Cross funds must have seemed like a windfall to the young institution, which had been founded during wartime and had received little tangible support from the Liberal government that was in power in the province at the time.

In addition to providing funds to the institutions to stimulate the creation of new pro-grams in public health nursing, the Canadian Red Cross Society provided financial aid to students who wanted to attend programs initiated under their sponsorship (King, 1970, p. 70). These actions were met with enthusiasm, and continued increases in enrolment ensured the survival of most of the universities after the three-year period of institutional grants had ended. Not surprisingly, these certificate courses became the first in a series of such courses that were offered by the universities and also led to the development of degree programs in most of the institutions. However, these developments in 1920 were preceded by years of effort on the part of nurses to secure advanced preparation. King (1970) notes,

> The first documentation concerning efforts to establish a university nursing program in Canada appeared in 1905 when a memorandum was submitted by the Graduate Nurses' Association of Ontario to the University of Toronto requesting the university "to offer a course of training and education of nurses." (p. 70)

In 1918, Dr. Helen MacMurchy, a physician and the first editor of *The Canadian Nurse*, wrote to the presidents of the universities to urge them to encourage estab-lishment of nursing programs at their institutions (MacMurchy, 1918). Although the influence of such communication remains a matter of speculation, it is reasonable to assume that it at least made administrators of higher education more aware of the needs and issues in nursing education. As one author concluded: "One of the most significant developments during the period from 1910 to 1930 was the growth of positive attitudes toward university education for nurses" (Allemang, 1974, p. 137).

The one exception to the lasting success of the stimulus provided by the Red Cross for establishment of university nursing education was the public health nursing certificate program begun at Dalhousie University, which was also the first of its kind to be initiated (Tunis, 1966). The program at Dalhousie was short-lived and, for financial and perhaps other reasons, did not survive after 1922. Although Dalhousie's program was the first to be initiated through Red Cross funds, the nature of the support differed in that it consisted of direct funding of students rather than institutional grants and was thus far less substantial than that given to other universities during those same years. It took until 1949 for Dalhousie University to finally establish a school of nursing (Twohig, 1998).

THE 1920S AND THE 1930S

During the 1920s, several new five-year, nonintegrated degree programs similar to the program at the University of British Columbia were initiated. The University of Western Ontario established a program in 1924, followed by one at the University of Alberta in 1925. At the request of the Grey Nuns, the Université de Montréal began offering courses to nurses in 1923. These beginnings led the Grey Nuns in 1934 to fund the Institut Marguerite d'Youville in Montreal, as an affiliated school to the Université de Montréal. In 1962, the institut became the Faculté des sciences infirmières (Faculty of Nursing) of the Université de Montréal. By establishing a nonintegrated degree program at their institut, the Grey Nuns became the leaders of nursing education in the French world. Indeed, they offered the first university nursing program available in French on the entire planet. It is clear that the sisters had been influenced by the developments at UBC and that because they owned and operated hospitals in western Canada they were well aware of continental trends in nursing education (Paul, 1994; Cohen, Pepin, Lamontagne, & Duquette, 2002). Finally, the University of Toronto experimented throughout the 1920s and 1930s with a new model of a diploma program that evolved into the integrated degree program. This model is discussed later in this chapter.

The 1920s were productive years, during which adequate financial support had been available to support programs and expansion into new fields. During this period, nursing entered the university scene in Canada with the development of programs in six universities. However, growth and expansion in these institutions after 1929 was limited because of the general lack of economic resources. The early 1930s were difficult for Canadian universities, and the struggles of the school of Graduate Nurses at McGill University, which best exemplify these hardships, are presented in the next section. There are frequent references to salary cuts that professors accepted rather than see colleagues lose their positions because of financial constraints. Evidence of the lack of growth in the decade after the stock market collapse was observed in all institutions, but particularly those in western Canada. Nonetheless, by the end of the decade things began to improve and the universities of Saskatchewan and of Ottawa introduced degree programs in 1938, followed by St. Francis Xavier University in 1939.

CRISIS AT MCGILL

The year 1929 spelled the end of a decade in which university nursing education in Canada improved by leaps and bounds. According to Allemang (1974), the stock market crash in the fall of 1929 and the economic depression that followed "brought unemployment and hardship to nurses" (p. 172). Nurses had experienced difficulties in securing employment before 1929, and because of the worldwide economic depression, the situation rapidly worsened. People could no longer afford to employ private-duty nurses, and private duty had been the most promising area of employment for graduate nurses (Gunn, 1933, p. 141).

For universities in general, the Depression meant a period of significant adjustment, which included reduced revenues, staff layoffs, and difficult working conditions. However, despite this adverse environment, enrolments continued to show generally slow but steady growth throughout the decade; perhaps because no employment was available for people who had completed their high school educations, many chose to remain in school. The impact of the Depression on an institution in Canada was determined to a large extent by the amount of external support it received from government and private sources.

The Depression was hard on McGill University. McGill received only token funding from its provincial government from the earliest times. As a private institution, its mandate was to raise funds from private sources to operate its programs or reduce the size of its enterprise. This mandate made financing difficult enough during prosperous times; during the lean years of the Depression, it became an onerous task. The School for Graduate Nurses at McGill was subjected to the impact of the financial crunch for more than a decade.

Helen Reid, a member of the first class to graduate from McGill, was a strong proponent of the establishment of a school of nursing at McGill because she felt this would give women another means of entering the university. Although she had originally envisioned a two-year degree course at McGill, in 1920 advice from Isabel M. Stewart, the Canadian-born professor of nursing at Teacher's College, Columbia University, suggested that "to attempt at present in any way to arrange for two-year courses would be a real injury to the undertaking" (Tunis, 1966, p. 22). The final announcement of the course reflected the intent to begin a degree program "in the near future" (Tunis, p. 22). After the Canadian-born nurse educator, author, and administrator from Yale University, Bertha Harmer, was appointed director of the school in 1928, the committee recommended "that a six-year undergraduate course leading to a degree be established at the School for Graduate Nurses" (Tunis, p. 42). It is reported that the attitude of the principal and vice-chancellor was encouraging: "When we establish the degree course we can promise that Miss Harmer's rank will be that of professor" (Tunis, p. 42).

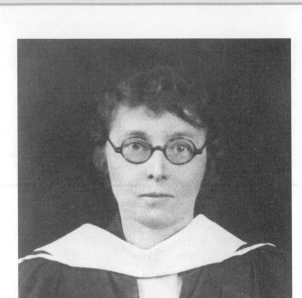

It was only through an unprecedented outpouring of financial support from alumni that Bertha Harmer, McGill's director of the School for Graduate Nurses, was able to maintain the school during the Depression.

Because there was reason for optimism, work went forward under Harmer's direction to develop a framework for the curriculum that would facilitate the transition to the degree program when it was established. Students could select from five new areas of focus, each of which could lead to a university diploma rather than a certificate after two years of study. To implement the new programs, four new faculty members were appointed for the 1929–30 academic year. Despite the optimism, however, the financial uncertainty under which the school operated after the termination of Red Cross funding in 1923 was a threat to its viability. To the new director this uncertainty must have been a continuing source of anxiety:

> *I have just returned to the office after a repeated attack of illness and had hoped to find a favourable decision of the Finance Committee awaiting me. At the risk of seeming to trouble you unduly I am writing to ask the decision of the Finance Committee in regard to our budget. I should not trouble you if it were not that so many important matters are depending on it. (Harmer, May 6, 1929)*

The undercurrent of suspicion toward nursing's place in the university environment surfaced again: "There are so many professors in the University who most cordially disapprove of schools of this kind. Their antagonism becomes more marked because of the necessity of reducing their salaries" (Currie, June 27, 1932).

A crisis was imminent, and the facts were given to Harmer by Sir Arthur Currie, the acting principal:

> *I quite agree with you that the School has had an increasing attendance, that it has done excellent work, and that the influence of its graduates on nursing and nursing education and administration has been most valuable. But there is the eternal question of finance. How are we to get the money to continue this School? (Currie, June 27, 1932)*

In the face of the university's economic difficulties due to the Depression, the school would not be permitted to continue to drain McGill's financial resources. It was given only one alternative to closure: it would have the opportunity to raise an endowment of $40,000 to provide for the annual operating expenses of $8,000, "which would keep it going for the next five years, in the hope that by that time financial conditions would be such that the expense of the School could be more readily provided for" (Currie, June 27, 1932).

The Alumnae Association and the Advisory Committee convened in joint session to consider the crisis that had beset the school and offered support for a national fundraising effort (Tunis, 1966). An appeal was sent to the presidents of all provincial nursing associations to assist with the campaign. In Harmer's (1932) words:

> *The nursing profession has many interested and grateful friends who appreciate the service which it renders, and it is quite right and just that they, in addition to the provincial and city government boards, and boards of hospitals and public health and welfare associations, should now be asked as individuals to contribute to the support of nursing education. (December 1, 1932)*

Support was also to be solicited from foundations, businesses, and corporations; however, the appeals to these organizations failed and the response was a great disappointment. "All was not lost, however, for the appeal to Canadian nurses did not go unheard and 'miraculously the money poured in. Within two months, more than $5,000 in cash was on hand and over $12,000 pledged'" (Tunis, 1966, p. 56).

The role of alumnae groups all over the country in ensuring the survival of the McGill School for Graduate Nurses was the critical factor in the resolution of the financial crisis that spanned more than a decade. In the process, the stature of nurses and nursing was raised, as nurses demonstrated a single-minded commitment to continuing the good work that had been started at McGill. It is clear from the documents that McGill administrators were surprised that nurse alumnae members and others would have sufficient interest or strength of purpose to donate funds so generously. Although the total amount raised never reached the goal of $40,000, about $20,000 was raised and applied to the operating costs of the school on an annual basis.

The fact that $20,000 was sufficient to see the school through ten difficult years was attributed to strict control over spending by school administrators (Tunis, 1966). An example of the nature of the commitment and dedication to the school is found in Harmer's report (1933) to the principal on the results of the first, and possibly the most important, phase of the campaign:

I am enclosing a statement showing results of the efforts of nurses to raise $40,000 to endow the School for the next five years. As it seemed hopeless, however, under present conditions, to raise this sum, efforts were concentrated on raising $8,000 in the hope that better times would enable us to raise an endowment later. Deducting my salary (my services were offered at the end of the year when it seemed the only hope of saving the School) left $5,000 as the objective. As the enclosed statement shows we have pledges for $5,597 for the next year, and $6,355.52 toward the next four years. (May 1, 1933)

In addition, many special lecturers in the program accepted reduced fees for their services or waived them altogether. Operating costs were lowered further when faculty members bought books for the library and supplies out of their own pockets (Tunis, 1966). Sir Arthur Currie's announcement (1933) that sufficient funds had been received in the first five months of the fundraising campaign to continue the school for one more year was a cause for rejoicing among faculty, alumnae, and friends of the school:

On the understanding that the Budget for the next year does not exceed the year just closing, and relying on the pledges outlined in your letter of May first, 1933, I shall recommend to the Board of Governors that the School for Graduate Nurses be continued for another year, that is, until June 30, 1934. (Currie, May 12, 1933)

The struggle was to be long, however, and neither Harmer nor Currie lived to see its conclusion. After Harmer's resignation and death in 1934, the continuing struggle for existence was carried on under the direction of Marion Lindeburgh as acting director until 1939 and as director thereafter. The stringent economies required that fewer courses be taught and that the two-year diploma programs were dropped in favour of one-year certificate programs (Tunis, 1966). The degree program had to be postponed until much later because program development priorities had to focus on retaining the programs that remained operational.

THE DEVELOPMENT OF AN EXPERIMENTAL SCHOOL OF NURSING AT TORONTO

It is ironic that at the very moment the McGill School for Graduate Nurses was served with notice of intent to terminate its programs by its administration, the University of Toronto School of Nursing received financial and philosophical encouragement to continue the innovative experiment with basic curriculum design that had begun in 1926, a program that was the vision of its director, Edith Kathleen Russell. This event had been preceded by many years of groundwork by Russell, and the grant was not the first the school had been awarded by the Rockefeller Foundation. The program established in 1926 and the improved one in 1933 were diploma rather than degree programs. Their importance for Canadian nursing was that they were radical departures from the existing philosophy of university education for nurses.

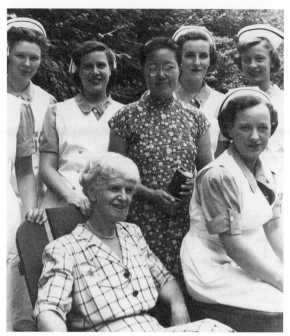

Kathleen Russell with students of the U of T School of Nursing, class of 1949. Russell is credited with developing the integrated nursing program and obtaining Rockefeller Foundation grants to establish it.

Russell, who came to the university early in the national development of higher education in nursing, was blessed with good health, a sound mind, and rare qualities of leadership. She had time to establish herself at the university and to develop her ideas about the pursuit of knowledge and truth as applied to nursing in the university setting. The credibility of the work accomplished and Russell's unique capabilities for leadership were remarkable. Ultimately, these factors augured well for the University of Toronto because, as Carpenter has indicated, "in the 30-year period ending in 1953, the Foundation supported the development of nursing education in 48 countries. The University of Toronto was the only Canadian university to receive this support" (1970, p. 94).

The proposal for the 1933 program, which also established the School of Nursing as an autonomous unit within the administrative framework of the university, allowing it to participate fully in university governance, was first submitted to the Rockefeller Foundation in 1929. The foundation agreed to support the project if support was also obtained from the university and the Ontario government, guarantees that were subsequently provided. The major feature of this 39-month program, which was unique from a developmental standpoint and made this curriculum model stand apart from the nonintegrated curriculum pattern, was the principle that the faculty of the school would assume total responsibility for students' education. Because the school was administratively independent from the hospital, new value was placed on clinical teaching. Student learning needs would no longer be put aside in favour of pressing hospital nursing service demands because students were not utilized in "staff" positions. They were viewed as learners, with the rights and responsibilities that accompany that role. The role of the faculty member in the clinical setting was one that was critical in facilitating the integration of theory and practice and fostering creative thinking and a questioning attitude (Carpenter, 1982). The function of the university school, as conceived by Russell (1956), was as follows:

> . . . to prepare professional women who, through studies in the humanities and social sciences, will grow in understanding and wisdom; with this education in the realm of human values they may approach with some degree of safety the work which is awaiting them. (p. 35)

🔍 CANADIAN RESEARCH FOCUS

Kirkwood, R. (1994). Blending vigorous leadership and womanly virtues: Edith Kathleen Russell at the University of Toronto, 1920–1952. *Canadian Bulletin of Medical History 11*(1), 175–205.

Using archival resources and interviews with former faculty members from the Faculty of Nursing at the University of Toronto, Kirkwood discusses how Kathleen Russell was expected to conform to the traditional feminine qualities of her time while showing the assertive leadership necessary to successfully promote university nursing education. This article will be of particular interest to students who wish to learn more about Russell and about gender issues.

NEW INITIATIVES AND INCENTIVES IN UNIVERSITY NURSING EDUCATION BETWEEN 1940 AND 1955

In 1940, as Canada became involved in World War II, the sluggish national economy improved because of the need for manufactured goods. The war also affected higher education. Education in the health sciences became a priority as the nation quickly recognized the need for health professionals to care for military personnel and the civilian population.

In the nursing profession, pressures arose from the conditions of returning prosperity in 1940 and, as these mounted, the balance between supply and demand reversed abruptly from what it had been during the 1930s. Where there had been oversupply, there was now a distinct shortage. With increasing prosperity, the return of the demand for private-duty nurses in both hospitals and homes was partially responsible for this turn of events, which placed the profession and health services in general in a tight squeeze. The economic conditions of the 1930s had forced many small hospitals to close their schools of nursing and hire from the large pool of unemployed nurses who would work for very low wages. By the end of the decade, general staff nursing in hospitals had become a major form of employment among nurses (Allemang, 1974). This contrasted sharply with the previous decade, in which there were few staff nurse positions in hospitals and graduate nurses generally sought employment as independent practitioners whose services were retained by families to care for ill family members in hospitals and homes.

Other factors that contributed to the development of the shortage included the wartime demands on a profession with a contribution to make:

> *Nursing administrators, supervisors, head nurses, teachers and public health nurses left their civilian positions for those of military service. These were key people in providing quality in nursing services and nursing education. Since bedside nursing care accompanied by supervision and ward teaching was considered the core of the curriculum, their loss was deeply felt.* (Allemang, 1974, p. 211)

Nurses were also needed in wartime industries, which generally offered better salaries and working conditions. For the most part, the shortages were most acute in rural areas for hospital and public health positions, as well as in special areas, such as tuberculosis sanitoria, isolation hospitals, and psychiatric institutions, where nurses were badly needed. In fact, the needs became so great and the possibilities for meeting them were so limited that a new category of health worker was created to fill the gap—the certified or registered nursing assistant or licensed practical nurse. Although some consideration was given to shortening nursing programs in Canada to meet specific needs related to war, this development never occurred because enough nurses volunteered for the armed services (Lindeburgh, 1942).

University schools of nursing soon began to reap benefits from federal interest in higher education, both from subsidizing the operations of the institutions and from its considerable response to the assistance requested by the professional organizations. Federal funds for nursing education, distributed through the CNA to the schools, amounted to $150,000 in 1942 and $250,000 each in 1943 and 1944. The program was maintained until the end of the war. Funds were then awarded through the provincial nurses' associations to the diploma and university schools of the provinces. In addition, the W.K. Kellogg Foundation initiated a program of fellowships in nursing and, between 1941 and 1959, granted $11,680 to institutions and agencies to be awarded to Canadian nurses for additional study. The university schools of nursing received the greater part of these funds so that they could upgrade the academic qualifications of their faculties. The fellowships were tenable in the United States and, during that period, there were no master's programs for nurses in Canada. The new funds, most of which were provided between 1941 and 1945, provided a stimulus to nursing education at a time when it was needed.

The W.K. Kellogg Foundation also made scholarship and loan funds available for students in programs at five universities between 1942 and 1944. Under this program, McGill University, l'Université de Montréal, the University of Toronto, and the University of Western Ontario each received $4,000, and Laval University received $6,000. For students seeking certificate or baccalaureate preparation, the Victorian Order of Nurses, a national agency that needed nurses with specific preparation in public health nursing, reactivated the bursary program initiated during the 1920s and discontinued in 1933. The Canadian Red Cross Society also made scholarships in public health nursing available (Tunis, 1966).

An awakened interest in nursing and nursing education in the postwar period led to the founding of new programs in nursing in several universities. Programs were initiated by Queen's University and McMaster University early in the decade (1941), by the University of Manitoba in 1943, by Mount St. Vincent University in 1947, and by Dalhousie University in 1949. Clearly, federal funds made available for schools and fellowship and bursary programs under the auspices of private foundations and agencies played an important role in the new developments. As in 1920, universities became aware of potential benefits from the sponsorship of nursing programs.

At McGill, the influx of additional funds was considerable and continuous. The courage and perseverance of those faculty, alumnae, and friends who had held out for the retention of the school through the long Depression and war years were rewarded. Their steadfast conviction that the school had a significant and critical function to fulfill at McGill was vindicated. The funds provided to the McGill School from the federal grant program administered by the CNA included "$2100 [in 1942], an amount that was increased to $6000 in 1943, and which by 1945 totalled $27,750" (Tunis, 1966, p. 73).

Nursing faculty at McGill were again able to entertain the idea of a degree program. Preparations began in 1941 for a five-year nonintegrated degree course and the first students were accepted in 1944. In 1945, the alumnae of the school disbanded their Special Finance Committee, but simultaneously revitalized earlier efforts to establish a Flora Madeline Shaw Endowment Fund to establish a chair in nursing (Tunis, 1966).

 ## DIPLOMA TO DEGREE: THE INCEPTION OF THE BASIC DEGREE PROGRAM AT THE UNIVERSITY OF TORONTO

The development of curricula in baccalaureate education for nursing has not been without difficulties. These have centred largely on contractual agreements between the university schools of nursing and hospitals and other agencies used for clinical experience. Brown (1948) cited two reasons to explain why these issues arose as major problems: the traditional outlook of the hospital, which viewed nursing education as service, and the meagre financial resources of many university schools and students. Probably the most influential event in the history of Canadian degree programs in nursing was the introduction of the basic degree program at the University of Toronto in 1942 that provided an alternative to the existing pattern of baccalaureate nursing education. In the integrated program, studies in the arts and sciences were combined with the nursing component. Courses were carefully planned and sequenced so that individual student development would be enhanced: "For the first time in a nursing undergraduate degree programme full authority and responsibility for the teaching of nursing rested in the university. . . . This simple fact, nonetheless, was a radical departure from existing degree programmes. . . ." (King, 1970, p. 72)

It is always difficult to break with tradition, and in nursing, the nonintegrated degree pattern had established its stepladder approach to nursing education well over 20 years before. In addition, the associated hospital programs had been entrenched for an even greater number of years. Effecting a change that made the basic degree program stand apart from its nonintegrated counterpart required a great leader. E. Kathleen Russell was such an individual as she exerted a profound influence on the thinking of her colleagues in nursing and was able to enlist the moral support of the Faculty of Medicine, the president of the University of Toronto, and the Rockefeller Foundation. In regard to her influence, Emory notes: "It has been said that greatness is attained through changing the course of events and changing them for always. If this be true, then in retrospect there can be detected in Edith Kathleen Russell's professional life and work an element of true greatness" (1964, p. 7).

A SECOND BASIC DEGREE PROGRAM BEGINS

In her study of basic degree programs in Canada, Bonin concluded: "The most salient driving forces which spurred the establishment of basic degree programs are key persons, especially Kathleen Russell and Gladys Sharpe, in two pioneering universities" (1976, p. 178). Four years after the introduction of the University of Toronto basic degree program, a second such program was developed at McMaster University under the direction of Gladys Sharpe. Sharpe was largely responsible for phasing out its predecessor, a degree and diploma program called Arts and Nursing, which had begun in 1941 at McMaster. At McMaster, the initiative of the Hamilton General Hospital had been important in developing the earlier affiliation between the hospital and the university, and the hospital continued to support the new program and its director. Similar support from an associated hospital had occurred in 1919 when the Vancouver General Hospital supported the establishment of the University of British Columbia School of Nursing. It was also evident that there was an extremely close working relationship between the Toronto General Hospital and the School of Nursing at the University of Toronto. In the early 1930s, consideration was given to combining the Toronto General nursing program with that of the University of Toronto (Carpenter, 1970).

REFLECTIVE THINKING

Reflect on the meaning of the evolution of university nursing education in Canada for the nursing profession.

REVISITING SURVEYS OF NURSING EDUCATION AND UNIVERSITY EDUCATION AND LOOKING TOWARD THE FUTURE

In the history of Canadian nursing education, periodic surveys have been undertaken by professional organizations and government to assess conditions and develop solutions to pressing problems. Kathleen Russell carried out a survey in New Brunswick that addressed the whole gamut of issues in nursing education in that province and had considerable impact on the thinking of nursing educators. The establishment of the School of Nursing at the University of New Brunswick in 1959 was a direct result of her recommendations about higher education in nursing in New Brunswick (Russell, 1956). Soon afterward, the CNA launched its Pilot Project for Evaluation of Schools of Nursing to assess readiness for a system of accreditation and published its report in 1960.

One of Mussallem's (1960) recommendations, "that a re-examination and study of the whole field of nursing education be undertaken" (p. vii), was implemented within a very short time. A royal commission was appointed by the federal government to investigate the problems and issues related to all aspects of the delivery of health care services in Canada. The report of that commission urged that ten more university nursing programs, under administratively autonomous schools of nursing, be established in Canada as soon as possible (Government of Canada, 1964). It also recommended elimination of nonintegrated basic programs at a time when admissions were 22% higher than admissions to integrated programs. The impact of this report was impressive, as only four years later "admissions to integrated programmes constituted 97% of all admissions to baccalaureate programmes" (King, 1970, pp. 178–79). In addition, the number of candidates seeking post-basic degrees after graduation from hospital or college diploma programs doubled during the same period. Schools of nursing made concerted efforts to increase maximum enrolment levels in response to the royal commission's recommendation despite limited space in clinical facilities:

> It is of the utmost importance that these schools be expanded in number to enable them to prepare approximately one-fourth of the total recruits to the nursing force. It is from this pool that the instructors, supervisors, administrators and other leaders in the profession must come. (Government of Canada, 1964, p. 67)

Since 1965 the ratio of diploma- to baccalaureate-prepared nurses has increased considerably from approximately 1 in 10 nationally in 1988, to 1 in 16 in 1993, and 1 in 21 in 1998 (CNA, 2001). In 2007, 35.5% of Canadian nurses in the workforce held a baccalaureate degree as their highest level of education (Canadian Institute for Health Information, 2008). In addition, all of the ten new university schools recommended by the royal commission were established. The number of university colleges, departments, schools, and faculties of nursing has continued to increase exponentially in support of the endorsement of the baccalaureate entry-to-practice position by the Canadian Nurses Association and provincial and territorial professional nursing associations. (Issues pertaining to entry to practice are considered in Chapter 19.) As baccalaureate nursing programs are becoming the norm in nursing education, the Canadian Association of Schools of Nursing (CASN) continues to champion higher education in nursing. In November 2008, CASN sponsored the Inaugural Nursing Education Summit, at which key stakeholders examined the relationship between nursing education and health human resources planning in Canada (CASN NES Summit Planning Committee & Pitters Associates Inc., 2009). It will be interesting to see the impact of this summit on nursing education during the next decade.

This cursory examination of events and trends important in the development of university-level education in nursing has revealed the changes in the nursing education system over time as well as the forces driving them. With the development of the discipline and the expansion of the knowledge base, concern about the appropriateness of the learning environment in part drove the desire for change. Widespread recognition that nursing remains one of the last sex-segregated professions has underscored injustices caused by differential treatment both of nurses and of the profession itself. Improvement in the status of women through attaining fundamental rights and privileges previously accorded only to men has led the profession to press for educational arrangements and advantages common in all other disciplines.

At the outset, nursing education was characterized by informal and on-the-job training. Hospital schools of nursing began to develop in 1874 and university schools in 1919. Community college nursing education programs, which were established in the 1960s, also offered diploma preparation. Today, the transition of basic nursing education to the university level is in full swing. Collaboration between colleges and universities to allow students the opportunity to study for a university degree in nursing is occurring across the country. There are many other arrangements to facilitate transfer of students from colleges to universities and to allow students this opportunity in both large and smaller centres across the country. Over time, there has been a progression in nurses' thinking about the means to educate members of the profession, guided from the beginning by concern for standards of education and practice leading to safe patient care.

CRITICAL THINKING QUESTIONS

1. What do you find most striking about the history of nursing education presented in this chapter? Why is this so?
2. If one day, once you have completed your nursing education, your school of nursing experiences serious financial difficulties similar to those encountered at the School of Nursing at McGill University during the 1930s, do you think you would be willing to help as graduates from McGill did? Please elaborate.

WEB SITES

Canadian Association of Schools of Nursing: http://www.casn.ca
The Mack Centre of Nursing Education Historical Plaque: http://www.ontarioplaques.com/Plaques_MNO/Plaque_Niagara67.html

REFERENCES

Allemang, M. M. (1974). *Nursing education in the United States and Canada, 1873–1950: Leading figures, forces, views on education.* Seattle: Doctoral dissertation, University of Washington.

Allen, M., & Reidy, M. (1971). *Learning to nurse: The first five years of the Ryerson nursing program* Ontario: Registered Nurses Association of Ontario.

Arpin, K. (1972). *Report of visit to the Association of Registered Nurses of Newfoundland.* St. John's: AARN.

Association of Nurses of the Province of Quebec. (1972). *CEGEP nursing education after five years.* Montreal: Author.

Baly, M. (1986). *Florence Nightingale and the nursing legacy.* London: Croom Helm.

Bonin, M. A. (1976). *Trends in integrated basic degree nursing programs in Canada: 1942–1972.* Ottawa: Doctoral dissertation, University of Ottawa.

Brown, E. L. (1948). *Nursing for the future.* New York: Russell Sage Foundation.

Burgess, M. A. (1928). *Nurses, patients and pocketbooks.* New York: Committee on the Grading of Nursing Schools.

Campbell, G. (1971). *Community colleges in Canada.* Toronto: McGraw-Hill.

Canadian Association of Schools of Nursing NES Summit Planning Committee & Pitters Associates Inc. (2009). *Nursing education summit report. Executive summary.* Ottawa: CASN.

Canadian Institute for Health Information. (2008). *Regulated nurses: Trends, 2003–2007.* Ottawa: Author.

Canadian Nurses Association. (1936). *A proposed curriculum for schools of nursing in Canada.* Montreal: Author.

Canadian Nurses Association. (1968). *The leaf and the lamp.* Ottawa: Author.

Canadian Nurses Association. (2001). *Education for registered nurses in a time of shortage.* Ottawa: Author. Retrieved on April 2, 2002, from www.cna-nurses.ca/pages.education/educationframe.htm.

Carpenter, H. M. (1970). The University of Toronto School of Nursing: An agent of change. In M. Q. Innis (Ed.), *Nursing education in a changing society* (pp. 86–108). Toronto: University of Toronto Press.

Carpenter, H. M. (1982). *Divine discontent: Edith Kathleen Russell—Reforming educator.* Toronto: Faculty of Nursing, The University of Toronto.

Cohen, Y. (2000). *Gertrude Elizabeth Livingston.* Dictionary of Canadian Biography Online. Toronto/Quebec City: University of Toronto/Laval University. Retrieved on May 8, 2010, from http://www.biographi.ca/009004-119.01-e.php?&id_nbr=7830&&PHPSESSID=ychzfqkvzape.

Cohen, Y., Pepin, J., Lamontagne, E., & Duquette, A. (2002). *Les sciences infirmières, genèse d'une discipline.* Montreal: Les Presses de l'Université de Montréal.

Committee on the Grading of Nursing Schools. (1934). *Nursing schools today and tomorrow.* New York: Author.

Currie, A.W. (1932, June 27). Letter to Dr. Helen R.Y. Reid. Financial crisis: 1933 to 1943 (Acc. 2432, File). Montreal, Quebec: McGill University Archive.

Currie, A. W. (1933, May 12). Letter to Bertha Harmer. Financial crisis: 1933 to 1943 (Acc. 2432, File). Montreal, Quebec: McGill University Archive.

Desjardins, E. (1971). *Heritage: History of the nursing profession in the province of Quebec.* Quebec: Association of Nurses of the Province of Quebec.

Emory, F. (1964, March 6). *Edith Kathleen Russell: An appreciation of her professional life and work.* (Acc. A-73011, mimeographed). Faculty of Nursing, University of Toronto.

Encyclopedia Britannica Online. (2008). Retrieved on September 12, 2009, from http://www.britannica.com.

Famous nurses in history. (Undated). "Gertrude Elizabeth Livingston." Guelph: The Sterling Rubber Company Ltd.

Gibbon, J. M., & Mathewson, M. S. (1947). *Three centuries of Canadian nursing.* Toronto: Macmillan.

Government of Canada. (1964). *Royal Commission on Health Services.* (Vol. I) (Emmett M. Hall, Chairman). Ottawa: Queen's Printer.

Gunn, J. I. (1933). Educational adjustments recommended by the survey. *The Canadian Nurse, 29*(3), 139–145.

Harmer, B. (1929, May 6). Letter to Dr. C.F. Martin. Financial crisis: 1933 to 1943 (Acc. 2432, File). Montreal, Quebec: McGill University Archive.

Harmer, B. (1932, December 1). Letter to presidents of provincial nursing associations. Financial crisis: 1933 to 1943 (Acc. 2432, File). Montreal, Quebec: McGill University Archive.

Harmer, B. (1933, May 1). Letter to Sir Arthur W. Currie. Financial crisis: 1933 to 1943 (Acc. 2432, File). Montreal, Quebec: McGill University Archive.

Healey, P. (1990). *The Mack training school for nurses.* Austin, TX: Unpublished doctoral dissertation, University of Texas.

Holt, M. (1936). Staffing with graduate nurses. *The Canadian Nurse, 32*(1), 5–10.

Jackel, S. (1985). *Women in Canadian universities: A historical overview. Keynote address to the Conference and Annual Meeting, Western Region, Canadian Association of University Schools of Nursing.* Edmonton, Alberta: University of Alberta.

King, M. K. (1970). The development of university nursing education. In M. Q. Innis (Ed.), *Nursing education in a changing society* (pp. 67–85). Toronto: University of Toronto Press.

Kirkwood, R. (1994). Blending vigorous leadership and womanly virtues: Edith Kathleen Russell at the University of Toronto, 1920–1952. *Canadian Bulletin of Medical History, 11*(1), 175–205.

Kirkwood, R. (2005). Enough but not too much: Nursing education in English language Canada 1874–2000. In C. Bates, D. Dodd, & N. Rousseau (Eds.), *On all frontiers: Four centuries of Canadian nursing* (pp. 183–196). Ottawa: University of Ottawa Press.

Letourneau, M. (1975). *Trends in basic diploma nursing programs within the provincial systems of education in Canada, 1964–1974.* Ottawa: Doctoral dissertation, University of Ottawa.

Lindeburgh, M. (1942). Important emergency measures. *The Canadian Nurse, 38*(12), 925–926.

Lord, A. R. (1952). *Report of the evaluation of the Metropolitan School of Nursing, Windsor, Ontario.* Ottawa: Canadian Nurses Association.

MacDermot, H. E. (1940). *History of the School of Nursing of the Montreal General Hospital.* Montreal: The Alumnae Association, Montreal General Hospital.

MacLaggan, K. (1965). *Portrait of nursing: A plan for the education of nurses in the province of New Brunswick.* Fredericton: New Brunswick Association of Registered Nurses.

MacMurchy, H. (1918). University training for the nursing profession. *The Canadian Nurse, 14*(9), 1284–1285.

Manitoba Association of Registered Nurses. (1968). *A position paper on nursing in Manitoba.* Winnipeg: Author.

McLean, C. D. (1964). *A report on the establishment of the Quo Vadis School of Nursing and the selection of the first class of students.* Toronto: Quo Vadis School of Nursing.

Mount Allison University. (2008). *About Mount Allison.* Retrieved on February 2, 2008, from http://www.mta.ca/about.html.

Murray, V. V. (1970). *Nursing in Ontario: A study for the committee on the healing arts.* Toronto: Queen's Printer.

Mussallem, H. K. (1960). *Spotlight on nursing education: The report of a pilot project for the evaluation of schools of nursing in Canada.* Ottawa: Canadian Nurses Association.

Mussallem, H. K. (1964). *A path to quality: A plan for the development of nursing education programs within the general educational system of Canada.* Ottawa: Canadian Nurses Association.

New Brunswick Association of Registered Nurses. (1971). *Position paper.* Fredericton: Author.

Nightingale, F. (1929). *Cassandra: An essay.* Old Westbury, NY: Feminist Press.

Paul, P. (1994). *A history of the Edmonton General Hospital: 1895–1970, "Be faithful to the duties of your calling."* Edmonton, AB: Unpublished doctoral dissertation, University of Alberta.

Registered Nurses Association of British Columbia. (1967). *A proposed plan for the orderly development of nursing education in British Columbia: Part One—Basic nursing education.* Vancouver: Author.

Rowe, H. R. (1967). *A study of transition in nursing education in Prince Edward Island.* Charlottetown: ANPEI.

Russell, E. K. (1956). *The report of the study of nursing education in New Brunswick.* Fredericton: Government of the Province of New Brunswick.

Saskatchewan Registered Nurses' Association. (1966). *Brief presented to the joint committee on higher education.* Regina: Author.

Schmitt, L. M. (1957). *Basic nursing education study: Report of the status of basic nursing education programs in Saskatchewan.* Regina: Saskatchewan Registered Nurses' Association.

Street, M. (1973). *Watch fires on the mountain: The life and writings of Ethel Johns.* Toronto: University of Toronto Press.

Study Committee on Nursing Education. (1971). *A study committee on nursing education.* New Brunswick: Department of Health.

Tunis, B. L. (1966). *In caps and gowns.* Montreal: McGill University Press.

Twohig, P. L. (1998). *Challenges and change—A history of the Dalhousie School of Nursing 1949–1989.* Halifax: Fernwood Publishing and Dalhousie University.

Weir, G. M. (1932). *Survey of nursing education in Canada.* Toronto: University of Toronto Press.

Wollstonecraft, M. (1787). *Thoughts on the education of daughters.* Clifton, NJ: A.M. Kelley.

Wollstonecraft, M. (1792). *A vindication of the rights of woman.* London: J. Johnson.

19

Entry to Practice: Striving for the Baccalaureate Standard

Marilynn J. Wood

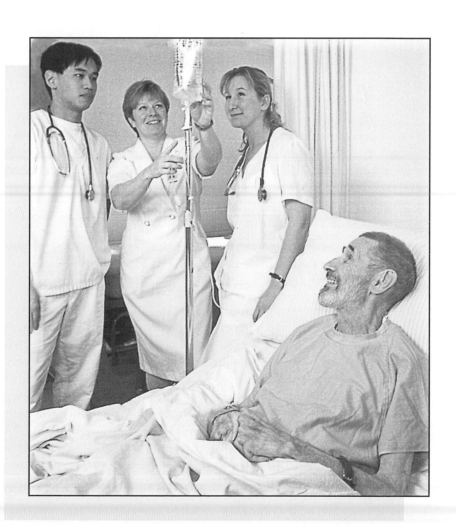

LEARNING OBJECTIVES

- To understand the issue of entry to practice in Canada.
- To appreciate the historical development of educational standards in Canadian nursing schools.
- To identify the current status of entry to practice in Canada.
- To appreciate how each provincial/territory has addressed the issue.

The baccalaureate degree as the minimum educational qualification for entry to the practice of nursing has been a highly controversial and hotly debated issue in the nursing profession (Besharah, 1981). Strong emotions have been generated in the entry-to-practice debate, because comprehensive restructuring of the educational system in nursing has been both perplexing and threatening to many. However, the discussion and debate stage of the "pros" and "cons" of the entry-to-practice position would appear to be almost a thing of the past as the movement to implement the baccalaureate standard has taken hold across the country. The steps that have been taken in the various provinces are outlined in this chapter.

Underscoring the movement to implement the entry-to-practice position is the clear fact that nurses' contributions to the promotion, maintenance, and restoration of health have made the nursing profession one that is held in public esteem. Nurses' contributions have also moved nursing to the threshold of the university because of the complexity of knowledge and skills required, and the fact that it is through the educational process that nursing students acquire the essential foundation for practice. It is thus necessary and important to understand and appreciate nursing as a complex, multifaceted process, embracing many roles and functions.

ENTRY TO PRACTICE: THE POSITION, ITS DEVELOPMENT, AND RATIONALE

The entry-to-practice position is often misunderstood. Many nurses believe it means that all nurses will be required to have a baccalaureate degree to maintain their practice. However, it actually refers to all those entering schools of nursing after the requirement changes. Those who will enter diploma nursing programs up to the time of implementation would not be required to have the baccalaureate credential. This approach, often termed "grandparenting," means that the new standard is phased in gradually, allowing ample time to make changes and adjustments in systems and resources. The right to practise nursing would not be jeopardized for those who qualified for practice prior to the year in which the change takes place.

More than three decades have passed since the first statement of the entry-to-practice position by the Alberta Task Force on Nursing Education (Government of Alberta, 1975). Since then a fundamental shift has occurred in the approach taken to the entry-to-practice position as endorsed by the Canadian Nurses Association (CNA) and the provincial nursing associations. In the late 1990s, Entry to Practice

2000 (EP2000) referred to the goal of attaining the baccalaureate standard for entry to practice by the year 2000. This goal was not achieved, but a great deal of progress was made across the country. Strategies to facilitate implementation of the policy commonly called EP2000 were developed at provincial and national levels by professional associations over the previous decade and a half. These were updated between 2001 and 2005. There has also been a concomitant increase in the demand for post-RN baccalaureate education by members of the profession qualified at the diploma level. Many nurses recognize a personal need for additional education and also that additional study may improve one's competitive position in relation to promotions, particularly at a leadership level.

The voice of the profession on this issue became an increasingly united one over time, as one provincial nursing association after another espoused commitment to the position that all new nurses entering the profession should be qualified at the baccalaureate level. Initial leadership came, however, neither from the profession nor from university faculties of nursing, but from a government-appointed committee established to study needs in relation to nursing education in the province of Alberta, the Alberta Task Force on Nursing Education. Although the Alberta government subsequently issued a denunciation of its committee's recommendation, stating that it did "not agree with making the baccalaureate degree a mandatory requirement for practice," the profession did not allow the matter to rest there (Government of Alberta, 1977, p. 6).

Discussion of the controversial document ensued among all interested parties immediately after its publication. The College and Association of Registered Nurses of Alberta (CARNA), prior to November 2005 known as the Alberta Association of Registered Nurses (AARN), issued an endorsement of the task force recommendations shortly thereafter (AARN, 1976). The year 2000 was subsequently suggested by the CARNA as a more realistic target date for implementation of the entry-to-practice position than the 1995 goal suggested by the task force (AARN, 1978, 1979). In Vancouver at the 1980 Biennial Convention of the Canadian Nurses Association, delegates debated a resolution to develop a statement on the minimum educational qualification needed to enter the profession. Following approval, the resolution became a priority for the 1980–82 biennium. Momentum began to grow with the establishment of a committee to study the issue, and articles appeared in *The Canadian Nurse* debating both sides of the question (Kerr, 1982; Rajabally, 1982). The decision to endorse the baccalaureate standard was taken by the CNA Board of Directors in February 1982 when the Report of the Committee was presented. Support was high, and the motion was carried unanimously. Delegates to the 1982 Biennial Convention in Newfoundland added further strength to the position by adopting a motion of support. Support for the position grew within the profession as the issues were debated in provinces that had not already adopted a position on the matter. Gradually, province by province, positions in support of baccalaureate entry to practice were taken. The enthusiasm and eagerness to reach the goal remained evident, as nurses from one end of the country to the other identified and developed mechanisms to ensure that logical, well-articulated, reasonable plans were made for its achievement. If they are to be successful, such plans must result in public policy commitments to the baccalaureate standard, as additional years of university-level nursing education for students require commitments to redistribute existing resources.

The question of why the issue of baccalaureate education for entry to practice (BETP) was supported so strongly by the nursing profession is often asked. The reason is to be found in the changing nature of practice and the knowledge necessary to engage in practice. Although the profession was accused of attempting to raise professional status through higher educational standards, this was not a just criticism. The profession agreed that achieving higher professional status does not constitute good and sufficient reason for implementing the baccalaureate standard for entry to practice. Nurses realize that the knowledge needed to practise nursing safely and effectively has mushroomed. Much of practice requires interdisciplinary cooperation and depth of knowledge not only of one's own discipline, but also those of the other members of the health care team. In addition, nursing has become increasingly specialized. Three decades ago, there were five or six distinct areas of hospital- and community-based practice. Today, there are upward of 30 different clinical nursing areas, each requiring mastery of a unique and specialized knowledge base.

The era of specialization in nursing arrived some time ago. No longer is it possible, if in fact it ever was, to graduate "a finished product." It is now accepted that a new nursing graduate is a beginning practitioner as are new graduates in other fields. Further, like other professionals, registered nurses must be lifelong learners. There is no way one can be master of all knowledge in nursing, either within the context of a program of basic nursing education or after graduation, when concentrating on a field of practice. The rapid rate at which care based on new knowledge is integrated into practice makes continuing education an individual, organizational, and professional responsibility to ensure that practitioners remain abreast of new developments in their areas of practice.

Advances in the health sciences have meant that today's programs of basic nursing education are hard-pressed to offer curricula that address the depth and breadth of theoretical content and related clinical experience for safe and effective practice. The impact of technology and changing roles requires the acquisition of appropriate knowledge and the development of new skills. The expansion of the knowledge required for competent practice and the range of responsibilities expected of nurses at all levels provide substantial rationale for the standard of educational preparation offered at a baccalaureate level. The movement of nursing education to the university level is also seen as a women's issue, for educational preparation at the level of complexity seen in male-dominated disciplines has long been the responsibility of the university.

REFLECTIVE THINKING

How would you address the criticism that movement to baccalaureate entry was a self-serving move on the part of nursing and is not in the best interest of the public?

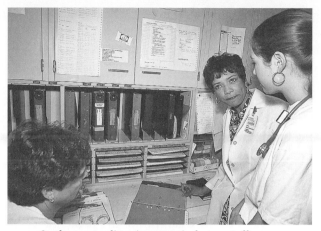

Student nurse listening attentively to a staff nurse.

STANDARDS OF NURSING EDUCATION: A HISTORICAL PERSPECTIVE

Florence Nightingale founded the first modern school of nursing in 1860 in conjunction with St. Thomas' Hospital in London. The idea was novel and soon became the model for the establishment of hospital training schools throughout Europe and America. However, in the translation of the model to North America, the idea of financial independence of the school of nursing was lost, and the new schools became dependent on hospitals to sustain them. The Nightingale school was an independent school supported by the Nightingale Fund, a substantial endowment resulting from gifts to support the success of her mission of caring for British soldiers during the Crimean War. Nightingale's reputation from her service in Crimea was such that her idea for a school of nursing was taken up readily and the nurses she prepared in her school were widely sought to lead new developments elsewhere.

Standards of education have historically been a primary concern of the nursing profession. There is considerable evidence that the quality of nursing education was one of the early issues addressed by professional organizations. During the 1920s and 1930s, after the successful resolution of the struggle to achieve nursing registration in each province, the profession became concerned with achieving higher educational standards through the development and adoption of a standard curriculum for schools of nursing. Undoubtedly these efforts, which were spearheaded by the CNA, did much to raise educational standards in schools of nursing (Weir, 1932). Although today the idea of a national standard curriculum may seem somewhat strange and rather prescriptive, undoubtedly there was a need for this kind of guidance because educational standards at the time were described as deplorable by many observers.

With the initiation of the first university degree program in Canada for nurses at the University of British Columbia in 1919 under the direction of Ethel Johns, a new era in nursing education began. Red Cross funding to six Canadian universities after

World War I encouraged the establishment and development of a variety of nursing programs in these institutions. They were the University of British Columbia, University of Alberta, University of Western Ontario, University of Toronto, McGill University, and Dalhousie University. Most began as certificate programs, and all eventually developed into degree programs. The first degree programs were based on the prevailing US model and were termed "nonintegrated programs." In such programs, the principle of university control over university courses and hospital control over the clinical nursing part of the program became firmly entrenched (Kerr, 1978).

In 1926, dissatisfied with the prevailing pattern of university degree programs in nursing, which she termed "an ill-arranged program of studies" (Russell, 1932, p. 87), Kathleen Russell, director of the Department of Public Health Nursing at the University of Toronto, set out to demonstrate that a nurse could be prepared in a much more effective and educationally sound manner by establishing the principle of university direction and control over all courses in the program. Although close cooperation with health care agencies was maintained, faculty who were responsible for clinical nursing education were employed by the university. A substantial Rockefeller Foundation grant was obtained to fund this innovative experiment in basic degree nursing education, resulting in the first integrated program in Canada at the University of Toronto in 1942. With its initiative to develop a basic integrated baccalaureate degree program in nursing in 1946, McMaster University became the second university in the country to do so.

In the formative years between 1940 and 1955, university schools of nursing became firmly established and began to accommodate ever-increasing numbers of students and administer increasingly large budgets. It is interesting that until 1965 no additional integrated degree programs besides those at Toronto and McMaster were established in any Canadian university. However, in 1964 the Royal Commission on Health Services was to change university nursing education dramatically and rapidly with recommendations that were highly critical of the existing system. Among the recommendations were those that proposed that ten more university nursing programs under administratively autonomous schools of nursing be established in Canada as soon as possible, and that nonintegrated basic degree programs in universities be eliminated. This came at a time when admissions to nonintegrated programs were 22% higher than admissions to integrated programs.

The impact of this report was impressive. Only four years following its publication, "admissions to integrated programmes constituted 97% of all admissions to baccalaureate programs" (King, 1970, pp. 78–79). The royal commission also recommended that baccalaureate programs "be expanded in number to enable them to prepare approximately one-fourth of the total recruits to the nursing force" (Government of Canada, 1964, p. 67).

MOVING BEYOND 2000

Although we have been dealing with questions involving standards of education in nursing since the profession became formally established in this country, today's issues are quite different. Everything has changed—the settings, conditions of practice, health needs and problems, beliefs about individual responsibility in health care, and performance expectations for nurses in all settings. This is not surprising because change is, after all, the inexorable reality of our existence.

Choices for the profession and its practitioners involve ways of influencing the direction of change in the manner most appropriate for the service rendered. Indeed, we have moved from questions of "why" and "what" to those of "how" and "when" in relation to the baccalaureate standard for initial entry to practice. The educational and service sectors are preparing for the changes that are occurring. The process of developing collaborative partnerships between diploma and degree programs to produce a baccalaureate-level practitioner is well underway across the country, but there is some distance to go before one could even say that the end is in sight. Creative new nursing education program models are being developed to implement the baccalaureate standard. Hospitals and other health care agencies, colleges, and universities are increasingly recognizing that they must become partners in planning and promoting an integrated system of nursing education that will benefit the health care consumers of the future.

The respective roles of the provincial and national nursing associations in the process of encouraging the implementation of baccalaureate entry to practice will undoubtedly continue to be critical factors in influencing opinion and action among health professionals and the general public. After the adoption of the entry-to-practice resolution by the Board of Directors in 1982, the CNA quickly moved to adopt a proactive stance on the issue. Committees were appointed to develop long-term goals and plans, discussion papers and annotated bibliographies on the subject, and strategies to achieve goals. CNA efforts were directed at encouraging member associations to develop specific plans for their provinces and territories. The five-year National Plan for Entry to Practice was adopted by the Canadian Nurses Association in March 1989. Professional nursing associations in all provinces and territories except Ontario are charged with legislative authority for the registration and discipline of nurses. In Ontario, the College of Nurses carries out regulatory functions for the profession. Except in Ontario and Quebec, the provincial nursing associations also have statutory responsibilities for nursing education. All are committed to improving standards of nursing education.

The grassroots campaign to implement the baccalaureate standard for entry to practice has taken place at the provincial and territorial level because that is where authority for health and education rests. Since the provincial and territorial ministries of education and health are charged with the responsibility for allocating resources for post-secondary education and for health personnel, the question of implementation of the entry-to-practice position is of vital concern at the provincial and territorial level.

Because of the complexity of determining costs of student education, conclusions based on inadequate information or comparisons have, in the past, led some to assume that exorbitant costs are associated with implementation of the baccalaureate standard, a conclusion the CNA has termed "unclear, unfounded, unwise and unwarranted" (CNA Staff, 1984, p. 1). It was concluded that there were no well-designed studies of the cost of nursing education in Canada and that "institutional costs per 'student year' or per 'student credit hour' or per 'student years of future graduates' might well have been lower in universities than in other institutions" (CNA Staff, 1984, p. 1). The CNA made it clear that the conclusion that a baccalaureate nursing program was more expensive than other types of nursing programs had no basis in fact, and that the actual situation might have been quite the reverse.

Nursing faculty in universities were articulate proponents of the baccalaureate standard for entry to nursing practice from the outset. The fact that academic units in nursing in universities were likely to sustain extensive change as a result of the tremendous impact of implementation did not deter faculty members from being proactive about the goal. It was clear also that all sectors of the nursing education enterprise would be dramatically affected by adoption of the entry-to-practice position.

Issues of concern continue to include availability of qualified faculty. Many university faculties of nursing have devoted considerable effort to assist faculty without doctoral degrees to achieve that level of preparation and, indeed, to go on to postdoctoral work. Recruitment of qualified faculty will continue to be a difficult issue for university schools as collaborative efforts take shape, for universities will be offering courses to a greater number of undergraduate students, and the need for a larger number of qualified faculty members to do this will be pressing. At the same time, universities are facing overall shortages of qualified faculty, as retirements are expected to exceed new hires over the next few years and there is keen competition for the best doctoral candidates.

It is thus evident that the preparation of faculty is a critical issue in relation to achieving baccalaureate entry to practice. Therefore, graduate programs strong in clinical and research preparation are key elements in expanding the ranks of well-prepared nursing faculty in universities. The development and expansion of university programs in nursing at the baccalaureate level cannot be accomplished without the infusion of considerable numbers of faculty prepared at the master's and doctoral levels.

Master's programs have been established in most regions of the country. However, whether or not there is sufficient capacity in existing master's programs is a matter that is open to debate. The CNA (CNA Staff, Winter 1992–93, p. 2) has pointed out in its newsletter on nursing education that "the rate of growth in admissions [to master's programs in nursing] has not kept pace with the growth in applications." While applications to master's programs went up 50% between 1987 and 1991, admissions rose only 24% in the same period. It has further been observed that while there were 12 master's programs for 262,288 registered nurses in Canada employed in nursing in 1991, there were 16 master's programs in social work for 48,591 social workers (CNA Staff, Winter 1992–93, p. 2).

Although the development of doctoral programs in nursing was slow to get started, development and expansion of programs has occurred relatively rapidly since the establishment on January 1, 1991, of the first official program at the University of Alberta. Other programs followed in rapid succession at the University of British Columbia (September 1991), McGill University and l'Université de Montréal (a joint program; fall 1993), the University of Toronto (fall 1993), McMaster University (fall 1994), the University of Calgary (1999), and the University of Western Ontario (2002). Since then, programs have been started at Dalhousie University, the universities of Laval and Sherbrooke in Quebec, and the University of Victoria.

Although admission quotas are still relatively small, enrolment in doctoral programs in nursing is growing steadily. Whether there is sufficient capacity for student positions in the doctoral programs remains a concern because of the increasing role of the university in nursing education. Strong and productive graduate programs will be essential in all approaches to implementing the entry-to-practice position.

The effect of program expansion on health care agencies will be considerable. A key factor will be partnership in the planning and development processes. Health care reform initiatives across the country have already meant dramatic changes in care environments, including roles of nurses. It will be essential for universities to ensure that there is meaningful participation by health care agencies in the plans for development of new goals, for program changes, and in the teaching and learning process. There are many ways in which working together can be fostered, including the use of joint appointments, secondment arrangements, shared projects, and organizational structural changes to foster partnership for mutual benefit. Many university schools and faculties of nursing are working collaboratively with health care agencies in these kinds of activities, as well as in others.

There is evidence that students are enrolling in existing baccalaureate programs at increased rates. From 1985 to 1988, admissions to basic baccalaureate programs climbed 31%. In the same period, full-time enrolment in post-RN baccalaureate programs decreased by 0.6%, while part-time enrolment rose by 24.4% (CNA Staff, 1989). In 1993, CNA statistics reported that university enrolments in baccalaureate programs in nursing were relatively constant at a figure between 5,000 and 6,000 students in the years from 1987 to 1991 (CNA Staff, Spring 1993, p. 3).

Expansion and development in baccalaureate programs in universities has taken place gradually, with the number of baccalaureate students rising steadily as degree programs became available to students across the country. Students in basic and post-RN baccalaureate programs made up 29.3% of all nursing students enrolled in Canada in 1991, while the comparable figure for 1981 was 26.3% (CNA Staff, Spring 1993, p. 3). Overall, the percentage of nurses in the workforce with baccalaureate degrees has been slowly rising, due to the increases in enrolment in university programs. The percentage rose from 17.9% in 1996 to 22.7% in 2000 (CNA, 2002). This is a large increase for a period of four years, and it represents the increased numbers of students graduating from baccalaureate programs, particularly in those provinces where collaborative programs are in place. In 1999, for the first time, the number of baccalaureate graduates surpassed the number of diploma graduates (CNA, 2002).

Although this may seem like very slow progress toward achieving the entry-to-practice position, it must be recognized that there are large and populous regions of the country that are not served well with opportunities for students to pursue baccalaureate education in nursing. In 2005, all nursing students in Ontario entered into baccalaureate degree programs, so this percentage will rise even more quickly. In the meantime, the movement to implement the entry-to-practice position has gained momentum across the country.

PROVINCIAL AND TERRITORIAL DEVELOPMENTS

THE FIRST STEPS

The transition of the Vancouver General Hospital School of Nursing from diploma nursing education to baccalaureate nursing education through a collaborative effort with the University of British Columbia and the enrolment of the first class in the newly structured program in September 1989 were the first of many such joint ventures to be implemented (CNA Connection, 1989b). Planning for this merger began in 1988, and plans were quickly translated into action to allow the program offered by the University of British Columbia School of Nursing to be extended to the Vancouver General Hospital School of Nursing site, with all subsequent students being admitted to the four-year program (CNA Staff, June 1991, p. 3). Unfortunately, the merger collapsed in 1995, when the Vancouver Hospital, during a period of fiscal restraint, withdrew its financial support from the UBC School of Nursing, thus requiring UBC to cut its enrolment drastically.

Planning began in 1985 in Alberta for an innovative arrangement between the University of Alberta Faculty of Nursing and Red Deer College that resulted in the implementation of a collaborative model for a four-year baccalaureate program in nursing. This collaboration between a community college and a university to award a degree was the first such model of its kind in the country when the first students enrolled in the program in September 1990. In this unique arrangement, all courses throughout the four-year program were offered on the Red Deer site. This collaborative model was extended to include the diploma schools of nursing at the University of Alberta Hospitals, Grant MacEwan College, the Misericordia Hospital, and the Royal Alexandra Hospital. Students at those sites were enrolled in the program in September 1991. This effort was unique in that all diploma schools in Edmonton, including the hospital schools and the college program, were integral partners in the collaboration from the outset.

In 1995, the Hospital Schools of Nursing were formally closed by the Alberta government, which meant that the collaborative program was then handled exclusively by the two colleges and the University of Alberta. In 1996, the colleges in Grande Prairie and Fort McMurray (Keyano) joined the collaboration and began offering the degree program at their sites. This was a turning point for Central and Northern Alberta, as now all nursing students entered a degree program in this region. All sites, except the University of Alberta, were required to offer a diploma-completion exit from the degree program, as the Alberta government would not support the baccalaureate entry-to-practice position. However, as the collaborative program developed, more than 80% of students selected the degree option. The CARNA approved a resolution requiring the baccalaureate degree for entry to practice in Alberta by 2004, but later changed this goal to the year 2010. The political climate in Alberta has always made it difficult to upgrade educational standards, particularly in a field that is primarily made up of women.

CANADIAN RESEARCH FOCUS

Tschannen, D., & Kalisch, B. (2009). The effect of variations in nurse staffing on patient length of stay in the acute care setting. *Western Journal of Nursing Research, 31*(2), 153–170.

This study took place in two midwestern US hospitals. The hypothesis was that greater nurse staffing is associated with an earlier discharge of patients from acute care.

"Greater nurse staffing" was made up of several variables, including education and expertise of nurses. Nurses in the study were both RNs and LPNs and largely had more experience than theoretical knowledge. Findings from this study support a significant association between patient length of stay and nurse staffing indicators. Expertise was a negative predictor and hours per patient day was a positive predictor of a shorter length of stay. The authors believe that unit staffing levels must include more nurses who have both experiential and theoretical knowledge in order to achieve optimum patient outcomes.

COLLABORATION BETWEEN DIPLOMA AND DEGREE PROGRAMS INCREASES

In Calgary, government approval of the conjoint program between the University of Calgary Faculty of Nursing and the two diploma schools of nursing at Mount Royal College and the School of Nursing at Foothills Hospital allowed for implementation of the program in September 1993 (CNA Staff, Summer 1993, p. 1). The government of Alberta announced early in 1994 that all hospital diploma schools of nursing in Alberta would be closed and their programs transferred to the general education system. Although this involved a 50% cutback in the resources of the hospital diploma schools in Edmonton and Calgary, it meant that there was a transition of student spaces to the University of Alberta and Grant MacEwan College in Edmonton and to the University of Calgary and Mount Royal College in Calgary (subsequently affiliated with Athabasca University and now offering its own Bachelor of Nursing program). The fact that collaborative programs had been operating for two and a half years in Edmonton and for one year in Calgary meant continued smooth operation of courses and continuation of programs.

A collaborative program between the University of Lethbridge and two colleges (Medicine Hat College and Lethbridge Community College) was initiated in 1995. The University of Lethbridge had previously had a small post-RN program, and diploma programs were in place at the two colleges. This collaboration was not without problems, primarily because of the fiercely independent nature of the two communities of Lethbridge and Medicine Hat. Disagreements between the college at Medicine Hat and the university led to the separation of Medicine Hat College from the collaboration. Medicine Hat College now collaborates with the University of Calgary to provide a degree option for students in nursing. The University of Lethbridge and Lethbridge Community College continue to offer a collaborative degree program.

Although Alberta provided early leadership in the move to baccalaureate education for nurses, it has become one of the last provinces to actually implement this ideal. In the early 2000s when the shortage of nurses was becoming apparent, the provincial government opened up additional seats for diploma students through Grant McEwan College, ostensibly to provide opportunities for rural students to enter nursing. This was a distinct setback to the movement toward BETP for Alberta.

British Columbia has moved to implement the baccalaureate degree for entry to practice over the last few years. All diploma programs in BC have been phased out. This move represents the culmination of many years of effort by nursing leaders in BC.

Early on in the move to upgrade nurses' education, nursing educators in BC developed a collaborative program between the University of Victoria and several colleges—Camosun, Cariboo, Malaspina, and Okanagan. As it was anticipated from the outset that degree-granting power would eventually be given to Okanagan and Cariboo University Colleges, a different arrangement was developed between these institutions and the University of Victoria, where the university worked with college faculty offering the courses throughout the four years. Although Malaspina College is also a university college, its participation initially took the form of offering some post-RN courses. At present, Malaspina has begun to offer the full program to both post-RN and continuing students. The University of Victoria has also taken on some additional partners—Langara College, North Island College (first students admitted September 1993), and Selkirk College (first students admitted September 1994). Two additional colleges, Douglas College and Kwantlen University College in Vancouver, admitted their first students in September 1996. The collaborative initiatives at the basic baccalaureate integrated program level were the logical extension of the University of Victoria's initial development of its post-RN program on the campuses of Okanagan and Cariboo colleges further to the 1987 provincial government resolution to increase access to postsecondary education (CNA Staff, March 1992, p. 3).

Other developments in British Columbia have taken place at the University of Northern British Columbia. This is a relatively young institution with a nursing program that has collaborated with several colleges, including Northern Lights Community College and the College of New Caledonia. A third college, Northwest College, had initially been a partner in this consortium, but did not admit students in September 1994 as originally planned. A collaborative, four-year curriculum was developed in a relatively short time because the three colleges already had a common curriculum and there was considerable support from the colleges for moving to a baccalaureate curriculum. The university did not receive adequate government funding to maintain a critical mass of faculty, and it was overly dependent on support from the College of New Caledonia. However, because of the commitment of the two institutions, the program has survived and is well supported by the community.

In Saskatchewan, a collaborative baccalaureate program is offered by the University of Saskatchewan College of Nursing and the Saskatchewan Institute of Applied Science and Technology (SIAST). The program is offered at University of Saskatchewan campuses in Saskatoon and Regina, as well as the Kelsey and Wascana campuses of SIAST. There are no diploma programs in Saskatchewan.

The earliest collaborative initiative that was implemented in Manitoba in 1991 developed into a consolidated effort by 1994. The four-year baccalaureate degree program in nursing that was developed was offered at the University of Manitoba and, beginning in

1991, at the Manitoba Health Sciences Centre. At the latter site and at the St. Boniface site, which joined the collaboration in 1992, one year of the program was added per year until all four years were operational. As the initiative was implemented and in view of the changing health care context and health care reform, a consolidated arrangement was developed so that blended teaching teams at the various sites were being used to avoid duplication of effort (Bramadat, personal communication, September 2, 1994). In the late 1990s, diploma programs were closed out briefly and a single baccalaureate program was directed by the University of Manitoba. However, diploma education was reinstituted in 1999 by a new government and continues to be offered through Red River College.

In 1998, the College of Nurses of Ontario recommended that the education for entry to practice be the bachelor's degree by January 2005. This recommendation was endorsed by the provincial cabinet on April 12, 2000. As a result, all diploma and university schools of nursing in Ontario began developing collaborative programs to meet the new requirement by 2005. This has been a complex undertaking because of the numbers of institutions involved in nursing education. There were 22 colleges and 14 universities involved in developing the current collaborative degree programs in nursing. Currently, 35 Ontario institutions offer baccalaureate degree programs in nursing, and the degrees are given by 15 universities, including the University of New Brunswick. It has been a monumental task to accomplish this in such a short time, and the Ontario nurses involved in the planning and implementation are to be commended.

In Quebec, the Collèges d'Enseignement Général et Professionnel (CEGEP) system of preparation allows for two years of preparation in the college system, followed by three years at the university level, leading to a degree in nursing. The colleges still offer diploma programs in nursing, and the graduates of these are eligible for licensing. The Quebec government required that by 2000 all universities (nine) and colleges (42) work together to plan a five-year program in nursing. The government then formed a committee, chaired by the deputy minister of education, to work out a master plan for nursing education. The resulting five-year program is now available as a collaborative program among colleges and universities. Also, post-RN programs are offered by a number of Quebec universities. Sadly, however, in 2006, 80% of newly registered nurses came from a college (diploma) program. In addition, of Quebec nurses who completed their certification exam in the years 2001 to 2006, 72.7% of those who come from CEGEP had not continued into a degree program (Diane Morin, personal communication, 2008). Because Quebec is the province with the largest number of nurses in the country, the continuation of diploma education there has a major impact on the profession in Canada.

In 1989, the baccalaureate degree became the minimum entrance requirement for nursing practice in New Brunswick. Baccalaureate degrees in nursing are offered by the University of New Brunswick and the Université de Moncton at seven sites across the province.

Initiatives in Nova Scotia resulted in an initial collaboration between Dalhousie University and two diploma programs in that province. A program involving the three institutions began in the fall of 1995, when the two diploma programs (Victoria General Hospital–Camp Hill Medical Complex and Yarmouth Regional Hospital School of Nursing) closed. Basic nursing education in Nova Scotia now requires a baccalaureate degree and programs are offered by Dalhousie University and St. Francis Xavier University. Diploma education in Nova Scotia was phased out during the late 1990s.

In Newfoundland, Memorial University collaborates with the St. John's Centre for Nursing Studies and the Western Regional School of Nursing in Corner Brook to provide a four-year baccalaureate program. There have been no diploma programs in Newfoundland since the early 1900s.

The announcement in 1988 of the decision by the government of Prince Edward Island to "phase out diploma education in favour of a degree program" (CNA Connection, 1989a) was the culmination of many years of effort on the part of nurses in Prince Edward Island to secure a baccalaureate program of nursing in their province. It is obviously more complex to envision implementing the baccalaureate degree as the basis for entry to practice in a large, populous province with many schools of nursing than it is in a small one, such as Prince Edward Island. However, the model established by the province of Prince Edward Island was an important one for the nation.

In the Northwest Territories, a degree program in nursing is offered by Aurora College, in collaboration with the University of Victoria. The former diploma program offered by the college has been phased out. In Nunavut, Dalhousie University has offered a degree program in partnership with Nunavut Arctic College since 1999. Formerly, students in this program obtained a diploma from Nunavut Arctic College after three years, allowing them to practise in hospital settings. However, this credential has been phased out, and the current basic program is a four-year degree program. The picture in the first near-decade of a new century is still fraught with unsolved problems, yet much progress has been made. In 2008, British Columbia, Saskatchewan, Ontario, New Brunswick, Nova Scotia, Prince Edward Island, Newfoundland, the Northwest Territories, and Nunavut all have progressed to baccalaureate entry to practice. Only three provinces, Quebec, Alberta, and Manitoba, continue to offer diploma programs in nursing. This is a vast improvement over the situation five years ago. The tasks ahead are difficult and challenging. However, a cursory glance through the pages of nursing history confirms that the road has never been easy. Nursing is at this educational crossroads today because there have been leaders with vision and courage who developed and found support for wise initiatives. Unity of purpose and action has characterized what the nursing profession has accomplished in moving toward successful achievement of its educational goals. The rationale for implementation of the baccalaureate standard for entry to practice can only be understood and accepted on the basis of the nature and range of knowledge and skills required to practise nursing and the right of the health care consumer to receive care from a well-prepared professional nurse. In the end, it is likely that the success of the transition to the baccalaureate entry-level standard will be achieved through the efforts of nurses at all levels and in all settings who were convinced of the importance of the issues involved and who worked tirelessly to make it happen.

CRITICAL THINKING QUESTIONS

1. Why is the issue of educational entry to practice important to nurses and nursing in Canada?
2. What are the major societal factors that may have contributed to the difficulties encountered by Canadian nursing educators in their efforts to upgrade the entry to practice to the baccalaureate level?

WEB SITES

Canadian Association of Schools of Nursing: www.casn.ca

REFERENCES

Alberta Association of Registered Nurses (AARN). (1976). *The response of the Alberta Association of Registered Nurses to the Government of Alberta's position paper on nursing education.* Edmonton: Author.

Alberta Association of Registered Nurses (AARN). (1978). *Position paper on nursing.* Edmonton: Author.

Alberta Association of Registered Nurses (AARN). (1979). *Position paper on nursing.* Edmonton: Author.

Besharah, A. (1981). When will the shouting start? *The Canadian Nurse, 77*(3), 6.

Bramadat, E. (September 2, 1994). *Personal communication.* University of Manitoba.

Canadian Nurses Association (CNA). (2002). Highlights of 2000 nursing statistics. Retrieved on May 9, 2002, from http://www.cna-nurses.ca/_frames/resources/statsframe.htm.

CNA Connection. (1989a). Baccalaureate education comes to PEI. *The Canadian Nurse, 85*(3), 10.

CNA Connection. (1989b). VGH School joins UBC. *The Canadian Nurse, 85*(2), 12.

CNA Staff. (1984). *Entry to practice bulletin.* Ottawa: Author.

CNA Staff. (1989). *Entry to practice newsletter, 5*(3), 1–3.

CNA Staff. (June 1991). VGH/UBC prepare for third year of collaboration. *Edufacts,* 1–4.

CNA Staff. (March 1992). University–college collaboration in BC. *Edufacts, 2*(1), 1–4.

CNA Staff. (Winter 1992–93). Do we have enough master of nursing programs? *Edufacts,* 1–4.

CNA Staff. (Spring 1993). Tracking enrolments. *Edufacts,* 1–4.

CNA Staff. (Summer 1993). Calgary Conjoint Nursing Program. *Edufacts,* 1–4.

Government of Alberta. (1975). *Report of the Alberta Task Force on Nursing Education.* Edmonton: Author.

Government of Alberta. (1977). *Position paper on nursing education: Principles and issues.* Edmonton: Author.

Government of Canada. (1964). *Royal Commission on Health Services.* Ottawa: Queen's Printer.

Kerr, J. C. (1978). *Financing university nursing education in Canada from 1919 to 1976. Doctoral dissertation.* Ann Arbor, MI: University of Michigan.

Kerr, J. C. (1982). The shouting starts. *The Canadian Nurse, 78*(2), 42–43.

King, M. K. (1970). The development of university nursing education. In M. Q. Innis (Ed.), *Nursing education in a changing society* (pp. 67–85). Toronto: University of Toronto Press.

Morin, D. (2008). Personal communication.

Rajabally, M. (1982). We have seen the enemy. *The Canadian Nurse, 78*(2), 40–42.

Russell, E. K. (1932). The teaching of public health nursing in the University of Toronto. In *Methods and problems of medication education* (pp. 82–88). New York: Rockefeller Foundation.

Tschannen, D., & Kalisch, B. (2009). The effect of variations in nurse staffing on patient length of stay in the acute care setting. *Western Journal of Nursing Research, 31*(2), 153–170.

Weir, G. M. (1932). *Survey of nursing education in Canada.* Toronto: University of Toronto Press.

Credentialing in Nursing

Janet C. Ross-Kerr

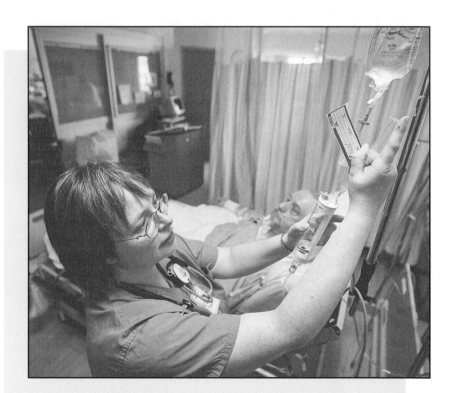

LEARNING OBJECTIVES

- To describe the major credentialing mechanisms used in nursing.
- To appreciate the efforts of nurses to secure legislation for regulation of nursing through registration.
- To describe the meaning of registration and licensure in the professional nursing context.
- To explain why mandatory licensure is important for the nursing profession.
- To outline the movement to allow nurse practitioners to practise in Canada.
- To identify the reasons for specialization in nursing
- To explain the program to recognize nursing specialties developed by the Canadian Nurses Association.

The study of credentialing in nursing is illuminating, for it draws attention to the growth and development of nursing as a profession. The relation of credentialing to professionalization can be seen in what has been referred to as "the natural history of professionalization," a history that is both recognizable and sequential in nature:

> There is a typical process by which the established professions have arrived. . . . [They] begin doing the work full time and stake out a jurisdiction; the early masters of the technique or adherents of the movement become concerned about standards of training and practice and set up a training school, which, if not lodged in universities at the start, makes academic connections within two or three decades; the teachers and activists then achieve success in promoting effective organization, first local, then national. . . . Toward the end, legal protection appears; at the end, a formal code of ethics is adopted. (Wilensky, 1964, p. 144)

The presence of a specialized knowledge base is fundamental to the processes and mechanisms of credentialing in nursing. The perception of the defining characteristics of this knowledge determines identification and acceptance of a field as a profession, including elements such as the following: (1) the knowledge and skills are abstract and consist of principles considered relevant to everyday situations; (2) there is a belief that the specialized knowledge will produce positive results when applied to real problems; (3) those in the profession are involved in developing and applying the knowledge base and in providing expert opinion in difficult cases; and (4) the knowledge and skills are complex, and only a few have the ability to acquire them (Goode, 1960). In a historical sense, Canadian nurses recognized early in the twentieth century that the knowledge and skills fundamental to the profession were important and that unqualified and unskilled practitioners could harm clients for whom they cared. They concluded that not only was it important to ensure that nurses were graduates of recognized schools of nursing, but also that professional standards were needed to regulate nursing education and practice.

Hospitals in Canada did not need to be encouraged to establish schools of nursing in the late nineteenth and early twentieth centuries. They all sought to emulate the successful Nightingale model in Britain and to ensure an adequate number of staff members as well as a qualified and inexpensive staff. However, this design was the antithesis of what

Nightingale intended, as her school was supported by the Nightingale endowment and was financially and administratively independent. Thus, evidence of graduation from a school of nursing was the earliest form of credentialing. The period during which this occurred was also characterized by a concerted drive by nursing leaders to secure legislation for registration of nurses to ensure that the educated would be differentiated from the uneducated for the protection of the public.

In a general sense, credentialing issues are similar today, although the nature and extent of the knowledge and skills that must be acquired to practise nursing have changed. The need for recognizing standards in programs, knowing the meaning of a certificate, securing qualified staff for many areas of specialization, establishing standards at the national level, and ensuring that practitioners update knowledge and maintain competence throughout their careers are important areas for discussion and study. However, questions pertaining to protection of the public from unscrupulous, unqualified, and unskilled practitioners are fundamental to credentialing processes and mechanisms.

CREDENTIALING MECHANISMS

The International Council of Nurses has referred to credentialing as "a term applied to processes used to designate that an individual, programme, institution or product have met established standards set by an agent (governmental or non-governmental) recognised as qualified to carry out this task" (Styles & Affara, 1997), which means recognizing the individuals who have met the established standards in particular areas by awarding credentials. Thus, individuals who have knowledge and skills in a certain area are distinguished from those who do not have such skills. Describing credentialing as a system of checks and balances seems appropriate. Nursing has two main credentialing mechanisms: professional and educational. On the professional side, registration and licensure are awarded to individuals for practice of the profession. In this chapter, the focus will be on professional credentialing mechanisms, as educational mechanisms are dealt with in detail in other sections of this book (Chapters 19 and 21).

THE MOVEMENT TO SECURE LEGISLATION FOR REGISTRATION

The drive for registration of nurses occurred early in the development of the profession in Canada. This was the issue that brought nurses together in professional organizations. The formation of the first national and international organization for nurses in 1893, the American Society of Superintendents of Training Schools for Nurses of the United States and Canada, was followed by the foundation of the Nurses' Associated Alumnae of the United States and Canada in 1896. The purpose of the latter organization was "to secure legislation to differentiate the trained from the untrained" (CNA, 1968, p. 35). Both organizations were initially headed by one of the most important nursing leaders of the time, Isabel Hampton Robb, a Canadian nurse from Ontario who was the first superintendent of nurses at the Johns Hopkins Hospital in Baltimore, Maryland.

These groups stimulated the formation of many other professional nursing organizations at the local, regional, and national levels in the United States and Canada, all of which worked to complete the groundwork necessary for the passage of legislation to regulate nursing in the provinces. The publication of the *American Journal of Nursing* in 1900 and *The Canadian Nurse* in 1905 helped the cause.

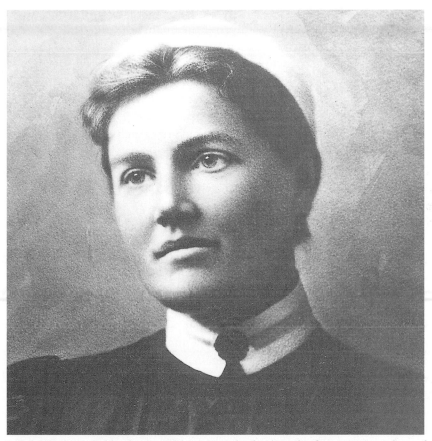

Isabel Hampton Robb, the Canadian nurse who became the first superintendent of nurses at Johns Hopkins Hospital in Baltimore, Maryland, in 1889.

The American and Canadian groups separated as activity intensified, and it was evident that the battle for passage of the legislation had to be fought regionally. In Canada, it was spearheaded in the provinces because the *British North America Act* of 1867 provided that the legislatures of each province be given exclusive right to make laws in relation to health and education. The Canadian Society of Superintendents of Training Schools for Nurses emerged in 1907, followed by the Provisional Society of the Canadian National Association of Trained Nurses in 1908. The first president of both groups was Mary Agnes Snively, a graduate of Bellevue Hospital in New York who had headed the School of Nursing at Toronto General Hospital since 1884 (CNA, 1968).

From the beginning, there have been valid reasons for requiring registration. Professional registration and licensure make the benefits that accrue from the services of a highly skilled group available to society and protect society from those who are not highly skilled, as well as from those who might knowingly misuse their knowledge and skills to the disadvantage of the populace. In each province in Canada, local graduate nurse groups joined forces to become provincial nurses' associations and sought legislation for registration of nurses. These nurses believed that registration acts that set standards for training schools would also improve the quality of care.

Two powerful social forces influenced the drive for legislation for the registration of nurses. The first was the consciousness-raising regarding women's rights, which was part of the movement for the enfranchisement of women. The second was that nurses' services were especially valued during World War I when the wartime need for nursing care both on the battlefront and behind the lines was great. During this period of worldwide social upheaval, nursing and nurses became very much valued, as so many nurses volunteered for war service and served with dedication and valour. The worldwide influenza pandemic between 1916 and 1918 further drove home the need to recognize the qualifications of nurses as essential to protecting the health of the populace. The passage of legislation in every province over a 12-year period may have been facilitated by these factors and represented general recognition of the need for a system to ensure that nurses were qualified.

There was considerable activity for a number of years before legislation was first passed in 1910, when Nova Scotia passed an act that made registration voluntary and allowed nongraduate nurses to register. Subsequent acts in other provinces were more restrictive regarding the standards incorporated into the legislation. Minimum standards for admission and curricula in schools of nursing were set, as were rules governing registration and discipline of practising nurses. Ontario was the last province to approve legislation for nursing because of a lobby against the legislation led by hospitals whose administrators feared that educational standards for maintaining schools could not be met. Opposition also arose from nurses who felt they could not meet the qualifications. These objections were overcome or overruled, and legislation was passed in that province in 1922 (Sabin, Price, & Sellers, 1973).

In all provinces except Alberta, the initial legislation gave the provincial nursing association the responsibility for administering the legislation. In Alberta, the *Registered Nurses Act* was passed in 1916, and uniform registration examinations were instituted in 1919. This statute was unusual because it placed nursing education under the aegis of the senate of the University of Alberta. A chronology documenting the process of securing registration in each of the provinces is presented in Table 20.1.

REGISTRATION AND LICENSURE

Registration allows the profession to maintain an official roster of member nurses. To be named on a register, a nurse must be a member in good standing of the organization incorporating the statutory responsibility for registration. Under permissive registration,

TABLE 20.1	Chronology of Legislation Regulating Nursing in Canadian Jurisdictions		
PROVINCE	DATE LEGISLATION FIRST ENACTED	CURRENT STATUS OF LEGISLATION	DATE MANDATORY LEGISLATION FIRST ENACTED
British Columbia	1918	Mandatory	1988
Alberta	1916	Mandatory	1983
Saskatchewan	1917	Mandatory	1900
Manitoba	1913	Mandatory	2001
Ontario	1922	Mandatory	1991
Quebec	1920	Mandatory	1973
New Brunswick	1916	Mandatory	1984
Nova Scotia	1910	Mandatory	1985
Prince Edward Island	1922	Mandatory	1972
Newfoundland	1931	Mandatory	1953
Northwest Territories and Nunavut	1976	Mandatory	1975
Yukon Territory	1994	Mandatory	2004

Sources: Good, S.R., & Kerr, J.C. (Eds.). (1973). *Contemporary issues in Canadian law for nurses* (p. 189). Toronto: Holt, Rinehart & Winston of Canada; Prowse, A.J. (1983). *Nursing legislation in Canada: An overview for health services administrators* (pp. 10–28; 36–41). Unpublished master's thesis, University of Alberta, Edmonton: Department of Health Services Administration; College of Nurses of Ontario. (2005). *The Regulated Health Professions Act.* Retrieved on April 28, 2008, from http://www.cno.org/docs/policy/41052_RHPAscope.pdf; Registered Nurses Association of the Northwest Territories and Nunavut. (2008). *Legislation.* Retrieved on April 1, 2008, from http://www.rnantnu.ca/Legislation/tabid/55/Default.aspx; *Regulated Health Professions Act,* 1991, S.O. 1991, c. 8; and Yukon Registered Nurses Association. (2008). *Nursing practice—registration.* Retrieved on April 1, 2008, from http://www.yrna.ca/nursingpractice/registration/indexreg.html. *Registered Nurses Act,* S.M. 1999. C. 38.

the legislation protects only the title of the registered nurse; that is, a person may practise nursing without being registered, but may not use the initials RN. In acts that provide for mandatory registration, the nature of the service provided by the profession is defined. This means that those who do not meet the requirements of the legislation may not practise nursing. Title is protected, as in permissive acts, but the definition of nursing and the restriction of practice as it applies to registered nurses are the critical features that differentiate the two forms of legislation.

Requirements for initial registration are similar in all provinces. An applicant must be a graduate of an approved school of nursing. Minimum standards for nursing education are established by an approval body. In all provinces except Ontario and Quebec, the approval body is the professional association. In Ontario, the *Health Disciplines Act* and the *Regulated Health Professions Act, 1991*, granted authority for approval and monitoring of diploma programs to the Ministry of Training, Colleges and Universities and to the Council of Ontario University Programs in Nursing (COUPN), and the university senate or governing council (for university programs). Subsequently, COUPN delegated its authority to approve university nursing programs to the Canadian Association of University Schools of Nursing (CASN) (Council of Ontario University Programs in Nursing, 2008). Accreditation of the university nursing program thus denotes approval. In Quebec, the Ministry of Higher Education and Science holds responsibility for monitoring diploma programs in the Collèges d'Enseignement Général et Professionnel (CEGEP). University programs in nursing are monitored by the individual universities.

The terms "registration" and "licensure" have different meanings, although they are used interchangeably in some situations. As previously noted, registration refers to the listing of a member in good standing of an organization on the roster of members. Licensure refers to the granting by a government body of the exclusive right to practise a profession to a member in good standing. In provinces where registration is mandatory, the same process may also be described as licensure. Practice of the profession by any person who has not been granted such a right is prohibited and punishable by law.

THE CASE FOR MANDATORY LICENSURE

Licensure laws were designed to protect the public from unethical and incompetent practitioners, not to protect the nursing profession from competition. The only justifiable reason for adopting legislation to guarantee professionals exclusive right to practise is to protect the public from unqualified and incompetent practitioners. The legislation cannot and must not bestow a special benefit on people who have completed a certain educational program and demonstrated designated qualifications where there is no public protective component.

In recent years, there has been public concern about self-rule by professional groups, the fear being that power may be exercised in the interest of the profession. The thrust of the consumer movement is to present challenges in areas in which the consumer interest may not be protected. The health care field is no exception in such efforts. This phenomenon, and the fact that it is not easy to change existing legislation that governs professional groups, explains why it was difficult for provinces and territories to replace their original permissive legislation with mandatory statutes. Mandatory licensure has been achieved by emphasizing the need to assure the public that licensed nurses have met an appropriate standard of practice, as determined by the profession.

All Canadian nursing jurisdictions have now achieved legislative provision for mandatory registration of nurses. The presence of a statutory definition of the scope of nursing practice is an important feature of legislature in jurisdictions with mandatory licensure. Nurses' functions are delineated more explicitly when a definition of nursing practice is incorporated into the statute. The potential for overlap with functions performed by other health care workers that exists in mandatory jurisdictions may be addressed through specific exemptions or by extending rights only to health care workers practising by virtue of other statutes.

In 1991, Ontario enacted legislation affecting all health care professions. This legislation, the *Regulated Health Professions Act* (RHPA), provides for the regulation of 23 professional groups under 21 individual professional acts. Each individual act describes a scope of practice and allows for restrictive use of title. To ensure public protection, however, the RHPA identifies 13 controlled acts that may be performed only by specific registered members as identified in the individual act. In this manner, it is the activity that is licensed, not the individual provider (College of Nurses of Ontario, 2005). Alberta also passed omnibus legislation for the health professions and proclaimed the registered nurses' schedule in 2005. The scope of nursing practice is incorporated into the statute as previously, and the legislation also provides for the practice of restricted activities as authorized in the regulations (Government of Alberta, 2008).

Registration and licensure ensure a minimum level of safe practice at the time of initial registration. Those registered are eligible for re-registration annually if practice requirements are met and there is no evidence of unsafe practice. New knowledge is continually introduced to the field, and the individual must maintain and extend competence to meet the changing requirements. The nursing profession has wrestled with the problem of maintaining competence in an effort to demonstrate public accountability. The merits of mandatory versus permissive continuing education programs have been debated at length. In most provinces, mandatory continuing education has been rejected in favour of requiring a certain number of days of employment within a specified time and a record of satisfactory practice as evidence of current knowledge and skills.

The move toward offering refresher courses for those who have been out of practice, upgrading programs, and providing opportunities for continuing education has become an integral and essential part of the nursing education system, as those who practise a profession must incorporate a commitment to lifelong learning. The nurse has a legal and ethical duty to maintain competence. In the event that a nurse's conduct is questioned by a patient, the practitioner may be called upon in a hearing of peers or in a court of law to provide evidence that reasonable effort has been expended to attend continuing education seminars and workshops to maintain competence in practice. Recently, some provinces have moved to incorporate mandatory continuing education as part of the continuing registration process. The intent here is protection of the public interest by ensuring that nurses maintain their knowledge and skills throughout their careers. The continuing competence program of the College and Association of Registered Nurses of Alberta is based on a self-reflective model requiring self-assessment, learning goals and progress toward meeting goals as a part of the yearly renewal process (College and Association of Registered Nurses of Alberta, 2008).

REFLECTIVE THINKING

Explore the importance to public health and safety of legislation to regulate the practice of nursing.

NURSE PRACTITIONERS

The nurse practitioner (NP) movement began in Canada in the 1960s, spurred on by advances in health care leading to evolving nursing roles, increasing specialization in nursing, and a developing shortage of family physicians. The first program for "outpost nurses" at Dalhousie University began in 1967, and led to similar programs at other Canadian universities jointly sponsored by faculties of nursing and medicine, but operated separately from ongoing degree programs in nursing. However, the graduates of the programs found themselves working in a legislative vacuum and for the most part were employed in northern and remote areas. Those who worked in cities were employed under physician supervision. Several studies made the expanded role of the nurse a priority in the 1970s (Boudreau, 1972; Hastings, 1971; *Canadian Nurse,* 1973). Responding to the perceived need for programs, university nursing programs began to develop courses in the 1980s, in health assessment at the undergraduate and graduate levels, and to discuss developing advanced nursing practice programs at the master's level. Gradually, more of these programs became available and began to replace existing programs as student demand for them increased.

In the late 1990s, a movement to develop legislation gained momentum in order to allow nurse practitioners to work under legal authority. For the most part, legislation has taken the form of amendments to the legislation for registered nurses in each jurisdiction. The expanded scope of practice allowed under each piece of legislation varies somewhat from jurisdiction to jurisdiction, but generally includes assessment of health status leading to diagnosis of disease, ordering of diagnostic and screening tests, and prescribing medications (Canadian Nurses Association & Canadian Institute for Health Information, 2006).

⚲ CANADIAN RESEARCH FOCUS

Forchuk, C., & Kohn, R. (2009). Prescriptive authority for nurses: The Canadian perspective. *Perspectives in Psychiatric Care, 45*(1), 3–8.

In this unique discussion of the evolution and status of prescriptive authority for nurses in Canada, the linkage to the development of advanced nursing practice is underscored. The authors note that prescriptive authority is a "work in progress," because legislation to enact it is not yet universal across the country. However, the initial form of legislation according prescriptive authority to nurses with specialized preparation hinged on the availability of medical practitioners, while more recent legislation tends not to make that requirement. The authors further outline facilitators and barriers to putting prescriptive authority into place in any particular jurisdiction.

SPECIALIZATION IN NURSING

The tremendous change in the nature and scope of nursing practice in Canada in this century has taken place almost imperceptibly, but it has been an evolution with a profound effect on health care and society. It has become increasingly difficult to master the knowledge required for practice in every area in which nurses function. The burgeoning increases in knowledge in the health care field have led to specialization in just about every area of nursing, a change that has raised questions about ensuring competence in those practising in specialized areas.

The medical profession itself is highly specialized. The movement toward specialization in medicine has been strong and, to a certain extent, has influenced nursing. Although there has been an attempt to place more value on the role of the general practitioner in medicine, more physicians are specializing. Given the tremendous increase in medical knowledge, this trend is not surprising. Nursing is also influenced by tremendous increases in knowledge in every area of practice, and the outcome has been the development of discrete and increasingly complex nursing specialties.

Transfer of functions from medicine to nursing is also of interest. Many functions that were previously restricted exclusively to medical practice have been redefined as nursing responsibilities. Although this is primarily a task-oriented approach to practice in an area in which functions overlap, it is important because the changes in medical practice that produce the changes in nursing practice are immediately apparent. It is also important to recognize that (1) transfer of functions among the health professions is an ongoing process; and (2) there will always be an overlap of functions among professions. With increases in knowledge, skills, and functions, the nurse is in a pivotal position in the delivery of health care. The nurse of today assumes roles and functions that were expected of the general medical practitioner of yesterday. In fact, the general practitioner of yesterday might be overwhelmed at the complexity of nursing roles of today!

The reasons for the trend toward specialization in the nursing profession are the increase in knowledge and the corresponding increase in skill needed for sound judgement and decision making. There is an almost constant demand for nurses who have expertise in highly specialized areas, so nurses must recognize their specialized skills and value the knowledge they require.

RECOGNITION OF SPECIALIZATION

Specialized practice is referred to as a focus upon a certain feature of nursing that could be age, health problem, medical diagnosis, environment of care, or the type of care (Canadian Nurses Association, 2002). Specialization has become an important phenomenon in nursing practice. Canadian nurses initially sought certification from programs in the United States to demonstrate knowledge in their areas of practice. At the 1980 CNA Biennial Convention, the CNA Board passed a resolution to study the feasibility of developing certification examinations in major nursing specialties. Consideration of the issues involved led the CNA to develop a policy statement on credentialing in nursing and to make a commitment to facilitate the development of certification in nursing specialties (CNA, 1982).

Guidelines for a certification mechanism were adopted, and a certification program was designed (CNA, 1986a). The process involved designation of a specialty for certification, development of a certification examination by the Canadian Nurses Association Testing Services (CNATS), and certification of individuals. The CNA differentiated those acquiring certification in this manner from the clinical nurse specialist, who is designated as a nurse with advanced preparation in a clinical area at the master's level (CNA, 1986b).

The issues presented by specialization and certification seem to be those in which the national association is to provide leadership. Since membership in specialty groups tends to be reasonably small, it is unlikely that the cost of developing a quality program could be borne by a province. Also, reciprocity would be an issue if different programs were developed in each province. Because specialization and certification are not part of basic preparation for practice (regulated by provincial or territorial legislation pursuant to the jurisdiction of provinces and territories as designated in the *Constitution Act*), development of programs at the national level appears to be the most appropriate and reasonable course of action.

The development of the CNA Advisory Council "to provide a forum for discussions between the Council and the CNA board of directors on health and nursing issues" (*CNA Connection*, 1989b, p. 10) enabled special-interest groups to address the CNA. The approach to the certification process taken by the CNA is broad: "The designation process applies to an area of nursing rather than to a group or an association, and the process may be initiated by any group of nurses that is able to provide evidence that a specific nursing area meets the required criteria" (*CNA Connection, 1989b*, p. 10).

REFLECTIVE THINKING

Discuss the advantages to nurses in specialty areas of nursing of the following: first, the CNA certification mechanism, and second, specialty programs offered by Canadian universities at the master's degree level.

In 1981, the CNA agreed to develop a certification examination for the Canadian Council of Occupational Health Nurses, which had received a grant to develop this program. They hired the CNATS to create the examination. Consultation services relative to the development of the examination were offered "on the understanding they would join the CNA certification program when it became a reality" (*CNA Connection*, 1989a, p. 7). However, the disappointing announcement was made that "following discussion and correspondence between CNA and the Canadian Council of Occupational Health Nurses Inc., the process of integrating the occupational health nursing examination into the CNA certification program has been suspended" because the occupational health nurses "would like more time to consider integration criteria, and [have] suggested waiting until at least 1991 to begin the process" (*CNA Connection*, 1990, p. 14).

At that point, the CNA decided that groups that had been scheduled to enter the certification program after the Canadian Council of Occupational Health Nurses would be accommodated first (*CNA Connection*, 1990). Thus, the first specialty groups to complete a certification program were nephrology nursing and neuroscience nursing. However, in March 1992 occupational health nursing was integrated into the CNA certification program, bringing the total number of specialty areas available for certification to three. Other specialty groups quickly followed suit, and by 2010 there were 19 such groups involved with and endorsing the CNA certification program. (See Table 20.2 for information about certification programs offered by the CNA.)

Meanwhile, demand for still other certification programs continued to grow, and the CNA recognized the need to expand the existing program. Based on recommendations of an ad hoc committee, the CNA Board of Directors reaffirmed its commitment to certification by adopting a plan for the accelerated expansion of the program. The

TABLE 20.2 Certification Programs in Nursing Specialties Offered by the Canadian Nurses Association

NAME OF SPECIALTY	NATIONAL NURSING SPECIALTY ASSOCIATIONS	DESIGNATION	OFFICIAL DATE PROGRAM ESTABLISHED
Cardiovascular Nursing	Canadian Council of Cardiovascular Nurses	CCN(C)	2001
Community Health Nursing	Community Health Nurses Association of Canada	CCHN(C)	2006
Critical Care Nursing	Canadian Association of Critical Care Nurses	CNCC(C)	1995
Critical Care–Pediatric Nursing	Canadian Association of Critical Care Nurses	CNCCP(C)	2003
Emergency Nursing	National Emergency Nurses' Affiliation Inc.	ENC(C)	1994
Enterostomal Therapy Nursing	Canadian Association for Enterostomal Therapy	CETN(C)	2008
Gastroenterology Nursing	Canadian Society of Gastroenterology Nurses and Associates	CGN(C)	2004
Gerontology Nursing	Canadian Gerontological Nurses Association	GNC(C)	1999
Hospice Palliative Care Nursing	Canadian Hospice Palliative Care Association	CHPCN(C)	2004
Medical-Surgical Nursing	Canadian Association of Medical and Surgical Nurses	CMSN(C)	2009
Nephrology Nursing	Canadian Association of Nephrology Nurses and Technologists	CNeph(C)	1993
Neuroscience Nursing	Canadian Association of Neuroscience Nurses	CNN(C)	1991
Occupational Health Nursing	Canadian Occupational Health Nurses Association	COHN(C)	1992
Oncology Nursing	Canadian Association of Nurses in Oncology	CON(C)	1997
Orthopedic Nursing	Canadian Orthopedic Nurses Association	ONC(C)	2006
Perinatal Nursing	Association of Women's Health, Obstetric and Neonatal Nurses—Canada	PNC(C)	2000
Perioperative Nursing	Operating Room Nurses Association of Canada	CPN(C)	1995
Psychiatric/Mental Health Nursing	Canadian Federation of Mental Health Nurses	CPMHN(C)	1995
Rehabilitation Nursing	Canadian Association of Rehabilitation Nurses	CRN(C)	2006

expanded certification program offers certification to any specialty area with 10,000 or more nurses employed in that area in Canada, an approach that would provide the CNA with sufficient financial support to continue expanding the program. The program has grown exponentially until by 2009, there were 15,225 nurses certified across the 14 nursing specialties (CNA, 2009).

Although the development of its certification program has taken time and has had its share of challenges, the CNA has successfully brought special-interest groups into the mainstream of professional association activities by establishing the process, developing an advisory council of representatives from specialty associations, and creating a position on the CNA Board of Directors for a representative from this group. The profession has been strengthened by these initiatives, and it is likely that such efforts will continue as more specialty groups become part of the certification program.

CRITICAL THINKING QUESTIONS

1. How did early Canadian schools of nursing established by hospitals in the late nineteenth and early twentieth centuries differ from the Nightingale model?
2. Describe the forces driving the establishment of legislation to regulate nursing.
3. Describe the way in which specialists in various areas of nursing are recognized.

WEB SITES

Canadian Association of Advanced Practice Nurses: http://www.caapn.com/
Canadian Nurses Association Certification Program: http://www.cna-nurses.ca/CNA/nursing/certification/default_e.aspx

REFERENCES

Boudreau, T. J., (Chairman) (1972). *Report of the Committee on Nurse Practitioners.* Ottawa: Health and Welfare Canada.

Canadian Nurse (1973). The expanded role of the nurse: A joint statement of CNA–CMA. *Canadian Nurse, 69,* 23–25.

Canadian Nurses Association. (1968). *The leaf and the lamp.* Author, p. 35.

Canadian Nurses Association. (1982). *Credentialing in nursing: Policy statement and background paper.* Ottawa: Author.

Canadian Nurses Association. (1986a). *CNA's certification program: An information booklet.* Ottawa: Author.

Canadian Nurses Association. (1986b). *Statement on the clinical nurse specialist.* Ottawa: Author.

Canadian Nurses Association. (2002). *Advanced nursing practice: A national framework.* Ottawa: Author.

Canadian Nurses Association. (2009). *Certification Bulletin.* April 7, 2009. Retrieved on October 12, 2009, from http://www.cna-aiic.ca/CNA/documents/pdf/publications/Cert_bulletin_7_April_09_e.pdf.

Canadian Nurses Association & Canadian Institute for Health Information. (2006). *The regulation and supply of nurse practitioners in Canada: 2006 update.* Retrieved on April 2, 2008, from http://secure.cihi.ca/cihiweb/dispPage.jsp?cw_page=PG_571_E&cw_topic=571&cw_rel=AR_1263_E#full.

CNA Connection. (1989a). *The Canadian Nurse, 85*(1), 7.

CNA Connection. (1989b). *The Canadian Nurse, 85*(9), 10.

CNA Connection. (1990). *The Canadian Nurse, 86*(1), 14.

College and Association of Registered Nurses of Alberta (CARNA). (2008). *Continuing competence: Program description.* Retrieved on April 2, 2008, from http://www.nurses.ab.ca/Carna/index.aspx?Web StructureID=1048.

College of Nurses of Ontario. (2005). *The Regulated Health Professions Act.* Retrieved on April 28, 2008, from http://www.cno.org/docs/policy/41052_RHPAscope.pdf.

Council of Ontario University Programs in Nursing. (2008). *Approval process documentation.* Retrieved on April 2, 2008, from http://ohs.cou.on.ca/_bin/home/coupn/publications.cfm.

Forchuk, C., & Kohn, R. (2009). Prescriptive authority for nurses: The Canadian perspective. *Perspectives in Psychiatric Care, 45*(1), 3–8.

Good, S. R., & Kerr, J. C. (Eds.), (1973). *Contemporary issues in Canadian law for nurses.* Toronto: Holt, Rinehart & Winston of Canada.

Goode, W. J. (1960). Encroachment, charlatanism, and the emerging professions: Psychology, sociology and medicine. *American Sociological Review, 25,* 903.

Government of Alberta. (2008). *Health Professions Act.* Retrieved on April 2, 2008, from http://www.qp. gov.ab.ca/Documents/acts/H07.CFM.

Hastings, J. E. G. (1972). *Community health centres in Canada: Report of the Hastings Committee.* Ottawa: Canadian Public Health Association.

Prowse, A. J. (1983). *Nursing legislation in Canada: An overview for health services administrators. Unpublished master's thesis, University of Alberta.* Edmonton: Department of Health Services Administration.

Registered Nurses Association of the Northwest Territories and Nunavut. (2008). *Legislation.* Retrieved on April 1, 2008, from http://www.rnantnu.ca/Legislation/tabid/55/Default.aspx.

Regulated Health Professions Act, 1991, S.O. 1991, c. 8.

Sabin, H., Price, D., & Sellers, B. (1973). Nursing: What it is and what it is not. In S. Good, & J. C. Kerr (Eds.). *Contemporary issues in Canadian law for nurses* (pp. 63–82). Toronto: Holt, Rinehart & Winston of Canada.

Styles, M. M., & Affara, F. A. (1997). *ICN on regulation: Towards 21st century models.* Geneva: Author. Retrieved on May 132010, from http://www.icn.ch/images/stories/documents/publications/fact_sheets/ 1a_FS-Credentialing.pdf1997.

Wilensky, H. L. (1964). The professionalization of everyone. *American Journal of Sociology, 70*(2), 143–144.

Yukon Registered Nurses Association. (2008). *Nursing practice—registration.* Retrieved on April 1, 2008, from http://www.yrna.ca/nursingpractice/registration/indexreg.html.

21 The Growth of Graduate Education in Nursing in Canada

Marilynn J. Wood and Janet C. Ross-Kerr

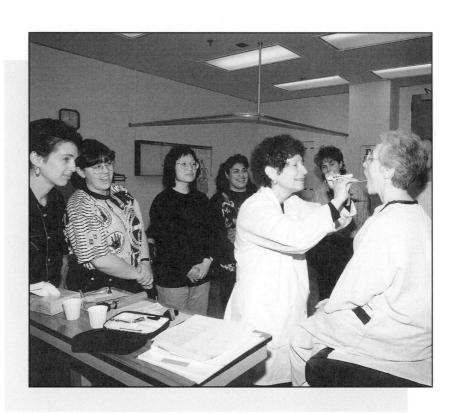

LEARNING OBJECTIVES

- To appreciate the development of graduate education in Canadian nursing over time.
- To understand the process of establishing master's degree programs in Canadian universities.
- To appreciate the growth over time of enrollment in master's programs.
- To describe the process of developing the faculty resources for graduate programs.
- To appreciate the process of preparing to undertake doctoral education.
- To understand the development of doctoral programs in Canada over time.
- To appreciate the growth of doctoral programs since the 1990s.
- To understand the need for postdoctoral programs to facilitate research development.

The first half-century of university education in nursing in Canada might be termed the "era of the undergraduate basic degree program." The development of graduate education has become an identifiable thrust in recent years, with achievement of improved access to master's degree programs (Figure 21.1). In 2009, doctoral programs in nursing were well established and growing, with 13 programs operating. Increased research activity in nursing has occurred as a result of a rapidly growing pool of nurses with preparation in research and the wider availability of funding for nursing research investigations. This development goes hand in hand with, and is a necessary condition for, establishment of graduate education in nursing. Most of the research in any field takes place in university settings, and teaching research methods are an important facet of graduate education. Approval of new programs by universities is unlikely to occur without evidence of substantial research activity and the doctoral degree as a standard qualification for faculty appointment.

THE ROOTS OF GRADUATE EDUCATION IN NURSING

Although the primary educational problems confronting the profession in the 1940s and 1950s centred on issues of quality in baccalaureate and diploma nursing education, the critical need for nursing leaders prepared at the master's and doctoral levels was recognized. In her study of the needs and resources for graduate nursing education in Canada, Hart (1962) observed that

> an increasing number of Canadian nurses recognized that graduate education was necessary to qualify for other specialized functions besides teaching. Canadian nurses had enrolled in programs leading to the master's degree to prepare for positions such as administration, supervision and consultation. Canadian nurses secured preparation for the specialized functions in nursing education as well as in nursing service in hospitals and health agencies. In spite of increasing demands for graduate education, by the time the study was undertaken there was still no provision for graduate study in nursing in Canada. (p. 51)

Hart (1962) concluded that the need to leave the country to pursue graduate study meant that relatively few Canadian nurses were qualified for leadership positions. Good (1969) concurred with this assessment ten years later: "Canadian nurses too have

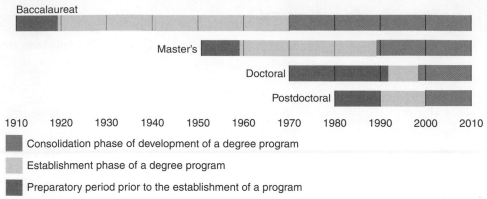

FIG 21.1 Chronology of the Growth and Development of University Degree Programs in Nursing in Canada.

followed the pattern of study abroad for graduate education. The country of focus was, and still is, the United States of America" (pp. 3–4).

The Canadian Nurses Association (CNA) was in the forefront of developments and strongly supported the call for graduate programs in nursing. Its Committee on Nursing Affairs reported to the 31st Biennial Convention in 1962:

> *We should promote immediately an assessment of present facilities, both university and clinical, in order to ascertain what is needed by way of the expansion of university nursing education. . . . On the principle that one can never go wrong with an investment in human beings, a crash program for the development of qualified faculty for Canadian schools of nursing should be undertaken by CNA. . . . CNA might also interest itself in giving some leadership to the development of graduate programs in nursing education, especially in terms of the pooling of university resources in particular specialties (CNA, 1962, pp. 23–25).*

The Committee on Nursing Education also made the following recommendations:

- Programs in nursing at the baccalaureate level should be expanded.
- The director of the school of nursing should be a nurse with preparation at a master's level and should have the necessary qualifications to assume the responsibility for administration of the school.
- All nurses responsible for teaching nursing students should have professional and academic preparation at least at the baccalaureate level and have demonstrated professional competence.
- Programs should be developed at the master's and doctoral level to prepare nurses who will be qualified as nursing specialists and for administration, consultation, research, and teaching (CNA, 1962, p. 46).

Thus the focus of the profession was broadened to include graduate education as a necessary adjunct in the quest for quality in basic professional education.

As was the case when baccalaureate programs were in their incipient stages, the first thrust was to develop fellowship programs to prepare nurse faculty to take on the responsibilities associated with graduate education. Hart (1962) reported that in 1957

> *a few unrestricted scholarships and fellowships were found to be available for graduate study in Canadian colleges and universities. Some scholarships were available specifically for nurses and other members of the health professions. . . . If programs for graduate study were available in Canada, it is likely that students in the nursing field would utilize such scholarship and fellowship aid. (p. 47)*

However, the Kellogg Foundation fellowship program, which spanned two decades, provided a much needed source of funds for graduate students who had to incur the expenses associated with taking up residence in a foreign country to find appropriate educational opportunities at the graduate level (Table 21.1).

In 1962, the Canadian Nurses Foundation (CNF) was formed with the assistance of a grant of $136,639 from the W.K. Kellogg Foundation for the establishment of a fellowship program for study at the master's and doctoral levels and for research assistance for nurses. The CNF has completed its first mandate admirably. Between 1962 and 2002, a total of 755 graduate fellowships were awarded: 494 for study at the master's level and 261 for doctoral work. The total amount given for fellowship awards over this 40-year period of the fund was $3,004,109 (Table 21.2). It should be noted that the CNF has been very active in fundraising and that provincial and territorial professional associations have been regular and substantial donors, and many individuals, institutions, and businesses have contributed funds. Owing to problems in maintaining the size of the fund in the first decade of its existence, the Research Committee of the CNF "formulated plans for developing nursing research in Canada but unfortunately, due to lack of funds, these could not be implemented" (Imai, 1971, p. 90). The CNF later initiated a program of research grants. The first such grant was one given to the Canadian Association of University Schools of Nursing (CAUSN) for a research project on accreditation of university schools of nursing. With the establishment of the Ad Hoc Research Committee in 1983, the CNF Board of Directors initiated a program of research grants, which, although small, has been important in encouraging nurses to undertake research.

THE ESTABLISHMENT OF MASTER'S DEGREE PROGRAMS

The efforts of the University of Western Ontario (UWO) to develop a one-year diploma program in nursing service administration led to the establishment of a master's level program in that area, one that became the first graduate program in nursing in Canada (Overduin, 1970). In 1957, when the president of the university, Dr. G.E. Hall, applied for Kellogg funding to implement the diploma program that had received the approval of the university senate as early as 1956, he

TABLE 21.1	W.K. Kellogg Foundation Grants to Canadian University Schools of Nursing and Selected Other Agencies, 1940–1981		

ORGANIZATION	TYPE OF GRANT	DATE	AMOUNT OF GRANT ($)
Alberta			
University of Alberta, Edmonton	Fellowships in nursing	1949–1954	10,862
British Columbia			
University of British Columbia, Vancouver	To aid in establishing nursing education, curricula leading to RN licensure, baccalaureate, master's, and doctoral degrees		333,225
	Fellowships in nursing	1974–1977	18,032
Vancouver Metropolitan Health Department	Fellowships in nursing	1946	675
Manitoba			
University of Manitoba, Winnipeg	Fellowships in nursing	1941–1949	2,815
New Brunswick			
New Brunswick Association for Registered Nurses, Fredericton	Fellowships in nursing	1953	715
University of New Brunswick, Fredericton	To aid in establishing a degree program in basic nursing	1958–1965	198,857
	To help establish a program of continuing education in nursing	1958–1961	17,504
Ontario			
Canadian Nurses Association, Ottawa (for Province of Ontario)	Fellowships in nursing	1950	1,493
McMaster University, Hamilton	Fellowships in nursing	1948–1954	19,787
	To help establish a graduate education curriculum in nursing	1973–1978	290,935
Quebec			
McGill University	Development of a master's degree program for non-nurse graduates	1981	86,279

Source: Annual reports of the W.K. Kellogg Foundation, 1940–1978.

requested $100,000 from the Foundation . . . $50,000 of which was slated for the "intensive development" of the new DNSA program—the Foundation indicated its willingness to support the school of nursing in its educational efforts in nursing administration. It supported the development of a master's program in Canada, to be supported by the Foundation over a five-year period just as it had done earlier in American universities. (Overduin, 1970, p. 84)

| TABLE 21.2 | Canadian Nurses Foundation Fellowship Awards, 1962–2002 |

YEARS AWARDS GIVEN	NUMBER OF MASTER'S AWARDS	NUMBER OF DOCTORAL AWARDS	TOTAL AMOUNT AWARDED ($)
1962–1963	9	1	11,700
1963–1964	12	-	31,000
1964–1965	8	3	35,700
1965–1966	6	2	27,250
1966–1967	11	3	37,175
1967–1968	11	2	36,700
1968–1969	15	2	52,550
1969–1970	16	1	42,100
1970–1971	14	5	56,537
1971–1972	11	2	32,500
1972–1973	12	2	36,200
1973–1974	9	1	31,000
1974–1975	3	1	13,500
1975–1976	5	1	17,900
1976–1977	8	0	21,900
1977–1978	12	2	35,500
1978–1979	12	2	37,800
1979–1980	9	4	61,500
1980–1981	5	5	34,000
1981–1982	4	3	15,000
1982–1983	15	6	37,208
1983–1984	12	5	37,700
1984–1985	9	6	32,500
1985–1986	9	2	36,000
1986–1987	7	5	44,000
1987–1988	6	6	45,000
1988–1989	8	9	65,000
1989–1990	17	14	122,000
1990–1991	18	14	126,000
1991–1992	14	17	129,340
1992–1993	15	15	124,500
1993–1994	17	14	128,000
1995–1996	26	16	177,799*
1996–1997	25	11	151,800*
1997–1998	25	13	161,800*
1998–1999	21	16	156,300*
1999–2000	24	18	255,300* **
2000–2001	12	22	270,850* **
2001–2002	22	10	235,500* **
Total	494	261	3,004,109

Sources: Personal communication with Eileen Mountain, assistant to the secretary-treasurer, Canadian Nurses Foundation, April 21, 1978; Bette Anne Smith, assistant to the secretary-treasurer, Canadian Nurses Foundation, April 23, May 15, 1987; Bev Campbell, executive director, Canadian Nurses Foundation, March 4, 1994; and Gaye Flower, scholarship coordinator, Canadian Nurses Foundation, June 27, 2002.
*total includes some baccalaureate awards
**total includes 2nd- or 3rd-year CHSRF funding to some candidates

A brief was prepared and submitted to the Kellogg Foundation.

[It] showed that Western met all the requirements set by the Foundation, described in detail the programs and courses offered by the school of nursing, and a projected budget for a five-year period indicating the cost of five major areas which would be supported by the Foundation: the master's program, and project of case-writing in administration, two fellowships per year to be granted during each year of the grant—each fellow to receive $2000 per year for each year of her two-year program, an annual seminar for senior nursing executives, and continuing education for faculty. (Overduin, 1970, p. 84)

Although it is reported that $142,000 was awarded by the foundation for the establishment of this program (Overduin, 1970; University of Western Ontario [UWO] School of Nursing, 1967–68), Kellogg records indicate that $128,618 was in fact expended between 1959 and 1965 "to help establish a program of graduate education in nursing service administration" (W.K. Kellogg Foundation; cited in Kerr, 1978, p. 261) (see Table 21.1). Planning for the implementation of the new program began in March 1959, and "on October 30, 1959, the Senate approved the first year of the program, and the entrance requirements" (Overduin, 1970, p. 85). Of note was the recognition that "the great need for research, especially research in appraising nursing care and service, was instrumental in the decision that a student would be required to produce a thesis" (Overduin, 1970, p. 85).

At McGill University, much progress had occurred since 1944, when the baccalaureate degree program was established. The transition to the integrated program occurred in 1957. However, planning for a master's level program began even earlier:

Research in nursing at McGill had been urged in Miss Green's report of 1953. The following year students in the second year degree programme undertook small research projects under the direction of staff members. Miss Chittick began to press for the creation of a Master's programme in nursing at the School for Graduate Nurses. (Tunis, 1966, p. 11)

After a resolution was passed at the 1958 CNA convention expressing the need for opportunities for graduate study in nursing in Canadian universities, "at McGill a two-year program leading to a degree of M.Sc. (Applied) was drawn up for approval by the Faculty of Graduate Studies and Research" (Tunis, 1966, p. 112). Senate approval, in principle, was received in September 1959, and again the Kellogg Foundation provided financial support to make the program plans operational with a grant of $195,000 over five years (Tunis, 1966). This brought the total amount of Kellogg Foundation assistance to McGill for the development of curricula to $221,252 between 1946 and 1967 (see Tables 21.1 and 21.3). Once again in the vanguard of developments in university nursing education in Canada, the W.K. Kellogg Foundation expressed its rationale for the assistance. "Graduate programs in Canadian universities are greatly needed. Better teachers of nursing produce better practitioners and, hence, improve patient care" (W.K. Kellogg Foundation, 1966, p. 56).

There was a considerable lapse of time after the early activity in the establishment of master's programs at the UWO and McGill University sponsored by the Kellogg Foundation grants. However, demonstrations had begun, and it was up to the institutions

TABLE 21.3	Kellogg Foundation Support (in Dollars) for Development of Master's Degree Programs in Nursing in Canada*						
YEAR	UNIVERSITY OF BRITISH COLUMBIA	UNIVERSITY OF WESTERN ONTARIO	MCMASTER UNIVERSITY	UNIVER- SITY OF TORONTO	MCGILL UNIVER- SITY	CNA	TOTAL
1959		19,233					19,233
1960		24,453					24,453
1961		25,406			48,159		73,565
1962		24,427			22,812	13,920	61,159
1963		25,948			28,209	27,717	81,874
1964		17,985			26,672	27,837	72,494
1965					14,567	69,668	84,235
1966					21,425		21,425
1967					18,499		18,499
1968				34,852			34,852
1969				28,159			28,159
1970							0
1971				72,006			72,006
1972				28,968			28,968
1973			135,143				135,143
1974	76,838		79,798	8,738			165,374
1975	131,316			75,436			206,752
1976	84,337		46,984				131,321
1977	40,734		20,936		108,797		170,467
1978			8,074		111,673		119,747
1979					159,884		159,884
1980					186,586		186,586
1981					23,830		23,830
1982							0
Total	333 225	137,452	290,935	248,159	771,113	139,142	1,920,026

*Since 1982 no grants have been made for Canadian health projects, as new guidelines have restricted grants outside the United States to Latin America and southern Africa only.
Source: Annual Reports of the W.K. Kellogg Foundation, 1959–1982.

to obtain their own resources if they wished to initiate graduate programs in nursing. Given the historical reluctance of universities to approve the development of new and costly graduate programs requiring ongoing and increasing operating expenditures, it is not surprising, particularly in the absence of financial inducements, that five years passed before another program was established. The year 1966 witnessed the inception of the graduate program at l'Université de Montréal, the first master's program in the French language in the world, and in 1968 a program was developed at the University of British Columbia (Good, 1971).

The W.K. Kellogg Foundation again offered support for development in master's programs with an award of $178,000 to the Faculty of Nursing at the University of Toronto "to establish a graduate program to prepare clinical nurse specialists" (W.K. Kellogg

Foundation, 1971, p. 28). In her annual report to the president, Dean Helen Carpenter (1970) describes the nature of the program in its first year of operation:

> The Master's Degree programme embodies specialization, mastery in depth of a specific area of knowledge, independent and critical study, and research. The purposes of the course are to make available advanced preparation for leadership roles in selected areas of nursing, and to advance nursing knowledge and skills through analytical study and investigation. Opportunity is provided for the students to acquire knowledge from nursing and the related sciences to provide the rationale for the management of complex health problems. (p. 74)

Another indication of interest in innovative developments in nursing curricula in Canada is the foundation support, granted in 1973 for a five-year period, to the School of Nursing at McMaster University for an "interdisciplinary graduate program to prepare clinical nurse specialists in primary and ambulatory care" (W.K. Kellogg Foundation, 1975, p. 19). This program award was for $290,196. An excerpt from the foundation's annual report (W.K. Kellogg Foundation, 1974) discusses the nature of this unique program:

> Foundation funds are helping the Division of Health Sciences of McMaster University, Hamilton, Ontario, develop an interdisciplinary graduate program to prepare nurses for advanced clinical practice in primary and ambulatory care. Students may choose clinical practice in maternal child health, family practice, or rehabilitation. Every attempt is made to include a true interdisciplinary experience, with members of several health professions learning together about issues in the delivery and management of health care. Nursing students will work with a physician preceptor during their clinical experience. The physician preceptor will also work with medical residents and will relate to both groups toward effective interdisciplinary clinical practice. (pp. 10–11)

Although the master's program at the University of Alberta, established in 1975, did not receive external funding, it derived substantial benefit from the development of the master's in Health Services Administration program in 1968. This program was initiated under the auspices of the Western Canadian Council on Education of Health Personnel, with a Kellogg Foundation grant of $212,250 for a five-year period (W.K. Kellogg Foundation, 1970). This program incorporated a stream for nursing administrators and paved the way for the 1975 development of the Master of Nursing program by providing for a joint appointment between the Division of Health Services Administration and the Faculty of Nursing and by developing a strong research thrust in the program. Both developments were assets to the Faculty of Nursing and facilitated the development of its master's program in 1975.

At the University of British Columbia (UBC), the initiation of the master's program took place initially without external funding. However, five years later, a large W.K. Kellogg Foundation grant was awarded to the School of Nursing "to aid in establishing nursing education curricula leading to registered nurse licensure, baccalaureate, master's and doctoral degrees" (W.K. Kellogg Foundation; cited in Kerr, 1978, p. 259) (see Table 21.1). Although the basic elements of such a ladder-system approach were developed before the termination of the grant in 1977, the doctoral part of the program was not established during the five-year time frame. Noteworthy, too, is the fact that UBC dropped the ladder concept before the end of the decade to concentrate on its basic and post-RN baccalaureate and master's programs. Another development in the availability of master's programs was the establishment of the first program in the Atlantic area at Dalhousie University in 1975.

Documentation of Kellogg Foundation support for the initiation of graduate programs on an annual basis between 1959 and 1982 provides a clear picture of financial resources expended by the foundation in the first phase in the development of graduate education in nursing in Canada (see Table 21.1). The resources, which were awarded to the CNA for the establishment of the CNF and are also included as CNF awards for graduate study, were a critical factor in the development of the faculty resources needed to offer graduate programs in Canada.

EXPANSION OF MASTER'S PROGRAMS IN NURSING

A great deal has occurred since the first master's programs were developed at the University of Western Ontario in 1959 and at McGill University in 1961 (see Table 21.4). The first programs offering study in clinical content areas were developed, beginning with

TABLE 21.4	Establishment of Master's Degree Programs in Nursing

INSTITUTION	DATE PROGRAM ESTABLISHED
Faculty of Nursing, University of Western Ontario	1959
School of Nursing, McGill University	1961
Faculté des sciences infirmières, l'Université de Montréal	1966
School of Nursing, University of British Columbia	1968
Faculty of Nursing, University of Toronto	1975
Faculty of Nursing, University of Alberta	1975
School of Nursing, Dalhousie University	1975
Faculty of Nursing, University of Manitoba	1979
Faculty of Nursing, University of Calgary	1981
School of Nursing, Memorial University of Newfoundland	1982
College of Nursing, University of Saskatchewan	1986
École des sciences infirmières, l'Université Laval	1991
School of Nursing, University of Ottawa	1993
School of Nursing, Queen's University	1994
School of Nursing, University of Windsor	1994
School of Nursing, McMaster University	1994
Faculty of Nursing, University of New Brunswick	1995
École des sciences infirmières, l'Université de Moncton	1998
Centre for Nursing and Health Studies, Athabasca University	2000
School of Nursing, Laurentian University	2003
Faculty of Health, York University	2004
Faculty of Community Services, Ryerson University	2004
Faculté de médecine et des sciences de la santé, Université de Sherbrooke	2005
l'Université du Québec à Chicoutimi, Outaouais, Rimouski and Trois-Rivières	2006

the program at l'Université de Montréal in 1966. The program at the University of British Columbia was begun in 1968. In the 1970s, three more new master's programs were established at the University of Toronto (1970), Dalhousie University (1975), and the University of Alberta (1975). As the impact of the slow growth and retrenchment of the early 1970s began to subside, three new master's degree programs in nursing appeared. These were located at the University of Manitoba (1979), University of Calgary (1981), and Memorial University of Newfoundland (1982). In 1986, another new master's program was initiated in the west, at the University of Saskatchewan. Further developments in the evolution of master's degree programs in nursing occurred in the first half of the l'université of the 1990s, when programs were established at l'Université Laval (1991), the University of Ottawa (1993), the University of Windsor (1994), and at Queen's University (1994). In the latter part of the 1990s, new master's programs were implemented at the University of New Brunswick (1995) and at Université de Moncton (1998).

Several more new master's programs have been added in the early 2000s. These programs are now in place at York University, the University of Victoria, Athabasca University, l'Université de Sherbrooke, Ryerson University, and l'Université de Moncton. l'Université du Québec now has a joint master's program at four sites. These are l'Université du Québec en Outaouais, l'Université du Québec à Trois-Rivières, l'Université du Québec à Rimouski, and l'Université du Québec à Chicoutimi (C. St. Pierre, personal communication, 2007).

The above statistics do not include interdisciplinary programs in which nursing may be one discipline of several that offer a master's degree program. Such programs have existed for some time and include the University of Alberta's Master of Health Services Administration program and McMaster University's interdisciplinary Master of Health Sciences program.

ANALYSIS OF ENROLLMENT TRENDS IN MASTER'S PROGRAMS

Considerable growth has occurred in master's programs since 1959, when the total enrollment at the University of Western Ontario was two students (Overduin, 1970) or since the 1960–61 academic year, when the combined enrollment at the UWO and McGill University was 16. In the next five years, total enrollment grew by 56%. In the next five-year interval, three more programs were established, and there was an increase of 675 in total enrollment (see Table 21.5). During this time, programs that offered study in a clinical content area were developed, beginning with the program at l'Université de Montréal in 1966. An analysis of early trends in the development of graduate education in nursing prompted one author to speculate on the reasons that Canadian nurses were still travelling to the United States for graduate study instead of enrolling in the new Canadian programs:

1. Historical precedent
2. More and better-qualified nurse faculty
3. Greater variety in programming

TABLE 21.5	Enrollment Changes in Master's Programs in Canadian Universities from 1965–1966 to 2006–2007

YEAR	TOTAL ENROLLMENT	PERCENTAGE CHANGE IN ENROLLMENT FROM YEAR TO YEAR
1965–1966	37	Base Year
1966–1967	51	28
1967–1968	56	9
1968–1969	79	29
1969–1970	73	-8
1970–1971	112	35
1971–1972	151	26
1972–1973	159	5
1973–1974	172	8
1974–1975	177	3
1975–1976	203	13
1976–1977	244	17
1977–1978	278	12
1978–1979	263	-6
1979–1980	304	13
1980–1981	345	12
1981–1982	381	9
1982–1983	381	0
1983–1984	526	28
1984–1985	524	0
1985–1986	699	25
1986–1987	632	-9.6
1987–1988	729	13.3
1988–1989	674	-7.6
1989–1990	783	13.9
1990–1991	847	7.6
1991–1992	829	-.02
1992–1993	904	6.3
1993–1994	784	-13.3
1994–1995	860	9.7
1995–1996	936	8.8
1996–1997	1,052	12.4
1997–1998	1,182	10.9
1998–1999	1,204	13.1
1999–2000	1,362	1.3
2000–2001	1,159	-14.9
2001–2002	1,802	55.4
2002–2003	1,706	-5.3
2003–2004	2,494	46.2
2004–2005	2,476	-.07
2005–2006	2,706	.09
2006–2007	2,981	10

Notes:
1. Prior to 1991, data collected were from January to December.
2. 1991 data were collected for the period ending July 1991.
3. 1992 data were collected for the period January to December 31, 1992.
4. Totals include part-time and full-time students.
Source: From annual statistical collection on university nursing students and faculty profiles collected by the Canadian Association for University Schools of Nursing and prepared by the Canadian Nurses Association, 1975–2000. From the CASN Student and Faculty Survey data: 2000–2004, 2004–2005, and 2006–2007.

At that time, US universities offered advanced study in five to eight clinical content areas, as well as in the functional specialties, whereas only one Canadian master's program offered study in a clinical area; the majority offered functional specialization (Good, 1969, p. 7).

Also interesting are enrollment trends since 1965. Erratic changes characterize the first five-year period, probably because of the smaller aggregate numbers on which the calculations are based, and because of the beginnings of retrenchment, as growth was replaced by shortfalls in enrollments nationally. The year 1969–70, when four programs were operational, was the only one of the decade in which there was a decrease in enrollment over the previous year. The next year saw a 35% increase, and a 26% increase occurred in 1971–72. In the period between 1970 and 1976, three more new master's programs were initiated, and total enrollment grew by 47%. For the academic years from 1971 through 1975, enrollment increases were lower, ranging from 3 to 8%, representing a slow but steady increase in student numbers and increased access to programs made possible by the addition of two programs after 1969–70. In 1975–76 there was a larger overall increase—about 13%—in the total enrollment figures. The new programs accounted for the larger percentage increase. Exponential increases occurred over the next decade with the addition of new programs and increases in the size of existing ones. By 1993, total enrollment in master's programs had reached 904, and by 1999–2000 there were 1,491 students enrolled in master's programs in Canada. Demand was apparent as more students applied for admission than could be accommodated in programs.

By 2005, the impact of the nurse practitioner programs can be seen as enrollments had increased sharply over the five years from 2000. New master's programs have been added, and most of these include a nurse practitioner option. Athabasca University, as an example, was one of the first to offer a nurse practitioner option that began as an Advanced Graduate Diploma in 1996, and in 2002 became an option in the Master of Nursing program.

In Ontario, a one-year program leading to certification as a Primary Health Care nurse practitioner became available to registered nurses in the early 2000s. The Ontario government funded the program through 2004. Education for the practitioner role was provided by a consortium of 10 Ontario universities. The program does not lead to an advanced degree, but rather a certificate enabling advanced practice. The curriculum was developed collaboratively by the consortium of participating schools. Over the years since this program began, the majority of Ontario university nursing schools have added a nurse practitioner option to their master's degree programs. This has led to a marked increase in enrollments in master's programs in Ontario and also to the development of several new master's programs.

In Quebec, the province requires 75 credits of master's level coursework for designation as a nurse practitioner. Programs are currently in operation at McGill, Laval, and Montreal, with Sherbrooke, Outaouais, Chicoutimi, Rimouski, and Trois-Rivières opening programs in the fall of 2008.

At the present time, the majority of Canadian master's programs in nursing offer a nurse-practitioner option in addition to a traditional thesis program. These programs vary greatly in their focus and intensity, but they represent a national movement toward advanced practice at the master's level.

ANALYSIS OF ENROLLMENT TRENDS IN DOCTORAL PROGRAMS

With the establishment of the first doctoral program in nursing at the University of Alberta on January 1, 1991, followed in September 1991 by the implementation of a second program at the University of British Columbia, nursing students no longer had to study in other disciplines or be admitted as special-case doctoral students in nursing. Programs at the University of Toronto and a joint program between McGill University and l'Université de Montréal were initiated in the fall of 1993, and a fifth program commenced at McMaster University in September 1994. The University of Calgary initiated a doctoral program in nursing in 1999, and Dalhousie University planned to begin a program in 2003. As doctoral programs have become established, enrollments have begun to climb. The first students were enrolled in doctoral programs in nursing between 1976 and 1988, and by 2000 enrollment across the country had reached 151. By 2005, there were 327 students registered in doctoral programs in nursing (see Table 21.6).

The number of Ph.D. programs has doubled since 2002, and now stands at 13. During the years from 1999 to 2005, there were 137 graduates with Ph.D. in Nursing degrees from Canadian universities. This is a significant number, yet is far from sufficient in being able to meet the need for faculty members across the country, and the need to strengthen the research base in nursing.

TABLE 21.6	Enrollment Changes in Doctoral Programs in Canadian Universities from 1987 to 2007		
YEAR	TOTAL ENROLLMENT	YEAR	TOTAL ENROLLMENT
1987–1988	2	1997–1998	112
1988–1989	6	1998–1999	146
1989–1990	6	1999–2000	174
1990–1991	8	2000–2001	125
1991–1992	8	2001–2002	161
1992–1993	18	2003–2004	271
1993–1994	35	2004–2005	327
1994–1995	48	2005–2006	390
1995–1996	62	2006–2007	358
1996–1997	97		

Notes:
1. Prior to 1991, data collected were from January to December.
2. 1991 data were collected for the period ending July 1991.
3. 1992 data were collected for the period January to December 31, 1992.
4. Totals include part-time and full-time students.

Source: From annual statistical collection on university nursing students and faculty profiles collected by the Canadian Association for Schools of Nursing (CASN) and prepared by the Canadian Nurses Association, 1975–2000 and available on the CASN Web site for 2000–2005, and the CNA Web site for 2005–2007.

REFLECTIVE THINKING

What would the outcome be for nursing if graduate education were not available in nursing and nurses continued to go to other disciplines (education, sociology, etc.) as they did in the past, for advanced degrees?

DEVELOPING THE FACULTY RESOURCES FOR GRADUATE PROGRAMS

The element that constitutes the most essential resource in successfully operating a graduate program is its faculty. Securing faculty members with the requisite skills to offer such a program is the most critical and difficult task. This was recognized earlier by Kathleen Russell (cited in Carpenter, 1970) as she laid the foundations of the basic baccalaureate degree program at the University of Toronto:

> *Among the criteria established for faculty positions were: the capacity for independent and creative thought and critical analysis, a broad concept of nursing, a university degree representing sound, general education in the humanities, and preparation for teaching. As nurses with these qualifications were difficult to find, fellowships were secured to assist those selected to undertake additional study and to broaden their understanding of nursing through travel and observation in other countries. (p. 93)*

Although skills such as creative thinking and critical analysis, complemented by a broad knowledge of nursing and research skills, can be learned in other than formal university settings, Stinson (1977) observed the following about the development of research skills: "One must consider the point that a great deal about research can be learned from participating in increasingly more complex projects" (p. 29). However, she also notes that "it is only in the rare instance that sound research preparation and high research productivity can occur in the absence of substantial amounts and kinds of formalized instruction" (Stinson, 1977, p. 29).

University nursing administrators have experienced difficulty in securing suitably qualified faculty for teaching in university programs. This was a major concern during the formative years in the establishment of baccalaureate programs, and there were times when schools were forced to operate with fewer staff than was desirable because of unfilled faculty positions. Supply and demand questions aside, there is still the leadership connection—that is, whether administrators of university schools were sufficiently perceptive and aggressive in recognizing the necessary skills and in encouraging their development in faculty members who showed promise.

Fellowship programs for faculty development have been available since the 1920s. In the early years, these were, for the most part, under the sponsorship of private foundations and were earmarked for faculty development. They were also often awarded directly to the institutions to offer to suitable candidates. However, in the late 1950s, public funds became available from federal sources administered through the provinces.

With the establishment of the CNF, fellowship funds for graduate study also became available from that source. Although they have been used to a great extent for faculty development, the new funds were not specifically earmarked for this purpose and have also been used for graduate preparation of nurses for practice, educational, and administrative settings.

The dearth of prepared faculty prompted Good (1969) to conclude that "the void in qualified nurse faculty in Canada has deterred development of Canadian graduate nurse education, and subsequent nursing research" (p. 8). The situation in 1960–61, shortly after master's programs were first initiated, was that among faculty teaching in university schools, 58% held baccalaureate degrees and 38% held master's degrees (Mussallem, 1965):

> *Although the academic qualifications of faculty in university schools of nursing are higher than those for hospital schools, it should be recognized that university instructors are teaching at the baccalaureate level and their preparation should be beyond that of their students. (p. 84)*

The situation changed slowly throughout the next decade as more master's programs became available, and by 1970–71, 1.43% of faculty in university programs held doctoral degrees, 44% held master's degrees, and 49% held baccalaureate degrees. In the five-year period ending in 1975–76, there was evidence of additional progress, as 3.74% held doctoral degrees, 31.28% held master's degrees, and 58.02% held the baccalaureate qualification (Statistics Canada, 1976). In 1980, Larsen and Stinson (1980) conducted a national survey to learn the number of nurses holding doctoral degrees. Of the 81 qualified at the doctoral level, 69% were employed in universities. A 1989 update of these statistics indicated that 257 held doctoral degrees; of these, 79% were employed in universities (Lamb & Stinson, 1990, p. 9). By the year 2000, the majority of faculty teaching in universities with graduate programs held doctoral degrees. This continues to be the case in 2009.

PREPARING TO ESTABLISH DOCTORAL PROGRAMS IN NURSING

In 1975, at the Fourth National Nursing Research Conference held in Edmonton, Alberta, a group of participants interested in facilitating the establishment of doctoral programs in the country held an informal meeting to discuss how this might be accomplished. Other discussions were held at national nursing meetings, and in 1976, a resolution was passed at the CNA Biennial Convention directing the association to provide leadership in the quest to establish doctoral education in Canada. Through a joint initiative of the CNA, CNF, and CAUSN, a national seminar on doctoral education in nursing was convened in 1978. The W.K. Kellogg Foundation provided funding for the seminar, which brought together deans and directors of university schools of nursing and deans of graduate studies at those institutions to consider issues in planning for the establishment of doctoral education in Canada. The meeting produced a commitment to establishing one or more Ph.D. programs in nursing (Zilm, Larose, & Stinson, 1979).

This was the first public recognition of the need to develop one or more programs in this country. As had happened when access to baccalaureate and later master's programs was limited, Canadian nurses emigrated to the United States to take advantage of the educational programs there. Some never returned to Canada, as they were offered attractive positions in the United States.

Another initiative at the national level was the establishment of the Working Group on Nursing Research in 1982 by the Medical Research Council (MRC). This occurred as the result of efforts by the CNA to document the low level of nursing research funding provided by the national granting councils. Although the smallest funding body, the National Health Research and Development Program (NHRDP), provided limited funding, funds were not specifically designated for nursing; many other disciplines depended on NHRDP for the major share of their funding. Also, although both the MRC and the Social Sciences and Humanities Research Council (SSHRC) stated that nursing was included among the disciplines that could be funded, nurses had difficulty getting either council to review nursing proposals. Consequently, few nursing proposals had been funded by either body. The Working Group was created to address these difficulties. Final recommendations in the Report of the Working Group in 1985 addressed the need to assist in creating opportunities for the establishment of doctoral nursing programs. Also addressed was the need to designate nursing research for funding within the Medical Research Council (MRC, 1985).

A special initiative to develop nursing research was established in 1988 jointly by the MRC and the Nursing Health Research Development Program (NHRDP), using the model developed for medicine and science, in which career funding is provided to outstanding candidates with proven track records. These funded scientists are then expected to develop others within their research programs. Unfortunately, there were too few outstanding candidates who could be funded under this system; in many of the smaller universities, there were none. Nursing faculty members, with the exception of a few unique individuals, had not developed the necessary track records to qualify. Many reasons can be cited for this situation: heavy teaching loads, lack of access to research funding, and an emphasis on service and teaching within faculties across the country, to name a few. The first round of this joint program resulted in funding of six individuals spread across the country. Members of the nursing profession were outraged at this outcome, believing it was merely a token effort at assisting with the development of research capacity in nursing.

A second round of this competition was held in 1989, but the result was more meagre than the first, as only three institutions received funding. The NHRDP/MRC program was then suspended for an evaluation, which took nearly three years to complete. When the results were reviewed at the MRC and the NHRDP, it was decided to hold one last round of the competition. This last round received significantly better proposals than did the first rounds, according to members of the review committee. It appears that the impact of the funding of those first scientists and scholars had created a new beginning for nursing research in Canada. Looking back from the vantage point of 2009, this effort on the part of the major funding agencies to build research capacity in nursing was quite successful.

The broadening of the mandate of the MRC to include health research in 1994 was an initiative that they had struggled with for many years. The exclusive focus of MRC on biomedical research had excluded many disciplines involved in health research, including nursing. Nursing research was clearly included as eligible for funding under this broadened mandate. This and the development of the Canadian Institutes of Health Research in 1999 completely changed the picture for nursing research in Canada.

Today, the picture for nursing research is vastly different than it was ten years ago. Efforts by the Canadian Nurses Association to secure targeted funding for nursing research were largely unsuccessful, as nursing was put under the umbrella of health services research. Although nursing competes on a level field with other disciplines for these funds, it is often difficult to secure grants for clinical nursing research that may not meet the criteria for clinical trials. However, there have been significant gains in funding for nursing research in a few centres (see Chapter 9).

THE ESTABLISHMENT OF DOCTORAL PROGRAMS

After the Kellogg National Seminar in 1978, McGill University and l'Université de Montréal prepared a joint submission for a cooperative, bilingual Ph.D. program, but several factors prevented its approval when it was proposed in 1980. The University of Toronto developed an arrangement with the Institute of Medicine whereby nurses could be admitted to the Ph.D. program offered by that unit to pursue studies in nursing. This arrangement included some Faculty of Nursing input in the program and allowed nurses to take a program more closely related to their own discipline.

In 1980, the Council of the Faculty of Nursing of the University of Alberta approved the development of a proposal for a Ph.D. program. Consequently, a proposal was developed and approved by that Faculty Council by 1985 and was approved by the Board of Governors of the university in 1986. The program was funded by the Alberta government on January 1, 1991, which allowed the admission of students to the first Ph.D. program in nursing in Canada (see Table 21.7).

A second doctoral program in nursing was implemented at the University of British Columbia in September 1991. Two additional programs began in the fall of 1993 at the University of Toronto and a joint program at McGill University and l'Université de Montréal. In the fall of 1994, a fifth program got under way at McMaster University, and in 1998 a program was implemented at the University of Calgary. Dalhousie University began a doctoral program in 2003, which brought the total number to seven programs. Since 2003, doctoral programs have been initiated by five more universities: the University of Victoria, the University of Western Ontario, the University of Ottawa, l'Université Laval, l'Université de Sherbrooke, and Dalhousie University.

In the late 1990s, a number of special-case students had been admitted to McGill University and the University of Alberta prior to the funding of bona fide Ph.D. programs. The first graduate to receive a Ph.D. in nursing from a Canadian university was a special-case student, Francine Ducharme, from McGill, who graduated in the fall of 1990. In the early 2000s, the School of Nursing at the University of Victoria offered a "Ph.D. by

TABLE 21.7	First Doctoral Programs in Nursing in Canada: Historical Overview	
INSTITUTION	DATE PROGRAM ACCEPTED FIRST STUDENTS	PRECEDED BY A SPECIAL CASE ARRANGEMENT
Faculty of Nursing, University of Alberta	January 1, 1991	Yes
School of Nursing, Faculty of Applied Sciences, University of British Columbia	September 1, 1991	No
Faculty of Nursing, University of Toronto*	September 1, 1993	No*
School of Nursing, Faculty of Medicine, McGill University/Faculté des sciences infirmières, l'Université de Montréal	September 1, 1993	Yes
School of Nursing, Faculty of Health Sciences, McMaster University	September 1, 1994	No
Faculty of Nursing, University of Calgary	September 1, 1998	No

*The Faculty of Nursing at the University of Toronto had some involvement in a doctoral program established in the Institute of Medicine. Prior to the establishment of their own nursing program, a number of University of Toronto nurses enrolled in and graduated from the institute's program.

Special Arrangement," an individualized Ph.D. program of studies similar to the special-case arrangements developed in other universities, including McGill and Alberta, prior to the establishment of their Ph.D. in Nursing programs (School of Nursing, University of Victoria, 1995). This program has now been implemented by the University of Victoria as a Ph.D. in Nursing program. Doctoral education has become much more accessible to nurses in Canada since the inception of the first program. Research in nursing is likely to continue to grow with the preparation of doctoral candidates having expertise in research.

The purpose of doctoral education is to prepare scholars and scientists who will develop knowledge for their discipline. In nursing, this knowledge provides the basis for practice and is therefore inextricably entwined with practice. It also informs health policy and provides the basis for educating future nurses. To be able to contribute at this level, students must have a good grasp of the discipline of nursing: its history, philosophy, research, and practice.

US doctoral programs have been around for about 100 years and underwent enormous expansion in the 1970s and 1980s. There are currently more than 80 universities with doctoral nursing programs in the United States. Most programs require a minimum of 30 credits of course work, followed by a supervised research project. The model they have developed has most courses being required for all students, with some flexibility in elective courses to meet students' individual interests and needs. Students typically do not require a faculty supervisor until their course work is completed and they are ready to begin the research. This model has the advantage of being able to accommodate large numbers of students taking course work and the disadvantage of postponing socialization of students into research roles until they are well into their course of study.

In Canada, there was a deliberate effort to provide a more research-intensive experience for doctoral students. The Canadian programs are remarkably similar in their goals, and all provide a major emphasis on research training, using at least to some extent the apprenticeship model. There is a continuum of flexibility in course requirements, varying from none to 18 credits. In most programs, students are assigned to a faculty supervisor upon admission, and a program of study is approved by the supervisor or, in some cases, a supervisory committee. The intent is for the course requirements to be individualized to meet that student's needs and to support the research the student will be doing.

From the standpoint of research training, the apprenticeship model is still unsurpassed. Students should expect to be involved in their faculty supervisor's research program. The more deeply students are involved with ongoing research, the better their socialization into research and scholarship will be, and the better prepared they will be to launch an academic career upon graduation.

CANADIAN RESEARCH FOCUS

Acorn, S., Lamarche, K., & Edwards, M. (2009). Practice doctorates in nursing: Developing nursing leaders. *Canadian Journal of Nursing Leadership, 22*(2), 85–91.

Shenke, J. (2006, October 30). Nursing doctorate programs changing the face of health care, US. *Medical News Today.* Retrieved on November 2, 2006, from http://www.medicalnewstoday.com/medicalnews.php?newsid=55298.

American universities and colleges are expanding the number of programs offering doctoral degrees in nursing practice (Shenke, 2006). The focus in the US is on improving patient safety concerns in areas such as

- Clinical research in antibiotic practice, to reduce postoperative infections
- Electronic health records linked to nurse-managed clinics, to improve access and continuity of care
- Preparing community clinics to respond to natural disasters or pandemics as well as terrorist attacks

This movement by American nurses, as well as similar movements in Australia and the United Kingdom, has led to discussion and debate in Canada as to whether doctoral degrees in nursing practice should be offered by Canadian universities.

In Canada, the only doctoral degree available at the present time is the Ph.D., which focuses on training for a career in research. The doctorate in nursing practice (DNP) focuses on the preparation of leaders for clinical practice, health policy, and clinical research. Acorn, Lamarche, and Edwards (2009) advocate the development of both Ph.D. and DNP degrees in Canada to advance nursing knowledge and provide leadership in health care. They argue that individuals whose goals are to undergo education aimed at providing leadership in nursing and health care must currently take positions in Ph.D. programs whose primary focus is on research training. Opponents to the DNP are concerned that practice doctorates will reduce enrolments in Ph.D. programs and weaken the research mandate of the profession because of limited resources available to support graduate education in nursing. This is an ongoing debate.

POSTDOCTORAL EDUCATION IN NURSING

Postdoctoral education in nursing is still relatively new, although this form of socialization to the academic world has been common in other disciplines for decades. The Canadian Institutes of Health Research agency offers postdoctoral fellowships to students whose research falls under the mandate of one of the institutes. The Social Sciences and Humanities Research Council also offers postdoctoral fellowships. The Canadian Nurses Foundation offers postdoctoral fellowships, as does the Canadian Council of Cardiovascular Nurses. In addition, there are postdoctoral funds available within the regional training centres.

Postdoctoral fellowships provide Ph.D. graduates with the opportunity to develop their research programs beyond the completion of the dissertation research. Typically, a new Ph.D. graduate will submit an application outlining a proposed research agenda for one to three years under the supervision of an established researcher. Candidates are encouraged to seek opportunities in settings other than the one in which they studied for the Ph.D. to expand their opportunities into a new intellectual environment. Funding for a "post-doc" allows the new graduate to continue research development activities prior to assuming the full responsibilities of an academic appointment. Although postdoctoral funding covers research activities, no regular teaching activities are allowed during this time.

Those who aspire to work as career scientists in research will find that postdoctoral funding is essential. These individuals will use their fellowship time to present and publish the results of their doctoral dissertations and to undertake new research activities, as well as to acquire grants for the next phase of their research. These are the essential components of a career scientist application, which would be the next step.

Postdoctoral educational opportunities in nursing are essential if graduates of the new doctoral nursing programs are to have an opportunity to develop ongoing research programs as they take up academic appointments in universities. Experience has shown that new Ph.D. graduates require support from more experienced researchers, as well as the time to plan their research and to submit research proposals to funding agencies. If they have the opportunity to work on a collegial basis with established researchers, they are much more likely to be successful when they take up their appointments in faculties and schools of nursing. Given the time and resources that have been invested in the brightest and the best, it would seem worthwhile to set up neophyte researchers for success.

CRITICAL THINKING QUESTIONS

1. Why do you think graduate education is important to nursing?
2. The difficulty encountered by university schools in establishing doctoral programs in nursing might be similar to difficulties encountered by the pioneers in other professions. What might these be, and how were they similar to or different from those in other professions?

WEB SITES

Canadian Association of Schools of Nursing: www.casn.ca
Canadian Nurses Association: www.nurses-cna.ca

REFERENCES

Canadian Nurses Association. (1962). *Folio of reports 1962*. Ottawa: Author.

Carpenter, H. M. (1970). The University of Toronto School of Nursing: An agent of change. In M. Q. Innes (Ed.), *Nursing education in a changing society* (pp. 86–108). Toronto: University of Toronto Press.

Good, S. R. (1969). *Submission to the study of support of research in universities for the Science Secretariat of the Privy Council*. Ottawa: Canadian Nurses Association and Canadian Nurses Foundation.

Good, S. R. (1971). *Submission to the Association of Universities and Colleges of Canada*. Calgary: University of Calgary.

Hart, M. E. (1962). *Needs and resources for graduate education in nursing in Canada*. Unpublished doctoral dissertation. New York: Teacher's College, Columbia University.

Imai, H. R. (1971). Professional associations and research activities in nursing in Canada. In *National Conference on Research in Nursing Practice*. Vancouver, School of Nursing: University of British Columbia.

Kerr, J. C. (1978). *Financing university nursing education in Canada: 1919–1976*. Unpublished Ph.D. dissertation. Ann Arbor, MI: University of Michigan.

Lamb, M., & Stinson, S. M. (1990). *Canadian nursing doctoral statistics: 1989 update*. Ottawa: Canadian Nurses Association.

Larsen, J., & Stinson, S. M. (1980). *Canadian nursing doctoral statistics*. Ottawa: Canadian Nurses Association.

Medical Research Council of Canada. (1985). *Report to the Medical Research Council of Canada by the Working Group on Nursing Research*. Ottawa: Author.

Mussallem, H. K. (1965). *Nursing education in Canada*. Ottawa: Queen's Printer.

Overduin, H. (1970). *People and ideas: Nursing at Western 1920–1970*. London, ON: University of Western Ontario

School of Nursing, University of Victoria. (1995). *PhD by special arrangement: Brochure (pp. 1–5)*. Victoria, BC: Author

Statistics Canada. (1976). *Nursing in Canada: Canadian nursing statistics, 1976*. Ottawa: Author.

Stinson, S. M. (1977). Central issues in Canadian nursing research. In B. LaSor, & M. R. Elliott (Eds.), *Issues in Canadian nursing* (pp. 3–42). Toronto: Prentice-Hall Canada.

Tunis, B. (1966). *In caps and gowns*. Montreal: McGill University Press.

University of Western Ontario. (1967–68). Calendar. London, ON: Author.

W. K. Kellogg Foundation. (1966; 1970; 1971; 1974; 1975). *Annual Report*. Battle Creek, MI: Author.

Zilm, G., Larose, O., & Stinson, S. (1979). *PhD (nursing)*. Ottawa: Canadian Nurses Association.

22

Career Development in Nursing

Marilynn J. Wood and Janet C. Ross-Kerr

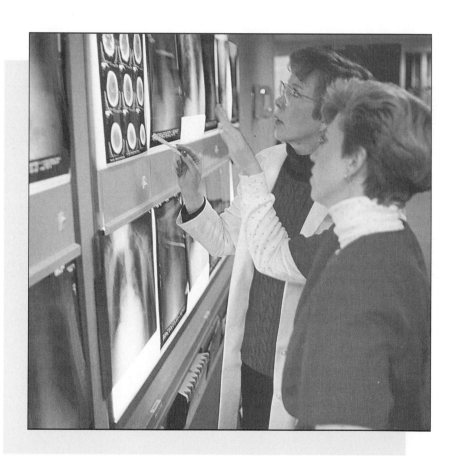

LEARNING OBJECTIVES

- To describe the clinical roles of Advanced Nurse Practitioners and Clinical Nurse Specialists.
- To identify how you would organize a job search indicating its component parts.
- To explain what should be taken into consideration in preparing for an interview with a prospective employer.
- To delineate the various types of research opportunities for nurses at various levels of education.
- To describe the activities aspiring nurse researchers need to undertake to succeed in building a research track record.
- To explain how an individual desiring graduate preparation would go about selecting a graduate program in nursing.

Although nursing was one of the first professions to open up to women in the nineteenth century, historical factors have intervened to hinder the view of nursing as a bona fide career for women. Looming large among these factors has been a paternalistic view of nursing as women's work and gender stereotypes relative to women's roles in society. In the meantime, nursing has been seen as a desirable career attracting not only women, but also an increasing number of men to its ranks. Nurses have taken on a wide range of roles both within the profession and in the larger health care field as advance practice nurses, managers, directors, vice-presidents, and presidents. Many have moved through their careers easily and without conscious planning to assess their abilities, determine their goals, and identify strategic directions to reach their goals. Increasingly, nurses are being encouraged to take the time to look at some of these issues and to become involved in thinking about their careers and how they would like their career paths to unfold. Donner and Wheeler (2009) have identified a career planning and development model that identifies the kinds of activities that can be undertaken to rationalize career planning and help the individual to take appropriate directions in the future.

There are unlimited opportunities in the profession for nurses who are entering practice. Despite cycles of downsizing followed by nursing shortages, there continue to be opportunities for those who have the right skill set and are eager to learn and explore new roles. The current environment fosters expansion of nursing roles and restructuring of traditional roles and responsibilities of all the health care professions.

Most nurses enter the profession because they want to provide nursing services to the public. Some will be satisfied to continue to hold staff nursing positions in a health care or other agency for the duration of their careers and may not look for advancement. However, whether or not one seeks career advancement, maintaining one's skills and furthering one's knowledge are essential to every nurse's success and should be part of a career plan. Opportunities for advancement in clinical practice include the positions of advanced practitioner, nurse practitioner, clinical specialist, and clinical educator. All involve graduate education and a specific area of specialization.

An awareness of the issues involved in career advancement, including selecting a graduate program and searching for a suitable position, will help nurses take the risks and make the professional transitions necessary to a successful career. Aside from an individual's aspirations, it is important to understand the processes involved in making sound decisions in relation to career opportunities.

BUILDING A CLINICAL PRACTICE CAREER: PATHWAY TO SUCCESS

A career in clinical practice is one of the most rewarding paths a nurse can take. Opportunities are in abundance, as health care and nursing have so many facets to be explored. Nurses who elect to build their careers in the practice arena must become expert practitioners over time. Career options in nursing require planning and preparation, since choices often involve narrowing the focus from general practice into a more specialized role. There have been efforts in the past to develop tools to help nurses assess their interests and skills in order to make good choices in their career progression. One such tool was the Nursing Career Preference Inventory (Hefferin and Kleinknecht, 1986). Unfortunately, this tool has not been updated, and no others could be found to take its place in the current nursing context. Nurses must depend on advice from mentors and their own practice experience to help them make appropriate career choices (Block, Claffey, Korow, & McCaffrey, 2005).

The two major categories of nurses in advanced clinical roles are Advanced Nurse Practitioners and Clinical Nurse Specialists (CNS). Both of these roles will enable nurses to spend their careers directly helping clients to improve their health and quality of life, as well as assisting clients to deal with threats to their health and well-being.

According to the Canadian Nurses Association (CNA), Advanced Nursing Practice (ANP) is an umbrella term, describing an advanced level of nursing practice requiring in-depth nursing knowledge and skill to meet the health needs of patients. These two roles (CNS and ANP) evolved from different perspectives and were influenced by different factors. The CNS role arose to meet institutional needs for support of nurses involved in managing complex patients and improving quality of care. The ANP role, on the other hand, came out of the need for nurses to assume expanded roles in areas where medical care was lacking—that is, in rural and northern areas. This role was extended to meet the needs of patients and families in tertiary-care hospitals because of the reduction of medical residents, particularly in Ontario, during the 1980s to 1990s. However, this role is not established in all jurisdictions in Canada.

In 2005, the CNA organized a dialogue on ANP, in which nursing leaders, experts on Advanced Nursing Practice, and nurses in ANP roles participated. The dialogue resulted in the development of some recommendations related to ANP. These include the following:

- An important goal is to ensure that ANP roles are well integrated into the health care system in order to facilitate increased access to quality health care, reduced waiting times, and rapid responses to pandemics and other health emergencies.

- Pan-Canadian coordination in the health care field in the areas of human resource planning, education, and regulation is key to effectively introducing, developing, and sustaining ANP roles in Canada.
- Nurses must work collaboratively with other health care providers to ensure the best possible health services for Canadians.

The Clinical Nurse Specialist role has evolved into one requiring master's degree preparation in a clinical area of specialization. Nurses in these roles often serve as consultants to other nurses in the health care system to solve problems related to patients with complex health issues. The ANP, on the other hand, provides direct care to patients in their area of specialization. Regardless of the professional direction taken, every nurse will apply for a position of employment at some time. Here the needs are to understand the type of work for which one is qualified, to be able to engage in honest self-appraisal, and to be prepared to present oneself in the best possible light to a prospective employer. It is also essential, following an employment interview, to be able to critically analyze both employer expectations and the context of the prospective work environment. The "right" decision will be based on the suitability of the position to one's abilities and the likelihood of personal satisfaction in carrying out the responsibilities of the job. Further, the nurse must bear in mind that every position provides basic experience that will increase knowledge and understanding in a particular clinical area. Since every position is by nature career building, employment opportunities should be selected for their appropriateness in enhancing experience as well as their ability to advance the nurse within the profession.

CANADIAN RESEARCH FOCUS

Chambers, P. (2009). Designing the nursing career you want. *AAACN Viewpoint, 31*(2), 4–5.

This author has made an appeal to nurses to exert "personal leadership" in planning their nursing careers. Chambers cites studies of human behaviour and career planning and makes the point that career planning is about being accountable to oneself. Citing the need for personal honesty, she exhorts nurses to take time to dream, then assess their strengths, personality, and job preferences in order to make positive career decisions. The most important element in career development is that nurses should ensure they look for challenging professional work environments in order to avoid stress and possible burnout.

THE WORK SEARCH

In approaching the search for suitable employment, nurses must be able to recognize positions that will be a good fit with their interests, values, and skills. Beginning the job search well in advance enables one to build some knowledge of the range of positions available. This allows the nurse to apply for those positions that offer the best opportunities to use knowledge and skills, and will consequently result in a high level of job satisfaction. Students looking for an entry level position following graduation from a nursing program should begin many months before they expect to be available for work.

THE PLAN OF ACTION

Organization is often the key to success in looking for a position (Donner & Wheeler, 2009; Alberta Human Resources & Employment, 2002). At the outset, it is helpful to draw up an outline of what needs to be done and then proceed through this plan in a logical manner. The first step is to identify what is being sought in a work situation, and then to specify skills and aptitudes needed for such work. The work search should then focus on a particular type of position that will be congruent with the applicant's abilities and interests, sufficiently remunerative, and conveniently located.

Self-appraisal is a central part of the process. Those looking for challenging and satisfying positions should be honest with themselves in acknowledging what they like, and want, to do. Self-appraisal also includes honest and critical evaluation of one's level of knowledge and skills, such as technical skills and knowledge in a particular area; problem-solving, organizational, and communication skills; leadership skills; creativity; and personal qualities such as capacity for responsibility, attitude toward work, intrinsic motivation, flexibility, and so on. Student organizations offer an opportunity to learn through dialogue with other students at various levels throughout the local educational program as well as regionally and nationally. In nursing, the ability to work with people is extremely important, and thus skill in communicating with others and establishing rapport with patients will be of singular interest to prospective employers.

 REFLECTIVE THINKING

Identify one career goal of your own, and outline a strategy for moving toward achieving it.

THE RÉSUMÉ

At this point it is useful to develop a résumé that lists information such as the following:

- Personal data including name, address, telephone, and e-mail contact information
- Degrees and certificates obtained, along with colleges and universities attended, major areas of study, and awards or other recognition achieved
- Previous employment experience and contact information for previous employers; titles of positions held, responsibilities assumed, and ways in which the applicant demonstrated skills
- Volunteer experience, interests, or memberships in organizations related to the profession
- Other skills, such as ability to speak and read other languages
- Names of personal references, including those who have supervised or have a good knowledge of the applicant's work

One can present a résumé in a variety of formats: chronological, functional, or a blend of these two approaches. Each style of résumé has advantages and disadvantages. Since the functional type describes skills without reference to the situations in which they were gained, this approach may not be appropriate for all applications. It is probably better to use a chronological approach or one that includes features of both chronological and functional résumés.

Drafting the résumé is the next step. It should be kept as straightforward and clear as possible. While a lengthy résumé may be acceptable for academic positions, for clinical practice positions, one- or two-page résumés are recommended. It is a good idea to have one or two other individuals with excellent writing and editing skills read the résumé, and to read and edit it several times oneself. It is essential to avoid spelling or grammatical errors in presenting a résumé to a prospective employer. If an individual has one or more breaks in work history due to family responsibilities, these should be explained in the résumé.

If applying for a position by mail, the applicant should include a covering letter with the résumé. The letter should engage the attention of the employer, briefly present the applicant's skills and achievements, and provide information that is appropriate in relation to the position sought. The covering letter should reflect both the applicant's personality and qualifications for the position. A well thought-out and well-written résumé can go a long way toward impressing an employer.

INITIAL CONTACT

Work searches may require extensive research on positions available in the nurse's area of interest. Many people send out résumés in large numbers to prospective employers. It is not wise to send out résumés without having been invited to do so. It is better to make personal contact with a prospective employer by telephone initially, and then to send a résumé if invited to do so. In the covering letter, the applicant would remind the employer that the résumé was requested by the employer. The objective at this point is to gain an interview. A polite follow-up call a few days after sending the résumé is always in order to find out if it was received and to ask whether an invitation to interview for the position will be extended.

THE INTERVIEW

An interview is an opportunity for applicants to present themselves favourably to a prospective employer. Since applying for a position is competitive, there is an advantage in arriving well prepared. It is wise to find out in advance the names and positions in the organization of those who will conduct the interview. It is also a good idea to ask for a copy of the job description beforehand. Information on the organization may be gathered (via the Internet or other sources) to gain some understanding of the organization. Employers are often impressed with the initiative of applicants who have done some work to learn about the organization for which they hope to work. It is also important to explain any breaks in work history if these were the result of family responsibilities. If the interview is conducted by telephone, steps should be taken to ensure that the conversation will not be interrupted.

Applicants should anticipate the questions that interviewers might ask. Questions about strengths and weaknesses are common. Identifying these in advance will enable an applicant to discuss them confidently.

An interview is a two-way street: it presents an opportunity for an employer to learn about a prospective employee, and it also allows an applicant to learn about the organization and the specific position. Applicants should try to learn as much as possible about the employment situation. It is a good idea to decide in advance the information one hopes to obtain about a position and to come to the interview with prepared questions.

First impressions are important. Arriving for the interview about 20 minutes early is advisable. Appearance, communication skills, and politeness are qualities that the employer will be observing. It is permissible to ask, at the conclusion of the interview, about the selection process for the position, if the interviewer has not given this information.

Even when a position is not offered, an interview should be viewed as a learning experience. It is also important to learn to handle rejection. Often, a rejection can be turned to one's advantage by asking why the position was offered to the successful applicant. There are always areas for future improvement; carrying out a post-interview analysis of what went right and what went wrong can be very helpful. A positive attitude during a work search will help the applicant through what may seem a long and frustrating experience. The nurse needs to focus on the objective of finding a position that is exciting and rewarding and that will lead to future career opportunities.

MENTORING

An essential element in career development, mentoring is often an elusive experience that many people never find. A good mentor–mentee relationship is a rare happening, yet it is believed to be the one factor that ensures success for upwardly mobile professionals. It can smooth the pathway for novices and save them untold hours, weeks, and years of struggle.

A mentorship is a close relationship in which the new employee can ask any question and discuss any topic without censure. The mentor, who will be senior in the profession or organization to the mentee, facilitates the novice's entry into the system by explaining the expectations of the role and the intricacies of the culture. The mentor is a role model as well as a counsellor, modelling successful behaviours for the role to which the novice aspires.

Many talented people have built successful careers without the benefit of a mentor. People who are pioneers rarely have mentors, since by nature they are breaking new ground. However, most people will find progress made significantly easier through the mentoring process. Watson (2000) has analyzed support from mentors in clinical settings. His work represents one of the few studies that have been done on the subject of mentoring. However, the literature in this area is increasing, and Andrews and Wallis (1999) have published a review of relevant literature on mentoring in nursing.

True mentoring is considered by many to be an intangible relationship that cannot be orchestrated, but rather must happen spontaneously. This expectation increases the difficulty of promoting mentoring within an organization, since mentorship may not be subject to management strategies such as delegation or assignment. Nevertheless, even if true mentorship is elusive, parts of the mentoring relationship can be fostered and utilized within an organization to promote both the development of staff and the expectation that senior members of the community will mentor junior ones. Thus, mentorship can become part of the organizational culture.

Senior members can be asked by leaders in the organization to oversee the progress of junior members and to advise them about appropriate ways to succeed in the system. Junior members can seek out several senior people who can advise them about different aspects of the job. This gives the junior person a variety of alternatives to use in planning career advancement.

Whether a nurse aspires to a career in clinical practice, research, management, education, or another field, mentorship is one key to success. An organization that can capture this ideal and make it work will be well on the way to creating a positive and supportive workplace.

REFLECTIVE THINKING

What does mentoring mean to you? Identify a significant mentor(s) in your life.

BUILDING A RESEARCH CAREER: PATHWAY TO SUCCESS

A career in research is an exciting prospect. Imagine being at the centre of a team in which new ideas are generated, better ways of doing things are tested, and knowledge is built. It is one of the most rewarding ways to spend one's life as a nurse. The nurse researcher of today works in an interdisciplinary team in which issues related to nursing and health are addressed by scientists from the perspectives of the various disciplines involved. A project such as promoting independence in seniors might be designed by a team that includes nurses, psychologists, physicians, anthropologists, exercise physiologists, and dietitians.

In the years ahead, many opportunities will be available to nurses wishing to be researchers. Those who identify research as an area of interest early in their training can make choices throughout their education and initial practice to facilitate research development. In the past, nurses have frequently had to wait until mid-career or later to consider research as an option. Because of the commitment of time and effort needed to become a researcher, this delay has been a disadvantage, leaving new researchers only a few years to contribute after their research training.

As with any other plan to advance in the profession, choosing a research career will require postgraduate education. Such preparation is even more crucial than it is for other career paths in nursing, as preparing for research entails acquiring a whole new set of skills in addition to those required to be a nurse.

OPPORTUNITIES FOR UNDERGRADUATE STUDENTS

Undergraduate nursing programs provide many opportunities for gaining an idea of what it would be like to work in research. Students who think they might be interested should test their interest and aptitude by taking advantage of these opportunities.

In all university schools of nursing and in many college programs, there are faculty members who undertake research. These faculty members frequently receive grants to offset the cost of research and can hire students as research assistants. Experience as a research assistant may involve all aspects of the research process, from assisting with the creation of grant proposals, to data collection, data entry and analysis, and writing articles to report the results. Some schools encourage students to select a research project instead of a clinical or management experience to meet course requirements. In other cases, students are assigned to a faculty research program specifically to gain hands-on experience as part of a nursing research course.

Most provinces offer opportunities for summer studentships in research, for which an undergraduate student may apply, along with a faculty supervisor. These are funded in various ways by agencies such as the Alberta Heritage Foundation for Medical Research, by provincial ministries of health, or by universities themselves. The purpose of summer studentships is to introduce outstanding undergraduate students to career opportunities in research by giving them an educational experience in an active research program, often as part of a multidisciplinary team.

Students typically collect data from research subjects; they often conduct interviews and participate in collecting physiological data from subjects (e.g., blood pressures, weights, tests of muscle strength, measurements of body mass index). Others may carry out systematic literature reviews on an assigned topic and develop a paper or presentation from this work. Still others learn to enter and clean data, run statistical tests on the computer, and master a variety of software programs used in research. These experiences help students to clarify whether a career in research appeals to them. Studentships also assist nursing schools in identifying excellent students with the potential for advancement in research. These people are then actively recruited for graduate school.

In the past, most nursing graduate schools did not welcome students who had recently completed an undergraduate program, believing that several years of experience were needed to prepare for graduate work. This view is now considered outdated. Forward-thinking graduate programs recruit at least some of their students directly from undergraduate programs. This change is supported in part by the new Regional Training Centres, funded by the Canadian Health Services Research Foundation, which have as their major goal the building of research capacity in each of the centre areas. These centres actively promote the building of research capacity by providing opportunities for students who are selected from undergraduate programs to progress through graduate programs and postdoctoral fellowships. These nurses will be the researchers of the future.

With a baccalaureate degree in nursing and some research experience, it is possible to find a position in nursing research at the level of research assistant or associate, project coordinator, or data collector. A more central role in the research team requires further preparation.

BUILDING A TRACK RECORD IN RESEARCH

Research is a competitive business. All researchers find themselves in competition for scarce funding throughout their careers. Nurses who aspire to research careers must begin as early as possible to build a track record that will help them to succeed.

Success in research requires creativity, intelligence, and commitment. Graduate programs, granting agencies, awards and scholarship committees, universities, and private foundations all consider these characteristics to be demonstrated by the following indicators:

- Grades
- Research experience
- Publications
- Grants
- Awards
- Recommendations
- Research plans

These indicators are used to award entry to graduate school, grant dollars, academic positions, and scholarships. The criteria are weighted differently, depending on the circumstances. For instance, publication might be considered desirable for a novice researcher but will be required for more senior applicants.

In most competitions for funding, whether for a research grant, a scholarship, or salary support, the criteria listed above provide the basis for ranking candidates. In some cases, additional criteria might be considered, such as oral presentations or interviews that offer applicants scope for personal expression. It is not enough just to have a brilliant idea; a prospective research candidate must also be able to inspire decision makers with the assurance of success. Because success in the past is the most dependable indicator of future success, this criterion will always count heavily with decision makers.

For most aspiring researchers, the first opportunity to accumulate some indicators of success (other than grades) is in an undergraduate program in which students are encouraged to gain research experience and present or publish their work. Faculty in undergraduate programs should be alert to finding students with research potential. They should identify them early and make sure the students are aware of enrichment opportunities that will help them succeed. There is general agreement among nurses about the importance of research in the development of nursing as a discipline. It is therefore a responsibility of all nurses to make the building of research capacity in nursing a priority.

When making decisions regarding experiences and opportunities that arise during graduate school, students should always keep the indicators of success in mind, and set priorities accordingly. Every student should expect to publish papers written to meet course requirements and should apply for awards and scholarships whenever possible, not only for financial need. Every research activity undertaken should have the potential to provide an opportunity to write for publication. These are important goals that faculty supervisors and students should plan together, thus maximizing the graduate school experience to enhance the likelihood of future success.

CHOOSING A GRADUATE PROGRAM

Every province in Canada now has graduate programs in nursing. A complete listing can be obtained from the Canadian Association of Schools of Nursing (CASN, formerly CAUSN), giving admission criteria and information about the faculty. Nurses who have decided on a career in clinical practice should choose a program with a strong clinical base, with faculty members who are actively involved in clinical practice. Many universities now offer nurse practitioner programs, most at the master's level. In the future, there may be opportunities to enroll in a clinically based doctoral program in Canada. At CASN, there is ongoing discussion about making this an option for students.

Nurses who have decided on a research career should choose one of the universities in Canada that has a doctoral program, since a Ph.D. is the minimum requirement for a research career. Most require students to complete a master's program first, but some allow baccalaureate graduates to enter directly into a doctoral program. Information about these programs, including course requirements, residency, and funding opportunities, can be found on the universities' Web sites. Some of the factors to look for in a graduate program include the following:

- Track records of key graduate faculty
- Success rate of graduate students
- Match between research underway in the school or clinical practice of faculty and the student's interest area
- Library and computer resources available to students
- Opportunities for "apprenticeship" in a research-intensive environment and/or an outstanding clinical practice setting
- Availability of funding for graduate students

Good clinical settings that support the development of excellence in practice can be found in conjunction with many of the graduate programs across Canada. University health centres can often provide excellent clinical experience for graduate students in a variety of clinical specialties. Nurses interested in Advanced Practice should seek out facilities where opportunities are provided for community-based and/or acute-care experiences. Settings where nurses can function as members of interdisciplinary teams provide good experience for students. For example, the University of Ottawa has a Nursing Best Practice Research Unit (NBPRU), a collaborative project between the university and the Registered Nurses' Association of Ontario, where leading-edge practice is carried out and evaluated. This is a setting in which evidence-informed practice is a primary focus, and where students can practise along with skilled practitioners in several disciplines. Best practice guidelines are developed and tested in settings such as an NBPRU.

Most universities now have interdisciplinary research centres built around research areas such as perinatal research, gerontology, or nursing work–life balance. These centres bring together researchers from several disciplines who work together to address issues arising from the research area. Research centres often have career scientists at the hub who provide leadership to the interdisciplinary teams. Team members will include academic researchers, clinicians, clinical researchers, and students from a number of disciplines. Sometimes a research centre operates in partnership with government, the health care system, or both. These can be found on the Web sites of individual universities.

Research centres can be the best environment for students to learn about research. Graduate students will have a rich environment, replete with colleagues from both nursing and other disciplines, resources (intellectual and fiscal), support from a variety of mentors, and the opportunity to develop their own interests and skills while contributing substantively to the research program of the centre. The interdisciplinary nature of the environment prepares students for the world at large, as the Canadian Institutes of Health Research are established on an interdisciplinary model. The presence of a research centre focused on the potential student's area of interest is a heavily weighted "plus" when deciding on a graduate school. The nursing research centres at the University of Alberta include

- International Institute for Qualitative Methodology
- Knowledge Utilization Studies in Practice
- Women's Health Research Unit
- Institute for Philosophical Nursing Research

The University of Toronto's nursing research centres include

- Randomized Controlled Trials Unit
- Nursing Health Research Unit

Not every university lists nursing research centres on their Web sites, but this does not mean there are not research centres on campus involving nursing researchers. The Web site for the University of Manitoba, for example, lists 37 research centres or institutes. Nursing researchers are involved in several of these centres, such as

- Centre on Aging
- Institute of Cardiovascular Sciences
- Manitoba Centre for Health Policy

Centres that are affiliated with the University of Manitoba and represent partnerships with the health system in Manitoba are the Diabetes Research and Treatment Centre and the Spinal Cord Research Unit. It is possible for nurses to collaborate on research in these centres as well. The Web sites of all the major universities in Canada contain this type of information, which can be very helpful in the process of selecting the most appropriate graduate program.

If possible, prospective students should visit the campus of the potential graduate school and interview key informants about the program. These might include students, research faculty, clinical specialists and graduate program administrators. For students wishing to develop a clinical specialty area, there must be faculty practising in that area who can supervise graduate students. For doctoral students, one or more potential supervisors must be available in the area of the student's research interest. An applicant must take the time to outline a tentative area of research interest prior to visiting the school. This outline gives a focus to the ensuing interviews and enables the prospective student and the faculty to assess whether a good match is likely. The outline will no doubt change as the student becomes more familiar with the chosen field and becomes aware of other opportunities.

Not every applicant can travel to on-site interviews before making a decision. Good decisions can still be made, however, based on data from Web sites; e-mail discussions with research faculty, graduate students, and administrators; and telephone interviews. No one should make a commitment to a school without first gathering as much information as possible. Whenever there is a local research conference, prospective graduate students can attend to meet researchers from the school in which they are interested.

FINANCING GRADUATE EDUCATION

In spite of the change toward encouraging nurses to enter graduate school at an early age, most are at least five years beyond the baccalaureate degree before they begin. Many nurses received their basic education in diploma programs and therefore have re-entered the educational system as post-diploma students in a baccalaureate program. For these students, not only has time been lost, but often they have not considered research or advanced practice as an option prior to re-entering the system. Post-diploma students frequently continue their education to advance on the job within the health care system. Left with student loans to repay, mortgages, and children, they may not see a viable way to become full-time graduate students. The result is that most graduate students enter the system as part-time students. This presents a difficult issue for the development of research capacity, when the best research training occurs in the context of an apprenticeship model.

The issue for schools of nursing revolves around helping students who apply to graduate programs to sort out the factors related to funding and to make good choices. There is no question but that future career scientists need to be full-time students for at least part of their graduate programs in order to qualify for funding opportunities that will increase their chances of success after graduation. At the same time, a stint of full-time study allows them to be immersed in research long enough to get a good grounding in the operation of a research program.

There are unprecedented sources of funding available today from the federal granting agencies in Canada to support graduate education in nursing. To qualify, however, the applicant must be a full-time student, working with a supervisor whose research is recognized as excellent. Some of the awards available to students are substantial; together with allowable extra teaching or research funding that can be arranged by faculty, these awards will provide students with a decent salary, enabling most to commit to full-time study. The key issue is to identify students with potential for success, link them with supervisors who will help them to get funding, and arrange whatever "top-up" funding is allowed or required to enable these students to succeed.

Most universities maintain recruitment funds to attract the very best graduate students. A proactive strategy for student recruitment is a must for any faculty desiring to be competitive. Once these outstanding students are recruited, the next step is to get them funding to continue, preferably from a federal source. One of the indicators of excellence in a graduate program is the number and proportion of students who hold awards from granting agencies outside the university. This is an important question to ask when applying to a graduate school.

Other sources of funding for graduate students are found within the university, in faculty research grants and from teaching and research assistantship funds. Teaching assistantships (TAs) are available in most faculties, and graduate students commonly teach undergraduates in most university departments. This is good experience, as well as a useful source of income. Research assistantships (RAs) are also part of most university budgets, but these may be limited in number. Usually RAs are a learning experience in which the student is assigned to assist a faculty member in research. Funded research projects are yet another source of funding, and require the student to carry out part of the research, often data collection, under the supervision of a project director.

These sources of funding all provide students with an alternative to maintaining a position outside the university, which often takes priority over educational goals.

GETTING THE MOST OUT OF GRADUATE EDUCATION

Graduate programs are meant to provide advanced knowledge in the discipline and to increase skill levels in practice and research. They often focus on the development of leaders, whether advanced practitioners, teachers, policymakers, managers, or researchers. In a practice discipline like nursing, undergraduate programs prepare graduates for beginning practice, providing both the necessary knowledge and skills. Graduate programs focus not only on building the knowledge base beyond the beginning level, but also provide the skills for advanced practice and for knowledge development through research and theory building.

In Canada, master's programs have evolved to the point where they focus primarily on advanced practice, with some attention to leadership and management. These programs require students to specialize in an area of practice, rather than attempt to increase skills and knowledge in all areas of nursing. Doctoral programs provide the opportunity to focus even more specifically on an area for research and knowledge development. Skills developed in doctoral programs relate mainly to research and theory building.

U.S. graduate programs are much more course-based than their Canadian counterparts. Master's programs are typically one to two years in length and require both course work and advanced practice. Courses tend to be in the clinical specialty area, theory, and research, and are often designed to meet requirements for specialty certification from the professional association. Doctoral programs also have extensive course requirements in such areas as philosophy, theory, clinical specialization, research, and cognate areas related to the research.

Canadian programs also offer specialization at the master's level and opportunities for advanced practice. They tend, however, to have fewer practice hours and fewer specialty courses than the U.S. programs and are not coordinated with requirements for specialty certification to any great extent. Since there are just a few Canadian specialty certification programs in Canada, most master's programs have not incorporated completion of a clinical specialty certification as part of the program. However, some Canadian master's programs do have such arrangements with some of the specialty certification programs in the United States. Doctoral programs in Canada tend to be more flexible, focusing more on the student's specific research needs than do the U.S. programs. The Canadian programs are heavily dependent on the apprenticeship model.

Once into a graduate program, students with goals for research development will find many opportunities to develop particular skills and areas of knowledge. Most important, however, is finding appropriate mentoring within the faculty. Mentoring is a critical element in the apprenticeship model, as students learn by working alongside faculty members in research and practice. As students become acquainted with the resources available in the faculty, they will find a number of individuals who can provide mentorship for different purposes.

The first year of a program should provide opportunities to investigate all potential resources. Social functions for faculty and students are a good place for networking, as are research presentations, information sessions, brown-bag lunches, conferences, and faculty meetings. Important also are opportunities to communicate with other students, particularly those who are farther along in the program. This is one area in which the full-time student has a definite advantage over the part-time student, who may be on campus only to attend classes. There are sources of information available to all students through the faculty's Web site, newsletter, and bulletin boards. These are important ways to track what is happening that might provide opportunities to develop.

Opportunities for development are particularly rich within research centres, since graduate students in the centre share a common area of interest and work closely with the research faculty. Students in a research centre have access to any faculty or staff within the centre. This access makes networking easier than it is for students in the larger faculty. Advanced practice students may not have this same opportunity to interact in a smaller group with experts in their field of interest.

POSTDOCTORAL STUDIES

The idea of a postdoctoral fellowship following completion of a Ph.D. program is still new for nurses. Historically, the doctoral degree was considered sufficient preparation for a research career. It is still considered so in some disciplines, particularly in the humanities, but other disciplines such as science and medicine have used the postdoctoral fellowship as an essential piece of research training for decades.

In the science model, students play a valuable role in the professor's laboratory. Graduate students take on a piece of the research as their own thesis project, but they also work alongside the professor and others to carry out the work of the entire research program. Postdoctoral students typically move to another laboratory for a period of one to three years to continue their development in a different intellectual environment and to attempt to set up an independent research program. Universities and industry recruit and employ postdoctoral fellows to fill academic and research positions. Often there is keen competition among postdoctoral fellows for the best jobs, but there is also keen competition among employers for the best postdoctoral opportunities. Failure to find a research position has meant, in some disciplines, working as a research associate in a laboratory or in some cases leaving the discipline altogether to find a job.

There has long been a shortage of doctorally prepared nurses to fill jobs in education and research. Students in doctoral programs have been recruited to start work in nursing schools and in clinical or management positions before they have finished their programs. Many faculty members were hired with master's degrees and were persuaded by their deans to go on for a Ph.D. Often, these faculty continued to work, full- or part-time, throughout the Ph.D. program. Such nurses are likely to be older than graduate students in other disciplines and to have family and other commitments that make it difficult for them to leave the workforce for a period of several years to complete a Ph.D. and postdoctoral fellowship. Theirs is a very different career trajectory from that of their colleagues in science. Although the scene has started to shift in nursing, this is still the predominant picture in most graduate programs.

Across North America, since the 1960s, the majority of the graduates of doctoral programs have assumed academic positions without the benefit of postdoctoral fellowships. Many of these graduates were not successful in launching research programs following their Ph.D. training. Since the main purpose of doctoral education is to train researchers, this has been a sad waste of talent. Numerous explanations have been offered for this problem. Some of these include heavy teaching loads in nursing programs; scarcity of role models; unrealistic expectations for productivity in research, teaching, clinical practice, and community service; and lack of good mentoring available to new academics. Today, however, the expectation for faculty members at research-intensive universities is that they will complete a postdoctoral fellowship in a recognized research institution prior to taking up a university appointment. In the short time this practice has been in place, it has made a tremendous difference in the development of research capacity in faculties of nursing.

A postdoctoral fellowship provides protection from competing priorities, particularly in teaching and clinical practice, since obligations in these areas will be either greatly reduced or absent altogether. A fellowship gives the new graduate time to focus on research prior to assuming all the responsibilities of a full-time academic.

In Canada, the shift to postdoctoral fellowships as the expectation for Ph.D. graduates has taken place since the doctoral programs began in the 1990s. The first graduates of the new Canadian programs in the early 1990s succeeded in obtaining funding for postdoctoral fellowships, and the movement began with them. Several of these early graduates have gone on to become career scientists with salary awards from federal sources. They, in turn, have developed successful research programs and are now supervising graduate students.

What is the outcome of a successful postdoctoral fellowship for the individual researcher? It varies somewhat depending on the goals of the researcher, but there are a few common outcomes that should be attained.

- *Publications:* Each postdoctoral fellow should expect to publish two to three articles per year while holding a postdoctoral fellowship. At least one of these articles should come from the Ph.D. thesis. Others will relate to work done during the postdoctoral fellowship. For instance, the research unit in which the fellowship is carried out will provide opportunities for fellows to get experience writing articles for publication from data already in place within the unit. Often these articles are jointly written by several team members.
- *Grants:* A major goal for the postdoctoral fellow involves obtaining research grant funds to support beginning development of a program of research.
- *Skill development:* The postdoctoral fellowship is a time for continued development in research techniques and skills. Instrument development and refinement, new analytical techniques, and discussion and debate of methodologies, whether quantitative or qualitative, are examples of the possibilities.
- *Network of colleagues:* The postdoctoral fellow expects to expand the network of colleagues beyond that already developed during the doctoral program. This is done in a variety of ways, including attending conferences, visiting other research centres, online discussions with experts in the field, and receiving and providing feedback on research and publications.

CAREER SCIENTISTS

Following a postdoctoral fellowship, the next phase in a research career is a beginning-level career science position. In Canada, this is a grant-supported position wherein all or part of an individual's salary is provided by the granting agency to the employer (university or other research institution) to ensure that the incumbent can spend the majority of time in direct research activities.

There are many sources of funding for career scientists. Some examples include the Ontario and Quebec ministries of health, which provide funding for career scientist awards, as does the Alberta Foundation for Medical Research. These provincial awards are intended to equip young researchers to compete for national awards. A career award from the Canadian Institutes of Health Research provides salary funding for five years at a time, renewable for good productivity. Career scientists are reviewed on a regular basis and must be judged to be meeting the terms of their awards for funding to continue.

Career scientist awards are progressive in nature, with the expectations for productivity and excellence increasing at each level. Scientists are judged on the quality of their research; their grants, publications, and presentations; awards and recognition; and the accomplishments of their students and associates. This is a demanding career. Research scientists are hard-working, dedicated individuals living competitive lives for whom risk taking is a normal everyday activity. However, a research career is also very rewarding with many positive attributes, not the least of which is the opportunity to make discoveries that improve the human condition.

CRITICAL THINKING QUESTIONS

1. Describe the various types of résumés and in what circumstances each would be appropriate.
2. What kinds of things are normally important considerations for employers in interviewing a prospective candidate for a position in nursing?
3. What types of activities are important in building a track record for a nurse pursuing a career in research?

WEB SITES

Canadian Association for Nursing Research: www.canr.ca/
Canadian Association of Schools of Nursing: www.casn.ca/en/

REFERENCES

Alberta Human Resources and Employment. (2002). *The job seeker's handbook*. Edmonton: Author.

Andrews, M., & Wallis, M. (1999). Mentorship in nursing: A literature review. *Journal of Advanced Nursing, 29*(1), 201–207.

Block, L. M., Claffey, C., Korow, M. K., & McCaffrey, R. (2005). The value of mentorship within nursing organizations. *Nursing Forum, 40*(4), 134–140.

Chambers, P. (2009). Designing the nursing career you want. *AAACN Viewpoint, 31*(2), 4–5.

Donner, G. J., & Wheeler, M. M. (2009). *Taking control of your career: A handbook for health professionals*. Toronto: Elsevier.

Hefferin, E. A., & Kleinknecht, M. K. (1986). Development of the nursing career preference inventory. *Nursing Research, 35*(1), 44–48.

Watson, S. (2000). The support that mentors receive in the clinical setting. *Nursing Education Today, 20*, 585–592.

23 Monitoring Standards in Nursing Education

Marilynn J. Wood

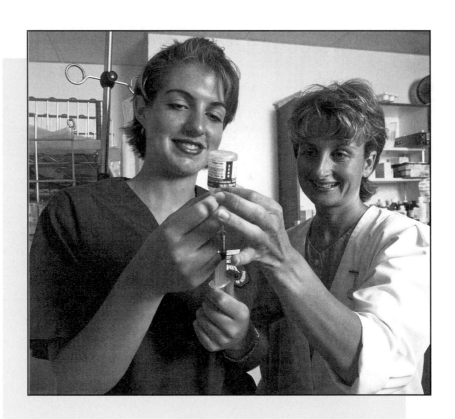

LEARNING OBJECTIVES

- To understand the importance of standards in nursing education.
- To differentiate between approval and accreditation of programs.
- To understand the process of accreditation by CASN.
- To appreciate the complexities of financing accreditation.
- To identify the benefits of maintaining standards.

Nursing education programs in Canada were originally developed in hospital schools of nursing, primarily for the purpose of staffing the hospitals. This was the standard means of staffing, regardless of the size of the hospital. Indeed, some hospitals admitted as few as 10 to 12 students per year, even in the 1950s. The only registered nurses in the hospitals were the head nurses, supervisors, and the director of nursing. Nursing students received instruction from a few nurses, who taught such courses as anatomy, physiology, and nursing arts (basic procedures) in the classroom, and from physicians, who taught courses about diseases and medical or surgical treatments. The only clinical supervision was provided by head nurses and supervisors.

Schools of this nature proliferated in the early part of the twentieth century and continued into the 1940s and early 1950s, despite the recommendation of the Weir Report in 1932 that nursing education be organized and administered separately from the hospitals. This independent pattern of organization was promoted by Florence Nightingale in the nineteenth century. Nursing leaders, such as Isabel Hampton Robb and Mary Adelaide Nutting, recognized the need for a system to monitor standards of education and worked for nurses within the professional nursing organizations to assume the monitoring role. Their goal was to devise a system requiring approval for new nursing programs, standards for existing schools of nursing that were equal to the new schools, and regular inspection of all programs to ensure that standards continued to be met.

NURSING EDUCATION STANDARDS

Standards in nursing education are delineated by knowledgeable nurse educators who have expertise in the practice of nursing and in methods of education. Standards range from minimal to ideal, depending on the purpose for which they are defined. There are two basic mechanisms for monitoring educational programs: approval and accreditation. Accreditation promotes excellence in nursing education programs, while provincial approval of nursing education programs is a regulatory and legislative requirement that focuses on standards of practice, ethics, and competencies demonstrated by new nursing graduates. Accreditation is a peer review process whereby institutions or programs are assessed and measured using a set of predetermined criteria that, if met, connote a basic level of quality.

Approval is a mandatory process, and minimum standards are established by a body authorized by provincial legislation or regulations pursuant to that legislation. Accreditation, voluntary and national or international in scope, measures institutions against criteria established by the accrediting body to promote quality. Accreditation of educational programs exists in many professions, but government approval and monitoring of programs are unique to nursing. No other profession is governed by legislation that regulates the content and conduct of educational programs; however, nursing is the only profession that has not required university-level preparation for entry to practice. This latter factor may explain how the practice of governments setting standards for approval of nursing education began, since universities have traditionally set their own standards and have resisted any attempts from governments to interfere with their autonomy. Standards for nursing education were set with the goal of ensuring that the safety of the public would be protected. Even with baccalaureate education as the basis for entry to nursing across Canada, it will be difficult to change the existing pattern of provincial approval of nursing programs, now entrenched in each province and territory.

The purpose of any credentialing mechanism is to protect the public and ensure accountability to consumers. In nursing education programs, not only are the students assured that the program they have chosen will prepare them appropriately to practise as nurses, but the public is assured that the school produces nurses who meet the standard expected of new graduates of nursing education programs. Because any system of credentialing benefits those who are credentialed, whether institutions or individuals, a system of checks and balances within the credentialing mechanism is necessary to ensure that the public is protected. In approval and accreditation, standards provide the checks and balances that ensure that the practitioners prepared in nursing education programs are competent to enter the practice of professional nursing.

APPROVAL OF PROGRAMS IN NURSING EDUCATION

In Canada constitutional responsibility for education and health care rests with the individual provinces. Consequently, policies and mechanisms for monitoring standards in nursing education are defined by each province. This responsibility is delineated in legislation that regulates the conduct of educational programs, whether the programs are conducted in universities, colleges, or other institutions of learning. In all provinces except Ontario and Quebec, the responsibility for defining and monitoring standards in nursing education is assumed by the provincial nursing association. Although specific mechanisms for defining standards and the process for approval of basic nursing programs may vary among provinces, the profession controls the educational standards for the admission of new practitioners to the profession (see Chapter 3).

In Alberta, responsibility for approval of nursing programs was formerly given to the Universities Coordinating Council (UCC), which, under the terms of the *Universities Act,* has ultimate responsibility for defining and monitoring standards for all postsecondary education in the province. However, in 1998 new legislation was enacted in Alberta governing all health professions, and now the responsibility for nursing education has been given to the College & Association of Registered Nurses of Alberta (CARNA; formerly known as the Alberta Association of Registered Nurses [AARN]). The responsibility for program approval and monitoring has been assigned to an independent committee of

CARNA, called the Nursing Education Program Approval Board (NEPAB). NEPAB has been carrying out program approval functions since 2001, but with the proclamation of the new act in 2005, it now operates under its own standards and policies. Standards for nursing education in Alberta are based on the CARNA entry-to-practice competencies.

In Ontario, the *Regulated Health Professions Act* was passed in 1991 as was the *Nursing Act* and 20 other individual professional acts. These acts protect the public by governing the practice of health care providers. The College of Nurses of Ontario (CNO) fulfills the registration and discipline functions for registered nurses and registered nursing assistants in that province. Before 2005, approval of Ontario's 22 diploma programs was the responsibility of CNO. Because all nursing education programs now fall under a university, the CNO voted in September 2000 to designate CASN accreditation to supplant program approval in Ontario. This regulation came into effect in 2005.

Monitoring and approval of the basic baccalaureate degree programs in universities is one of the major responsibilities of the Council of Ontario University Programs in Nursing (COUPN), a member of the Health Sciences Council of the Council of Ontario Universities. COUPN has delegated its authority for program approval and monitoring to the Canadian Association of Schools of Nursing (CASN; formerly known as the Canadian Association of University Schools of Nursing [CAUSN]). This means that all university degree programs must be accredited by CASN in order to be approved by the province (CAUSN, 1992, p. 12). In 2000, Ontario ratified a recommendation from the College of Nurses that education for entry to the practice of nursing be the baccalaureate degree, now in effect since the year 2005.

In Quebec, all postsecondary education, including nursing education programs, is governed by the Ministry of Higher Education and Science. There has been no mechanism for approval of nursing programs, but a mechanism for approval is being developed for the diploma programs of the Collèges d'Enseignement Générals et Professionnels (CEGEP). University nursing programs are subject to the approval process required of all educational programs in their respective universities and are also entitled to seek accreditation from CASN.

Thus, primary responsibility for approval of nursing education programs is delegated to the provincial nursing association in all provinces except those previously mentioned. One can expect considerable differences in the systems for regulation and monitoring because of the variety and number of nursing education programs. All provinces now have at least one university nursing program. Prior to 1988, Prince Edward Island was an exception, with only one diploma program; however, "on November 9, 1988, a provincial government decision to phase out diploma nursing education in favour of a degree program was announced . . . a move supported by the professional nursing association, nurses' unions, employers and educators alike" (*CNA Connection*, 1989, p. 10). With the official opening of the baccalaureate degree in September 1992, Prince Edward Island became the first province in Canada to achieve the goal of a baccalaureate degree as the minimum preparation for entry into nursing.

Nursing education in community colleges exists in all provinces and territories except Newfoundland, New Brunswick, Nova Scotia, and Prince Edward Island. Hospital schools of nursing, which were initially the only type of nursing education program in all provinces, no longer exist in any of the provinces. The phasing out of these programs began in the 1970s, when the governments of Ontario, Quebec, and Saskatchewan closed their hospital schools. The remaining provinces with hospital schools phased them out during the late 1980s and early 1990s. There were never hospital schools in the territories, but formerly there were college diploma programs in both the Northwest Territories and Nunavut. In 2004, these two territories joined forces to form the Registered Nurses Association of the Northwest Territories and Nunavut. The Board of Directors of this association has the authority to approve nursing programs.

The standards for nursing education programs in each province and territory cover areas such as administration and general organization, philosophy, and objectives; faculty; students; curriculum; educational resources and facilities, records, and reports; and evaluation. In most cases, provincial associations have based their standards for education on the beginning competencies they have designated as required of entry-level practitioners. Approval must be obtained to establish a new program in nursing, and monitoring for continued approval occurs at regular intervals. Approval must also be obtained to eliminate a nursing program.

The approval process involves submitting a report, or self-study, based on the provincial standards for nursing education. This will be followed by a visit by persons designated by the authorized body to assume this responsibility. A review team always includes one or more qualified registered nurses who report their recommendations to the appropriate body. In universities, programs are also required to meet the university's own standards for academic programs. Universities usually have their own review processes to determine whether programs meet these standards.

Although the approval mechanism in all provinces is designed to ensure compliance with minimum standards, it is important that the standards and the process by which they are implemented ensure that nursing students are adequately prepared to enter practice. Delineating adequate preparation for entry is the subject of much debate and has always been a major issue in nursing education. In the days when almost all nursing students were prepared in hospital schools of nursing and each hospital recruited its own graduates, few questions were asked about the adequacy of preparation. The "inbreeding" that resulted from this system may have fostered obedience and strict adherence to the status quo. At that time, the emphasis was on procedures and technical preparation as opposed to the broader education that was encouraged after the initiation of university nursing programs. It has been difficult for some nurses in practice settings to accept the fact that graduating students are novices, not expert practitioners, as tended to be the perception regarding new graduates in the past. However, such an attitude was unrealistic because new graduates, even then, had much to learn. No other profession expects expert performance from newly graduated practitioners. What the public and the employer of a new graduate do have the right to expect is safe practice, a very different concept from expert practice.

Another issue in the approval process pertains to the delineation of minimum standards. Who decides what constitutes the minimum, and what standards are considered more than minimum? It is important that standards be defined by well-prepared, competent nurses. There is no doubt that the ideal in all provinces is to have the authority for this important regulatory mechanism remain with the professional associations. One exception may be Ontario, where the CNO, rather than the Registered Nurses' Association of Ontario (RNAO), has the responsibility for registration and discipline.

At the present time, all provinces and territories except Quebec have designated the baccalaureate degree to be the basic educational credential for nursing at some point in time. The question of whether all programs should be under the same approval mechanism will continue as long as there is more than one type of program preparing students for entry-to-nursing practice. This will no longer be an issue when the goal of a required baccalaureate degree for entry to practice is attained.

Another problem that is prevalent in imposing regulatory mechanisms is avoiding rigidity in the standards and allowing for flexibility within the system. It is important that standards be defined broadly enough to allow for differences and creative approaches while maintaining basic accountability to the public and to the students, who are direct consumers of nursing education.

ACCREDITATION OF NURSING EDUCATION PROGRAMS

No system for accreditation of nursing education programs was present in Canada until 1986, when the Canadian Association of University Schools of Nursing approved the establishment of an accreditation program for university nursing programs after devoting 12 years to the development of an accreditation program. The major impetus for the program was that nursing was one of the few health sciences educational programs that did not have a system for accreditation. French (1982) states:

> In 1972 CASN was designated as the accrediting agency for university programs in nursing. In 1974 CASN established a committee on accreditation to develop a program of accreditation for university based programs in nursing. Recognizing the need for a method to stimulate the development of educational programs that are responsive to societal needs, and the dangers inherent in the accreditation process, CASN demanded a program that would support and promote change. The criteria on which the accreditation process was to be based had to reflect attributes of change and development. The major objective of the program of accreditation was to ensure that the educational programs were preparing the quality of practitioner required to deal effectively with existing and future health problems. Through the process of accreditation, institutions would be encouraged to engage in a process of self-evaluation, i.e., to study the goals of its educational program(s) and the means of attaining those goals. (p. 2)

From 1974 to 1984, the CASN Committee on Accreditation examined existing programs of accreditation, including the National League for Nursing (NLN) accreditation program in the United States, which had existed since 1952. The American accreditation program was conducted from 1939 to 1952 by the National League for Nursing Education, precursor of the NLN. The model for the Canadian accreditation process was proposed by Allen (1977) and adopted by CASN as the criteria by which programs would be evaluated. The model is built around the following three qualities: (1) *relevance* to the trends in society that have an impact on the health needs of the community; (2) *accountability*, defined as the extent to which the program teaches students that the primary responsibility in nursing is to the patient; and (3) *relatedness*, or the extent to which parts of the program support and build on other parts, thereby promoting the achievement of goals. Subsequently, a fourth criterion, *uniqueness*, was adopted. It was defined as "the extent to which a program capitalizes on the resources within its particular setting" (CAUSN, 1978, p. 3).

The CASN Committee on Accreditation developed procedures for applying these criteria in the process of accreditation. A number of university nursing programs across Canada were involved as test sites in developing standards and instruments. Thus, the program of accreditation for university-based nursing programs evolved over 12 years before being accepted for general implementation by the CASN Council in June 1986. This accreditation program was launched in May 1987 (Kirkwood & Bouchard, 1992). These standards were revised in 1995. Subsequently, the Task Force on Accreditation was appointed by CASN to review the program and recommend changes. With the advent of collaborative programs in Canada, it was difficult to apply the standards and procedures of the accreditation programs to these new models without some revision. In 2005, a revised accreditation program was implemented by CASN. Although the program has a new framework and expanded standards, the basic philosophy remains the same.

CASN implements its accreditation function through its Accreditation Bureau, whose members are elected and/or appointed by CASN Council according to the bylaws governing the bureau. The bureau is a standing committee of CASN, and functions within established CASN policy and guidelines. It is the decision-making body for accreditation decisions, and it reports to the council. The ten members of the Accreditation Bureau are shown in Box 23.1.

Currently, there are 91 nursing programs in Canada, many of which are collaborations between colleges and universities: there are 17 in British Columbia, 11 in Alberta, 3 in Saskatchewan, 4 in Manitoba, 36 in Ontario, 9 in Quebec, 2 in New Brunswick, 3 in Newfoundland, 3 in Nova Scotia, 1 in Prince Edward Island, 1 in the Northwest Territories, and 1 in Nunavut. By 1994, 12 programs had been reviewed and accredited either for a three- or seven-year period (McBride, 1994). By 2002, this number had increased to 30. Initially, most of the programs seeking accreditation were in Ontario, Quebec, and Nova Scotia, the three provinces in which accreditation is part of the program-approval mechanism. In 2009, 52 of these programs were accredited by CASN. New baccalaureate degree programs have the option of being reviewed for candidacy while still in a developmental stage. At the present time, two new programs have taken advantage of this opportunity and have been granted candidacy status. All additional programs have declared their intention to go through the accreditation process over the next ten years. Many of these are re-accreditation reviews (CASN, 2008b).

Within CASN's framework, "accreditation has two main purposes: (1) the support and improvement of standards of baccalaureate and graduate nursing programs in CASN member institutions; and (2) the recognition of programs that have been

---

BOX 23.1 Membership of the CASN Accreditation Bureau

Membership

The Accreditation Bureau consists of ten members:

- Five members, with full-time faculty positions in CASN member schools, elected by CASN Council;
- One representative of a service agency nominated by the Canadian Nurses Association;
- One academic representative nominated by the Association of Universities and Colleges of Canada;
- One community representative selected by CASN Executive Committee;
- One regulatory body representative selected by CASN Executive Committee; and
- One consumer (student/graduate) representative, nominated by CASN member schools, and appointed by CASN Executive Committee.

  Other responsibilities and roles are outlined below:

- The CASN president and executive director are non-voting ex officio members of the Accreditation Bureau;
- The chair is elected each year; any voting member may be nominated to stand for election as the chairperson; the chairperson is elected by the members who hold full-time faculty appointments with a CASN member school;
- The Accreditation Bureau chair is an ex officio member of the CASN Board of Directors;
- Nurse faculty members must be currently involved in baccalaureate or graduate programs in nursing, have a minimum education of a master's degree in nursing or equivalent degree, and have five years' teaching experience in a baccalaureate or graduate program in nursing;
- No member of CASN Council shall be appointed to the Accreditation Bureau;
- Accreditation Bureau members sign commitment forms and comply with CASN Conflict of Interest Guidelines, May 2004;
- At least five members of the Accreditation Bureau shall be able to read documents in both French and English;
- Members should have experience or knowledge of standards and quality improvement; and,
- Management support is provided by the Accreditation director and program officer.

Term of Office

The term of office is three years, and a member can be re-appointed or stand for election for a second term, with the exception of the regulatory body representative.

The term of office for the regulatory body representative is two years for one term only.

Source: Canadian Association of Schools of Nursing (CASN). (2008a). *Accreditation Bureau*. Retrieved on January 29, 2008, from http://www.CASN.ca/content.php?doc=49.

---

reviewed and have met specific standards" (*CASN Newsletter*, 1989, p. 1). CASN's policy is that "once a member unit has received notice from the Board of Accreditation concerning its accreditation status, and has had opportunity to respond, and if no appeal is pending, then it becomes public information and it is published in the *CASN Newsletter*" (CAUSN Council, 1989), and added to the CASN Web site. Thus, accreditation status will become known to recipients of the *CASN Newsletter*, including all member institutions and all individual members of the four regional chapters of CASN: Atlantic Region (ARCASN), Quebec Region (QRCASN), Council of Ontario University Programs in Nursing (COUPN), and Western Region (WRCASN), and to all who access the Web site. The information published on the CASN Web site to date identifies 52 universities that have been reviewed and accredited, but not whether for a three-year or seven-year period (CASN, 2009). There is no indication of a denial of accreditation. For many years, there was no stated means of providing information about the accreditation status of schools to prospective students, to guidance counsellors, or to nurses interested in earning a baccalaureate degree in nursing, in spite of the decision of the CASN Council in 1990 that such information should be in the public domain. The CASN Web site had previously contained no information indicating which programs were accredited, nor did it have a mechanism to advise prospective students of this information. This situation has now been rectified, and the outcome of the accreditation process is published on the CASN Web site. There is still no indication of schools that may have been denied accreditation, but at least prospective students can see whether their schools of choice are currently accredited.

In the United States, where the National League for Nursing and now Commission for Collegiate Nursing Education have been responsible for accreditation of all nursing programs from 1952, the listings of accredited programs have appeared regularly in the official publications of these organizations. As with CASN, however, these lists include only accredited programs and do not provide information as to whether programs not listed have failed to meet required standards or simply did not seek accreditation, which is a voluntary process. McCloskey (1985) and others question whether the concept of public accountability is actually fulfilled when accreditation bodies publicize only programs that have been accredited and do not release information about those that have not been.

⌕ CANADIAN RESEARCH FOCUS

Molzahn, A.E., & Purkis, M.E. (2004). Collaborative nursing education programs: Challenges and issues. *Canadian Journal of Nursing Leadership, 17*(4), 41–55.

Orchard, C. (2004). Commentary: The case for national standards. *Canadian Journal of Nursing Leadership, 17*(4), 54–55.

Collaborative Nursing Education Programs bring unique issues to the process of monitoring the quality of educational programs. However, monitoring the quality of these programs has provided a distinct challenge for the CASN accreditation program. The collaborative programs themselves have identified many of the challenges they have faced in maintaining the quality of the degree collaborations. Often these stem from the differing cultures, priorities, goals, and aspirations of the colleges and universities that have entered into collaboration.

Molzahn and Purkis (2004) have identified the major issues and offer strategies to address these stemming from their experience in collaboration in British Columbia. The differing cultures of universities and colleges can present significant issues, most of which stem from the traditional values of universities that promote scholarship and research and the strong focus of colleges on providing access to opportunity. These issues can present themselves in the form of difficulties in agreeing on admission criteria and standards for progressing through the program. Even when these issues are resolved through contractual agreements, universities have tended to view the collaboration as deleterious to the university's reputation.

Strategies recommended to enhance collaboration include clear legal agreements between institutions and ensuring that mutual expectations are clearly addressed in advance. Agreement on evaluation and review processes to monitor and demonstrate quality is also critical. In this area, the accreditation program can provide strong support to help the collaborative partners to manage difficulties within their own institutions as they strive to maintain a high level of quality in their programs.

Orchard (2004) has stressed the importance of national standards to insure that programs meet the current and future needs for nursing practice across the country. She recommends evaluation research to determine the success of the collaborative programs. To date, this has not been undertaken by the nursing profession.

FINANCING ACCREDITATION

Financing the accreditation program has been a major concern. In 1977, CASN submitted a proposal to the W.K. Kellogg Foundation for possible funding; however, support was not obtained. The foundation was approached again in 1979, but by 1980, there were strong indications that support would not be forthcoming. Consequently, CASN proceeded with plans for implementing the program, and a special annual fee, assessed to all university nursing programs, was kept in reserve to support the accreditation program. When the accreditation program was implemented in 1987, thus completing a review of the first nursing program to seek accreditation, a specific fee for the review had not been established. Therefore, a fee was charged based on the amount of involvement with each nursing program (J. Bouchard, personal communication, April 25, 1990). However, it became obvious that additional funding was needed. In November 1989, CASN Council approved a fee of $3,000 to be instituted in the 1989–90 academic year and to be increased to $4,500 for 1990–91 and 1991–92. Once the initial reserve had been exhausted, the CASN Council stated that the accreditation program would be a cost-recovery program, which is how it now operates. CASN charges a standard fee for the accreditation program to be carried out, plus an additional fee for each collaborating partner institution. In addition, the school pays the costs of travel and lodging for the review team (CASN, 2008c).

The cost of the program is sometimes felt to compete with other priorities the school might have, such as costs related to the development of graduate programs, including the development of doctoral programs in nursing that began as recently as January 1991; development of research in nursing to advance nursing knowledge and improve practice; and development of exemplary nursing practice in settings where students learn to nurse and faculty continue to practise and conduct research. Another issue is the amount of time required for a faculty or school to conduct a self-study and for faculty participation in the visitation and review processes for programs other than their own. Time thus expended is not available to pursue other goals. French (1984) stated:

> A program of accreditation had to facilitate, not impede the achievement of these goals. Accreditation was to be conducted with a minimum of effort, cost and time. It was to promote the interest of the educational consumers and the public. Educational primacy and the portability of educational qualification were identified as basic objectives of accreditation. (p. 3)

Thomas, Arseneault, Bouchard, Coté, and Stanton (1992) reported that the schools that completed the evaluation tools designed to evaluate the accreditation process indicated that "the self-study process was found to be very time-consuming . . . even though it increased awareness and stimulated discussion about the programme among faculty and students" (p. 41). Thomas and Arseneault (1992) concur that the self-study is time-consuming and increases faculty workload and stress but is also rewarding because it fosters self-development and reinforces issues that have already been recognized.

The programs that have not yet undergone accreditation will have to decide whether they will do so, since it is a voluntary option and not a mandatory requirement such as approval. The $3,000 accreditation fee for 1989–90 was increased to $4,500 for 1990–91, to $5,000 in 1993, and $7,000 in 2005. If it becomes a fiscal decision, it may be based on the availability of financial resources and time to do the self-study, or on other factors, such as the benefits of having accreditation status within the system of higher education. There is no doubt that an accreditation system encourages self-study and peer review by faculty and staff of an institution. Self-study and peer review can also be achieved through internal review, which is a common practice in most universities across Canada. In fact, internal reviews may be conducted every five years; in these cases, thought must be given to the number of times the self-study process and the review procedure can reasonably be carried out within a single academic unit. Thomas et al. (1992) indicated:

> It is difficult at this time to evaluate the long-term financial feasibility of the accreditation pro-gramme, given the variability in the number of programmes requesting reviews, particularly during times of budgetary constraint in postsecondary institutions. Financial viability must be monitored. The potential for multiple three-year reviews could affect the feasibility of the existing program. (p. 44)

Nor is it known whether universities will be able to afford the time required for the actual process if they seek accreditation and if faculty members choose to be involved in the peer-review process of accreditation in other institutions. This commitment to the process of assessing quality is shared by other professions within universities, so that when there are other health disciplines present, accreditation for nursing will usually be accepted as an important part of professional education. At present in Canada, the survival of the accreditation program is virtually assured by the number of provinces that now require accreditation in lieu of program approval.

REFLECTIVE THINKING

How could the process of accreditation be streamlined and made more financially viable, without giving up the goal of quality?

OTHER ISSUES REGARDING ACCREDITATION

Many issues other than cost are related to accreditation in general and to accreditation in nursing education in particular. One benefit claimed by supporters of accreditation is that it facilitates transfer of students from one institution to another. This may be true in the United States, where there are thousands of colleges and universities, including private ones, but it may not be true in Canada. Knowledge of accredited programs may help a student select a transfer institution, but transferability of courses depends on the equivalence of courses in the institutions and the student's achievement in these courses. In Canada, the low number of private institutions and the geography of the country discourage frequent transfer.

McCloskey (1985) questions the extent to which accreditation helps prospective students decide which institution to attend. She notes that most students are unaware of accreditation status, and that it is doubtful that guidance counsellors in high schools use this information. Whereas accreditation status may have relevance for prospective students in the United States, where there are more than 500 accredited baccalaureate nursing programs from which to choose, it is questionable whether this would apply in Canada, where there are 92 baccalaureate degree programs located in public colleges and universities that are sometimes required to give preference to residents from their own provinces.

One of the stated goals of CASN's accreditation program is to raise the standards of nursing education in Canada. The question of whether accreditation promotes quality is difficult to answer because of problems in measuring quality. Young (1976) states, "Accreditation has never defined 'quality of education' except in terms of numbers of PhDs produced, books published, grants received, and the like; the validity of these criteria has never been demonstrated" (p. 622). The task of evaluating the accreditation process was delegated by the CASN Council to the Accreditation Bureau. Criteria for evaluation were identified and defined, as were sources of data for each criterion and the data collection instruments. The committee completed an evaluation in the mid-1990s, and a revision of the criteria was undertaken, reducing some of the reporting requirements and streamlining others. CASN's purpose was to assess the validity of the four criteria selected for the accreditation process, as well as the validity and reliability of the instruments used to collect data. Another review, held in the early 2000s, resulted in a major revision of the accreditation program in order to bring it up to date with changes in nursing education across the country.

An important question that is often raised is the effect of accreditation on research productivity within the faculty, which is important in university nursing programs. In the past, faculty members have tended to devote more attention to teaching and curriculum development than to research. Unless the criteria emphasize and require research, the process of accreditation may not help promote it, as evidenced by events in the United States for many years. In fact, U.S. participants in accreditation have reported that the time and effort devoted to accreditation impeded the progress of research. The difficulties lie in the amount of time required by the self-study and visitation processes, and the time required for faculty to serve as visitors and review board members. This time could have been devoted to research. This issue has not been raised by Canadian nursing education programs.

There are many issues still to be addressed. Can accreditation programs promote research? If an accreditation program does not promote research and the application of research findings in teaching and practice, can one say that it is promoting quality in nursing education? Will accreditation help programs obtain what they need? This is considered a potential benefit by some proponents of accreditation who assume that if the accreditors note a deficiency and the recommended action to correct it requires infusion of resources, this will influence the administration to grant funding. Although this may occur in some cases, in times of financial constraint it may not.

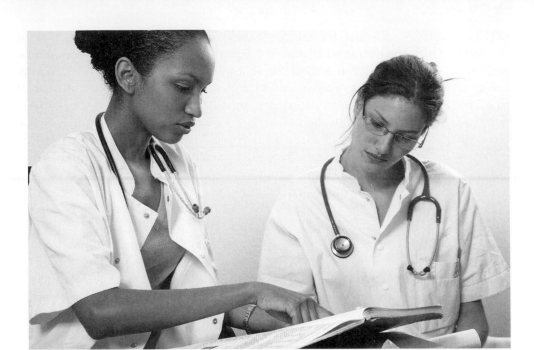

Whether the accreditation program will be or should be extended to involve graduate education in nursing, as well as baccalaureate education, is another issue to be addressed in Canada. The issue of accreditation of graduate programs has been brought to the CASN Council for discussion on more than one occasion. Members have approved the idea of accreditation of graduate programs; however, no steps have yet been taken to include graduate programs in the accreditation process. In the United States, master's degree programs in nursing have been part of the accreditation process for many years; however, faculty involved in doctoral education have strongly resisted any extension of accreditation to the doctoral level. To date, their resistance has been effective in preventing movement in this direction. Will the same issue arise in Canada with the development of doctoral education in nursing? Only time will tell. It makes sense that accreditation should apply to programs preparing students for practice (as it does in other disciplines), whether this be at the undergraduate, master's, or doctoral level.

CONCLUSION

It is important to have standards for nursing education and a system to monitor the achievement of standards and promote quality in nursing education. The accreditation process has been accepted as the best means to achieve this goal in professional programs. There is an accreditation process in place for most health professions, including medicine, and this is supported by universities as a justifiable expense. There is still a question in Canada as to whether the university nursing education units that make up the membership of CASN can afford to support and be involved in several systems of monitoring, the approval process in provinces where university programs are monitored, intra-institutional evaluation programs where they exist, and the accreditation process, in addition to meeting the obligations to which all university faculty members are subject. At present, however, the accreditation program appears to be surviving financially, perhaps in part due to the increase in membership in CASN brought about by the collaborations with colleges.

The goal of accreditation, to promote excellence, depends on the extent to which the process influences standards of education. One of the hazards may be that continual upgrading of standards may result in unrealistic expectations. This is a concern in other professions as well (Mar, Rakowski, & Wetle, 2008). There is a need to focus on student outcome criteria as a more valid index of educational quality because the criteria have tended to be structure-process oriented, dealing more with the teaching-learning environment than with the actual learning that takes place. A study within social work has examined self-efficacy as a means of measuring student outcome within educational programs (Holden, Barker, Rosenberg, & Onghena, 2007). Within nursing, there is a move to focus on entry-to-practice competencies as an outcome of educational programs (CARNA, 2008) to avoid the tendency to measure process variables within programs. Accountability to the public is of vital importance in any credentialing mechanism. This involves the development and maintenance of programs that the public expects will prepare practitioners who can deliver a high level of care. In addition, accountability involves the credentialing body. This organization must function in a transparent way so that the integrity of the system is protected. If the public is to be served, there must be a means to maintain standards and to demonstrate and assess accountability.

CRITICAL THINKING QUESTIONS

1. Why should nursing education programs be subject to approval and monitoring when other programs, such as education, are not?
2. How does accreditation benefit nursing students, present and future?

WEB SITES

Canadian Association of Schools of Nursing: www.casn.ca
Canadian Nurses Association: www.nurses-cna.ca

REFERENCES

Allen, M. (1977). *Evaluation of educational programmes in nursing.* Geneva: World Health Organization.
Bouchard, J. (1990). Personal communication, April 25, 1990.
Canadian Association of Schools of Nursing (CASN). (2008a). *Accreditation Bureau.* Retrieved January 29, 2008 from http://www.CASN.ca/content.php?doc=49.
Canadian Association of Schools of Nursing (CASN). (2008b). *Accredited Schools/Programs.* Retrieved on January 25, 2008, from http://www.casn.ca/content.php?doc=47.

Canadian Association of Schools of Nursing (CASN). (2008c). *Accreditation*. Retrieved on February 26, 2008, from http://www.casn.ca/content.php?sec=5.

Canadian Association of Schools of Nursing (CASN). (2009). *Accreditation*. Retrieved on October 2, 2009, from www.casn.ca/en/54.html.

Canadian Association of University Schools of Nursing (CAUSN). (1978). *Development of a method to promote growth and change in university schools of nursing and nursing in general*. Ottawa: Author.

Canadian Association of University Schools of Nursing (CAUSN). (1992). *Anniversary report*. Ottawa: Author.

Canadian Association of University Schools of Nursing Council. (1989). *Minutes of meeting of November 17*.

CASN Newsletter/ACEUN—Bulletin d'Information. (1989, September). pp. 1–4.

CNA Connection. (1989). Baccalaureate education comes to PEI. *The Canadian Nurse*, 85(3), 10.

College and Association of Registered Nurses of Alberta (CARNA). (2008). *Continuing Competence Program*. Retrieved on January 20, 2008, from http://www.nurses.ab/CARNA.

French, S. (1982). Design for accreditation of educational programs in nursing. In M. S. Henderson (Ed.), *Recent advances in nursing no. 4: Nursing education* (pp. 81–102). London: Churchill Livingstone.

French, S. (1984). *The development of an accreditation program for university programs in nursing in Canada*. Document submitted to Canadian Association of University Schools of Nursing.

Holden, G., Barker, K., Rosenberg, G., & Onghena, P. (2007). Assessing progress toward accreditation raised objectives: Evidence regarding the use of self efficacy as an outcome in the advanced research concentration curriculum. *Research on Social Work Practice*, 17(4), 456–465.

Kirkwood, R., & Bouchard, J. (1992). *"Take counsel with one another": A beginning history of the Canadian Association of University Schools of Nursing, 1942–1992*. Ottawa: Canadian Association of University Schools of Nursing.

Mar, V., Rakowski, W., & Wetle, T. (2008). Retaining program diversity in undergraduate public health education. *Journal of Public Health Management and Practice*, 14(1), 3–5.

McBride, W. (1994). (1994, Summer). Executive director's message. *CASN Newsletter*, 2–3.

McCloskey, J. C. (1985). Accreditation of nursing education: An overview and issues. In J. C. McCloskey & H. K. Grace (Eds.), *Current issues in nursing* (2nd ed, pp. 507–524). London: Blackwell Scientific Publications.

Molzahn, A. E., & Purkis, M. E. (2004). Collaborative nursing education programs: Challenges and issues. *Canadian Journal of Nursing Leadership*, 17(4), 41–55.

Orchard, C. (2004). Commentary: The case for national standards. *Canadian Journal of Nursing Leadership*, 17(4), 54–55.

Thomas, B., & Arseneault, A. (1992). Organizing your school for accreditation. *Canadian Journal of Nursing Research*, 24(2), 58–59.

Thomas, B., Arseneault, A., Bouchard, J., Coté, E., & Stanton, S. (1992). Accreditation of university nursing programmes in Canada. *Canadian Journal of Nursing Research*, 24(2), 33–48.

Young, K. E. (1976). Issues in accreditation. *Nursing Outlook*, 24(10), 622–624.

CANADIAN AND INTERNATIONAL NURSING

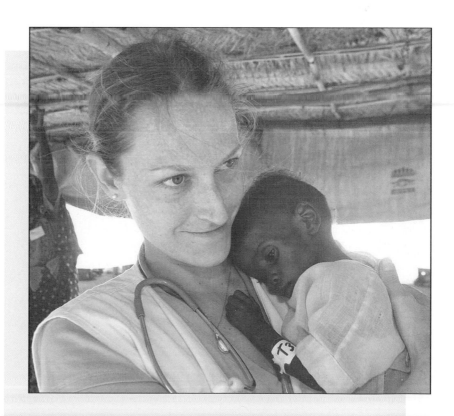

Laura Cobey in the Darfur region of Sudan while serving with Médecins Sans Frontières (MSF) Holland.

24 International Nursing: Looking Beyond Our Borders

Richard Splane and Verna Splane

Updated by Judith Shamian and Jane L. MacDonald

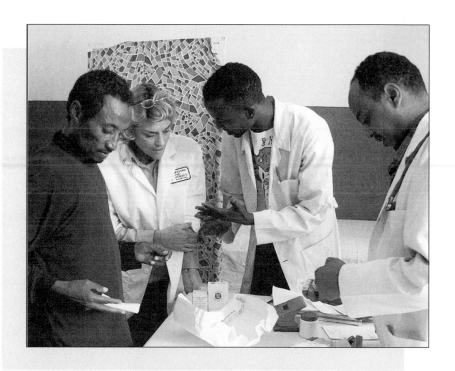

A nurse conducts a clinical mentoring session with Ethiopian male nurses in Mekele, Ethiopia.

LEARNING OBJECTIVES

- To describe the impact that the key international health-related events that have occurred since 2000 have had on health systems and health status globally.
- To discuss the impact that recent international nursing events have had on the evolution of the nursing profession.
- To identify and discuss the major issues and factors that have influenced the evolution of the Canadian health care system since 2000.
- To identify and discuss the major issues and events that have affected the nursing profession in Canada since 2000.
- To discuss the contribution of several Canadian international nursing initiatives.

This chapter provides an extensive update to the chapter on International Nursing written by Richard Splane and Verna Huffman Splane in the previous edition. Comments and additions started with the year 2000. Major global events have continued to shape the international health and nursing agenda. It is critical that Canadian nurses understand the implications for nursing practice here in Canada, as well as appreciate the potential contribution that Canadian nurses make to the global health agenda.

MAIN INTERNATIONAL HEALTH-RELATED ISSUES AND EVENTS SINCE 2000

PANDEMICS

Awareness of the need to plan for, and expect, global and national pandemics has become more acute since 2000. The combination of international travel and new and emerging diseases is important for all health workers to understand. Nurses are often the first health providers to encounter someone with possible pandemic symptoms, and they therefore need to be acutely aware of presenting symptoms, national and international protocols, and international travel advisories and restrictions.

Canada has experienced several infectious disease outbreaks that have led to system-wide reform and have had international repercussions. In particular, SARS (Sudden Acute Respiratory Syndrome) surprised both Canada and the international community in 2003. The disease first occurred in China and was brought to Canada by a woman from China. SARS taxed both the coordination and capacity of the Canadian health care system and prompted much reform of the system at the national and provincial levels. SARS highlighted the great need for coordinated international disease surveillance systems. For Canada, it highlighted the weakness of our public health system.

The World Health Organization (WHO) has identified other acute respiratory diseases of concern (particularly those with pandemic potential—for example, avian flu) for targeted international focus. The WHO is now in the process of completing teaching modules to assist grassroots health workers worldwide in recognizing and managing cases of acute respiratory diseases of concern.

Most recently, the WHO declared a global pandemic of the H1N1 virus. This pandemic was a new strain of the influenza virus and began in late April 2009 with a rash of cases in Mexico. It then spread to other countries around the globe, including Canada. On June 11, 2009, the threat to global health was determined to be significant, and the WHO raised the level of alert to a Level 6. This is the highest level declared by the WHO and implied that community level outbreaks, in at least one other country in a different WHO region from the original outbreak, had taken place. Throughout the summer, the WHO and national health agencies continued to carefully monitor this quickly evolving global health situation.

A second wave of H1N1 began in September 2009. Mass immunization campaigns were implemented in all provinces and territories. This wave tapered off by January 2010. A total of 428 deaths occurred in Canada, with over 8000 people admitted to hospital—1500 of these to Intensive Care Units. Globally there were approximately 14,300 deaths. The role of the Public Health Agency of Canada in coordinating information and connecting with their provincial counterparts was evident during this pandemic.

Some key issues were highlighted during this pandemic including: vaccine production, availability and procurement; organization and roll out of mass public health campaigns; communication and coordination at all levels; and ethical issues relating to vaccine distribution and prioritizing

MIGRATION AND CHANGING DEMOGRAPHIC PATTERNS

During the twenty-first century, the migration of people globally is increasing (see Figure 24.1). This migration is both internal to countries and between countries. In many cases, this movement is due to wars and violence (e.g., Sudan, Ethiopia, Colombia); in other cases, it is due to environmental factors (floods, droughts, tsunamis, hurricanes); and in still more cases, economic factors are the cause (from the South to the North; from Canada to the United States). For example, the out-migration of poor people in New Orleans following Hurricane Katrina has changed the face of that city.

These migration patterns are changing the demographics of countries globally and Canada specifically. Between 1994 and 2004, Canada had the second-highest rate of population growth among the G8 countries (Statistics Canada, 2005). However, more than half of Canada's growth now comes from immigration, and this is changing the face of Canada. For example, Chinese citizens now make up Canada's largest visible minority group, followed by South Asians and Blacks (Canadian Nurses Association [CNA], 2006) (see Figure 24.2). This increasing racial diversity brings the international context and issues much closer to home and to our health care system.

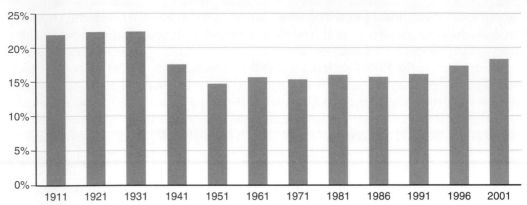

FIG 24-1 Immigrants as a percentage of the population, Canada. (Source: Canadian Labour and Business Centre. (2003). *CLBC Handbook: Immigration Skills and Shortages.* Section A: Trends in Immigration (p. 2). Retrieved on October 20, 2009, from http://www.clbc.ca/files/Reports/IHB_section_a.pdf.)

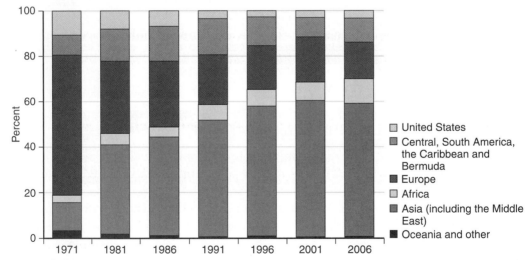

FIG 24-2 Region of birth of recent immigrants to Canada, 1971–2006. (Source: Statistics Canada. (2006). *Immigration in Canada: A portrait of the foreign-born population, 2006 Census* (p. 9, Fig. 2). Retrieved on October 20, 2009, from http://www12.statcan.ca/census-recensement/2006/as-sa/97-557/pdf/97-557-XIE2006001.pdf.)

WARS AND VIOLENCE

Since 2000, various countries have experienced increased violence. Iraq and Afghanistan are at the top of Canadians' awareness. However, other countries and regions, such as Sudan with the Darfur tragedy, Colombia with its continuing internal violence, and the continued tensions in the Middle East, remain the concern of many people worldwide. In addition, the continued dehumanizing acts of violence directed particularly toward women and children are a huge cause for concern. For example, the use of rape as a weapon of war as documented by Amnesty International (2004) and the recruitment of child soldiers in various countries around the world have been viewed in the past decade as degrading and in violation of the rights of children. In 2007, at a meeting in Paris sponsored by the Government of France and UNICEF, representatives of 58 countries committed themselves to putting an end to the unlawful recruitment and use of children in armed conflicts. The Paris Principles continue to be signed by other countries worldwide (United Nations, 2007).

HIV/AIDS

HIV/AIDS continues to be one of the most significant global population issues. Although the incidence of HIV globally is starting to level off and the number of new infections has fallen, there were still (in 2007) 33.2 million people living with HIV, 2.5 million people who were newly infected, and 2.1 million who died of AIDS in the world. The sub-Saharan region of Africa, while seeing a significant reduction in new HIV infections since 2001, remains the region most affected—almost 68% of the global total is from this region (WHO Media Centre, 2007).

A recent report released by UNICEF (2006) estimates that by 2010, 15.7 million children in sub-Saharan Africa will have lost at least one parent due to AIDS. This figure could account for as much as 12% of all the region's children.

The impact on families and health systems in that region is enormous. The drop in life expectancy in some African countries is astounding and primarily due to the impact of HIV/AIDS. In Zimbabwe, for example, life expectancy plunged from 56.6 years in 1990 to 33.9 years in 2002 (Africa Policy E-Journal, 2007).

INTERNATIONAL TOBACCO CONVENTION

May 21, 2003, was a historic day for global public health. At the 56th World Health Assembly, the WHO's 192 member states unanimously adopted the world's first public health treaty, the WHO Framework Convention on Tobacco Control. Negotiated under the auspices of the WHO, this new treaty is the first legal instrument designed to reduce tobacco-related deaths and disease around the world. The treaty required countries to impose restrictions on tobacco advertising, sponsorship and promotion; establish new packaging and labelling of tobacco products; establish clean indoor air controls; and strengthen legislation to clamp down on tobacco smuggling (WHO, 2003).

GLOBAL INFLUENCES

The World Trade Center bombing on September 11, 2001, and subsequent global terrorist attacks (Bali in 2002 and Spain in 2004) have changed the way we interact in the global community and in Canada. Increased air travel security, more restricted travel between countries (e.g., the need for Canadians to have a passport to travel to the United

States), and a heightened awareness of security issues, have all been products of this increased vigilance in the international community. Health professionals in Canada have needed to become more aware of international issues and regulations, and health issues.

CLIMATE CHANGE AND CLIMATE EVENTS

Climate and the environment are now top of mind for many politicians and bureaucrats. The effects of global warming have been seen in Canada in the ice storm of 1997 and internationally in the tsunami of 2004 in South Asia, Hurricane Katrina in 2005 in New Orleans, and droughts in 2005 in sub-Saharan Africa. Awareness of environmental responsibility and the effects of increased environmental degradation is important for the nursing community. The international awareness of the disproportionate use of energy in the north compared with the south has called for international treaties such as the Kyoto Accord (2005), which has the objective of reducing greenhouse gases caused by climate change. At this writing, Canada has not ratified the Kyoto Accord and is instead proposing its own greenhouse-gas reduction plan. The effects of environmental pollution are increasing. Windsor, Toronto, Montreal, and Vancouver are Canadian cities where the ozone air quality objective is exceeded an average of 10 or more days in the summer (meaning these cities will have smog alerts) (Environment Canada, 2007).

The WHO recognized the importance of the environment and in 2008 declared the theme for World Health Day as "Protecting Health from Climate Change." This raises the profile of health dangers posed by global climate variability and change. The theme was selected because of the overwhelming evidence showing that climate change presents growing threats to international public health security—from extreme weather-related disasters to the wider spread of such vector-borne diseases as malaria and dengue (WHO, 2008c).

UNITED NATIONS MILLENNIUM DEVELOPMENT GOALS

In 2000, the United Nations (UN) member states agreed on eight Millennium Development Goals (MDGs) with targets to be achieved by 2015. Three of the eight directly relate to health: reduction in child mortality; improved maternal health; and combating HIV/ AIDS, malaria, and other diseases. Of the remaining five goals, at least three strongly relate to health. The Millennium Development Goals (UNDP, 2008) can be seen in Table 24.1.

A road map has been developed globally to work to attain these goals, and Canada is active in the global push to achieve these goals.

INTERNATIONAL DISEASE SHIFT

During this decade, the incidence of chronic disease has grown remarkably both in Canada and internationally. According to the Chronic Disease Prevention Alliance of Canada (CDPAC), chronic diseases are the leading causes of death and disability worldwide and in Canada, and about two-thirds of total deaths are due to chronic diseases (CDPAC, 2008). Internationally, it is a similar picture. The WHO recognizes that chronic diseases are the leading cause of

| TABLE 24.1 | United Nations Millennium Development Goals |

GOAL	TARGETS
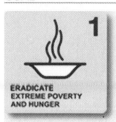

Eradicate Extreme Poverty and Hunger | Target 1. Halve, between 1990 and 2015, the proportion of people whose income is less than $1 a day
Target 2. Halve, between 1990 and 2015, the proportion of people who suffer from hunger |
|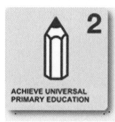

Achieve Universal Primary Education | Target 3. Ensure that, by 2015, children everywhere, boys and girls alike, will be able to complete a full course of primary schooling |
|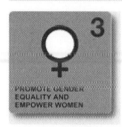

Promote Gender Equality and Empower Women | Target 4. Eliminate gender disparity in primary and secondary education, preferably by 2005, and in all levels of education no later than 2015 |
|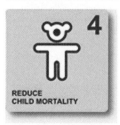

Reduce Child Mortality | Target 5. Reduce by two-thirds, between 1990 and 2015, the under-five mortality rate |

Continued

TABLE 24.1	United Nations Millennium Development Goals—cont'd

GOAL	TARGETS
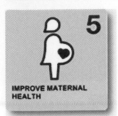 Improve Maternal Health	Target 6. Reduce by three-quarters, between 1990 and 2015, the maternal mortality ratio
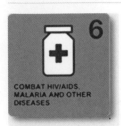 Combat HIV/AIDS, Malaria and Other Diseases	Target 7. Have halted by 2015 and begun to reverse the spread of HIV/AIDS Target 8. Have halted by 2015 and begun to reverse the incidence of malaria and other major diseases
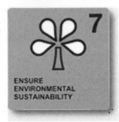 Ensure Environmental Sustainability	Target 9. Integrate the principles of sustainable development into country policies and programs and reverse the loss of environmental resources Target 10. Halve, by 2015, the proportion of people without sustainable access to safe drinking water and basic sanitation Target 11. Have achieved by 2020 a significant improvement in the lives of at least 100 million slum dwellers
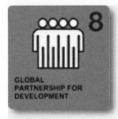 Global Partnerships for Development	Target 12. Develop further an open, rule-based, predictable, nondiscriminatory trading and financial system (includes a commitment to good governance, development, and poverty reduction both nationally and internationally) Target 13. Address the special needs of the Least Developed Countries (includes tariff- and quota-free access for Least Developed Countries' exports, enhanced program of debt relief for heavily indebted poor countries [HIPCs] and cancellation of official bilateral debt, and more generous official development assistance for countries committed to poverty reduction) Target 14. Address the special needs of landlocked developing countries and small island developing states (through the Program of Action for the Sustainable Development of Small Island Developing States and 22nd General Assembly provisions) Target 15. Deal comprehensively with the debt problems of developing countries through national and international measures in order to make debt sustainable in the long term

TABLE 24.1	United Nations Millennium Development Goals—cont'd
GOAL	**TARGETS**
	Target 16. In cooperation with developing countries, develop and implement strategies for decent and productive work for youth
	Target 17. In cooperation with pharmaceutical companies, provide access to affordable essential drugs in developing countries
	Target 18. In cooperation with the private sector, make available the benefits of new technologies, especially information and communications technology

Source: United Nations Development Programme. (2006). *UN Millennium Project: Millennium Development Goals: Goals, targets, indicators.* Retrieved on October 21, 2009, from http://www.unmillenniumproject.org/goals/gti.htm. Copyright © United Nations Development Programme, 2001.

mortality worldwide, representing 60% of all deaths (see Figure 24.3 and Figure 24.4). Out of the 35 million people who died from chronic disease in 2005, half were under the age of 70 and half were women. In fact, 80% of chronic-disease deaths now occur in low- and middle-income countries (WHO, 2008a). Unfortunately, in addition to the climbing incidence of chronic disease in low- and middle-income countries, communicable diseases and diseases of poverty, like tuberculosis, continue to remain important causes of morbidity and mortality.

REFLECTIVE THINKING

1. Discuss the impact that the 2003 SARS epidemic and the 2009 H1N1 pandemic had on health systems both nationally and internationally.
2. What factors influence the attainment of the United Nation's Millennium Development Goals?

MAIN INTERNATIONAL NURSING ISSUES AND EVENTS SINCE 2000

THE WORLD HEALTH ORGANIZATION

In 2002, the WHO recommended a framework on collaborative action to support countries in enhancing the capacity of nursing and midwifery services to contribute to national health goals. *Strategic Directions for Nursing and Midwifery Services* recommended five Key Result Areas (KRAs) for concentration of effort between 2002 and 2008 (WHO, 2002):

KRA	Focus
KRA 1	Health planning, advocacy, and political commitment
KRA 2	Management of health personnel for nursing and midwifery services
KRA 3	Practice and health system improvement
KRA 4	Education of health personnel for nursing and midwifery services
KRA 5	Stewardship and governance

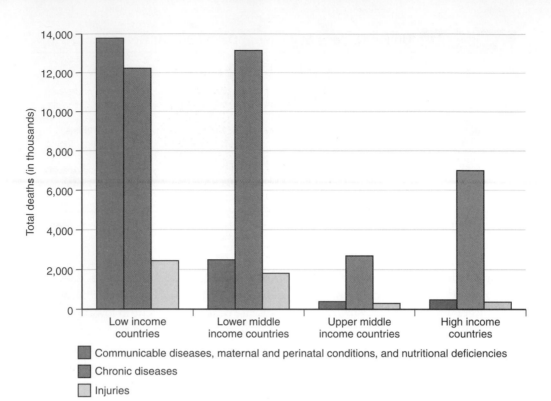

FIG 24-3 Projected deaths by major cause and World Bank income group, all ages, 2005 (Source: WHO & Public Health Agency of Canada. (2005). *Global Report: Preventing chronic diseases: A vital investment* (Part 1: Overview, p. 4). Retrieved on October 20, 2009, from http://www.who.int/chp/chronic_disease_report/part1/en/index2.html.)

In the KRAs, the WHO also recognized the importance of nursing and midwifery involvement in senior policy discussions.

New Director General and Refocus on Primary Health Care

In 2006, Dr. Margaret Chan was appointed to the position of director general of the WHO, succeeding Dr. Lee Jong-Wook, who was director general from 2003 to 2006. Dr. Gro Harlem Brundtland finished her term in 2003.

Dr. Chan is calling for renewed emphasis on Primary Health Care (PHC) as an approach to strengthening health systems around the world. Nurses and midwives form the backbone of the PHC system, and both deliver the majority of care and provide the leadership in managing the system.

In her report to the 122nd session of the WHO executive board in January 2008, Dr. Chan states: "I believe we will not be able to reach the health-related Millennium Development Goals unless we return to the values, principles and approaches of primary health care" (WHO, 2008b).

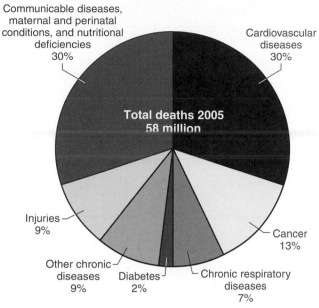

**Total deaths 2005
58 million**

Communicable diseases, maternal and perinatal conditions, and nutritional deficiencies 30%

Cardiovascular diseases 30%

Injuries 9%

Other chronic diseases 9%

Diabetes 2%

Chronic respiratory diseases 7%

Cancer 13%

FIG 24-4 Projected main causes of death, worldwide, all ages, 2005. (Source: WHO & Public Health Agency of Canada. (2005). *Global Report: Preventing chronic diseases: a vital investment* (Part 2: The Urgent Need for Action, p. 38). Retrieved on October 20, 2009, from http://www.who.int/chp/chronic_disease_report/part2_ch1/en/index.html.)

The basic principles of PHC were defined in the Alma Ata agreement sponsored by the United Nations in 1978. The *Alma Ata Accord* also laid the groundwork for the current emphasis on Social Determinants of Health (WHO, 1978). The original basic principles of PHC (CNA, 2003) included the following:

- Public participation
- Health promotion
- Appropriate skills and technology
- Accessibility
- Intersectoral collaboration

WORLD HEALTH ASSEMBLY ENDORSEMENT OF THE ISLAMABAD DECLARATION ON STRENGTHENING NURSING AND MIDWIFERY

The World Health Assembly (WHA) is the overall decision-making body for the WHO. It meets once a year and is attended by delegations led by the ministers of health from all of WHO's 192 member states, including Canada. Its main function is to determine the policies of the organization. In May 2006, the WHA endorsed Resolution WHA59.27, which reaffirmed the crucial contribution of the nursing and midwifery professions to health systems and the health of people they serve. Following this WHA endorsement, a global consultation on nursing and midwifery was held in March 2007 in Islamabad, Pakistan. The WHO, the International Council of Nurses (ICN), and the International Confederation of Midwives coordinated this consultation. It resulted in the *Islamabad Declaration on Strengthening Nursing and Midwifery* (WHO, 2007b), which recommended urgent action in three areas:

- Scaling up nursing and midwifery capacity
- Maintaining skill mix of existing and new cadres of workers
- Implementing positive workplace environments

INTERNATIONAL COUNCIL OF NURSES

The International Council of Nurses (ICN) is a federation of national nurses' associations (NNAs), representing nurses in more than 128 countries. Founded in 1899, ICN is the world's first and widest-reaching international organization for health care providers. Operated by nurses for nurses, ICN works to ensure quality nursing care for all, sound health policies globally, the advancement of nursing knowledge, and the presence worldwide of a respected nursing profession and a competent and satisfied nursing workforce. In Canada, the CNA is the official member of the ICN. The three goals of ICN (ICN, 2008a) are to:

- bring nursing together worldwide;
- advance nurses and nursing worldwide; and
- influence health policy.

Leadership for Change Program

In 1996, the ICN developed the Leadership for Change program. The goal of this program is to prepare selected nurses for management and leadership in health system reform, with the specific aim of enhancing their contribution to the health services through appropriate and proactive leadership strategies. Nurses in more than 60 countries have gained the knowledge, skills, and strategies that they need to take leadership roles in nursing and health systems, build partnerships, and improve health care. The ICN has a strategic partnership with the WHO to foster leadership and management capacities of nurses and midwives globally (ICN, 2008b).

International Centre for Human Resources in Nursing

The International Centre for Human Resources in Nursing (ICHRN) was established in 2006 by the ICN and the Florence Nightingale International Foundation. The centre is dedicated to strengthening the nursing workforce globally through the development, ongoing monitoring, and dissemination of comprehensive information, standards and

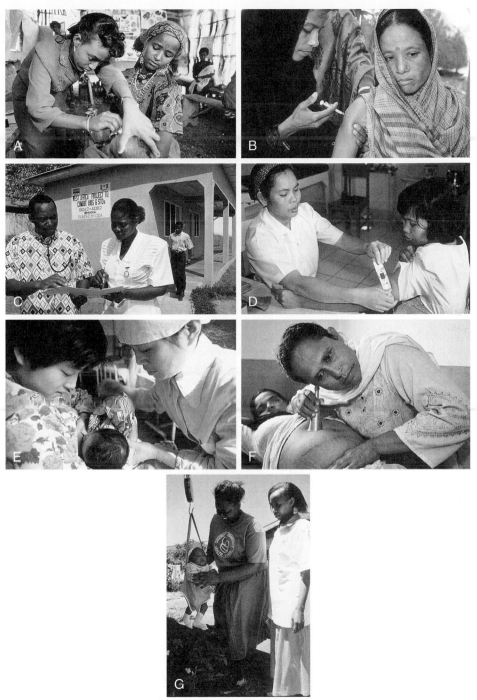

International Council of Nurses advocates: nurses and the world. **A,** Ethiopia; **B,** Bangladesh; **C,** Ghana; **D,** Indonesia; **E,** China; **F,** Pakistan; and **G,** Kenya.

tools on nursing human resources policy, management, research, and practice. The mission of the ICHRN is to improve the quality of patient care through advancing nursing and health care services. The ICHRN has produced valuable global research on health human resources in nursing (ICHRN, 2006).

CHIEF NURSES

Several of the recent WHA resolutions call for the appointment of government Chief Nurses. Chief Nurses can contribute to health and policy development and implementation that strengthens the health of citizens and the contribution that nursing makes to it. Dr. Jean Yan, the Chief Nursing Scientist for WHO, has strongly supported the appointments of Chief Nurses in each of the WHO member countries. Having Chief Nurses in each member country increases understanding and cooperation among member countries and leads to better nursing cohesiveness. We are seeing gradual uptake of member countries. While some countries always had a government Chief Nurse, others are putting those positions in place. Canada introduced the position of Executive Director Nursing Policy, Health Canada in 1999. Dr. Judith Shamian was the first appointed to the position, followed by Sandra MacDonald-Rencz.

COMMONWEALTH NURSES FEDERATION

The Commonwealth Nurses Federation (CNF) is a working group formed under the umbrella of the Commonwealth Ministers of Health (of which Canada's minister of health is a member). It was founded in 1973 and is a federation of national nurses' associations in Commonwealth countries. It is involved in the promotion of high standards of professional practice. The objectives of the CNF (Commonwealth Secretariat, 2008; CNF, 2007) are to:

- influence health policy throughout the Commonwealth
- develop nursing networks
- enhance nursing education
- improve nursing standards and competence
- strengthen nursing leadership

THE LILLIAN CARTER CENTER FOR INTERNATIONAL NURSING

The Lillian Carter Center for International Nursing (LCCIN) has as its mission the improvement of the health of vulnerable people worldwide through nursing education, research, practice, and policy. The LCCIN focused on enhancing the impact of nursing globally through targeted international academic exchanges; partnerships fostering scholarship; creation of a forum for exploration of issues relating to the global supply, demand, distribution, and quality of the nursing workforce worldwide; and through increasing access to relevant training and education (Emory University, 2008). The focus of the LCCIN is to strengthen the capacity of the Government Chief Nursing Officers with whom they are working.

In 2006, the LCCIN hosted the biennial Global Government Chief Nursing Officers (CNOs) Institute. This meeting focused on managing key challenges facing CNOs globally. Over 100 CNOs from around the world, including Canada, attended this meeting.

In addition to facilitating communication between CNOs, the LCCIN also facilitates interdisciplinary communication. Prior to the CNO Institute, the LCCIN hosted a pre-forum workshop focusing on the public health response to health emergencies and influenza pandemics. Both Chief Nursing Officers and Chief Medical Officers (CMOs) attended this workshop.

Following the CNO Institute, the Global Government Health Partners Forum 2006 took place. This year's focus was The Breaking Point—Human Resources for Health. Both CNOs and CMOs from over 100 countries participated. The goal of the forum was the formation of partnerships among health leaders within and across national boundaries to improve the health of individuals and communities worldwide.

FOCUS ON HEALTH HUMAN RESOURCES (HHR)

HHR is an urgent issue for health care systems worldwide. In Canada, the Canadian Nurses Association (CNA) identified that, according to a 2004 OECD study, Canada had the highest relative nursing shortage of the six countries examined, at 6.9% of the present workforce. The CNA goes further to state that if we continue with past workforce utilization patterns of registered nurses (RNs), Canada will experience a shortage of 78,000 RNs by 2011 and 113,000 RNs by 2016 (CNA, 2005a).

This HHR situation is of global concern, and the nursing profession has known for a long time that this crisis was coming. According to a report published in 2004 by the ICN, "The scarcity of qualified health personnel, including nurses, is being highlighted as one of the biggest obstacles to achieving the Millennium Development Goals (MDGs). . . . Nurses are the "front line" staff in most health systems, and their contribution is recognised as essential to meeting these development goals and delivering safe and effective care" (ICN, 2004, pp. 4–6).

This shortage of nurses is particularly acute in many countries in Africa—particularly sub-Saharan Africa, where AIDS has had a dramatic impact on the nursing workforce. In the ICN work, there is an estimate of a shortfall of more than 600,000 nurses just in the sub-Saharan countries (ICN, 2004, p. 5).

The ICN document identified three critical challenges related to nursing shortages:

- The impact of HIV/AIDS
- Internal and international migration of nurses
- Achieving effective health-sector reform and reorganization

The other important issue influencing the HHR shortage is the gender factor—in most countries, over 90% of the HHR workforce is female. According to the ICN report,

"The challenges facing the nursing workforce are interlinked with the challenges of ending gender bias and discrimination in society and in employment" (ICN, 2004, p. 7).

REGULATORY AND ASSOCIATION CHANGES IN THE EASTERN BLOC COUNTRIES

During the communist regime, the Eastern Bloc countries did not have stand-alone nursing regulatory bodies or clear legislative frameworks to govern the nursing profession. Over the last two decades, many of these countries have been developing new government structures, policies, and processes. Currently, most of the former Eastern Bloc countries have established nursing councils. Countries such as Poland, Bosnia, Russia, and others have benefited from support from Canadian nursing leaders in their journeys.

 REFLECTIVE THINKING

1. What impact do global demographics and migration have on the profession of nursing?
2. What role do nurses play in health-system reform?

 MAIN NATIONAL HEALTH ISSUES AND EVENTS SINCE 2000

HEALTH SYSTEM REORGANIZATION AND REFORM

Nationally, Canada has been grappling with political and health issues similarly identified in the international environment. Some of the most important issues are highlighted below.

Primary Health Care (PHC)

Canadians, too, have recognized that access to adequate and appropriate primary health care is critical to a well-run health care system. However, access to health providers at the PHC level is becoming more difficult. For example, according to the College of Family Physicians of Canada, five million Canadians are without a family doctor (College of Family Physicians of Canada, 2007). Without first-line access to the health care system, Canadians who do not have a family doctor will need to find other PHC resources to deal with their urgent (and not so urgent) care needs. This may mean going to the Emergency Department for issues that do not really require the resources available in an acute-care setting.

Various solutions are being proposed to deal with this problem of access. Increasing the number of general practitioners is one; however, there are other options, including increasing the number of registered nurses and nurse practitioners; creating and implementing models of interdisciplinary practice (like community health centres and family health teams); and looking at system-wide solutions such as regionalization.

In an effort to encourage and support PHC in Canada, the federal government supported the Primary Health Care Transition Fund, which provided $800 million to the provinces and specific projects to support PHC reform in Canada. Each province and territory is experimenting with its own solutions to create more accessible and integrated PHC programs (Government of Canada, 2007).

The broad framework of PHC laid out in the *Alma Ata Declaration* has also provided a basis for the inclusion of and emphasis on the social determinants of health in PHC. This includes the importance of self-care and community involvement in the attainment of health goals (Public Health Agency of Canada, 2004).

Regionalization

During the first decade of the new millennium, most provinces have regionalized their health care systems. This has involved amalgamating various services at the acute care, primary health care, public health, and home care levels in an effort to provide a more coordinated and responsive system.

Financing Debate

The debate in Canada continues over public-private funding of the health care system. Several seminal events have placed this debate in the public eye:

- The Supreme Court of Canada ruled in 2005 on the *Chaoulli-Zeliotis v. Government of Quebec* case that Quebec citizens have the right to purchase private insurance to pay for medically necessary health care services when wait times are unreasonably long (Attorney General of Quebec, 2005; CUPE, 2005).
- In 2005, the Canadian Medical Association discussed the topic of privatization of health care at its Annual General Council. Several resolutions were discussed at this council that supported increasing private health insurance in Canada if the health system is not responding appropriately (CMA, 2005).
- The Canadian Nurses Association and its constituent members, the Provincial Registered Nursing Associations, have continued in their public and vocal support of a publicly funded and delivered health care system (CNA, 2004).

HEALTH CARE COMMISSIONS

In order to examine more closely the health care systems in Canada and provide recommendations for how to move forward, several health commissions have been completed at both the federal and provincial levels since 2000. There is much synergy across these reports and commissions concerning coordination, integration, client involvement, financing, and providing care at the appropriate level and by the appropriate person. The most significant commissions and committees include the following:

- *Quebec's Health Review* (2001) (The Clair Commission)
- *Final Report of the Commission on Medicare* (2001) (The Fyke Report)

- *The Mazankowski Report* (2001) (Premier's Advisory Council on Health)
- *Commission on the Future of Health Care in Canada (2002)* (Romanow Commission)
- *The Health of Canadians—The Federal Role* (2002) (Standing Senate Committee on Social Affairs, Science and Technology, and chaired by Senator Michael Kirby)
- *Out of the Shadows at Last: Transforming Mental Health, Mental Illness and Addiction Services in Canada* (2006) (Standing Senate Committee on Social Affairs, Science and Technology, and chaired by Senator Michael Kirby)

PUBLIC HEALTH

SARS

Following the outbreak of SARS in 2002, the federal minister of health established the National Advisory Committee on SARS and Public Health, chaired by Dr. David Naylor, then Dean of Medicine at the University of Toronto. The Naylor Report (Public Health Agency of Canada, 2003) was released in October 2003 and recommended urgent changes in Canada's health protection and promotion systems. The Naylor Report identified several systemic deficiencies. It focused particularly on the capacity to detect, prevent, and manage outbreaks of infectious diseases. One critical component identified in the report was the lack of adequate, appropriate, and coordinated communication between the various levels of health authority and health practice. In Ontario, the independent Commission to Investigate the Introduction and Spread of SARS was created in June 2003. Its purpose was to investigate how the SARS virus came to the province, how the virus spread, and how it was dealt with. Its findings were released in 2007 (Government of Ontario, 2007). Particularly relevant to nursing is that various recommendations for the safety of health care providers were made in each of these reports.

INCREASED FOCUS ON PUBLIC HEALTH AND THE CREATION OF THE PUBLIC HEALTH AGENCY OF CANADA

The Naylor Report also recommended the creation of a national health protection and promotion agency working at arm's length from the government. The Public Health Agency of Canada (PHAC) was created in 2004 (Health Canada, 2004) with the mandate to focus on

- preventing chronic diseases, including cancer and heart disease,
- preventing injuries, and
- responding to public health emergencies and infectious disease outbreaks.

HOME AND COMMUNITY CARE

Home and community care has become more prominent in the national health agenda over the past few years. Home and community care services support people to live as independently as possible in the community. According to the Public Policy Forum on the Future of Home Care in Canada held in March 2007, the demand for home and community care services has been increasing dramatically in recent years. Approximately 850,000 Canadians received home care services in 2002. Despite a 60% increase in the number of home care recipients, only 3.5% of total public health expenditures went toward home care (Public Policy Forum, 2007).

 REFLECTIVE THINKING

1. Why is home and community care becoming more important in the Canadian health care system?
2. Reflect on the experience with SARS and the role nursing plays in such an outbreak.
3. Reflect on the public-private financing discussion in Canada. How do you think the health care system should be financed?

 # MAIN NATIONAL NURSING ISSUES AND EVENTS SINCE 2000

HEALTH HUMAN RESOURCES

Nursing health human resources is a critical issue in Canada. How many nurses is the right number? Although this is difficult to answer, there is general consensus that Canada needs to be graduating more nurses. According to a study done in 2002 by the CNA, if we continue with past workforce utilization patterns of registered nurses (RNs), Canada will experience a shortage of 78,000 RNs by 2011 and 113,000 RNs by 2016 (CNA, 2008b).

INTERNATIONALLY EDUCATED NURSES

The nursing workforce around the world has become increasingly mobile. As a result, there are growing numbers of internationally educated nurses seeking registration and employment in Canada (CNA, 2005c).

In 2004, the Health Human Resource Strategies Division of Health Canada supported the development of the Internationally Educated Nurses (IEN) taskforce. Various nursing and government organizations participated in this taskforce. A report by the CNA in 2005 identified various issues relating to the integration of IENs into the workforce. Language and culture remain two of the biggest barriers for IENs in integrating into the health care system. Lack of jurisdictional coordination is also a factor for IENs wanting to be registered in Canada (CNA, 2005b).

OFFICE OF NURSING POLICY (HEALTH CANADA)

The Office of Nursing Policy (ONP) was created at Health Canada in 1999. The first executive director was Dr. Judith Shamian. The current executive director is Sandra MacDonald Rencz. The ONP has been active in creating liaisons among all nurses (registered nurses, licensed practical nurses, and registered psychiatric nurses) in Canada. It has focused its initiatives on the health of nurses, recruitment and retention issues, interdisciplinary practice, and leadership. The ONP is present at many policy tables within the federal government. It has also been active in international circles. In 2002, a WHO forum on health human resources was hosted by Canada. The executive director has attended the World Health Association Meeting as part of the Canadian delegation. Currently, the ONP is involved in the HHR and leadership agenda at WHO globally, and particularly in the WHO African region.

CHIEF PROVINCIAL NURSING OFFICERS

Chief Nursing Officers (CNOs) occupy the highest governmental position in nursing within a province or territory. In 2008, the following provinces had Chief Nursing Officers: Prince Edward Island, Newfoundland, Nova Scotia, New Brunswick, Quebec, Ontario, Saskatchewan, and British Columbia. Manitoba and Alberta have nurses in Human Resources Advisor positions. Nunavut has tried to recruit a CNO, to no avail. The Northwest Territories and Yukon Territory do not have Chief Nursing Officers. CNOs play an important role in positioning nursing issues within government. They also have an important role to play in bringing the many nursing voices together for both policy and advocacy.

CANADIAN NURSES ASSOCIATION

The Canadian Nurses Association (CNA) is a federation of 11 provincial and territorial nursing associations and colleges representing more than 133,714 registered nurses. It is the national professional voice of registered nurses, supporting them in their practice and advocating for healthy public policy and a quality, publicly funded, not-for-profit health system. The CNA has four focus areas: nursing policy, public policy, regulatory policy, and international.

The CNA is the official Canadian representative to the ICN. In fact, CNA was created in 1908 to allow for membership in the ICN, and it was the fourth national nursing association to join ICN. One Canadian has been an ICN president (Alice Girard), four have been ICN vice-presidents (Helen Glass, Helen Evans, Alice Baumgart, and Eleanor Ross), and CNA's former executive director, Judith Oulton, is currently ICN's executive director (CNA, 2008a).

International Health Partnerships
Table 24.2 shows some recent international health partnerships that Canada has formed with other organizations worldwide.

Influencing Policy: A Workshop for Nurses
In 2005, the CNA developed and has now delivered in Canada, Russia, South Asia, Latin America, and Southern Africa, the Influencing Policy workshop. The purpose of this workshop is to help nurses understand the basic principles and features of healthy public policy, and how they can become involved in the public policy process. A Train-the-Trainer Tool Kit has also been developed to support global colleagues.

TABLE 24.2 International Health Partnerships

PARTNERSHIP NAME	DATES	FOCUS	PARTNER COUNTRIES
Strengthening Nurses, Nursing Networks and Associations Programs (SNNNAP)	2007–2112	This program is funded through the Canadian International Development Agency (CIDA) with the objectives of <ul><li>building the capacity of national nursing associations and networks,</li><li>enhancing collaboration between nurses from Canada and developing country partners, and</li><li>increasing the understanding of global health issues among Canadian nurses.</li></ul>	Currently there are projects in El Salvador, Ethiopia, Indonesia, Nicaragua, Southern Africa, and Vietnam
The Canada–South Africa Nurses HIV/AIDS Initiative	2003–2008	This initiative funded by CIDA aims to improve the health and health care of those infected and affected by HIV by increasing the capacity of nurses to deliver high-quality HIV and AIDS services in South Africa.	The Democratic Nursing Organization of South Africa is CNA's partner
The Ethiopian Nurses and Needle Stick Injury Research Project	2006–2008	CNA and the Ethiopian Nurses Association were awarded this grant to improve nurses' occupational health and safety, particularly as it relates to the heightened risk of exposure to blood-borne pathogens. This is part of a CIDA project funding that addresses HIV/AIDS issues in developing countries.	It is being carried out collaboratively with the Canadian Society for International Health and the Canadian Association of Nurses in AIDS Care, as well as the Zambia Nurses Association.
Canada–Russia Initiative in Nursing	2004–2008	This project is strengthening the capacity of the Russian Ministry of Health and the Russian Nurses Association for creating conceptual, regulatory, organizational, and educational frameworks.	It is being carried out collaboratively with Grant MacEwan College and Capital Health in Edmonton, Alberta.

Ethical Recruitment

Ethical recruitment of internationally educated nurses by Canadian health care organizations has been hotly discussed over the past decade. The CNA supports ICN's Ethical Nurse Recruitment Policy, which was developed in 2001. ICN and its member associations firmly believe that quality health care is directly dependent on an adequate supply of qualified and committed nursing personnel, and supports the evidence that links good working conditions with quality service provision (CNA, 2001).

2020 Document

In 2005, Health Canada and the Office of Nursing Policy at Health Canada provided support to CNA to critically examine the state of nursing in Canada and globally, consult with Canadians, and produce possible scenarios predicting the state of nursing and the health care system in 2020. The document *Toward 2020: Visions for Nursing* is the product of that consultation. During 2006 and 2007, extensive presentations and discussions were held across Canada (CNA, 2006).

To mark the celebrations for CNA's 100th anniversary in 2008, and to build on the momentum from the 2020 document, the CNA launched the Vision for Change Campaign, which emphasizes that CNA offers practical solutions, new thinking, and innovation in the health care system (CNA, 2008c).

CANADIAN FEDERATION OF NURSES UNIONS (CFNU)

Delegates to CFNU's 2005 convention voted to create the CFNU International Solidarity Fund. One-half of the annual fund revenue will go to assisting workers to obtain the right to health. In addition, CFNU will pursue long-term partnerships in developing countries with unions representing nurses and other health care workers (CFNU, 2008).

CANADIAN HEALTH SERVICES RESEARCH FOUNDATION/CANADIAN INSTITUTE OF HEALTH RESEARCH (CHSRF) NURSING RESEARCH FUND

The Nursing Research Fund (NRF) was created in 1999 to support nursing research in Canada. For example, the Canadian Health Services Research Foundation/Canadian Institute of Health Research Chair Awards are 10-year awards that fund mid-career leaders in applied health services and nursing research to train graduate students, act as mentors for new researchers, build national networks, and conduct research. The NRF also supports the Nursing Care Partnership Fund for research on nursing care, and the CADRE program, which addresses short-term and long-term capacity building for applied health services and nursing research (CHSRF, 2006).

REGISTERED NURSING ASSOCIATION OF ONTARIO (RNAO)

In 1999, the RNAO launched the Nursing Best Practice Guidelines Program. There are currently 29 published guidelines as well as a toolkit and educator's resource to support implementation. Examples of guidelines include the following: healthy work environments, women abuse, asthma, breastfeeding, smoking cessation, and wound care. Some of the guidelines are available in French. Nurses in many different practice settings have used these guidelines worldwide (RNAO, 2008).

WHO COLLABORATING CENTRES

The Global Network of WHO Collaborating Centres for Nursing and Midwifery Development is an independent, international, not-for-profit, voluntary organization. It is made up of 39 WHO Collaborating Centres worldwide (WHO, 2007a). There are two WHO Collaborating Centres in Canada:

• McMaster University (Hamilton, Ontario): WHO Collaborating Centre for Nursing Development for Primary Health and Educational Development
• University of Alberta (Edmonton, Alberta): WHO Collaborating Centre for Nursing and Mental Health

The mission of these 39 collaborating centres is to maximize the contribution of nursing and midwifery in order to advance Health for All in partnership with WHO and its member states, member centres, NGOs, and others interested in promoting the health of populations.

The network carries out advocacy and evidence-informed policy activities within the framework of WHA and regional resolutions and the WHO Programs of Work.

INTERNATIONAL RESEARCH COLLABORATIONS AT UNIVERSITIES

Many Canadian universities and Faculties of Nursing are active in international research projects. Nursing students and faculty members have numerous opportunities to become involved in international health.

REFLECTIVE THINKING

1. Reflect on the role that Canadian partnerships have had in international settings—what do you think are the most important elements of a successful collaboration?
2. In your opinion, what are the most important factors that influence nursing recruitment and retention?
3. Why do you think the position of Chief Nursing Officer is important?
4. What are the two biggest barriers for Internationally Educated Nurses who are entering the Canadian workforce?

CANADIAN RESEARCH FOCUS

International nursing research is underway in Australia, New Zealand, and Canada on the implications of nurse turnover. A Canadian research team is a partner in this international research. The pan-Canadian research project, entitled "Understanding the Costs and Outcomes of Nurses' Turnover in Canadian Hospitals," is intended to provide new evidence about the incidence of nurse turnover, its predictors, and associated system costs. It will also examine its impact on patient and nurse outcomes. The goal of this study is to identify the extent, costs, and predictors of nurse turnover in Canada. Concerns have frequently been expressed about the shortage of nurses and the issue of turnover, yet data to support effective policies is lacking. The research is supported by the Canadian Institutes of Health Research, and co-sponsors are Linda O'Brien-Pallas, Gail Tomblin Murphy, and Judith Shamian. For a copy of the paper, please visit http://www.nursingturnover.ca/

SUMMARY

Canada plays an important role in the international nursing community. We are strong members of ICN and WHO and have led the way with nursing research on working conditions and Health Human Resources. Canada also plays an important role in supporting the global health and nursing agenda through its participation in the WHO, the World Health Assembly, the ICN, and through the many grassroots non-governmental organizations involved in international health and development issues.

CRITICAL THINKING QUESTIONS

1. Discuss the impact that the changing global demographics and changing migration patterns have on global health.
2. The WHO has declared that primary health care is the way to attain truly sustainable and appropriate health care systems. Why is the role of the nurse so critical in PHC?
3. Access to a primary care practitioner is a problem for many Canadians. What are some solutions to this crisis?
4. What role should nursing organizations play in health system reform?
5. What skills and knowledge do Canadian nurses need to work effectively in international settings?

REFERENCES

Africa Policy E-Journal. (2007). *Africa: Life expectancy.* Retrieved on February 14, 2008, from http://www.africaaction.org/docs00/life0006.htm.

Amnesty International. (2004). *Sudan: Rape as a weapon of war in Darfur.* London, UK: Amesty International. Retrieved on February 10, 2008, from http://www.amnesty.org/en/library/info/AFR54/084/2004.

Attorney General of Quebec. (2005) *Chaoulli v. Quebec* (Attorney General), [2005] S.C.J. No. 33. Retrieved on January 20, 2008, from http://www.canlii.org/en/ca/scc/doc/2005/2005scc35/2005scc35.html.

Canadian Medical Association. (2005). *Privatization if necessary: Not necessarily privatization.* Ottawa: CMA. Retrieved on February 8, 2008, from http://www.cma.ca/index.cfm?ci_id=10028034&la_id=1.

CDPAC. (2008). *Confronting the epidemic of chronic disease.* Ottawa, ON: CDPAC. Retrieved on February 14, 2008, from http://www.cdpac.ca/content.php?doc=1.

CFNU. (2008). *Nurses Voice,* May/June 2007. Ottawa: CFNU. Retrieved on February 9, 2008, from http://www.nursesunions.ca/media.php?mid=518.

CHSRF. (2006). *Nursing research fund.* Ottawa: CHSRF. Retrieved on February 15, 2007, from http://www.chsrf.ca/nursing_research_fund/chairs_e.php.

CNA. (2001). *Position Statement: Ethical nurse recruitment.* Ottawa: Author. Retrieved on January 20, 2008, from http://www.cna-aiic.ca/CNA/documents/pdf/publications/psrecruit01Jan_2001_e.pdf.

CNA. (2003). *Primary Health Care: The time has come.* Ottawa: Author. Retrieved on February 9, 2008, from http://www.cna-nurses.ca/CNA/documents/pdf/publications/NN_PrimaryHealthCare_Sept_2003_e.pdf.

CNA. (2004). *Building a stronger, viable, publicly funded, not-for-profit health system.* Ottawa: Author. Retrieved on February 10, 2008, from http://www.cna-aiic.ca/CNA/documents/pdf/publications/I_platform_e.pdf.

CNA. (2005a). *National planning for human resources in the health sector.* Ottawa: Author. Retrieved on January 18, 2008, from http://www.cna-aiic.ca/CNA/documents/pdf/publications/PS81_National_Planning_e.pdf.

CNA. (2005b). *News release: Navigating to become a nurse in Canada.* Ottawa: Author. Retrieved on February 7, 2008, from http://www.cna-aiic.ca/CNA/news/releases/public_release_e.aspx?id=177.

CNA. (2005c). *Position statement: Regulation and integration of international nurse applicants into the Canadian health system.* Retrieved on February 8, 2008, from http://cna-aiic.ca/CNA/documents/pdf/publications/PS79_Regulation_e.pdf.

CNA. (2006). *Toward 2020: Visions for nursing.* Ottawa: Author. Retrieved on January 15, 2008 from http://www.cna-aiic.ca/CNA/documents/pdf/publications/Toward-2020-e.pdf.

CNA. (2008a). *About CNA.* Retrieved on January 15, 2008, from http://www.cna-aiic.ca/CNA/about/default_e.aspx.

CNA. (2008b). *The nursing shortage: The nursing workforce.* Ottawa: Author. Retrieved January 21, 2008 from http://www.cna-aiic.ca/CNA/issues/hhr/default_e.aspx.

CNA. (2008c). *Vision for change.* Retrieved on February 15, 2009, from http://www.cna-aiic.ca/CNA/documents/pdf/publications/Vision_of_Change_e.pdf.

College of Family Physicians of Canada. (2007). *News release—The College of Family Physicians of Canada takes action to improve access to care for patients in Canada.* Retrieved on February 8, 2008, from http://www.cfpc.ca/English/cfpc/communications/news%20releases/2007%2010%2011/default.asp?s=1.

Commonwealth Nurses Federation (CNF). (2007). *About the CNF.* Retrieved on February 8, 2008, from http://mysite.wanadoo-members.co.uk/cnf.

Commonwealth Secretariat. (2008). *Commonwealth Nurses Federation.* Retrieved on February 8, 2008, from http://www.thecommonwealth.org/Internal/151814/151927/commonwealth_nurses_federation/.

CUPE. (2005). *Inside the Chaoulli Supreme Court Ruling.* Ottawa: Author. Retrieved on January 20, 2008, from http://cupe.ca/updir/rev_CONSOLIDATED.pdf.

Emory University. (2008) *Lillian Carter Centre for International Nursing.* Retrieved on February 8, 2008, from http://nursing.web.emory.edu/lccin/index.shtml.

Environment Canada. (2007). *Reducing Smog.* Ottawa: Government of Canada. Retrieved on January 28, 2008, from http://www.ns.ec.gc.ca/epb/ccme/smog.html.

Government of Alberta. (2001). *A framework for reform.* Edmonton: Author. Retrieved on January 20, 2008, from http://www.health.gov.ab.ca/resources/publications/PACH_report_final.pdf.

Government of Canada. (2002). *Quebec's Health Review: The Clair Commission.* Ottawa: Author. Retrieved on January 20, 2008, from http://dsp-psd.pwgsc.gc.ca/Collection-R/LoPBdP/BP/prb0037-e.htm.

Government of Canada. (2003). *Reforming health protection and promotion in Canada: Time to act.* Ottawa: Author. Retrieved on January 20, 2008, from http://www.parl.gc.ca/37/2/parlbus/commbus/senate/com-e/soci-e/rep-e/repfinnov03-e.htm.

Government of Canada. (2006). *Out of the shadows at last: Transforming mental health, mental illness and addiction services in Canada.* Ottawa: Author. Retrieved on January 20, 2008, from http://www.parl.gc.ca/39/1/parlbus/commbus/senate/com-e/soci-e/rep-e/rep02may06-e.htm.

Government of Canada. (2007). *Health care system—Primary health care.* Retrieved on February 8, 2008, from http://www.hc-sc.gc.ca/hcs-sss/prim/index_e.html.

Government of Ontario. (2007). *The SARS Commission.* Toronto: Author. Retrieved on February 9, 2008, from http://www.sarscommission.ca/.

Government of Saskatchewan. (2001). *Caring for Medicare: Sustaining a quality system.* Regina: Author. Retrieved on January 20, 2008, from http://www.health.gov.sk.ca/medicare-commission-final-report.

Health Canada. (2002). *Building on values: The future of health care in Canada.* Ottawa: Government of Canada. Retrieved on January 20, 2008, from http://www.hc-sc.gc.ca/english/care/romanow/index1.html.

Health Canada. (2004). *Public Health Agency of Canada.* Ottawa: Government of Canada. Retrieved on January 20, 2008, from http://www.hc-sc.gc.ca/ahc-asc/branch-dirgen/phac-aspc/index_e.html.

ICHRN. (2006). Introduction to the International Centre for Human Resources in Nursing. Geneva: Author. Retrieved on February 10, 2008, from http://www.ichrn.org/.

ICN. (2004). The global shortage of registered nurses: An overview of issues and actions (pp. 4–6). Retrieved on February 14, 2008, from http://www.icn.ch/global/shortage.pdf.

ICN. (2008a). *About ICN.* Geneva: Author. Retrieved on February 10, 2008, from http://www.icn.ch/abouticn.htm.

ICN. (2008b). *Leadership for change: General information.* Geneva: Author. Retrieved on February 15, 2008, from http://www.icn.ch/leadchange.htm.

Public Health Agency of Canada. (2003). *Learning from SARS: Renewal of public health in Canada.* Ottawa: Government of Canada. Retrieved on February 10, 2008, from http://www.phac-aspc.gc.ca/publicat/sars-sras/naylor/

Public Health Agency of Canada. (2004). *The social determinants of health: An overview of the implications for policy and the role of the health sector.* Ottawa: Government of Canada. Retrieved on January 18, 2008, from http://www.phac-aspc.gc.ca/ph-sp/phdd/overview_implications/01_overview.html.

Public Policy Forum. (2007). *The future of homecare in Canada: Roundtable outcomes and recommendations for the future* (p. 4). Ottawa: Author. Retrieved on January 27, 2008, from http://ppforum.ca/common/assets/publications/en/future_homecare_report_en.pdf.

RNAO. (2008). *Nursing Best Practice Guidelines.* Toronto: Author. Retrieved on January 29, 2008, from http://www.rnao.org/Page.asp?PageID=861&SiteNodeID=133.

Statistics Canada. (2005). *Canada's visible minority population in 2017.* (Cat. No. #91-541-XIE). Ottawa: Author. Retrieved on February 15, 2008, from http://www.statcan.ca/cgi-bin/downpub/listpub.cgi?catno=91-541-XIE2005001.

UNDP. (2008). *Millennium development goals (MDGs).* New York: United Nations. Retrieved on February 15, 2008, from http://www.undp.org/mdg/.

UNICEF. (2006). *Africa's orphaned and vulnerable generations: Children affected by AIDS.* New York: Author. Retrieved on February 15, 2008, from http://www.unicef.org/publications/files/Africas_Orphaned_and_Vulnerable_Generations_Children_Affected_by_AIDS.pdf.

United Nations—Office of the Special Representative of the Secretary-General for Children and Armed Conflict. (2007). *Paris principles.* New York: United Nations. Retrieved on February 10, 2008, from http://www.un.org/children/conflict/_documents/parisprinciples/ParisPrinciples_EN.pdf.

WHO. (1978). *Declaration of Alma Ata.* Geneva: Author. Retrieved on January 18, 2008, from http://www.who.int/hpr/NPH/docs/declaration_almaata.pdf.

WHO. (2002). *Nursing Midwifery Services: Strategic directions 2002– 2008.* Geneva: Author.

WHO. (2003). *The WHO Framework Convention on Tobacco Control.* Geneva: Author. Retrieved on January 20, 2008, from http://www.who.int/features/2003/08/en/index.html.

WHO. (2007a). Global network of WHO collaborating centres for nursing and midwifery. Geneva: Author. Retrieved on January 30, 2008, from http://www.whocc.gcal.ac.uk/.

WHO. (2007b). *Islamabad Declaration on strengthening nursing and midwifery.* Geneva: Author. Retrieved on January 18, 2008, from http://www.who.int/hrh/nursing_midwifery/declaration_Islamabad.pdf.

WHO. (2008a). *Chronic diseases and health promotion.* Geneva: Author. Retrieved on February 14, 2008, from http://www.who.int/chp/en/index.html.

WHO. (2008b). *Report to the Executive Board, 122nd session.* Geneva: Author. Retrieved on January 16, 2008, from http://www.who.int/dg/speeches/2008/20080121_eb/en/index.html.

WHO. (2008c). World Health Day 2008: Protecting health from climate change. Retrieved on January 18, 2008, from http://www.who.int/world-health-day/en/.

WHO Media Centre. (2007). *Global HIV prevalence has leveled off.* Geneva: WHO. Retrieved on January 18, 2007, from http://www.who.int/mediacentre/news/releases/2007/pr61/en/index.html.

25 Internationalizing Nursing in Canada: Perspectives in Nursing Practice and Education

Susan E. French

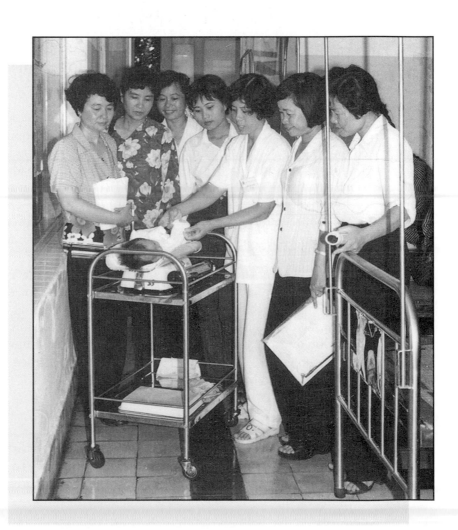

LEARNING OBJECTIVES

- To place the internationalizing of nursing in Canada within the context of human resource development in nursing.
- To describe and illustrate the strategies and activities whereby Canadian nursing practice and education have become internationalized.
- To identify key issues confronting nursing in Canada with respect to internationalizing of practice and education.
- To identify the relationship between issues in Canadian nursing and actions leading to increased internationalization of the nursing workforce.
- To illustrate how the contributions of nursing in Canada to the development of nursing globally are being recognized.
- To describe how the future generation of nurses is being introduced to nursing external to Canada.
- To distinguish between institutional support and institutional building interventions.
- To identify major challenges associated with the strategies for internationalizing Canadian nursing.

Countries differ with respect to the priority given to health, but globally, there is consensus that the health of a society's population is critical to its development. The outcome affects both the country's wealth and the quality of life of its citizens. The most important input into any health system is its human resources. In Canada, as in many other societies, nursing comprises the nation's largest group of health care providers. Nursing plays a pivotal role in the overall performance of health services and the achievement of health outcomes. Ensuring an adequate supply and appropriate utilization of nursing personnel with the necessary knowledge, skills, and motivation to meet present and future needs is a challenge within Canada and globally.

Internationalizing Nursing in Canada addresses how nursing is transcending our national boundaries and concerning itself with the development of nursing in other countries and how Canadian nursing is becoming international in character. This chapter will explore the internationalization of Canadian nursing from the perspective of education and practice. The activities will be placed within the health human resources development (HHRD) conceptual framework, with a focus on nursing. Major issues associated with internationalization will be identified.

HEALTH HUMAN RESOURCES DEVELOPMENT

Health human resources development (HHRD) is a process consisting of three major interrelated dimensions: *planning*, *production*, and *management*. To ensure an effective and efficient health system, all three dimensions need to be addressed (Hall & Majia, 1998). Planning for nursing is the process of estimating the numbers, mix, and distribution of nursing personnel, and the knowledge, skills, and attitudes needed to achieve predetermined health goals. It involves determining supply, requirements, and imbalances between supply and demand, now and in the future. The goal is to achieve the optimal number, mix, and distribution of nursing personnel at a cost a society can afford.

Planning is concerned with both quality and quantity and always involves choices; for example, level, type, and quality of health services to be provided and nursing personnel to deliver those services. It also encompasses health policy to guide the allocation of resources and efforts (Hall, 1988). The value placed on categories of health care providers, such as nurses, has an impact on the planning process. Globally, nursing is seen as women's work and is undervalued, especially in countries in which women have lower social status and less power than men. The development of nursing is influenced by three potent factors: power, gender, and the medicalization of health services (WHO, 1997). The influence of these factors starts at the planning stage.

Production is concerned with basic and post-basic education. It encompasses education from the diploma to graduate levels, and in schools, colleges, and universities. It involves identifying the potential applicant pool, recruitment and selection of students, attrition rates, number and type of graduates, numbers and qualification of faculty, faculty–student ratios, curricula, and coordination between graduates and their utilization (Hall, 1988).

Management is concerned with mobilization, motivation, development, and fulfillment of human beings in and through work. Recruitment into the workforce, employment, utilization, retention, turnover, attrition, motivation, evaluation, and continuing education are all dimensions of management (Hall, 1988).

STRATEGIES FOR INTERNATIONALIZATION OF CANADIAN NURSING

In the early years, much of the efforts of Canadian nursing in the international arena focused on production and management. More recently, greater attention has been given to planning and policy, and integrated approaches in which all three dimensions of NHRD are addressed. From its early beginnings, Canadian nursing has been cognizant of the importance of understanding nursing in other countries (Zilm, 2008). The development of nursing in other countries, globalization, and advances in technology, especially in the field of communications, are powerful forces shaping and internationalizing nursing in Canada today.

Strategies for internationalizing Canadian nursing may be categorized as *bringing in* or *reaching out*. Within the *bringing in* category, major activities or interventions are preparation of individual nurses, recruitment of foreign nurses, and enabling internationally educated nurses (IENs) to practise as nurses in Canada. Within the *reaching out* category, the major activities or interventions are international placements, faculty, practitioner and student exchanges, or both, and export of Canadian nursing expertise through the work of individual consultants or partnership projects aimed at building capacity through institutional strengthening. The categories are not mutually exclusive, and some projects have a number of activities cutting across categories.

PREPARATION OF INDIVIDUAL NURSES

Foreign students in educational institutions bring perspectives that enrich the educational and research programs and student life. The number of foreign students in nursing varies across level of program. Tuition in Canada is higher for foreign students than for Canadian students, and the majority of foreign students are from countries with a high level of socioeconomic development, such as the United States or countries in Western Europe or are sponsored by governments, foundations, or private donors. In the early years, many nurses were sponsored by organizations such as the World Health Organization (WHO), Rockefeller Foundation, or the Kellogg Foundation to prepare them to be potential leaders to develop nursing in their home countries. The extensive enrolment of foreign nurses in undergraduate nursing programs across the country from the 1940s to the 1980s produced many nursing leaders; for example, the late Dame Nita Barrows, a graduate from the University of Toronto, was not only a leader in the development of nursing in the Caribbean but also a leading worldwide authority in the areas of public health and health education. She later served as the governor-general of Barbados (Hezekiah, 2001).

Study in Canada is expensive and accessible to a limited number of nurses, content may not always be relevant, and graduates may not return to their home country, or may return but emigrate within a short time period. The loss to sponsoring countries of potential leaders is a tragedy. The development of indigenous programs is preferable because of their accessibility, relevance, retention, and sustainable development.

With the development of indigenous educational programs at the diploma and undergraduate levels or programs at this level becoming available through distance education, the focus shifted to graduate education or short-term training in specialty nursing services. More recently, the focus is shifting to doctoral and postdoctoral programs to prepare a cadre of nurses for senior positions in governments, health services, and education. Communication technology has increased accessibility of educational programs at all levels. Greater attention is being given to ensuring a high degree of relevancy in the educational experiences; for example, graduate students return home to conduct their research under the supervision of faculty based at the Canadian university. The value of graduate study within the same geographical region as the student's home country is being recognized; for example, in a partnership project between Memorial University of Newfoundland (MUN) and institutions in Vietnam, nurses from Vietnam were sponsored for graduate study in nursing in Thailand rather than bringing them to MUN. As with educational programs at the undergraduate level, the thrust has been to assist other countries in developing their own graduate programs.

RECRUITMENT

The educational capacity in Canada at all levels is unable to meet the increasing demands of health care and educational systems (CNA & CASN, 2007). A critical factor is the shortage of qualified teaching staff. The Canadian Association of Schools of Nursing

(CASN) has projected a need for 3,673 master's-prepared nurses annually (CNA & CASN, 2007). The number of master's graduates in 2004 was 418. In 2006, the overall number of nurses employed in nursing in Canada holding a master's or doctorate degree was only 3% (CIHI, 2007). The shortage will worsen with future retirements. The age of nurse educators employed in nursing is significantly higher in the 45 to 64 age group than in the total nurse workforce (CNA & CASN, 2007).

Recruitment of teaching staff from outside the country is viewed as enriching an academic community. Such recruitment is becoming increasingly common in nursing, especially for senior administrative positions; for example, the dean of the Faculty of Nursing, University of Toronto, and a former dean, Faculty of Nursing, University of Calgary, were recruited from Australia. To date, the recruitment has been reciprocal with countries comparable to Canada in their socioeconomic development and nursing. Active recruitment from outside can be expected to accelerate with the expanded need and retirement of current faculty. Canada is in a very advantageous position to recruit externally and could contribute to the depletion of essential and very limited nursing resources from countries that are unable to participate in reciprocal recruitment. Canada is among the countries that signed a code of ethics stating that it is inappropriate to actively recruit significant numbers of trained health care providers from countries experiencing a shortage (Halliwell, Shamian, & Shearer, 2004). At the same time, individuals are seen as having a right to migrate (International Council of Nurses, 1989).

Canadian nursing will be dealing with increased recruitment of its nurses with advanced degrees by other countries, such as the United States, Australia, and the United Kingdom for English-speaking nurses, and Switzerland and France for francophone nurses. The close geographical proximity of the United States, comparability of educational programs, and the ease of mobility for qualified nurses pose special challenges. For example, retention in Canada of doctoral-prepared nurses in light of the anticipated retirements from the professorial ranks in the United States, where the average ages of doctoral-prepared nurse faculty are 58.6 (professor), 55.8 (associate professor), and 51.6 years (assistant professor) (AACN, 2007).

INTERNATIONALLY EDUCATED NURSES (IENS)

The supply of Canadian-educated nurses is predicted to decrease due to the retirement of nurses in the "baby boomer" generation and the inability to provide sufficient numbers of Canadian-educated graduates. Availability of accurate data is limited, but large numbers of nurses are migrating from developing or unstable countries to more developed and stable countries such as Canada (Kline, 2003; Vujicic, Zurn, Diallo, Adams, & Dal Poz, 2004). Nursing is among the top 20 regulated professions for skilled migrants to Canada (MacKenzie, 2006). Canadian nursing researchers, such as Baumann, Blythe, Kotofylo, and Underwood (2004), are contributing to our understanding of the international nursing labour market. Most provinces have programs to increase the numbers of immigrants in designated professions, and health care providers such as nurses will most likely be included (Baumann, Blythe, Rheaume, & McIntosh, 2006). Few countries have the equivalent of registered practical nurses (RPN) and relatively few migrate to Canada (CIHI, 2007).

In 2006, IENs accounted for approximately 8% of the 250,976 registered nurses employed in nursing in Canada (based on information reported and not all nurses reported on location of graduation). That number has remained relatively constant since 2003 at 7% to 8%. Variations in number reflect the larger immigration patterns. Ontario and British Columbia have the highest percentage of nurses who graduated from a nursing program outside Canada: 12.2% and 15.4% respectively. Ontario with its large nursing workforce has the highest number of IENs—11,228 in 2006. Nurses from the Philippines (30.8%) and the United Kingdom (17.9%) account for the largest numbers of IENs in the Canadian nursing workforce (CIHI, 2007). The high percentage from the Philippines is consistent with that country's policy of facilitating migration of nurses. It is estimated that 85% of nurses from the Philippines are working internationally and represent a significant source of foreign currency for the country (Lorenzo, 2002, cited in Buchan, Kingma, & Lorenzo, 2005). There is a high probability that the percentage of IENs will rise; for example, in 2005, Ontario-educated nurses accounted for 34.1% and IENs accounted for 52.4% of new registered nurses entering the workforce in Ontario (Baumann et al., 2006).

A 2006 study of IENs in Ontario reported that an estimated 40% of the IEN applicants do not complete registration, and challenges existed at all stages in the process of entering Canada and gaining employment as professional nurses (Baumann et al., 2006). IENs bring a wealth of experience to Canadian nursing and add to the cultural diversity of the workforce. A 2006 study undertaken by the Ontario College of Nurses and York University's School of Nursing revealed that the IEN participants identified that nurses educated in Canada have a broader scope of practice, are more involved in clinical decision making, are more assertive with co-workers, have more responsibility for patients, are more respected by members of other health care professions, and the relationship between nurses and doctors is less hierarchical (College of Nurses of Ontario, 2007).

The Government of Canada and provincial governments, nursing organizations such as CASN, provincial regulatory bodies, and educational institutions are taking action to decrease the barriers and facilitate the process of entry into the professional role. For example, in Alberta, the Government of Canada is funding a pilot test of an innovative offshore assessment program aimed at expediting the licensure process (Health Canada, 2007). In Saskatchewan, the provincial government is funding a program offered by distance education allowing nurses to begin training in their country of origin prior to moving to Canada (Saskatchewan Institute of Applied Science and Technology, 2007). In Ontario, the provincial government funds a program dedicated to enabling IENs to practise and excel in the profession in the shortest possible time. Practice environments are providing assistance, such as mentoring programs, to enable IENs to familiarize themselves with the nursing role in Canada and to acquire specific knowledge and skills. No data are available on the impact of IENs on the education of future practitioners or nursing work-life.

⌕ CANADIAN RESEARCH FOCUS

The Nursing Health Services Research Unit (NHSRU), McMaster University School of Nursing

Baumann, A., Blythe, J., Kotofylo, C., & Underwood, J. (2004). *The International nursing labour market*. Hamilton, ON: McMaster University, Nursing Health Services Research Unit.

Baumann, A., & Blythe, J. (2008). Globalization of higher education in nursing. OJIN: The *Online Journal of Issues in Nursing, 13*(2). Retrieved from http://www.nursingworld.org/MainMenuCategories/ANAMarketplace/ANAperiodicals/OJIN/.

Blythe, J., Baumann, A., Rheaume, A., & McIntosh, K. (2009). Nurse migration to Canada: Pathways and pitfalls of workforce integration. *Journal of Transcultural Nursing, 20*(2), 202–210.

Since 2004, Baumann and associates have conducted a series of studies contributing to our understanding of the internationalization of the Canadian nursing workforce. The study on the international nursing labour market (Baumann, Blythe, Kotofylo, & Underwood, 2004) provided a global perspective on nursing workforce issues in Canada. The study to determine what helps or hinders IENs from entering the Ontario health care system identified factors contributing to success and failure of IENs to re-establish their professional careers in nursing in Canada (Blythe, Baumann, Rheaume, & McIntosh, 2009). That exploratory study showed that the IENs encountered obstacles at every step in the process, from the migration interview to integration into the workforce. Baumann and Blythe (2008), after a review of the globalization of higher education in nursing, present an argument for the necessity of international educational standards for nurses.

INTERNATIONAL PLACEMENTS AND/OR FACULTY, PRACTITIONER, AND STUDENT EXCHANGES

Course work addressing global health and experiential learning through international placements are the norm in many nursing programs. International placements offer an unparalleled opportunity for students to gain insight about the broad determinants of health, comparative health care systems, and nursing outside Canada, while contributing to the practice of nursing. In a number of instances, student placements are part of larger projects designed to assist in the further development of nursing in specific countries or regions, such as the Highlands of Hope project between McGill University School of Nursing and Tanzania, designed to strengthen nursing services in a remote area of Tanzania.

Increasingly, partnerships between a Canadian institution (nursing education and/or service) and one or more institutions in other countries promoting student, faculty, and practitioner exchanges are becoming the norm. Exchange programs provide opportunities for mutual learning and facilitate understanding of the determinants of health in a global context and acquisition of requisite knowledge and skills. Exchanges may focus on research and education, such as the scholarly exchange program between the University of British Columbia and Mahidol University, Thailand, or on a combination of education, practice, and research, such as McGill University and the McGill Health Sciences Centre exchange with the Second Military Hospital and University in Shanghai, PRC.

Trade agreements such as the North American Free Trade Agreement (NAFTA) between Canada, Mexico, and the United States of America, enacted in 1994, allows for enhanced job mobility of health care providers, including nurses. A highly relevant initiative is the North American Mobility Project between two university schools of nursing in Canada (Dalhousie University and the University of Prince Edward Island), two in the United States, and two in Mexico allowing exchange students to study factors shaping health care systems and individual patient care and health care systems and the impact of each system on the role and scope of nursing practice (Kuehn et al., 2005).

Exchange agreements between Canadian institutions and those in other countries reflect political and socio-economic changes occurring worldwide, such as the emergence of China as an economic force. Nursing in China has established relations with a number of Canadian institutions, such as the exchange agreement between the University of Saskatchewan and Fudan University, Shanghai, PRC. Exchange programs are most effective when the interests and skills of the personnel are matched. Outcomes include: on-going collaboration on issues of mutual interest, changes in education or practice, transfer and utilization of knowledge, careers in international health, or work in the host country. The process of acculturation takes approximately three months and, for short-term exchanges, is hardly complete prior to departure. Long-term exchanges are preferable but have implications for work and home life and have less universal appeal. Exchanges must overcome potential barriers such as timetabling of courses, language, regulations governing clinical practice, and financial costs.

CONSULTATION

Canadian nursing expertise is recognized worldwide. That expertise may be offered through private arrangements between the nurse consultant and the out-of-country organization, as part of the services offered by an organization, such as the Canadian Nurses Association consultants sponsored to provide assistance in the strengthening of professional nursing associations, or an integral part of international partnerships. The majority of university schools of nursing have faculty serving as consultants in countries in the North (e.g., Switzerland) and the South (e.g., South Africa). Canadian nurses have served as consultants to governments, professional organizations, donor agencies such the Canadian International Development Agency (CIDA) and Oxfam Canada; agencies such as Asian Development Bank and the World Bank, World Health Organization (WHO), and health and nursing services; and educational institutions. Canadian nurses are volunteers with humanitarian aid organizations, such as Médecins Sans Frontières.

Individual consultants contribute to the development of nursing education, services, and research as well as to health policy, health human resource development, and health services in general. The nature of the consultants' work reflects the changes residing in Canadian nursing. During the last two decades, there has been a significant increase in consultancies relating to nursing research and planning and policy. Advances in technology are facilitating the work of multi-site research teams.

PARTNERSHIPS

Partnerships are designed to improve the capacity of institutions to incorporate new knowledge, new experience, new technology, and new learning (Eyford, 1991). Interventions fall along a continuum ranging from institutional support to institutional building. The former requires minimal intervention on the part of the donor or partner, and little or no structural change in the partner institution. Projects that focus on, for example, education of faculty, curriculum design, learning modules, or evaluation methods fall into the category of institutional support, such as the collaborative educational project involving nursing and nutrition students at educational institutions in England, Finland, Sweden, and Estonia along with the Université de Moncton, Mount Royal College, and the University of Prince Edward Island. Institutional building projects are concerned also with the institution's mission and goals, management style, leadership, planning, potential to influence nursing, health policy formulation, implementation, or some combination of these. Institutional building is more time-consuming, involves more joint planning, and includes deliberate attention to institutional elements as distinct from the specific project focus (Eyford, 1991).

Institutional building is complex and not easily implemented (Robinson, 1993). The intent of projects needs to be worked through carefully in the planning stage, or problems may arise later. Sustaining the innovations associated with institutional capacity building requires knowledge, skills, and time. Capacity building helps to create and reinforce the ability of people and countries to carry out their own development. It emphasizes lifelong learning, education, and training that contribute to institutional improvement and an enabling environment that reinforces the benefits of education and training. Capacity building involves complex learning, adaptation, and attitudinal changes at the individual, group, organizational, and societal levels (Morgan, 1997). The University of Ottawa–China Yunnan maternal and child health project (Edwards & Roelofs, 2006) illustrates the complexity of institutional capacity building and the strategies used to support sustainability.

In the early years, the majority of partnerships fell along the institutional support end of the continuum identified by Eyford (French & Watters, 1993). Since the 1990s, the focus has moved to the institutional building end of the continuum and is moving beyond a focus on production and management to include planning and policy; for example, under the leadership of nursing at the University of Ottawa, a multidisciplinary team of 20 researchers and research users from six countries is engaged in strengthening nurses' contribution to health policy development and health systems reform in order to improve the effectiveness of HIV and AIDS policies and practices (Edwards & Roelofs, 2007).

Institutional support projects may be the forerunner of institutional building projects. For example, the Ministry of Health of Trinidad and Tobago and McMaster University School of Nursing project to prepare a critical mass of nurses with specialty preparation in oncology nursing evolved into a partnership with the University of West Indies to deliver the oncology program in Trinidad and to foster the development of local capacity and expertise to enable the university to offer the program independently by 2009.

The shift in focus is an indication of local governments recognizing the importance to their country of nursing human resource development, such as the project undertaken by the Faculty of Nursing, University of Manitoba, in partnership with the Ministerio de Salud Publica (MINSAP), Cuba, and the Society of Cuban Nurses (SCN). That project is addressing one of the top three priorities of the Cuban government; that is, health human resource development, specifically nursing. The project will enhance Cuba's capacity to provide relevant nursing education at the graduate level, strengthen nursing's capacity to conduct research and disseminate results, and through continuing education enhance the capacity of Cuban nurses to use evidence-informed and gender-sensitive knowledge in practice.

For Canadian institutions, the goal of strategic partnerships is viewed as a means of sharing and enhancing nursing knowledge and improving nursing and the level of health standards globally. The reciprocal nature of partnerships is highlighted in the vast majority of projects; for example, the College of Nursing, University of Saskatchewan's partnership with the Ministry of Health in Mozambique is directed toward strengthening the capacity of institutions in Mozambique to train health workers to work better with the communities they serve. Lessons learned contribute to the way health workers are trained at the University of Saskatchewan. This project is similar to many others in providing opportunities for students enrolled at the Canadian university to have international placements within the project.

Canadian nursing is becoming more oriented toward inter-professionalism, and the same trend appears in international partnerships. For example, the Memorial University of Newfoundland School of Nursing in conjunction with the School of Social Work is engaged in a project focusing on poverty reduction by improving social work and health in rural Vietnam. McMaster University School of Nursing in partnership with the newly established University of Sharjah developed a college of health sciences, including a department of nursing. McMaster School of Nursing provided overall leadership and academic expertise, including advice and support for the mission, goals, faculty recruitment, retention, and development; curriculum review and development; alumni and external relations; and academic governance. The college, including the Department of Nursing, became self-sustaining in 2002.

International partnerships may be influenced by the university's environment or unique role in global nursing, such as the UBC–India project. Similarly, the School of Nursing, Dalhousie University, has a formal partnership with the Nova Scotia Gambia Association (NSGA). Numerous opportunities are provided for faculty and students to work with the NSGA and The Gambia to promote health. Nursing in Quebec is providing leadership in furthering the development of nursing in francophone countries and those with large French-speaking regions, such as Switzerland. The academic, clinical, and regulatory expertise of nursing in Quebec was a driving force in the formation of an international organization dedicated to the further development of nursing knowledge, education, practice, and governance in francophone nursing globally.

BOX 25.1	Internationalizing in Practice: The UBC–Guru Nanak Partnership Project

Since 1998, the University of British Columbia School of Nursing has had the privilege of participating in a unique kind of partnership with the local Vancouver Punjabi Sikh community and its nongovernmental organization in Northern India's rural Punjab region. Among the ex-patriot Punjabi community in British Columbia there has been tremendous interest in facilitating development opportunities for the homeland. Bud Singh Dhaban, a local community elder who immigrated to Canada in 1959, has quietly led an extended initiative to enhance health and development in the Punjab through the education of young women, the provision of high-quality health care, and the advancement of cooperation among the various religious and political groups within the region. Since 1983, he and his many supporters and colleagues have steadily pressed forward with a vision to create a school for girls, to build a hospital, and more recently, to create a school of nursing. Recognizing that nursing education is a critical element in providing an educational opportunity for young women and in creating a new cadre of skilled health care professionals, leaders in the British Columbia community sought consultation and advice from the UBC School of Nursing. Their aim was to create a nursing education program that was capable of producing nursing graduates at a baccalaureate level and to work toward attaining baccalaureate education that would be recognized internationally.

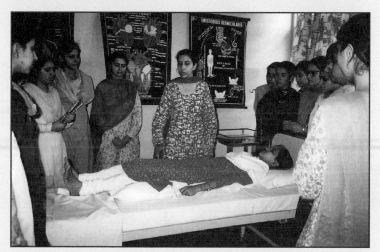

Lab practice at the Guru Nanak College of Nursing. The UBC School of Nursing and the Vancouver Punjabi community are collaborating to help to develop and support the school in rural India.

Over the past several years, the community has actively supported an intensive exchange of ideas, resources, and skills. Faculty from UBC have provided considerable professional development and curricular support to their colleagues at the Guru Nanak College of Nursing on site in Dhatan-Kaleran, Punjab. More recently, faculty and students from Guru Nanak College have spent time in Vancouver, gaining insight into expanded roles for nursing in an international context. Step by step, the curriculum is becoming stronger, the physical resources of the college are being built up, and the scholarly activity of the faculty members is increasing. In support of this evolving vision of what an educated nursing workforce can accomplish, the Canadian community partner (the Canada–India Education Society) has obtained CIDA funding for a primary health care project assessing the health needs and building the community capacity in 70 surrounding villages. With the continuing support of the UBC School of

Continued

BOX 25.1   Internationalizing in Practice: The UBC–Guru Nanak
Partnership Project—cont'd

Nursing team, Punjabi doctors, nurses, students, and faculty are beginning to experience scholarship in action and to appreciate the value of advanced education in improving the quality of health services at all levels in a larger context.

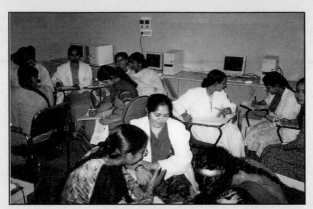

A faculty computer workshop at the college in Dhahan-Kaleran, Punjab.

An especially important aspect of this partnership has been the Partnership Advisory Committee, made up of UBC School of Nursing faculty members, local South Asian community leaders, and bicultural community nurses. Tackling the complexities of pedagogy and curriculum across the two distinct cultures might have been impossible without the context of teamwork, dialogue, and common purpose. The faculty members at the UBC School of Nursing have learned a tremendous amount from their partners about community building and fundraising. Social events bringing the university and community together regularly draw crowds of several hundred, celebrating the partnership project's successes and encouraging each other toward taking the next steps.

Sally Thorne

An emerging approach to institutional building is the establishment by a Canadian university of an overseas branch campus as a means of assisting another country to develop its nursing workforce and/or to promote the generation and utilization of nursing knowledge addressing global health and nursing issues in general and national or regional issues in particular. For example, in response to a request from the government of Qatar, the Faculty of Nursing, University of Calgary, has established a campus in Qatar to provide state-of-the-art education and research programs in nursing to assist Qatar to develop and retain a world-class nursing workforce. The programs delivered on the campus in Qatar are equivalent to those offered at the University of Calgary. Currently, the focus is on the undergraduate level, but eventually will include the provision of graduate programs at the master's and doctoral levels.

The significant role played by Canadian educational and service institutions has been recognized by the WHO. In 1989, the global network of WHO Collaborating Centres for Nursing and Midwifery Development was established to maximize the contributions of nursing and midwifery in the advancement of the "Health for All" agenda. The designation for each centre reflects specific area(s) of nursing expertise and significant international contributions. Two of the 40 centres are in Canada: McMaster University School of Nursing, designated in 1992 as the WHO Collaborating Centre for Nursing Development for Primary Health and Educational Development; and the Faculty of Nursing, University of Alberta, designated in 2004 as the WHO Collaborating Centre for Nursing and Mental Health.

ISSUES

The internationalization of Canadian nursing is an evolving process that reflects the growth of the profession in Canada and globally. International activities, especially those in the *reaching out* category, require resources. Successful partnerships require considerable effort to establish and maintain. Few, if any, educational or practice organizations have sufficient resources (human and financial) to allocate to international activities of any magnitude. The source of funding tends to drive international ventures. CIDA continues to be a source of funding but the trend is toward funding emanating from research agencies, external governments, organizations, or private donors. That trend has serious implications for countries with low socioeconomic development whose governments are not in a position or lack private sources to purchase Canadian nursing expertise.

If Canadian nursing is to make judicious use of limited resources, it will need to achieve a fine balance between efforts directed toward the further development of Canadian nursing and development of nursing in the global community. As nursing institutions in Canada confront the challenges of limited capacity and a growing gap between supply and demand, the benefits of internationalization will need to be articulated clearly and defended. The ethical dilemma associated with the recruitment of the nurses from poorer and less well-developed countries will become an issue as more and more actions are taken to facilitate migration to address the nursing shortages. Conversely, Canadian nursing will need to find means to ensure that the recruitment of its members by other countries does not result in a significant loss. As the mix of Canadian-educated nurses and IENs changes, the positive and negative implications of those changes on practice and education will need to be addressed.

REFLECTIVE THINKING

1. What factors should be considered before Canadian schools of nursing or nursing services use scarce resources to assist in the development of nursing outside of Canada?
2. What are the ethical dilemmas associated with recruitment of nurses from outside of Canada?
3. What are the advantages and disadvantages of having nursing students exposed to nursing and health services outside their own country?

CONCLUSION

Nursing in Canada has and continues to play a major role in the development of nursing worldwide and to benefit from those activities as well as from the global migration of nurses. Nursing's contributions are being recognized and valued, such as the requests for partnerships and exchanges, and the designation of two WHO collaborating centres in nursing. Nursing is building on its strengths and using a variety of approaches to contribute to all dimensions of nursing human resource development and global health. Current and future members are engaged in activities that will further their understanding of global health issues and the interdependency of nursing worldwide. There are challenges ahead, but Canadian nursing has demonstrated its commitment to internationalization.

CRITICAL THINKING QUESTIONS

1. What are the potential advantages and disadvantages for basic nursing education of the presence of a large number of IENs in the clinical sites?
2. What are the major arguments for bringing nurses to Canada to study in graduate programs in nursing? For not bringing them?
3. Increasingly, international projects are being supported by foreign governments or private individuals or organizations. What do you see as the major outcomes for international nursing of that trend?
4. International placements for students are common, but only a limited number of students participate. What do you think are the major factors that facilitate or hinder participation?

WEB SITES

WHO Collaborating Centres: http://www.int/collaboratingcentres/database/en or http://www.int/ collaboratingcentres/datbase/fr
WHO Collaborating Centre for Nursing Development for Primary Health and Educational Development, McMaster University, Hamilton, Ontario: http://www.mcmaster.ca/nursing/
WHO Collaborating Centre for Nursing and Mental Health, University of Alberta, Alberta: http://www.nursing.ualberta.ca
Nursing Health Services Research Unit, McMaster: http://www.NHSRU.com

REFERENCES

American Association of Colleges of Nursing (AACN). (2007). *Nursing faculty shortage. Fact sheet. Updated, October, 2007.* Author.

Baumann, A., & Blythe, J. (2008). Globalization of higher education in nursing. OJIN. *The Online Journal of Issues in Nursing, 13*(2). Retrieved on October 8, 2009, from http://www.nursingworld.org/ MainMenuCategories/ANAMarketplace/ANAperiodicals/OJIN/.

Baumann, A., Blythe, J., Kotofylo, C., & Underwood, J. (2004). *The International nursing labour market.* Hamilton, ON: McMaster University, Nursing Health Services Research Unit.

Baumann, A., Blythe, J., Rheaume, A., & McIntosh, K. (2006). *Internationally educated nurses in Ontario: Maximizing the brain gain. Human health Resources, Series Number 3* (2nd ed.). Hamilton, ON: McMaster University, Nursing Health Services Research Unit.

Blythe, J., Baumann, A., Rheaume, A., & McIntosh, K. (2009). Nurse migration to Canada: Pathways and pitfalls of workforce integration. *Journal of Transcultural Nursing, 20*(2), 202–210.

Buchan, J., Kigma, M., & Lorenzo, F. M. (2005). *International migration of nurses: Trends and policy implications. Issue 5. The Global Nursing Review Initiative.* Geneva, Switzerland: International Council of Nurses.

Canadian Institute for Health Information (CIHI). (2007). *Workforce trends of registered nurses in Canada in 2006.* Ottawa: Author.

Canadian Nurses Association & Canadian Association of Schools of Nursing (CAN & CASN). (2007). *Registered nursing education in Canada: 2004 snapshot.* Ottawa: Author.

College of Nurses of Ontario. (2007). The unique world of IENs. *The Standard* (Summer 2007), 2–14, 34.

Edwards, N. C., & Roelofs, S. M. (2006). Sustainability: the elusive dimension of international health projects. *Canadian Journal of Public Health, January–February,* 45–49.

Edwards, N. C., & Roelofs, S. (2007). Strengthening nurses' capacity in HIV policy development in Sub-Saharan Africa and the Caribbean: An international program of research and capacity building. *Canadian Journal of Nursing Research, 39*(3), 187–189.

Eyford, G. (1991). *Institution capacity building in academic settings.* Gatineau, PQ: Canadian International Development Agency.

French, S. E., & Watters, D. (1993). International activities of university schools of nursing in Canada. In S. E. French, J. Beaton, H. Fraser-Davy, & J. Bouchard (Eds.), *Canadian university nursing and international development* (pp. 53–80). Ottawa: Canadian Association of University Schools of Nursing.

Hall, T. L. (1988). Guidelines for health workforce planners. *World Health Forum, 9,* 409–413.

Hall, T. L., & Majia, A. (1998). *Health manpower planning: Principles, methods, issues.* Geneva: World Health Organization.

Halliwell, C., Shamian, J., & Shearer, R. (2004). Health human resources: A key policy challenge. *Health Policy Research Bulletin, 8*(May), 3–7. Ottawa: Health Canada.

Health Canada. (2007). *Off-shore assessment of internationally educated nurses (IENs).* Ottawa: Health Canada. Retrieved on October 8, 2009, from http://www.hc-sc.ca/ahc-asc/media/nr-cp/2007/2007_174_bk_e.html.

Hezekiah, J. (2001). *Breaking though the glass ceiling: The stories of three Caribbean nurses.* Mona, Jamaica: West Indies Press.

International Council of Nurses (ICN). (1989). *Recruitment of nurses from abroad.* Geneva, Switzerland: Author.

Kline, D. (2003). Push and pull factors in international nurse migration. *Journal of Nursing Scholarship, 35,* 107–111.

Kuehn, A., Chircop, A., Downe-Wambodt, B., Sheppard-LeMoine, D., Murnaghan, D., Elliott, J., & Cardenas, V. (2005). Exploring nursing roles across North American borders. *The Journal of Continuing Education in Nursing, 36*(4), 153–162.

Lorenzo, F. (2002). *Nurse supply and demand in the Philippines.* Manila, Philippines: Institute of Health Policy and Development Studies, University of Philippines.

MacKenzie, P. (2006, June 13). *Immigrant labour market integration.* Ottawa: Presentation to AUCC Policy Workshop.

Morgan, P. (1997). *The design and use of capacity development indicators.* Gatineau, PQ: Canadian International Development Agency.

Robinson, S. (1993). Institution partnerships: A strategy for sustainable development. In S. E. French, J. Beaton, H. Fraser-Davy, & J. Bouchard (Eds.), *Canadian university nursing and international development* (pp. 8–26). Ottawa: Canadian Association of University Schools of Nursing.

Saskatchewan Institute of Applied Science and Technology (SIAST). (2007). *Orientation to nursing in Canada for internationally educated nurses*. Saskatoon, SK: Author.

Vujicic, M., Zurn, P., Diallo, K., Adams, O., & Dal Poz, M. (2004). The role of wages in migration of health care professionals from developing countries. *Human Resources for Health, 2*, 1–14.

World Health Organization (WHO). (1997). *Strengthening nursing and midwifery: A global study (Rep. No. WHO/hrp/nur-Mid/97.2)*. Geneva: Author.

Zilm, G. (2008). Nurses associations: Their past, present and future. *Canadian Nurse, 104*(1), 44.

Index

Page numbers followed by *f* indicate figures; *t*, tables; *b*, boxes.

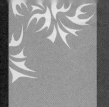

Photo Credits